Medical Genetics: Role of Genetics in Diseases and Disorders

Medical Genetics: Role of Genetics in Diseases and Disorders

Edited by Solomon Culver

hayle medical

New York

Hayle Medical,
750 Third Avenue, 9th Floor,
New York, NY 10017, USA

Visit us on the World Wide Web at:
www.haylemedical.com

ISBN: 978-1-63241-656-8

Printed in China.

Cataloging-in-Publication Data

Medical genetics : role of genetics in diseases and disorders / edited by Solomon Culver.
p. cm.
Includes bibliographical references and index.
ISBN 978-1-63241-656-8
1. Medical genetics. 2. Human genetics. 3. Genetic disorders. I. Culver, Solomon.
RB155 .M43 2019
616.042--dc23

Table of Contents

Preface IX

Chapter 1 **Chromosomal Minimal Critical Regions in Therapy-Related Leukemia Appear Different from Those of *De Novo* Leukemia by High-Resolution aCGH** 1
Nathalie Itzhar, Philippe Dessen, Saloua Toujani, Nathalie Auger, Claude Preudhomme, Catherine Richon, Vladimir Lazar, Véronique Saada, Anelyse Bennaceur, Jean Henri Bourhis, Stéphane de Botton and Alain Bernheim

Chapter 2 **Penicillamine Increases Free Copper and Enhances Oxidative Stress in the Brain of Toxic Milk Mice** 23
Ding-Bang Chen, Li Feng, Xiao-Pu Lin, Wei Zhang, Fu-Rong Li, Xiu-Ling Liang and Xun-Hua Li

Chapter 3 **Regulation of miR-146a by RelA/NFkB and p53 in ST*Hdh*^{Q111}/*Hdh*^{Q111} Cells, a Cell Model of Huntington's Disease** 37
Jayeeta Ghose, Mithun Sinha, Eashita Das, Nihar R. Jana and Nitai P. Bhattacharyya

Chapter 4 **Association of Coagulation Activation with Clinical Complications in Sickle Cell Disease** 58
Kenneth I. Ataga, Julia E. Brittain, Payal Desai, Ryan May, Susan Jones, John Delaney, Dell Strayhorn, Alan Hinderliter and Nigel S. Key

Chapter 5 **A Genome-Wide Association Study of Total Bilirubin and Cholelithiasis Risk in Sickle Cell Anemia** 67
Jacqueline N. Milton, Paola Sebastiani, Nadia Solovieff, Stephen W. Hartley, Pallav Bhatnagar, Dan E. Arking, Daniel A. Dworkis, James F. Casella, Emily Barron-Casella, Christopher J. Bean, W. Craig Hooper, Michael R. DeBaun, Melanie E. Garrett, Karen Soldano, Marilyn J. Telen, Allison Ashley-Koch, Mark T. Gladwin, Clinton T. Baldwin, Martin H. Steinberg and Elizabeth S. Klings

Chapter 6 **Isofagomine *In Vivo* Effects in a Neuronopathic Gaucher Disease Mouse** 77
Ying Sun, Huimin Ran, Benjamin Liou, Brian Quinn, Matt Zamzow, Wujuan Zhang, Jacek Bielawski, Kazuyuki Kitatani, Kenneth D. R. Setchell, Yusuf A. Hannun and Gregory A. Grabowski

Chapter 7 **Urinary Copper Elevation in a Mouse Model of Wilson's Disease is a Regulated Process to Specifically Decrease the Hepatic Copper Load** 89
Lawrence W. Gray, Fangyu Peng, Shannon A. Molloy, Venkata S. Pendyala, Abigael Muchenditsi, Otto Muzik, Jaekwon Lee, Jack H. Kaplan and Svetlana Lutsenko

Chapter 8 **The Role of Fibrocytes in Sickle Cell Lung Disease** 99
Joshua J. Field, Marie D. Burdick, Michael R. DeBaun, Brett A. Strieter, Ling Liu, Borna Mehrad, C. Edward Rose, Jr., Joel Linden and Robert M. Strieter

Chapter 9 **Applying Microsatellite Multiplex PCR Analysis (MMPA) for Determining Allele Copy-Number Status and Percentage of Normal Cells within Tumors** 110
Carles Garcia-Linares, Jaume Mercadé, Bernat Gel, Josep Biayna, Ernest Terribas, Conxi Lázaro and Eduard Serra

Chapter 10 **High-Content Chemical and RNAi Screens for Suppressors of Neurotoxicity in a Huntington's Disease Model** 119
Joost Schulte, Katharine J. Sepp, Chaohong Wu, Pengyu Hong and J. Troy Littleton

Chapter 11 **Losses of Both Products of the *Cdkn2a/Arf* Locus Contribute to Asbestos-Induced Mesothelioma Development and Cooperate to Accelerate Tumorigenesis** 132
Deborah A. Altomare, Craig W. Menges, Jinfei Xu, Jianming Pei, Lili Zhang, Ara Tadevosyan, Erin Neumann-Domer, Zemin Liu, Michele Carbone, Ilse Chudoba, Andres J. Klein-Szanto and Joseph R.Testa

Chapter 12 **A High Degree of LINE-1 Hypomethylation is a Unique Feature of Early-Onset Colorectal Cancer** 138
Marina Antelo, Francesc Balaguer, Jinru Shia, Yan Shen, Keun Hur, Leticia Moreira, Miriam Cuatrecasas, Luis Bujanda, Maria Dolores Giraldez, Masanobu Takahashi, Ana Cabanne, Mario Edmundo Barugel, Mildred Arnold, Enrique Luis Roca, Montserrat Andreu, Sergi Castellvi-Bel, Xavier Llor, Rodrigo Jover, Antoni Castells, C. Richard Boland and Ajay Goel

Chapter 13 **Bifunctional Anti-Huntingtin Proteasome-Directed Intrabodies Mediate Efficient Degradation of Mutant Huntingtin Exon 1 Protein Fragments** 150
David C. Butler and Anne Messer

Chapter 14 ***Hdac6* Knock-Out Increases Tubulin Acetylation but does not Modify Disease Progression in the R6/2 Mouse Model of Huntington's Disease** 161
Anna Bobrowska, Paolo Paganetti, Patrick Matthias and Gillian P. Bates

Chapter 15 **Underlying Factors Associated with Anemia in Amazonian Children: A Population-Based, Cross-Sectional Study** 172
Marly A. Cardoso, Kézia K.G. Scopel, Pascoal T. Muniz, Eduardo Villamor and Marcelo U. Ferreira

Chapter 16 **A New Drug Design Targeting the Adenosinergic System for Huntington's Disease** 180
Nai-Kuei Huang, Jung-Hsin Lin, Jiun-Tsai Lin, Chia-I Lin, Eric Minwei Liu, Chun-Jung Lin, Wan-Ping Chen, Yuh-Chiang Shen, Hui-Mei Chen, Jhih-Bin Chen, Hsing-Lin Lai, Chieh-Wen Yang, Ming-Chang Chiang, Yu-Shuo Wu, Chen Chang, Jiang-Fan Chen, Jim-Min Fang, Yun-Lian Lin and Yijuang Chern

Chapter 17 **Replication Study in Chinese Population and Meta-Analysis Supports Association of the 11q23 Locus with Colorectal Cancer** 193
Li Zou, Rong Zhong, Jiao Lou, Xuzai Lu, Qi Wang, Yang Yang, Jiahong Xia, Juntao Ke, Ti Zhang, Yu Sun, Li Liu, Yongping Cui, Haibing Xiao, Lei Chang, Ding Xia and Hua Xu

Chapter 18 **Clinical Characteristics and Disease Predictors of a Large Chinese Cohort of Patients with Autosomal Dominant Polycystic Kidney Disease** 202
Dongping Chen, Yiyi Ma, Xueqi Wang, Shengqiang Yu, Lin Li, Bing Dai, Zhiguo Mao, Lijun Sun, Chenggang Xu, Shu Rong, Mengjun Tang, Hongbo Zhao, Hongchao Liu, Andreas L. Serra, Nicole Graf, Shiyuan Liu, Rudolf P. Wüthrich and Changlin Mei

Chapter 19 **Integration of SNP and mRNA Arrays with MicroRNA Profiling Reveals that MiR-370 is Upregulated and Targets NF1 in Acute Myeloid Leukemia** 213
Laura García-Ortí, Ion Cristó bal, Cristina Cirauqui, Elisabet Guruceaga, Nerea Marcotegui, María J. Calasanz, Remedios Castello-Cros and María D. Odero

Chapter 20 **Retinal Neurodegeneration in Wilson's Disease Revealed by Spectral Domain Optical Coherence Tomography** 222
Philipp Albrecht, Ann-Kristin Müller, Marius Ringelstein, David Finis, Gerd Geerling, Eva Cohn, Orhan Aktas, Hans-Peter Hartung, Harald Hefter and Axel Methner

Chapter 21 **Loss of Polycystin-1 Inhibits Bicc1 Expression during Mouse Development** 230
Peiwen Lian, Ao Li, Yuan Li, Haichao Liu, Dan Liang, Bo Hu, De Lin, Tang Jiang, Gilbert Moeckel, Dahui Qin and Guanqing Wu

Permissions

List of Contributors

Index

Preface

A genetic disorder is a genetic condition caused due to abnormalities in the genome. Such conditions are either inherited or acquired. Acquired defects may be caused due to changes in the DNA or due to new mutations. Genetic disorders can be single-gene disorders or multiple gene disorders. Over 6000 diseases are caused due to single gene mutations. Genetic disorders can be complex and multifactorial, involving a number of different genes and highly influenced by the environment. The field of medical genetics is concerned with the diagnosis of genetic disorders and their management. Though there is no known cure for genetic disorders, not all genetic diseases are fatal. Therefore, providing a quality of life and maintaining patient autonomy is the chief objective of medical genetics. This book unravels the recent studies in the field of medical genetics. Also included herein is a detailed explanation of the role of genetics in the incidence of varied diseases and disorders. For all readers who are interested in medical genetics, the case studies included in this book will serve as an excellent guide to develop a comprehensive understanding.

All of the data presented henceforth, was collaborated in the wake of recent advancements in the field. The aim of this book is to present the diversified developments from across the globe in a comprehensible manner. The opinions expressed in each chapter belong solely to the contributing authors. Their interpretations of the topics are the integral part of this book, which I have carefully compiled for a better understanding of the readers.

At the end, I would like to thank all those who dedicated their time and efforts for the successful completion of this book. I also wish to convey my gratitude towards my friends and family who supported me at every step.

Editor

Chromosomal Minimal Critical Regions in Therapy-Related Leukemia Appear Different from Those of *De Novo* Leukemia by High-Resolution aCGH

Nathalie Itzhar[1,2,3], Philippe Dessen[1,2,4], Saloua Toujani[1,2], Nathalie Auger[1,2,3], Claude Preudhomme[5], Catherine Richon[4], Vladimir Lazar[3,4], Véronique Saada[3,6], Anelyse Bennaceur[3,6], Jean Henri Bourhis[6], Stéphane de Botton[6], Alain Bernheim[1,2,3]*

1 Institut de la Santé et de la Reherche Médicale U985, Génétique des tumeurs, Institut Gustave Roussy, Villejuif, France, **2** Université Paris XI, Paris Sud, Orsay, France, **3** Molecular Pathology, Villejuif, France, **4** Institut Gustave Roussy, Functional Genomics Unit, Institut Gustave Roussy, Villejuif, France, **5** Department of Hematology, Centre de Biologie-Pathologie, Centre Hospitalier Régional Universitaire de Lille, Lille, France, **6** Department of Hematology, Institut Gustave Roussy, Villejuif, France

Abstract

Therapy-related acute leukemia (t-AML), is a severe complication of cytotoxic therapy used for primary cancer treatment. The outcome of these patients is poor, compared to people who develop *de novo* acute leukemia (p-AML). Cytogenetic abnormalities in t-AML are similar to those found in p-AML but present more frequent unfavorable karyotypes depending on the inducting agent. Losses of chromosome 5 or 7 are observed after alkylating agents while balanced translocations are found after topoisomerase II inhibitors. This study compared t-AML to p-AML using high resolution array CGH in order to find copy number abnormalities (CNA) at a higher resolution than conventional cytogenetics. More CNAs were observed in 30 t-AML than in 36 p-AML: 104 CNAs were observed with 63 losses and 41 gains (mean number 3.46 per case) in t-AML, while in p-AML, 69 CNAs were observed with 32 losses and 37 gains (mean number of 1.9 per case). In primary leukemia with a previously "normal" karyotype, 18% exhibited a previously undetected CNA, whereas in the (few) t-AML with a normal karyotype, the rate was 50%. Several minimal critical regions (MCRs) were found in t-AML and p-AML. No common MCRs were found in the two groups. In t-AML a 40kb deleted MCR pointed to *RUNX1* on 21q22, a gene coding for a transcription factor implicated in frequent rearrangements in leukemia and in familial thrombocytopenia. In *de novo* AML, a 1Mb MCR harboring *ERG* and *ETS2* was observed from patients with complex aCGH profiles. High resolution cytogenomics obtained by aCGH and similar techniques already published allowed us to characterize numerous non random chromosome abnormalities. This work supports the hypothesis that they can be classified into several categories: abnormalities common to all AML; those more frequently found in t-AML and those specifically found in p-AML.

Editor: Anita Kloss-Brandstaetter, Innsbruck Medical University, Austria

Funding: IGR Taxe Apprentissage. The funders had no role in study design, data collection and analysis, decision to publish, or preparation of the manuscript.

Competing Interests: The authors have declared that no competing interests exist.

* E-mail: bernheim@igr.fr

Introduction

Therapy-related myeloblastic leukemia, including therapy-related myelodysplasia, (t-AML), constitutes approximately 10% of AML and has several characteristic features [1,2]. As the incidence of cancers increases, so does that of t-AML. Nowadays, thanks to treatment intensification, the cure rate of primary neoplasia has increased but these very treatments are also implicated in severe therapy-related hematological consequences.

Factors associated with the development of t-AML include prior cytotoxic therapy. Two different types of t-AML are to be distinguished. The first one is due to prior therapy with alkylating agents (AA) or radiotherapy [1,2,3,4]. It occurs generally after a latency period of 5 to 7 years. This kind of t-AML is often preceded by a preleukemic period of myelodysplasia (t-MDS). Approximately 90% of the patients with AA-related t-AML exhibit clonal chromosomal aberrations including monosomy or deletions on chromosome 5 and/or 7, or complex aberrations involving chromosome 3, 12, 17 and 21. Drugs that target topoisomerase II (ATII), such as etoposide and anthracyclines may induce the second type of t-AML [1,2,3,4]. It occurs in a median of 2 years and is not preceded by MDS. Cytogenetic analysis shows a high frequency of rearrangements of chromosome band 11q23 but also recurrent balanced rearrangements t(8;21), t(15;17) and inv(16) [1,2].

The prognosis is poor in t-AML, excepted in case of t(8;21), t(15;17) and inv(16) which follow the same course as p-AML and the karyotype is more frequently modified with at least 2 abnormalities or more.

p-AML are also heterogeneous entities, classified according to bone marrow cell morphology and karyotype with the recent addition of several gene mutations. AML was among the first diseases to be treated and monitored according to somatic acquired chromosomal abnormalities, including the first successful targeted treatment against a pathological gene product in AML3.

As t-AML appear to have a particular leukemogenesis pathway [3,4], the aims of this work were:

1) to analyze t-AML using high resolution array CGH in order to find genome region or even gene-specific copy number abnormalities (CNA) at a higher resolution than conventional cytogenetics; 2)

Table 1. Clinical, biological features and karyotype of t-AML patients.

Pts[1]	Age[2]/ Sex	Primary [3] - Cancer[3] -	PC Tt[4]	FAB[5]	Karyotype at diagnosis of t-AML	FISH[6]	p-AML Type[7]	AML Tt[8]	Allog.[9]	Survival> 12 month
t-1	71/F	Ovarian C.	Tax/SP/PSC833/Iressa	RAEB	57,XXX,+1,+4,del(5)(q15;q33)×2,−7,+8,+9, +13,+14,−17,+18,+19,−20,+22,+mar [4]	MLL WT	A	no	no	no
t-2	67/F	VLSL	Fluda/Chlorambucil	AML-M5	44, XX, 5q-, −7, −12, −14, −18, + der(12?) +mar [20]	MLL WT	A	no	no	dead at diagnosis
t-3	44/F	Breast C Lipo- sarcoma	Alk/AT II	AML-M0	46,XX,der(1)t(1;17)(p36;?),der(7) t(7;?)(p15;?),der(10)(7;10;17)(?;p11; q?21),der(17)(q11?),ins(17?) [11]	MLL ND	U	yes	yes	yes
t-4	45/F	Astrocy-, toma + skin T NHL	RT/BCNU/Alk/ AT II, Autograft	AML-M0	45,XX,dup(2)(q22;q34),-3p21, t(5;13)(p15;q14),t(6;8)(p21;q24),+i(7q) ,der(7)t(7;15)(q10;q10),der(12) t(12;17)(p13;q11),−15,−17 [18]	MLL WT	U	yes	no	no
t-5	72/M	Esophag. C	5FU/SP/RT/curie	RAEB	45,XY,add(1)(q41),−5,−7, +mar [11]/ 45,XY,add(1)q41,−5,−7, t(12;20?)(p12;q12),+mar [11]	MLL ND	A	no	no	no
t-6	44/M	Follicular NHL	ATII/Alk/Oncovin Alk/AT II/TBI/ Alk Fluda	AML	46,del(X)(q23),Y,der?(6),t(2;6)(q12; q21),−7,del(18?)(q12),add(20)(q12) but uncertain conclusion at diagnosis	MLL ND	A	no	no	no
t-7	73/M	Multiple myeloma	Alk/steroids/INF/ AT II/BCNU	AML + Myeloma	46-**47**,XY,−7,−8,+r+dm [20]	MLL ND	A	no	no	no
t-8	72/M	Follicular NHL	Alk/ATII/Fluda/ Chlorambucil, Rituximab/ Spleen RT	AML-M5	47,XY,del(7)(q21q32),+13 [11]	MLL ND	A	yes	no	no
t-9	69/M	Head and Neck C.	RT	AML-M5	45,XY, −7 [12]	MLL WT	A	no	no	no
t-10	57/M	Bladder Cancer	RT/SP	MDS	46,XY, [14]/46–47,XY,del(7q-) [5]	MLL ND WCP 7	A	no	no	no
t-11	62/M	Follicular NHL	Alk/ATII/INF/ MethylGAG Rituximab/skin RT	AML-M5	NA#	MLL ND	A	yes	no	no
t-12	63/M	NSCLC	AT II/SP/RT	AML	46 XY,t(8;21)(q22;q22) [1]/46 XY, t(8;21)(q22;q22),del(7)(q11q34) [13]	MLL ND	U	no	no	no
t-13	38/F	Breast Cancer	Alk/RT/ ATII/RT/AM	AML	46,XX,add(1)(q 3?) [25]	MLL ND	U	yes	no	no
t-14	25/F	Endometre cancer	Alk/AT II/SP, Actinomycine	AML-M4	47,XX, +8 [14]	MLL WT	U	yes	yes	yes
t-15	52/F	Breast Cancer	Alk/AT II/RT	biphenotypic AML-M4	48,XX,+8,t(9;22)(q34;q11),+17 [12]	MLL ND WCP 8 + WCP 17 BCR-ABL fus	U	yes	no	no
							T	yes	no	yes
							T	yes	no	yes
							T	yes	no	yes
t-19	55/F	Breast Cancer	Alk/ATII/RT/HT/ Tax	AML-M5	46,XX,t(9;11)(p21;q23) [21]	MLL ND	T	yes	no	no
t-20	61/F	Breast C.	Alk/AT II/RT/HT	AML-M5	46,XX,t(9;11)(p22;q23) [14]	MLL sep	T	yes	yes	no

Table 1. Cont.

Pts1	Age2/ Sex	Primary 3 - Cancer3 -	PC Tt4	FAB5	Karyotype at diagnosis of t-AML	FISH6	p-AML Type7	AML Tt8	Allog.9	Survival> 12 month
t-21	60/F	NHL	Alk/AT II, Autograft	AML-M5	46,XX,t(9;11)(p22;q23) [12]	MLL sep	T	yes	no	no
t-22	19/M	Osteo- sarcoma	Alk/AT II/SP	AML-M5	46,XY,t(9;11)(p21;q23) [8]/ 46,XY,t(9;11)(p21;q23),+8 [10]	MLL sep	T	yes	no	yes
t-23	22/F	HL	Alk/ATII/Bleo/ Oncov	AML-M5	46,XX,t(11;19)(q23;q13) [12]	MLL sep	T	yes	no	dead at diagnosis
t-24	44/F	Ovarian cancer	Tax/SP/AT II/ Iressa	biphenotypic AML	46,XX, [2]	MLL sep	T	yes	no	no
t-25	64/F	Ovarian cancer	Tax/SP/Iressa	MDS	46,XX [17]	MLL WT	U	no	no	no
t-26	51/F	Anal + Breast C	RT, Alk/AT II/RT	AML	46,XX [5]	MLL WT	U	yes	no	no
t-27	47/F	Breast C.	Alk/AT II/RT/HT	AML-M2	46,XX [20]	MLL WT	U	yes	no	U
t-28	54/F	Breast C	Alk/AT II/RT	AML-M1	46,XX [16]	MLL WT	U	yes	yes	yes
t-29	71/M	Prostatic cancer.	RT	AML	46,XY [20]	MLL WT	U	no	no	no
t-30	67/M	Head and Neck C.	AT II/SP/Bleo/RT	AML-M5	46,XY [21]	MLL WT	U	yes	no	no

1 = patients. 2 = age at diagnosis of AML. 3 = Primary cancer; NHL: Follicular non hodgkin lymphoma, NSCLC: Non small cell lung cancer, VLSL: Villositary lymphocyte splenic lymphoma. 4 = Primary cancer treatment; Alk: alkylating agent, RT: radiotherapy, AT II: anti-topoisomerase II, AM: anti-metabolite, brachy: brachytherapy, Clo: Chlorambucyl, Tax: taxane, Fluda: fludarabine, SP: platinium, Bleo: bleomycin, HT: hormonotherapy, INF: interferon, Rit: Rituximab, RT: Radiotherapy, TBI: Total Body Irradiation, Oncov: Oncovin, A: alkylating-agent-inducing type, T: anti-topoisomerase-inducing type, U: undetermined. 5 = FAB classification: biph = biphenotypic. 6 = FISH column: MLL WT = MLL Wild Type, MLL R = MLL rearranged, ND = Not Done. 7 = Type of t-AML; A: alkylant induced, T anti-topoisomerase-induced. 8 = AML treatment. 9 = Allograft as treatment.

#This patient had secondary MDS for several years before the leukemia, with transitory partial monosomy 7, that had disappeared a year later, two years later the t-AML appeared.

to delimitate minimal critical regions (MCR) in order to identify potential candidate genes induced by AA or ATII implicated in oncogenesis: 3) to perform a similar analysis for p-AML and 4) to compare these two AML entities in our series and in the literature.

Materials and Methods

Patients

The patients were studied according to protocols approved by the Institut Gustave Roussy (Villejuif, France) Ethics Committee. Between 1995 and 2007, 30 t-AML and 36 p-AML with various karyotype results were collected at disease onset. (table 1 and 2).

Cytogenetic analysis

Cytogenetic analyses were performed on metaphase spreads obtained from tumor, bone marrow or blood. In each case, 20 RHG-banded metaphases were analyzed when possible.

Fluorescence in situ hybridization (FISH) studies

A set of commercial probes was used to search for abnormalities such as WCP1, WCP2, WCP5, WCP7, WCP8, t(8;21) RUNX1-ETO fusion probes (fp), t(9;22)BCR-ABL (fp), MLL dissociation probes, WCP14, t(15;17) PML-RARA (fp), WCP17 (tables 1 and 2). They were used according to the manufacturer's protocol (Vysis® or Kreatech®).

Cell culture

Most samples were diagnosis bone marrow cells except for patients t-4, t-9, t-11, t-17, t-19, t-26 and p-33 derived from whole blood. After thawing, all t-AML samples were cultured for 24h (20% fetal calf serum in RPMI 1640 with antibiotics) without selecting CD34+ cells. The mononuclear cells were collected and washed before DNA extraction. Bone marrow was cultured in the same flask with the same media, to allow adherent cell proliferation in order to obtain constitutional fibroblasts from the patient. However, no adherent cells were obtained from this procedure. Pooled commercial DNA (Promega®) was thus used for all t-AML and p-AML work in order to maintain a homogenous process for the 64 AML.

Oligonucleotide aCGH

Tumor genomic DNA was isolated according to Qiagen protocols with modifications [5]. Samples containing more than 60% of blasts were chosen in order to analyze a majority of pathological cells. High-molecular-weight genomic DNA was extracted from the cell lines with a DNeasy extraction kit (Qiagen).

Patient leukemia samples were analyzed using 244 K micro-arrays (Agilent Technologies, Santa Clara, CA, USA). Only t-AML were processed as dye-swap pairs. In all experiments, sex-matched DNA from a pooled human female or male individual (Promega, Madison, WI) was used as the reference. Oligonucleotide aCGH processing was performed as detailed in the manufacturer's protocol (version 4.0; http://www.agilent.com). Data were extracted from scanned images using Feature extraction® software (version A.8.5.3, Agilent). Raw data text files from the latter were then imported for analysis into CGH Analytics® 3.4.40. Aberrations were detected with the ADM2

Table 2. Clinical, biological features and karyotype of the p-AML patients.

Patients	Age[1]/ Sex	FAB	Karyotype	FISH	Allograft	Survival duration > 12 months
p-1	68/F	M1	45,XX,−7	ND	No info	No info
p-2	34/M	M6	45,XY,−7	ND	no	no info
p-3	66/M	M1	48,XY,+8,+13	ND	No	Yes
p-4	54/F	M5	47,XX,+i(21q)	ND	Yes	Yes
p-5	32/M	M5	47,XY,t(2;14)(q21;q32),+4	wcp2, wcp14	No	No
p-6	44/F	M5	46,XX,der(5)t(1;5)(q32;q35),inv(9)(p12q13)[20]. ish(5p15,5q31)×2,add(5)(q35?)(wcp1+)	MLL WT, wcp1, wcp5,wcp17	No	No info
p-7	68/M	M5	46,XY,del(7)(q21q31),der(9)(WPC9+),?der(11)(q23)/46,XY[2]	MLL WT	No	No
p-8	25/F	M3	46,XX,t(15;17)(q22;q21)	PML-RARA fus		
p-9	46/F	M3	46,XX,t(15;17)(q22;q21)	PML RARA fus	No	No info
p-10	46/F	M3	46,XX,t(15;17)(q22;q21)	PML RARA fus	No	Yes
p-11	27/M	M3	46,XY,i(3)(p10),i(3q),t(15;17)(q22;q21)	PML RARA fus	No	Yes
p-12	47/M	M3	46,XY,t(15;17)(q22;q21)	PML RARA fus	No	No
p-13	73/M	M3	46,XY,t(15;17)(q22;q21)	PML RARA fus	No	Yes
p-14	35/M	M3	46,XY,t(15;17)(q22;q21)	PML RARA fus	No	Yes
p-15	57/M	M3	46,XY,t(15;17)(q22;q21)	PML RARA fus	No	Yes
p-16	54/M	M4	46,XY,t(16;16)(p13;q22)	CBFB sep	Yes	No
p-17	26/M	M4Eo	46,XY,t(16;16)(p13;q22)	ND	Yes	Yes
p-18	19/M	M2	45,XY,t(8;21)(q22;q22),del(9)(q31q34)	ND	No	Yes
p-19	37/M	M1	45,XY,t(9;11)(p22;q23),del(7)(p12;p21)	MLL sep	No	Yes
p-20	25/M	M1	46,XY,t(9;11)(p22;q23)	MLL sep	Yes	Yes
p-21	80/M	M1	46,XY[3]/50–53,XY,−1,−3,−4,−15?,−21,+7 to 10 mar	ND	No	No
p-22	42/M	M1	46,XY,t(3;5)(q25;q34),del(4)(q26),der(12)t(4;12) (q28?;p12),der(18)t(12;18)(p12;q21),mar?	WCP(3; 4) WCP(5; 12)	Yes	Yes
p-23	30/M	M5	46,XY,t(11;12)(q13;p13)[2]46,XY,id,der(1)t(1;1) (p16;q12)[1]/46,XY,id,der(7)t(1;7)(q12;q36)[1]/ 46,XY,id,der(9)t(1;9)(q12;p24)[2]46,XY,id,der(14) t(1;14)(q12;p10)[2]46,XY,id,der(20)t(1;20)(q12;p12) [1]46,XY,id,der(20)t(1;20)(q12;q13)[2]46,XY,id, der(21)t(1;21)(q12;q10)[3]	ND	No	No
p-24	71/M	M2	43–46,XY,−2,−5,−7,−16,+mar1,+mar2,+mar3, +mar4, variations	ND	No	No
p-25	63/F	M2	46,XX	ND	No	Yes
p-26	52/F	M2	46,XX	MLL WT	Yes	Yes
p-27	23/F	M2	46,XX	MLL WT	No	Yes
p-28	23/F	M5	46,XX	MLL WT	Yes	Yes
p-29	45/F	M5	46,XX	ND	No	No
p-30	73/F	M5	46,XX	ND	No	No
p-31	31/M	M0	46,XY	MLL WT	No	No info
p-32	75/M	M1	46,XY	MLL WT	No	No
p-33	41/M	M1	46,XY	MLL WT	Yes	No info
p-34	48/M	M2	46,XY	MLL WT	Yes	Yes
p-35	38/M	M2	46,XY	MLL WT	No	No
p-36	63/M	M4	46,XY	ND	No	No

1 = age at diagnosis of AML. FAB column: FAB classification. FISH column: MLL WT = MLL Wild Type; MLL sep = MLL rearranged (separated); PML-RARA fus = fusion of PML and RARA gene; WCP = whole chromosome paint; ND = Not Done.

Table 3. Germinal and immunoglobulin genes related CNVs.

Location	Some CNV genes	miRNA
Germinal CNVs		
−1p36.13 <16.71–17.14>	CROCC MSTP9 ESPNP	
−1q21.3 <150.82–150.84>	NLCE3C	
−1q23.3 <159.75–159.90>	FCGR2A FCGR2B FCGR3A HSPA6	
−1q44 <246.79–246.86>	OR2T34 OR2T10 OR2T11	
+/−3q29 <196.90–196.96>	MUC20	mir-570
+/−4q13.2 <69.05–69.16>	UGT2B17	
+5p15.33 <0.76–0.87>	ZDHHC11	
−6p25.3 <0.20–0.32>	DUSP22	
+/−6p21.2 <32.56–32.72	HLA-DQA1 HLA-DRB1 HLA-DRB5 HLA-DRB6	
+/−8p11.3 <39.35–39.50>	ADAM3A	
−10q11.22 <46.37–47.73>	ANXA8 PPYR1 GPRIN2 SYT15 ANTXRL	
+11q11 <55.12–55.20>	OR4P4 OR4C11 OR4S2 OR4C6	
+12p12 <19.36–19.46>	PLEKHA5	
+/−14q11.2 <18.62–19.49>	OR4K5 OR4K1 OR4N2 OR4K2 OR4Q3 OR4M1	
+/−15q11.2 <18.65–20.08>	BCL8 NF1P1 OR4N4 OR4M2	mir-1268
+/−15q14 <32.51–32.62>	GOLGABB	mir-1233
+/−16p11.2 <31.86–33.53>	TP53TG3 SLC6A10P HERC2P4...	mir-1826
+17q21.31 <41.52–41.57>	KIAA1267	
−17q21.31 <41.55–42.04>	NSF LRRC37A ARL17P1 KIAA1267 LRRC37A2	
−19q13.2 <48.20–48.43>	PSG1 PSG3 PSG6 PSG7 PSG11	
+/−22q11.23 <22.65–22.72	GSTT1.	
Immunoglobulin genes related CNVs		
−2p11.2 <89.10–89.26>	IGKC IGKV1-5 IGKV3D-15 IGKV1D-13 IGKV3-20 IGKV2-24	
+/−7p14.1<38.22–38.41>	TRGC2 TRGV5 TRGV7 TRGV9 STARD3NL	
+/−14q11.2 <21.43–22.04>	TRA@ TRD@ TRDV1 TRAV20 TRAJ17 TRAC	
−14q32.33 <105.13–106.00>	IGH@ IGHA1 IGHA2 IGHG1 IGHG2 IGHG4 IGHV4-31 C14orf81	

The CNVs are either lost or gained as indicated by a "−" or a "+". Locations on chromosomes are described according to the ISCN 2009 with slight modifications: sequence numbers are included between <> and expressed in Mb, with a resolution of 10kb. Column 2: coding genes included in the CNVs: Column 3; miRNA genes included in the CNVs.

algorithm and the filtering options of a minimum of 5 probes and abs(log2Ratio) >0.3. Aberration segments were individually reviewed using build 35, hg18 from the UCSC Genome browser [6]. Anomalies that were localized to regions with high-copy repetitive or GC-rich DNA sequences including telomeric regions were excluded. We defined gains and losses for the oligonucleotide dataset as a linear ratio ≥1.2 or ≤0.8 respectively. High and low-level amplification events were defined as a linear ratio ≥4 or between <2 and <4 respectively. The data are described in accordance with MIAME guidelines and have been deposited in ArrayExpress under accession number E-TABM-1014.

Results

Copy Number Variations (CNV)

As no paired DNA had been obtained, Copy Number Variations (CNV) were distinguished from Copy Number Abnormalities (CNA) based on various criteria: i) sequence size below 2 Mb; ii) the presence of repetitive identical breakpoints between patients; iii) the genes involved such as olfactory receptor genes, the NF1P1 locus or GSTT1 (chromosome 22) and iv) consultation of the Database of Genomic Variants [7]. Many Mendelian CNVs, that are present throughout the entire genome [8], were seen in the two AML samples (table 3). Together with classic genes, four microRNA embedded in CNV regions were found: mir-570 in 3q29 within MUC20, mir-1268 in 15q11 within NF1P1, BCL8 and olfactory receptors, mir-1233 in 15q14 within GOLGCABB, and mir-1826 in 16p11.2 within TP53TG3 HERC2P4 (table 3).

Deletions inside immunoglobulin gene (IG) clusters, consecutive to VDJ rearrangement were observed mainly in t-AML. These illegitimate recombinations were considered as acquired CNVs [5], characteristic of the malignant clone. In t-AML, four losses were located in 2p11 in IGLK and 9 in 14q32.3 in IGH. Two t-AML were bi-phenotypic acute leukemia (cases 2 and 7). In three cases (t-15, t-17 and t-25), both genes were rearranged (table 4). No relationships were observed with MLL or other translocations. In p-AML (table 5), only 2 rearrangements were observed: on IGLK (case p-21) and on IGH (case p-24). No rearrangement of IGLL on 22q11 was observed. The difference in the proportion of IG rearrangements in t-AML compared to p-AML was statistically significant with a $p<0.002$.

Table 4. Gains and losses CNA in t-AML and revised karyotype after aCGH.

Patients	Gains	Losses	Revised karyotypes
t-2	+14q11.2q12<24,09–26.24>[1.23]	−1q44<241.94–247.19>[0.61]	44,XX,**−1q44**,−5q14.3q35,−7,**−7q33q34,−12p11.2p13.2,**
	+14q12q13.3<29.52–35.74>[1.26]	−5q14.3q35<85.18–167.84>[0.58]	**−12p11.2q12,−12q13.1,−12q13.3q22,−12q23.3,**
	+14q21.1q21.2<41.52–44.69>[1.23]	−7pterp22.3<0.14–2.67>[0.65]	**−14q12,+14q12,−14q12,+14q12q13.3,**
	+14q21.3q22.1<47.25–52.51>[1.54]	−7p21.3<8.21–11.79>[0.64]	**−14q21.2,+14q21.1q21.2,−14q21.2,+14q21.3q22.1,**
		−7p15.2q14.3<27.40–33.28>[0.67]	**−18q11.1qter,−18q11.2q12.1,**
		−7p14.1q33<39.89–135.74>[0.63]	**−18q22.3q23**
		−7q33q34<135.74–137.48>[0.16]	
		−7q34qter<137.48–158.76>[0.60]	
		−12p13p11.2<11.27–25.37>[0.61]	
		−12p11.2q12<32.77–37.09>[0.65]	
		−12q13.1<47.09–49.44>[0.66]	
		−12q13.3q22<55.30–92.75>[0.63]	
		−12q23.3<105.58–107.51>[0.68]	
		−14q11.2<23.73–24.07>[0.70]	
		−14q12<26.25–27.10>[0.65]	
		−14q21.2<35.77–37.62>[0.66]	
		−14q21.2<44.69–45.26>[0.66]	
		−18q11.1q11.2<16.79–21.74>[0.59]	
		−18q11.2q12.1<21.74–24.41>[0.22]	
		−18q12.1q22.3<24.41–71.05>[0.59]	
		−18q22.3q23<71.06–71.76>[0.23]	
		−18q23<71.76–76.11>[0.59]	
t-24	+17q11.1qter<22.80–78.65>[1.39]	−2p11<89.65–91.05>[0.62]*	46,XX,t(11;?)(q23;?),**i(17)(q10),−19p13.3,+19p13.3**
	+19p13.3<4.96–6.82>[1.44]	−17pterp11.2<0.28–21.22>[0.63]	
		−19p13.3<0.21–4.96>[0.60]	
t-8	+13q11qter<18.36–114.10>[1.46]	−7q31.1q36.1<107.67–150.28>[0.55]	47,XY,**−Xp11.4,−7q31.1q36.1**,+13,**−21q22.1**
		−21q22.1<35.01–35.60>[0.11]	
		−Xp11.4<39.25–39.85>[0.16]	
t-13	+2p16.1p25.3<0.02–54.88>[1.46]	−1q42.3.q44<233.13–247.19>[0.53]	46,XX,**der(1)t(1;2)(q42.3;p16.1),−10q11.2**
		−10q11.2<45.53–47.97>[0.78]	
t-30		−2p23.3<25.31–25.60>[0.50]	46,XY,**−2p23.3**
		−14q32.3<105.96–106.00>[0.65]*	
t-15	+8pterqter<0.16–146.26>[1.31]	−2p11<88.98–91.05>[0.46]*	46,XX,+8,t(9;22)(q34;q11),+17
	+17pterqter<0.02–78.65>[1.31]	−4q31.2<146.62–146.67>[0.68]	
		−14q32.3<105.40–106.15>[0.34]*	
t-4	+2q14.3q32.3<128.11–193.87>[1.34]	−1p36.11<26.73–27.04>[0.64]	**46,**XX,**dup(2)(q14.3q32.3),**t(5;13)(p15;q14)
	+7q11.2q36.3<61.46–158.81>[1.65]	−1q43<237.92–238.50>[0.62]	**−5q31.3q32,**+i(7)(q10),**der(7)t(7;15)(q10;q21.3),**
	+12p12.1 p11.2<24.32–30.60>[1.37]	−5q31.1q33.1<142.91–148.19>[0.63]	**der(12)t(12;17)(p12.1;q11),+12p11.2p12.1,**
		−7p11.1p22.3<0.14–57.89>[0.65]	**−15pterq21.2, −17p11.2p13.3,−17q23.2**
		−12pterp12.1<0.05–21.96>[0.63]	
		−14q32.3<105.13–105.84>[0.68]*	
		−15q11.2q21.3<20.24–55.80>[0.65]	
		−17p13.3p11.2<0.02–22.07>[0.65]	
		−17q22<51.84–54.75>[0.64]	
t-16	+7p15.2<27.15–27.18>[1.33]		46,XX,**+7p15.2,+8q24.2q24.3,**inv(16)(p13;q22)
	+8q24.2q24.3<139.48–140.18>[1.46]		
t-23	+4q35.1q35.2<187.17–187.37>[1.49]	−14q32.3<106.21–106.25>[0.66]*	46,XX,**+4q35.1q35.2,**t(11;19)(q23;q13)
t-17	+7p15.2<27.15–27.18>[1.26]	−2p11<89.10–89.89>[0.70]*	**−3p12.3p14.1,+7p15,**t(15;17)(q22;q21)+
	+6q27<168.12–168.84>[1.20]	−3p12.3p14.1<69.07–79.19>[0.54]	.ish(PML;RARA)
		−14q32.3<105.85–105.89>[0.59]*	

Table 4. Cont.

Patients	Gains	Losses	Revised karyotypes
t-29		−14q32.3<105.94–106.00>[0.66]*	46,XY,−**21q22.1**
		−21q22.1<34.98–35.29>[0.59]	
t-3	+8q24.3<143.73–143.90>[1.50]	−14q32.3<104.96–105.22>[0.76]*	46,XX,**t(1;17)(p36;?),t(7;?)(p15;?),+8q24.3,**
			t(7;10;17)(?;p11;q21;?)
t-26	+2q11.2<98.43–98.63>[1.42]		46,XX,**+2q11.2**
t-12	+21q22.1qter<35.07–46.91>[1.19]	−7q22.1q36.3<101.85–158.79>[0.80]	46,XY,−7q21.2q36.3,t(8;21)(q22;q22),**+21q22.1qter**
t-9	+4p16.3<1.20–1.30>[1.38]	−7pterqter<0.14–158.76>[0.56]	45,XY,**+4p16.3,**−7
	+6q27<168.08–168.32>[1.50]		
t-11		−21q22.12<35.11–35.15>[0.68]	46,XY,**−21q22.12**
t-14	+7p15.2<27.15–27.18>[1.38]	−14q32.3<105.96–106.00>[0.60]*	47,XX,**+7p15**,+8,−17q11.2
	+8pterq24.3<0.16–142.23>[1.35]	−17q11.2<25.96–27.38>[0.72]	
	+8q24.3<142.23–145.81>[1.52]		
	+8q24.3<145.81–146.26>[1.35]		
t-1		−5q15qter<94.36–177.87[0.79]	57,XXX,+1,+4,del(5)(q15q33)×2,−7,+8,+9,+der(11),
			+13, +14,−17,+18,+19, −20,+22,+mar
t-5	+5p15.2p14.3<10.78–21.71>[1.27]	−3p14.1p12.3<69.67–80.18>[0.54]	**46,**XY,**−3p12.2p14.1,−5p15.2pter,**+5 p14.3p15.2,
	+5p13.3q11.2<31.24–53.59>[1.31]	−5pterp15.2<0.09–10.76>[0.57]	**+5p12q12.3,−5q12.3qter,−7p11.1p22.3,**
	+21q22.1<36.40–36.53>[1.60]	−5q12.3qter<65.23–180.64>[0.57]	**−7q21.3q32.1,−12p13.1p13.2,+21q22.1**
		−7pterp11.1<0.14–57.66>[0.57]	
		−7q21.3q36.3<97.13–158.76>[0.57]	
		−12p13.2p13.1<11.82–13.33>[0.62]	
t-10	+1q44<246.44–247.06>[1.32]	−7p22.2<3.02–3.12>[0.48]	46,XY,**+1q44,−7p22.2,−7q11.2,−7q21.3q22.1**
		−7q11.2<64.40–75.85>[0.77]	
		−7q21.3q22.1<97.69–101.88>[0.77]	
t-7	+9q34.3<135.98–139.80>[1.30]	−7pterqter<0.14–158.81>[0.79]	**45,**XY,−7,**+9q34.3,+12p13.1,**+**12p11.1,**−**12q11q12,**-
	+12p13.1<14.25–14.61>[1.36]	−12q12<36.73–42.14>[0.65]	**−12q13.1,+12q13.12q14.3,−17p11.2p13.3,**
	+12p11.1<31.55–34.64>[1.34]	−12q13.1<45.33–47.69>[0.68]	**−21q21.1q21.2,+21q21.2q21.3,−21q22.11q22.12,**
	+12q13.1q14.3<47.69–51.83>[1.42]	−17pterp11.3<0.02–21.23>[0.78]	**+21q22.12q23,−21q22.3**
	+12q14.1q14.3<58.80–64.31>[1.33]	−21q21.1q21.2<19.84–23.05>[0.65]	
	+21q21.2q21.3<23.17–30.35>[1.42]	−21q22.1<34.38–36.12>[0.66]	
	+21q22.1q22.3<36.20–43.01>[1.58]	−21q22.3<43.02–43.08>[0.65]	
t-6		−7pterqter<0.14–158.76>[0.70]	45,XY,t(2;6)(q12;q21),−7
t-22	+2p25.2<2.54–3.57>[1.37]		46,XY,**+2p25.3,**+8,t(9;11)(p21;q23)
	+8pterqter<0.16–146.26>[1.40]		
t-19	+7p15.2<27.15–27.18>[1.40]	No CNA	46,XX,+7p15.2,t(9;11)(p22;q23)
t-21	No CNA	No CNA	46,XX,t(9;11)(p22;q23)
t-20	No CNA	No CNA	46,XX,t(11;19(p22;q23)
t-18	No CNA	−14q32.3<105.94–106.00>[0.64]*	46,XX,t(15;17)(q22;q21)
t-25	No CNA	−2p11<89.10–91.05>[0.69]*.	46,XX
		−14q32.3<105.96–106.00>[0.61]*	
t-27	No CNA	No CNA	46,XX
t-28	No CNA	No CNA	46,XX

Column 2 and 3: The CNA are either lost or gained as indicated by a "−" or a "+"; locations on chromosomes are described according to the ISCN 2009 with slight modifications: sequence numbers are included between <> and expressed in Mb, with a resolution of 10kb; linear ratios are written between brackets after an "×"; CNAs with a linear ratio >2 (low level of amplification) or losses <0.25 are labeled in **bold** and ***italics***; "*" indicates CNA that are probably part of a rearrangement of the immunoglobulin genes. They have not been included in the synthetic karyotypes because they could be considered as an acquired CNV which is characteristic of monoclonal proliferation.

Column 4: In **bold** are new data or those modified by aCGH in the synthetic karyotypes; CNAs that were contiguous but whose ratios were not too different were fused to express overall chromosome abnormality for readability.

Table 5. Gains and losses CNA in p-AML and revised karyotype.

Patients	Gains	Losses	Revised karyotypes
p-24	+1p36.3<1.52–7.56>[1.26]	−2pterp22.3<0.02–32.60>[0.66]	**46,XY,+1p34.2p36.3,**−2pterp22.3,−2p14p13.3,
	+1q21q22<153.19–154.64>[1.67]	−2p14p13.3<68.01–71.72>[0.66]	−2q35qter,**+3p21.3, −3p21.3p22.2,+4p16.3,**
	+3p21.3<50.26–50.29>[2.54]	−2q35qter<219.02–242.39>[0.66]	−**5q14.2q33.3,−7p15.2p15.3,**−**7q11.2,**−**7q21.1q22.2,**
	+3p21.3<52.29–52.31>[4.00]	−3p22p21.3<38.35–49.66>[0.66]	**−7q31.3q36.3,+15q11.2,+15q22.2q26.2,**
	+4p16.3<0.99–1.65>[1.61]	−5q14.2q33.3<82.18–158.75>[0.61]	**+15q23,−15q26.2q26.3,−16p13.3q23.1,**
	+15q22.2q23<56.84.18–67.10>[2.05]	−7p15.2p15.3<19.64–26.31>[0.63]	**+16q23.3q24.3,−17p11.2q12,−17q21.31q21.3,**
	+15q23<67.44–68.37>[3.64]	−7q11.22q11.23<69.84–72.44>[0.65]	**+19p13.3p13.1, +20p12.3p13, +21q22.1q22.3,+22q13.1**
	+15q24.1<70.42–72.67>[2.89]	−7q21.12q22.2<87.65–105.96>[0.71]	
	+15q24.1q26.2<72.70–94.54>[1.30]	−7q31.32q36.3<123.35–158.81>[0.64]	
	+16q23.3q24.3<82.61–88.67>[1.8]	−14q32.3<105.60−105-70>[0.74]*	
	+19p13.3p13.1<0.64–19.72>[1.41]	−15q26.2q26.3<94.55–100.21>[0.75]	
	+20p12.3p13<0.27–9.14>[1.26]	−16p13.3q23.1<15.38–78.80>[0.74]	
	+21q22.1<33.30–37.23>[1.79]	−17p11.2q12<0.18–29.54>[0.65]	
	+21q22.1<37.24–38.54>[2.5]	−17q21.3q21.33<38.29–46.94>[0.66]	
	+21q22.1<38.54–39.38>[3.00]		
	+21q22.2q22.3<39.40–43.22>[2.18]		
	+21q22.3<43.23–46.89>[1.70]		
	+22q13.1<35.86 = 37.20>[1.33]		
p-21	+3p14.3p14.2<57.97–62.19>[1.48]	−1q21.1q44<147.21–247.19>[0.62]	50–53,XY,−1**q21.1q44,−2p24.3,**
	+3p14.2p14.1<63.60–64.29>[1.31]	−2p11.2<89.38–91.05>[0.61]*	−3**p12.1p14.1,+3p14.1,−3p14.1,+3p14.1p14.2,**
	+3p14.1<64.32–65.50>[4.61]	−2pterp24.3<0.02–16.22>[0.61]	**+3p14.2p14.3,−3p14.3p24.3,+3p11.2qter,**
	+3p14.1<66.40–67.67>[4.71]	−3 p24.3p14.3<0.03–57.40>[0.63]	**−4q22.1q27,−9q22.3q31.1,**
	+3p11.2qter<89.28–199.32>[1.35]	−3p14.2<62.20–63.58>[0.60]	**+21q11.2q21.1,**
	+21q11.2q21.1<14.29–17.97>[5.46]	−3p14.1<65.51–66.11>[0.60]	**+21q22.1qter**
	+21q22.1q22.3<38.27–43.54>[5.45]	−3p14.1p12.1<67.68–86.30>[0.67]	
	+21q22.3<43.59–45.12>[2.11]	−4q22.1q27<88.94–123.72>[0.61]	
	+21q22.3qter<45.12–46.91>[1.7]	−9q22.3q31.1<93.92–103.86>[0.63]	
p-22		−4q28.2q28.3<130,24–134,36>[0,55]	46,XY,t(3;5)(q25;q34),**del(4)(q28.2q28.3),**
		−12p12.1p13.2<11,40–21,20>[0,55]	der(12)t(4;12;18)(q28?;p12;q21)**,**
		−18q21.2<48,99–51,05>[0,55]	**−12p12.1p13.2,−18q21.2,−18q22.3q23**
		−18q22.3q23<69,56–76,03>[0,55]	
p-23	+1q23.2qter<158.48–247.17>[1.24]	No CNA	46,XY, t(11;12)(q13;p13)/46,XY,id,der(1)t(1;1)(p16;q12)/
			46,XY,id,der(7)t(1;7)(q12;q36)/
			46,XY,id,der(9)t(1;9)(q12;p24)/46,XY,id,
			der(14)t(1;14)(q12;p10)/46,XY,id,der(20)t(1;20)
			(q12;p12)/46,XY,id,der(20)t(1;20)(q12;q13)/
			46,XY,id,der(21)t(1;21)(q12;q10),+1q23.2qter
p-5	+4pterqter<0.06–191.02>[1.43]	No CNA	47,XY,t(2;14)(q21;q32),+4
p-32		−3p21.3p21.3<44,20–49,02>[0,59]	46,XY,**−3p21.3**
p-6	+1q32.1qter<201.31–247.10>[1.39]		46,XX,der(5)t(1;5)(q32;q35),inv(9)(p12q13)
p-1		−7<0.14–158.76>[0.61]	45,XX,−7
p-2	**+Xp22.2<15.95–16.61>[2.04]**	−7<0.14–158.76>[0.55]	45,XY,**+Xp22.2,**−7,−22q11.2
		−22q11.2<21.36–21.41>[0.52]	
p-7	+11q24.2qter<124.85–134.43>[1.23]	−7q31.2qter<115.49–158.78>[0.77]	46,XY,−7**q31.2q36.3, +11q24.2q25**
p-3	+8pterqter<0.16–146.25>[1.27]	−2p11.2<88.93–89.14>[0.69]*	48,XY,+8,+13
	+13pterqter<18.31–114.12>[1.28]		
p-18	No CNA	−8q21.3q22.1<93.15–94.17>[0.63]	46,XY,t(8;21)(q22;q22),**del(8)(q21.3q22.1),−9q12q31.1**
		−9q12q31.1<67.20–104.45>[0.62]	
p-13	+17q21.2<35.76–35.84>[1.49]	No CNA	46,XY,t(15;17)(q22;q21)**,+17q21.2**
p-4	+21q11.2qter<14.31–46.91>[1.77]	No CNA	47,XX,+i(21q)

Table 5. Cont.

Patients	Gains	Losses	Revised karyotypes
p-8	No CNA	No CNA	46,XX,t(15;17)(q22;q21)
p-9	No CNA	No CNA	46,XX,t(15;17)(q22 ;q21)
p-10	No CNA	No CNA	46,XY,t(15;17)(q22;q21)
p-11	No CNA	No CNA	46,XY,t(15;17)(q22;q21)
p-12	No CNA	No CNA	46,XY,t(15;17)(q22;q21)
p-14	No CNA	No CNA	46,XY,t(15;17)(q22;q21)
p-15	No CNA	No CNA	46,XY,t(15;17)(q22;q21)
p-16	No CNA	No CNA	46,XY,t(16;16)(p13;q22)
p-17	No CNA	No CNA	46,XY,t(16;16)(p13;q22)
p-19	No CNA	−14q32.3<105.02–105.04>[0.76]*	45,t(9;11)(p22;q23),del(7)(p12;p21)
p-20	No CNA	No CNA	46,XY, t(9;11)(p22;q23)
p-25	No CNA	−14q32.3<105.96–105.94>[0.61]*	46,XX
p-26	No CNA	No CNA	46,XX
p-27	No CNA	No CNA	46,XX
p-28	No CNA	No CNA	46,XX
p-29	No CNA	No CNA	46,XX
p-30	No CNA	No CNA	46,XX
p-31	No CNA	No CNA	46,XY
p-33	No CNA	No CNA	46,XY
p-34	No CNA	No CNA	46,XY
p-35	No CNA	No CNA	46,XY
p-36	No CNA	No CNA	46,XY

Column 2 and 3: The CNA were either lost or gained as indicated by a "−" or a "+"; the locations on the chromosomes are described according to the ISCN 2009 with slight modifications: sequence numbers are included between <> and expressed in Mb, with a resolution of 10kb; linear ratios are written between brackets after an "×"; CNAs with a linear ratio >2 (low level of amplification) or losses <0.25 are labeled in **bold** and ***italics***; "*" indicates CNA that are probably part of a rearrangement of the immunoglobulin genes. They are not included in the synthetic karyotypes as they could be considered as an acquired CNV characteristic of monoclonal proliferation.
Column 4: In **bold** are new data or those modified by aCGH in the synthetic karyotypes; CNAs that were contiguous but whose ratios were not too different were fused to express overall chromosome abnormality for readability.

Karyotypes and CNA

Karyotypes and aCGH were well correlated, with few exceptions. Ninety-six unbalanced chromosomal abnormalities previously undetected by mitotic karyotypes, were detected after high resolution aCGH (tables 1, 2, 4 and 5). Most of the additional abnormalities were too small to be detected by karyotypes. Some revealed masked rearrangements (Figure 1). In case t-1, the discrepancy between the karyotype and aCGH was probably due to a combination of hyperploidy, genetic heterogeneity and the presence of normal cells resulting in aCGH detection of only the del(5q).

In both groups of AML, 25 cytogenetically balanced translocations (table 1, 2 tables 4 and 5) did not show any cryptic rearrangement (gain or loss) at their breakpoint locations. In 5 cases (t-3, t-5, t-12, p-18, p-13), a CNA was found near the breakpoints. Patient t-3 was considered as having multiple balanced translocations that could not be further analyzed due to insufficient material. Patient t-5 had a poorly defined translocation implicating 12p and according to aCGH analysis, a small loss began in the middle of ETV6, suggesting a rearrangement of this gene. Patient t-12, had a standard t(8;21) and following "good practice" rules, no further investigation was initially performed. aCGH revealed a duplication of 21q22.1qter that was confirmed by FISH as another translocation or insertion on an unidentified chromosome. The unbalanced translocation breakpoint was 30 Kb centromeric to the 3′ end of RUNX1 suggesting a possible double event. Patient p-18, with a t(8;21) p-AML, had a 1Mb loss that included the first two exons of RUNXT1 on 8q21.3. Patient p13 had a t (15.17) accompanied by a small duplication of the telomeric part of RARA and of the TOP2A genes (table 5).

In some cases the confrontation between aCGH and the karyotype allowed us to better define the previously diagnosed rearrangements. In patient t-13, an add(1)(q3?) was found in the morphological karyotype. With aCGH, it was concluded that it resulted from an unbalanced translocation der(1)t(1;2)(q42.3;p16.1). The breakpoint was virtually cloned from the arrays: on 1q42.3<231.374>, it was sitting in the middle of PCNXL2, between exons 11 and 12. On 2p16.1<54.943>, it was lying in an EML6 gene in the vicinity of exon 12 of the gene. P-22, a primary AML with a t(3;5), had a loss of 10Mb of 12p13 secondary to a additional complex translocation encompassing ETV6 and CDKN1B (table 5).

t-AML

All patients (excepted three who had received radiotherapy alone) had been treated with multi-agent chemotherapy (AA and ATII) combined or not with radiotherapy. Thus, the type of induction mechanism was most of the time, deduced from the observed chromosomal abnormalities (table 1): 9 cases were probably AA induced, 9 were ATII-induced and in 12, the mechanism could not be determined because CNA categorization was indistinguishable between t-AML induced by AA or by ATII. The medium time elapsed between cancer therapy and the

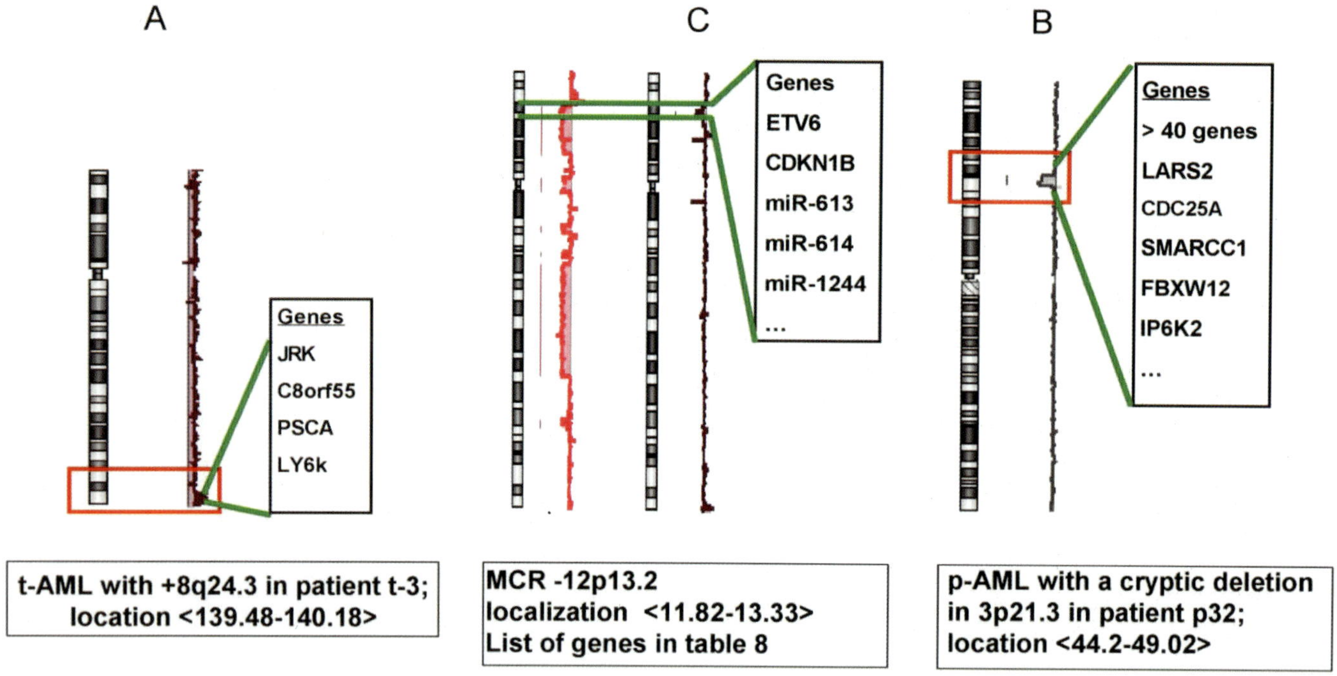

Figure 1. Details of critical rearrangements concerning MCRs. A = gain on 8q24.3 in a t-AML; B = loss of 12 p13 in t-AML (patients t-4 and t-5); C loss of 3p21.3 in a p-AML.

diagnosis of t-AML was 5.1 years, 2.3 years and 4.7 years respectively.

Twenty-five patients (80%) with 104 CNA exhibited 41 gains and 63 losses (table 4). The mean number per total case number was 3.46. Six patients with a normal karyotype had at least one CNA. Six patients (20%) had no CNA, 3 had a normal karyotype and the 2 others had a balanced translocation (one a t(15;17) and one a MLL rearrangement). The mean CNA length was 4.1Mb for the t-AML patients with at least an unbalanced rearrangement.

The twelve losses in the immunoglobulin genes (IG) on 2p11 and 14q32.3 were considered as a special category of CNA. Among the 8 patients with IG rearrangements, 2 had bi-phenotypic leukemia and the others had various forms of AML.

p-AML

Among 36 patients, 12 had a normal karyotype, 4 exhibited an anomaly on chromosomes 5 or 7. A t(15;17)(q22;q21), characterizing AML-M3, was present in 9 cases (table 2).

In p-AML, 64 CNAs were observed (table 5) with 30 losses and 34 gains while the mean number was 1.78. Twenty-two patients had no CNA, 11 had a recurrent balanced translocation while the 11 others had a normal karyotype. The mean number of CNA among p-AML patients with unbalanced rearrangements was 2.66. This value was due to 4 patients with very complex genomic rearrangements (>8 chromosomal abnormalities).

Minimal Critical Regions (MCR)

A MCR was defined as such if 2 cases or more shared a common genomic location. Twelve MCRs were observed in t-AML and eight in p-AML (table 6).

The size of MCRs was smaller in t-AML, with a minimum of 0.04 Mb compared to p-AML with a minimum of 0.95 Mb. The longest MCR in t-AML was 36.44 Mb, of the same order of magnitude as in p-AML where it was 45.69 Mb.

Unique CNA

These single cases were of various sizes, from 0.04Mb to 26.89 Mb. Most of them were small and not known as polymorphisms. They are detailed in table 7.

Discussion

The CNVs

As we were obliged to use a pool of normal DNA as a reference, Mendelian CNVs that are present throughout the entire genome [8], were revealed by the 244K aCGH (table 3). They were identified in the Toronto Database [7] in order to avoid including them in the analysis of somatic CNA. However, as a relationship between some CNVs and malignancy has already been suggested [9], several of them were retained in a separate table (table 3). For example a GSTT gene cluster was reported to be a susceptibility co-factor in cancer [10,11,12]. It is noteworthy that several miRNA, i.e. mir-570, mir-1268, mir-1233 and mir-1826 were found embedded in CNVs, with a possible multigene regulatory effect, as reported by Lin [13].

High resolution aCGH allowed us to study the whole set of IG gene rearrangements [5]. VDJ rearrangement in immunoglobulin genes (IG) has been described in AML [14,15] and associated with MLL rearrangements [16]. The two series of patients (t-AML *vs* p-AML), were found to be significantly different, with a p value of <0.002. The fact that a quarter (8/30) of t-AML exhibited a VDJ rearrangement suggests that the transformed cells are often multipotent in these diseases.

The CNAs

The acquired chromosomal abnormalities detected by morphological cytogenetics were quite similar in t-AML and p-AML. The CNA patterns were well correlated between the morphological cytogenetics and aCGH. Their frequency was increased after high resolution aCGH. Losses were more frequent than gains in both series. The number of CNAs was higher in t-AML (n = 104, mean

Table 6. Minimal Critical Region in the two groups of patients.

MCR (localization by aCGH)	Patients	Size (Mb)	Possible genes
t-AML			
−1q44 <241.94–247.19>	t-2, t-13	5.25	>25 genes among them SMYD3
−3p14.1p12.3 <69.67–79.19>	t-5, t-17	9.52	MITF FOXP1 EIF4E3 GRP27 PROK2 RYBP
			SHQ1 PPP4R2 PDZRN3 CNTN3 FAM86D
			FRG2C ZNF717 ROBO2 ROBO1
−5q31.3q33.1 <142.91–148.19>	t-1, t-2, t-4, t-5	5.28	ADRB2 DPYSL3 HTR44 POU4F3 PPP2R2B
			SPINK1 JAKMIP2 TCERG1 SPINK5 LARS
			RBM27 KCTD16 HMHB1 FBXO38 YIPF5
			SPINK7SCGB3A2 GPR151 PRELID2
			SH3RF2 PLAC8L1 STK32A SPINK6 SPINK9
+6q27<168.12–168.32>[1.50]	t-9, t-17	0.20	KIF25 FRMD1 HGC 6.1.1
−7p22.2 <3.02–3.12>	t-5, t-6, t-7, t-9, **t-10**	0.10	GNA12 CARD11
+7p15.2 <27,15–27,18>	t-14, t-16, t-17, t-19	0,03	HOXA6 HOXA7 HOXA9 HOXA10 miR-196b
−7q21.3 <97.69–101.88>	t-2, t-5, t-6, t-7, t-9,	4.19	NPTX2 LMTK2 BRI3 BAIAP2L1 BHLHB8 CUX1
	t-10		miR-86 miR-93miR-106b miR-548o
−7q33q34<135.74–137.48>	**t-2**, t-5, t-6, t-7, t-8, t-9	1.74	CHMR2 PTN DGK1 CREB3L2 miR-490
+8q24.3 <143.73–143.9>	**t-3**, t-14	0.17	PSCA LY6D JRK C8orf55 LY6K
			SLURP1 LYNX1 LYPD2
−12p13.2p13.1<11.82–13.33>	t-2, t-4, **t-5**	1.51	ETV6 CDKN1B CREBL2 EMP1 GPR19 LRP6
			GPRC5A HEBP1DDX47 MANSC1 GPRC5D
			KIAA1467 BCL2L14 DUSP16 APOLD1 GSG1
			HTR7P miR-613 miR-614 miR1244
+17q21.3 <22.80–78.65>	t-15, **t-24**	55.85	Whole 17q
−21q22.1 <35.11–35.15>	t-7, t-8, **t-11**, t-29	0.04	RUNX1
p-AML			
+1q21q22<153.19–154.64>	p-23, p-24	1.4	>25 genes EFNA4 R1AP1 DPM3
			YY1AP1 DAP3 ROBLD3 CCT3 CLK2
+1q32.1q44<201.31–247.19>	p-6, p-23	45.69	Numerous genes
−3p21.3<44.20–49.02>	p-21, p-24, p-32	5.18	>40 genes SMARCC1 NCKIPSD
−7q31.2q36.3<115.49–158.78>	p-1 and p-2, p-7	43.29	Numerous genes
−9q22.3q31.1<93.92–103.96>	p-18, p-21	9.81	>60genes FANCC XPA
Amp 21q21.1<14.29–17.97> [5.46]	p-4, p-21	3.78	LIPI ABCC13 RBM11 HSPA13 SAMSN1
			NRIP1 USP25 C21orf34 CXADR BTG3
			miR-99a miR-125b-2hsa-let-7c
Amp 21q22.2<38.27–43.54> [3 & 5.2]	p-4, p-21, p-24	5,25	DSCR4 KCNJ15 ERG ETS2 BRWD1
			other genes
+21q22.3qter<43.54–46.91>	p-4, p-21, p-24	7.49	>50 genes

Column 1, the location of the MCR that follows the rules of tables 4 and 5; the figures in brackets and in bold are the ratios of the amplified regions. Column 2, patients; the figures in bold indicate the smaller CNA.

number 3.5), than in p-AML (n = 69, mean = 1.9). The value found here is of the same order of magnitude than that reported elsewhere [17,18,19,20]. Subcytogenetic CNA were present in half of the t-AML with normal karyotypes (table 4) while only 1 case (p-32) was observed in p-AML (tables 5 and 7). These findings are in accordance with the role of cytotoxic drugs in oncogenesis in t-AML [4,21].

Twenty-five balanced translocations remained undetected (tables 4 and 5). No deletion or amplification at the breakpoint was observed in the five t-AML, nor in the two p-AML cases with rearranged MLL. The exceptions were two t(8;21) complex translocations resulting in detectable quantitative CNA at their breakpoints. In case t-12, a t-AML, a distal trisomy 21 began at the 5′ extreme part of RUNX1

Table 7. Single CNA of interest.

Patients	MCR unic cases	Size (Mb)	Possible genes
t-AML			
t-2	+14q22.1 <47.25–52.51>	5.26	>30 genes
t-2	−18q11.2q12.1<21.74–24.41>[0.23]	2.67	SS18 (Synovialosarcoma translocation) +7 other genes
t-2	−18q22.3q23<71.06–71.76>	0.69	TSHZ1 Colon cancer ag a zinc finger protein
t-13	−1q42.3.q44<233.13–247.19>	14.06	>100 genes
t-13	−10q11.2<45.53–47.97>	2.44	>20 genes
t-5	−12p13.2p13.1<11.82–13.33>	1.51	>20 genes ETV6 CDKN1B miR613 miR614 miR1244
t-22	+2p25.3 <2.54–3.57>	1.03	TSSC1 TTC15 ADI1 RNASEH1
t-14	−17q11.2 <25.96–27.38>	1.42	EVI2A EVI2B NF1 OMG SH3GLP2 SUZ12 CRLF3 C17orf79
			CENTA2 UTP6 C17orf42 ATAD5 RNF135 RAB11FIP4
			LRRC37B SUZ12P miR193a miR365-2
t-15	−4q31.2 <146.62–146.67>	0.05	SMAD1
t-30	−2p23.3<25.31–25.60>	0,10	DNMT3A miR1301
p-AML			
p-24	+3p21.3<50.26–50.29>[2.54]	0.03	GNAI2 SEMA3B
p-24	+3p21.3<52.29–52.31>[4.00]	0.03	NCLYTK miR135a-1
p-21	+3p14.1<64.32–67.67>[4.59]	1.94	LR1G1
p-18	−8q21.3q22.1<93.15–94.17>[0.63]	1.02	RUNXT1
p-22	−12p12.1p13.2<11.40–21.20>[0.55]	9.8	ETV6 CDKN1B among more than 20 genes
p-24	−17p11.2q12<0.18–29.54>[0.65]	29,36	multiple genes
p-24	+15q23<67.44–68.37>[3.64]	3.31	KIF23 RPLP1 TLE3 miR-629
p-22	−18q21.2<48.99–51.05>[0.55]	2.06	DCC and 4 other genes

Column 2: The CNA were either lost or gained as indicated by a "−" or a "+"; the locations on chromosomes are described following the ISCN 2009 with slight modifications: sequence numbers are included between <> and expressed in Mb, with a resolution of 10kb; linear ratios are written between brackets after an "×"; chromosomes with a linear ratio >2 (low level of amplification) or losses <0.25 are labeled in **bold** and *italics*.

(chr21:35.08). FISH studies showed a distal 21q unbalanced translocation on an unidentified chromosome in addition to the classic t(8;21) derivatives. In case p-18, a p-AML with a t(8;21), a 1Mb loss on 8q21.3 amputated the first 5′ exons of RUNX1T1, probably inactivating the ETO-AML1 chimeric gene on the der(21) and left the 3′ RUNX1T1 coding sequence intact in the AML1-ETO transcript on the der(8) [22]. This cryptic rearrangement allowed a "virtual cloning" of the t(8;21). The detailed molecular mechanisms of these rearrangements with an apparently identical t(8;21) seems to be different in these secondary and *de novo* leukemias.

MCR

In the present series, twelve MCRs were isolated in t-AML and 8 in p-AML (table 6). The size of MCRs was smaller in t-AML, with a minimum of 0.04Mb compared to 1.4 Mb in p-AML. There were 7 MCR of <2Mb in p-AML compared to only 1 in p-AML. The longest MCR in t-AML was 55 Mb, of the same order of magnitude as in p-AML where it was 45.69 Mb. A quarter of MCR contained sites for microRNAs (miRNAs). They have been shown to be involved in different biological processes, and in particular, hematopoiesis [23,24]. They are also described as behaving as tumor suppressor genes or oncogenes [25,26]. Few new studies have reported on molecular abnormalities implicating miRNAs that can be up- or down-regulated in AML [27].

Table 8 and table 9 present the MCR from the data reported in the literature [18,19,20,28,29,30,31,32,33,34]. Despite a certain amount of heterogeneity in the samples, the techniques, the genome constructs and other parameters, this table provides a global view of nearly 550 p-AML and 50 t-AML. It allowed us to clearly show the MCR and their frequencies.

When we compared the number of losses and gain in the "table" sample to those in the present series, a chi2 test showed that as they were not different, we could include them in the table. In all AML 123 MCR were losses and 51 were gains. In t-AML, 34 MCR were losses and 4 were gains while in p-AML 34 were losses and were 4 gains.

We will examine the lost and gained MCR found in our series together with the most specific or frequent MCR found in this table.

−1q

A small juxta-telomeric MCR loss in -1q44 was not reported in p-AML and does not seem to be very frequent (tables 8 and 9). Among more than twenty genes, SMYD3 is a histone methyltransferase that plays a role in transcriptional regulation as a member of an RNA polymerase complex. It is expressed in CD34 cells.

Table 8. Minimal critical regions in the literature including the present work: losses.

Chromosome abnormalities	All	p (%)	t (%)	consensus MCR location in Mb	References	Genes
1p36.2	6	6 (1)		7.81–7.89	A, D, E	PER3 UTS2
1p35.1	6	6 (1)		22.39–22.44	A, D, E	
1p34.2	3	3 (0.5)		42.07–42.45	A, D, E	KRC HIVEP3
1p31.3p31.1	3	2 (0.3)	1 (2)	67.07–69.95	A, D, E	WDR78 MIERS1 C1orf141 IL12RB2 SERBP1
						GADD45A GNG12 DIRAS3 GPR177 RPE65 DEPDC1
1q42.1	3	3 (0.5)		222.6–222.9	D	CNIH4 WDR26 CR625980 CNIH3
1q44	2		2 (4)	241.94–247.19	K	WDR64 EXO1 MAP1LC3C PLD5?CEP170 AKT3
						ZNF238 C1orf101 FAM36A EFCAB2 KIF26B
						SMYD3 TFB2M ADSS HNRNPU PPPDE1 AHCTF1
2p23.3	3	3 (0.5)		25.25–25.46	D, E	
2p23.1	3	3 (0.5)		30.29–30.95	A, D, E	
2q36.2	8	8 (1.4)		222.01–225.42	A, D, E	EPHA4 PAX3 FARSB MOGAT1 ACSL3 KCNE4 AP1S3
						WDFY1 SERPINE2 MRPL44 FAM124B CUL3 SCG2
3p26.3-p25.3	4	3 (0.5)	1 (2)	0–9.14	D, G	
3p26.3	4	3 (0.5)	1 (2)	14.96–16.15	A, D	
3p21.3	8	5 (0.9)	3 (6)	44.46–49.64	A, D, K	Numerous ZNF more than 30 genes
3p14.1p12.3	3		3 (6)	69.67–79.19	A, K	MITF FOXP1 EIF4E3 GRP27 PROK2 RYBP SHQ1
						PPP4R2 PDZRN3 CNTN3 FAM86D FRG2C ZNF717
						ROBO2 ROBO1
3q11.2q13.3	5	5 (0.9)		95.03–120.21	D, E	more than 30 genes
3q13.1q13.3	2	1 (0.2)	1 (2)	106.75–109.60	D	
3q13.3	3	2 (0.3)	1 (2)	117.78–118.40	D	
3q24q29	3	2 (0.3)	1 (2)	160.62–162.14	D	
3q24q29	3	2 (0.2)	1 (2)	164.51–165.39	D	SI SLITRK3 CR612557
4q24	7	7 (1.2)		106.1–106.72	A, D	TET2 PPA2 FLJ20184 INTS12 GSTCD
4q27q28	6	5 (0.9)	1 (2)	122.92–124.45	D	ADAD1 IL21 BBS12 FGF2 NUDT6 SPATA5 SPRY1
4q31.2	4		4 (8)	146.62–146.67	D, K	SMAD1
5q11.1	3	2 (0.3)	1 (2)	50.16–50.21	D	
5q11.2	3	3 (0.5)		51.79–53.66	D	
5q11.2	5	4 (0.7)	1 (2)	55.73–56.92	A, D	
5q11.2	4	3 (0.5)	1 (2)	57.49–57.79	A, D	
5q12.1	7	5 (0.9)	2 (4)	59.54–59.87	A, D, E	
5q13	14	10 (1.9)	4 (8)	82.72–84.65	A, D, E, J	VCAN HAPLN1 EDIL3
5q14.3q15	20	17 (3)	3 (6)	86.54–95.19	A, D, E, J	CCNH TMEM161B MEF2C CETN3 POLR3G
						RASA1 LYSMD3 GPR98 VLGR1 ARRDC3 NR2F1
						FAM172A POU5F2 ANKRD32 MCTP1 UNQ630
						TTC37 ARSK GPR150 RFESD RHOBTB3 GLRX
5q15q22.3	20	16 (2.6)	4 (8)	95.51–114.14	A, D, E, J	PCSK1 CAST ERAP1 ERAP2 LNPEP LIX1 2
						RIOK CHD1 PAM HISPPD1 NUDT12
						CR610784 RAB9P1 EFNA5 FBXL17 FER PJA2
						MAN2A1 TMEM232 TSLP WDR36 CAMK4
						STARD4 C5orf13 EPB41L4A APC SRP19
						ZRSR2 REEP5 DCP2 MCC YTHDC2 KCNN2
5q22.3q31.1	16	13 (2.3)	3 (6)	129.23–131.96	A, D, E, J	CHSY3 LYRM7 CDC42SE2 RAPGEF6 FNIP1 ACSL6
						CSF2 IL3 P4HA2 PDLIM4 IRF1 RAD50
5q31.1	21	12 (2.1)	9 (18)	133.52–134.26	A, D, E, H	PPP2CA CDKL3 UBE2B PHF15 SAR1B CAMLG
						DDX46 C5orf24 TXNDC15 PCBD2
5q31.3q33.1	19	11 (2)	8 (16)	142.91–148.19	A, D, E, J, K	HMHB1 YIPF5 PRELID2 GRXCR2 RBM27 POU4F3 LARS GPR151 PPP2R2B TCERG1 STK32A JAKMIP2

Table 8. Cont.

Chromosome abnormalities	All	p (%)	t (%)	consensus MCR location in Mb	References	Genes
						SPINK1 SPINK5 SPINK6 SPINK7 SPINK9 FBXO38
						HTR4 SH3TC2
5q33.3	14	10 (1.8)	4 (8)	156.39–156.51	A, D, E, J	
5q33.3	13	10 (1.8)	3 (6)	157.25–158.80	A, D, E, J	CLINT1 EBF1 RNF145 UBLCP1 IL12B
6p25.1p24.3	10	7 (1.2)	3 (6)	5.54–8.38	A, B, C, D	FARS2 NRN1 F13A1 LY86 MMD-1 Zep-1
						RREB1 SSR1 CAGE1 RIOK1 DSP BMP6
						TXNDC5 MUTEDEEF1E1
6p22.3p22.2	5	4 (0.7)	1 (2)	20.29–23.74	A, B, D	
6p22.2p22.1	6	5 (0.9)	1 (2)	24.15–26.16	A, B, D	DCDC2 KAAG1 MRS2 GPLD1 ALDH5A1 TTRAP
						ACOT13 GMNN FAM65B DKFZp686H12134
						HIST1H cluster TRIM38 HFE
6q24.1	2	1 (0.2)	1 (2)	140.6–142.5	D, F	
6q25.3	2	1 (0.2)	1 (2)	156.39–156.61	D	
7p22.2	7	1 (0.2)	6 (12)	3.02–3.12	D, K	CARD11
7p14.1	4	3 (0.5)	1 (2)	39.5–41.7	D, F	
7p12.2	2	2 (0.3)		50.18–50.45	D	IKZF1
7q21.1	4	3 (0.5)	1 (2)	85.41–86.44	A, C, E	
7q21.1	5		5 (10)	90.21–90.44	A, D	PFTK1
7q21.3q22.1	14	6 (1)	8 (16)	97.69–100.36	A, D, E, K	LMTK2 BHLHA15 TECPR1 BRI3 NPTX2
						TMEM130 TRRAP SMURF1 KPNA7 MYH16
						ARPC1A PDAP1 BUD31 PTCD1 CPSF4 ATP5J2
						ZKSCAN5 CYP3A4 TRIM4 COPS6 MCM7
						TAF6 GATS PILRB PILRA ZCWPW1 MEPCE
						FBXO24 GNB2 EPO mir-25 mir-93 mir-106b
7q31.3	16	15 (2.7)	1 (2)	121.7–123.9	B, D, F, J, K	PTPRZ1 LKR/SDH AASS FEZF1 CADPS2 RNF133
						TAS2R16 NDUFA5 ASB15 WASL HYAL4
7q33q34	22	15 (2.7)	7 (14)	135.74–137.48	B, D, E, J, K	CALD1 TMEM140 STRA8 WDR91
						CNOT4 NUP205 FAM180A TPN miR490
7q34	20	19 (3.4)	1 (2)	139.72–140.02	B, D, E, J, K	TBXAS1 PARP12 MST109 JHDM1D KIAA1718
7q35q36.1	16	16 (2.9)		146.12–148.2	B, D, E, J, K	CNTNAP2
7q36.1q36.2	16	15 (2.7)	1 (2)	152.02–152.80	A, B, D, E, J, K	MLL3 XRCC2 ACTR3B FABP5L3
8p23.2	3	2 (0.3)	1 (2)	3.48–3.58	A, D	
8p22p21.3	2	1 (0.2)	1 (2)	18.72–21.93	D	
8p21.2p12	2	1 (0.2)	1 (2)	24.40–36.30	D	
8q22.1	3	3 (0.5)		93.15–94.17	A, K	C8orf83
8q24.1	4	3 (0.5)	1 (2)	117.81–118.38	I	
8q24.1q24.2	4	3 (0.5)	1 (2)	126.54–129.58	A, D	
8q24.2	3	3 (0.5)		130.53–130.80	A, D	
8q24.2q24.3	3	2 (0.3)	1 (2)	131.51–146.26	A, D	
9p24.3p13.3	4	4 (0.7)		0.19–33.18	A, D, E	
9q21.3	5	4 (0.7)	1 (2)	82.37–84.44	B, C, D, E	
9q22.3q31.1	5	5 (0.9)		93.92–103.96	C, D, E, K	more than 30 genes
9q32q33.1	2	2 (0.3)		116.51–117.92	B, D	
10q23.1q23.3	4	4 (0.7)		87.93–90.77	C, D	
10q24.1q24.2	4	4 (0.7)		96.48–100.81	C, D	
11p15.5p15.4	8	7 (1.2)	1 (2)	2.48–3.35	B, C, D, E	KCNQ1 KCNQ1OT1 KCNQ1DN CDKN1C
						SLC22A18NAP1L4 PHLDA2 CARS

Table 8. Cont.

Chromosome abnormalities	All	p (%)	t (%)	consensus MCR location in Mb	References	Genes
						OSBPL5 C11orf36 MRGPRE
11q12.3q13.1	3	3 (0.5)		63.98–65.65	D	
11q13.1q25	4	4 (0.7)		67.25–134.24	B, D, E	
11q23.3	4	2 (0.3)	2 (4)	117.86–119.81	A, D, E	
12p13.3	4	2 (0.3)	2 (4)	0.06–4.05	D, E	
12p13.2	10	6 (1)	4 (8)	10.62–11.72	C, D, E, J	
12p13.2	12	10 (1.8)	2 (4)	11.2–12.70	C, D, E, F, J	
12p13.2p13.1	17	14 (2.5)	3 (6)	12.20–13.13	C, D, E, J, K	ETV6 BCL2L14 LRP6 MANSC1 LOH12CR1 AX748225 DUSP16 CREBL2 GPR19 CDKN1B APOLD1 DDX47 GPRC5A TVAS4 HEBP1
12p12.3	7	5 (0.9)	2 (4)	15.54–19.17	C, D, E, J, K	PTPRO EPS8 STRAP MGST1 LMO3 RERGL PIK3C2G CAPZA3
12q12	3	2 (0.3)	1 (2)	42.64–43.26	A, D	
12q13.1	2	2 (0.3)		46.06–46.30	A, D	
12q24.3	4	3 (0.5)	1 (2)	81.57–105.06	A, D, E	
12q24.3	3	2 (0.3)	1 (2)	121.28–122.73	A, D	
12q24.3	3	3 (0.5)		128.71–128.91	A, D, E	
13q14.3	8	7 (1.2)	1 (2)	49.63–50.51	C, D, E	
13q21.1	4	4 (0.7)		54.33–54.45	B, D	
16p11.1q12.1	20	20 (3.6)		35.06–50.12	D, G	VPS35 SHCBP1 ORC6L MYLK3 GPT2 DNAJA2 NETO2 ITFG1 PHKB ABCC12 ABCC11 LONP2 SIAH1 LONP N4BP1 CBLN1 HEATR3
16q21	24	23 (4.1)	1 (2)	57.56–58.96	B, D, G	GPR114 GPR56 GPR97 CCDC135 KIFC3 CNGB1 TEPP MMP15 CSNK2A2 GINS3 NDRG4 SETD6 CNOT1 GOT2
16q21	26	24 (4.3)	2 (4)	62.51–63.81	D, G, J	
16q22.3	25	22 (4)	3 (6)	70.76–71.46	D, G, J	VAC14 HYDIN FTSJD1 CALB2
16q22.3q23.1	26	26 (4.7)		73.30–73.57	G, H, J	BC042734
16q24.1	24	23 (4.1)	1 (2)	83.37–85.07	D, G, J	CDH13 HSBP1 MLYCD OSGIN1 NECAB2 MBTPS1 HSDL1 LRRC50 TAF1C ADAD2 KCNG4 USP10
16q24.3	26	26 (4.7)		87.30–87.37	G, J, K	FBXO31
17p13.2p13.1	22	16 (2.9)	6 (12)	4.01–8.20	A, D, J	TP53 NLRP1 NUP88 C1QBP XAF1 and more than 30 genes
17p12p11.2	7	5 (0.9)	2 (4)	14.74–19.35	A, D, E	
17p11.2	4	3 (0.5)	1 (2)	20.02–21.45	C, D, E	
17q11.2	44	39 (7.1)	5 (10)	26.49–27.52	A, D, E, G, H, J, K	NF1 EVI2A EVI2A
17q21.33	4	2 (0.3)	2 (4)	44.98–45.43	D, E	
17q21.33	3	3 (0.5)		46.22–47.56	D, E	
17q25.1q25.3	2	2 (0.3)		69.43–73.16	D	
18p11.32p11.31	14	12 (2.1)	2 (4)	1–4.62	D, G, J	C18orf2 METTL4 NDC80 SMCHD1 EMILIN2 LPIN2 MYOM1 MYL12B TGIF1 DLGAP1
18p11.23	17	16 (2.9)	1 (2)	7.42–7.58	G, H, J	PTPRM
18p11.22p11.21	5	4 (0.7)	1 (2)	9.03–13.81	D, H	
18q11.2	9	8 (1.4)	1 (2)	18.1–22.05	D, G	
18q11.2q12.2	21	18 (3.2)	3 (6)	21.74–33.13	D, G, K	CABYR OSBPL1A IMPACT HRH4 ZNF521 SS18 PSMA8 TAF4B CDH2 DSC3 DSC1 DSC2 DSG4 DSG3 DSG2 TTR RNF125 DTNA MAPRE2

Table 8. Cont.

Chromosome abnormalities	All	p (%)	t (%)	consensus MCR location in Mb	References	Genes
18q21.1	21	20 (3.6)	1 (2)	43.39–46.37	D, E, G, K	HAUS1 LOXHD1 PIAS2 SMAD2
18q21.2	22	20 (3.6)	2 (4)	50.21–51.05	D, E, G, K	RAB27B CCDC68
18q21.32	22	20 (3.6)	2 (4)	55.08–55.51	D, E, G, J, K	ONECUT2 FECH NARS ATP8B1
18q22.3	23	22 (4.0)	1 (2)	69.06–69.18	D, E, G, K	
18q22.3q23	4	2 (0.3)	2 (4)	71.06–71.76	E, G, J	FBXO15
19p13.3	3	2 (0.3)	1 (2)	0.21–1.81	A, D	
19q13.2q13.43	2	2 (0.3)		46.16–63.43	C, D	
20q11.2q13.1	2	2 (0.3)		34.59–43.45	E	more than 30 genes
20q13.1q13.3	2	2 (0.3)		43.85–55.73	E	more than 30 genes
21q22.12	11	7 (1.2)	4 (8)	35.11–35.15	A, D, K	RUNX1
21q22.3	3	3 (0.5)		44.70–45.09	D	

The first column lists the chromosomal losses and gains. The second lists the absolute number of each rearrangement (excluding a single rearrangement). The third and the fourth are the absolute numbers in p-AML and t-AML respectively and the percentage is indicated between parenthesis. The chromosomal location is listed. The references are indicated by letters: A [32], B [33], C [34], D [18], E [19], F [28], G [29], H [30], I [31], J [20], K present work. The last column lists the genes included in those MCR.

−3p

Two MCR were found. The most telomeric one on 3p21.3 was a 5.18 Mb recurrent loss covering more than 40 genes. It was found in p-AML (table 6, figure 1) but also in t-AML (tables 8 and 9).

A more centromeric 10Mb loss was found exclusively in t-AML. Both patients in the present work contributing to this MCR had been treated with RT and 5FU. PROK2, a prokineticin 2 isoform A precursor, is highly expressed in bone marrow [35] and could have chemokine-like activity [36]. Another gene, the SHQ1 homolog, expressed in CD34 cells has been purported to be required for the assembly of H/ACA small nucleolar and telomerase RNPs [35,37].

−4q

A specific loss in p-AML was found in 4q24 (table 8) including TET2, a tumor suppressor gene described in myeloid cancers [38].

A small loss of 4q31.2, exclusively in 8% of t-AML (tables 7 and 8) was found to delete the 5′ half of SMAD1. This protein mediates the signals of bone morphogenetic proteins (BMPs), which are involved in a range of biological activities including cell growth, apoptosis, morphogenesis, development and immune responses. It is expressed in BM cells (UCSC).

−5q

The 5q- region was fragmented in more than twelve groups. In p-AML, the most frequent regions were comprised between 86.54 and 114.14 Mb, with proximal and distal "spreading". This region contains the RASA1 gene which exhibits tumor suppressor activity on the RAS gene. RASA1 has been reported to be a CNA in breast cancers and a putative tumor suppressor gene [39]. PCSK1 may be implicated in malignancy [40]. APC and MCC genes are implicated in colorectal cancer. The more proximal area contains the AML/MDS region that Evers considered as a 5.2 Mb MCR [41].

Two MCR were observed in more than 10% of t-AML (table 8). Both were proximal to the previously reported 7.7 Mb 5q33.3 region [41]. The first MCR was located on 5q31 and was smaller than 1Mb. It contained several genes of interest such as CDKL3, an important regulator of cell cycle progression, UBE2B that is required for post-replicative DNA damage repair, and the helicase DDX46 which is highly transcribed in bone marrow.

The second 5.22 Mb MCR in 5q31.3q32, was delineated by the present work (table 6). Among the 29 genes it harbored, several are overexpressed in bone [35]. PRELID2 codes for a protein containing a PRELI/MSF domain. It is an evolutionary conserved gene [42,43]. TCERG1 is a transcription factor that binds RNA polymerase II, inhibits the elongation of transcripts from target promoters and regulates transcription elongation in a TATA box-dependent manner. LARS encodes a cytosolic leucine-tRNA synthetase, a member of the class I aminoacyl-tRNA synthetase family. FBXO38 is a F-box protein 38 isoform A that is overexpressed in early erythroid cells. FBXO32, a family member of these cells, is a PRC2-targeted gene [44]. POU4F3, a POU class 4 homeobox 3 is a member of the POU-domain family of transcription factors that is not expressed in bone marrow but in monocytes. Furthermore, another member of the POU gene family, POU4F1, has been recently described to be associated with AML exhibiting t(8;21) [45]. RBM27 is a zinc finger RNA-binding protein member of the family that includes RBM15, alias OTT, which is involved in the regulation of hematopoietic stem cells and is fused with MKL1 in the t(1;22) of AML7 and plays a major role in the pathogenesis of this disease [46].

Finding different MCR with a maximum frequency in p-AML and in t-AML suggests different oncogenesis pathways on this chromosome.

7p MCR

A 90kb MCR in 7p22.2 (table 6 and 8) had deleted he CARD 11 gene in t-AML. The CARD domains of this caspase have been shown to activate NF-kappaB and to induce the phosphorylation of BCL10 when expressed in CD34+ cells [47]. CARD 11, via the immune cell restricted complex CARD11-BCL10-MALT1, [48] is implicated in lymphoma.

In three t-AML cases, a gain of 7p15 concerned the homeogene cluster of HOXA6, HOXA7, HOXA9 and HOXA10 (Table 6). This area has not been described as a CNV [7]. The HOXA

Table 9. Minimal critical regions in the literature including the present work: gains.

Chromosome abnormalities	All	p (%)	t (%)	consensus MCR location in Mb	References	Genes
GAINS						
1q21.3q22	4	3 (0.5)	1 (2)	153.19–154.64	C, D, K	S100A8 S100A9 S100A13 S100A6 SNAPIN ILF2
						NPR1 INTS3 VLCS-3 GATAD2B TORC2 CREB3L4
						TPM3 HAX1 IL6R SHE UBE2Q1 ADAR CHRNB2
1q32.1	3	2 (0.3)	1 (2)	204.98–205.04	C, D	
1q32.1q44	6	5 (0.9)	1 (2.1)	235.00–235.10	A, B, K	BC016972 ?
3q26.3q29	2	2 (0.3)		182.99–133.31	E	more than 30 genes
4p13q12	2	2 (0.3)		42.30–58.23	B, D	
4q12q13.1	2	2 (0.3)		59.13–62.98	B, D	
4q28.3	2	2 (0.3)		132.8–136.7	B, G	
5p13.2q11.1	2	1 (0.2)	1 (2)	37.98–50.15	A, D	
5q11.2	3	2 (0.3)	1 (2)	51.21–54.12	A, D	
6q11.2q12	8	8 (1.4)		63.43–63.7	A, G	
6q27	3	2 (0.3)	1 (2)	168.12–168.32	D, K	MLLT4 avoir table 6
7p15.2	4		4 (8)	27.15–27.18	K	HOX genes
8q24.3	16	12 (2.1)	4 (8)	143.73–143.90	B, D, G, I, J, K	JRK PSCA LY6K C8orf55 LYPD2 SLURP1 LYNX1
						LY6D
9p21.3	2	2 (0.3)		21.5–23.4	F, G	
9q13q21.3	2	2 (0.3)		70.23–83.52	E	FXN APBA1 TJP2 SMC5 TRPM3 GDA TCM1 ANXA1
						RARB RFK GNA14 TLE4 TLE1
11q12.1q14.1	16	16 (2.9)		59.1–79.6	G	more than 50 genes
11q14.1	5	5 (0.9)		79.6–81.3	D, G	
11q24.2q24.3	31	31 (5.6)		126.53–130.23	D, E, G, J	KIRREL3 ETS1 FLI1 C11orf45 TP53AIP1 RICS
						BARX2 NFRKB PRDM10 APLP2 ST14 ZBTB44
12p13.33p11.21	13	13 (2.3)		0.1–32.7	E, G	no gene
13q12.11q13.1	3	3 (0.5)		19.9–31.7	G	
13q31.3	2	2 (0.3)		90.45–90.97	E	GPC5
15q21.1	3	3 (0.5)		46.52–47.36	B, D, E	
15q21.3q22.1	3	3 (0.5)		55.6–56.6	B, E, F	
15q23	5	5 (0.9)		67.44–68.37	B, E, J	SMAD3 AAGAB MAP2K5 LBXCOR1 PIAS1
15q26.q26.3	6	6 (1)		92.5–100.0	C, E, G	
17q12	6	4 (0.7)	2 (4)	32.82–33.20	C, D, E, J	TMEM132E
17q21.2q21.31	5	3 (0.5)	2 (4)	37.08–38.48	D, E, J	FBXO47 PLXDC1 FBXL20 MED1 CRKRS TCAP
						PGAP3 ERBB2 GRB7 IKZF3 GSDMB ORMDL3
						PSMD3 CSF3 MED24 THRAP4 NR1D1 MSL1 CASC3
						WIPF2 CDC6 RARA
19p13.3p13.12	13	13 (2.3)		2.19–14.11	D, G, J	
19p13.12p13.11	13	13 (2.3)		16.0–16.15	F, G, J	
19q13.31	2	2 (0.3)		49.2–49.9	D, F	
19q13.41	2	2 (0.3)		58.3–59.1	D, G	
20q11.1q11.21	3	3 (0.5)		28.2–30.5	E, G	
21q21.1	2	2 (0.3)		14.29–17.97	K	LIPI ABCC13 RBM11 HSPA13 SAMSN1 NRIP1
						USP25 C21orf34 CXADR BTG3
						miR-99a miR-125b-2 hsa-let-7c
21q22.2	18	18 (3.2)		38.65–38.85	C, D, G, J, K	ERG ETS2
21q22.3q	4	4 (0.7)		45.09–46.91	D, K	RRP1B PDXK RRP1 CSTB AGPAT3 TRAPPC10

Table 9. Cont.

Chromosome abnormalities	All	p (%)	t (%)	consensus MCR location in Mb	References	Genes
GAINS						
						TMEM1 PWP2 C21orf33 ICOSLG DNMT3L AIRE
						PFKL TRPM2 LRRC3 UBE2G2 SUMO3 PTTG1IP PBF
						ITGB2 ADARB1 COL18A1
22q12.3	13	12 (2.1)	1 (2)	33.90–35.32	D, G	LARGE
22q13.1q13.2	14	13 (2.3)	1 (2)	36.78–42.24	D, G	more than 30 genes
22q13.31q13.32	11	10 (1.8)	1 (2)	44.92–48.08	D, G	PRR5 ARHGAP8 PHF21B NUP50 UPK3A SMC1B
						ATXN10 WNT7B GTSE1 GRAMD4

The first column lists the chromosomal losses and gains. The second lists the absolute number of each rearrangement (excluding a single rearrangement). The third and the fourth are the absolute numbers in p-AML and t-AML respectively and the percentage is indicated between parenthesis. The chromosomal location is listed. The references are indicated by letters: A [32], B [33], C [34], D [18], E [19], F [28], G [29], H [30], I [31], J [20], K present work. The last column lists the genes included in those MCR.

family of genes encode HOX family transcription factors, which play an important role in the development of body segmentation and in the survival of hematopoietic stem cells. HOXA6 is directly implicated in the process of hematopoietic progenitor cell development. HOXA9, that can be fused with NUP98 in some AML [49], is fundamentally involved in the AML process in transgenic mice [50,51,52].

These genes belong to the HOXA5-11 cluster and are expressed throughout the CD34+ compartment [53,54]. The CD34+ level becomes important in AML due to the immature status of blastic cells.

As overexpression of Abd-B HOXA genes has been demonstrated in AML with a rearranged MLL [55], the gain of the HOXA cluster could be expected in case t-19 which had a t(9;11). The other t(v;MLL) did not exhibit this gain. The other two patients with such a gain (cases t-17 and t-14) had a t(15;17) and a +8 respectively. They were cytologically and cytogenetically different and had wild type MLL. The HOX gain was not detected in p-AML.

−7q

On 7q, the 11 MCR with a specificity for t-AML or p-AML were interlaced. Three MCR were reported in more than 10% of t-AML (table 8). The first one is 7q21.1 with a small region potentially implicating PFTK1, a member of a protein kinase family whose gain was recently shown to be involved in hepatocellular carcinoma cells.

The most frequent MCR in t-AML was 7q21.3q22.1 (tables 6 and 8). The number of genes present in this almost 3 Mb-long MCR prohibited extensive reviewing.

Three miRNA, mir-25, mir-93 and mir-106b were present in this deleted region (table 6 and table 8), regulating numerous genes. The miR-106b~25 cluster cooperates with its host gene MCM7 in cellular transformation both *in vitro* and *in vivo*, so that the concomitant overexpression of MCM7 and the miRNA cluster triggers prostatic intraepithelial neoplasia in transgenic mice [56]. MCM7 can be associated with CDK4 that may regulate the binding of this protein to the tumor suppressor protein RB1/RB. Among 30 genes, BRI3 appears to be overexpressed in BM-CD33+ cells. It seems to play a key role in TNF-induced cell death [57].

A defect in DNA repair was reported in TRRAP-deficient cells [58].

In 7q33q34, a 1.74Mb MCR had a low ratio in a patient (t-2), implying a probable double deletion, while the remaining ratio could have been due to the few normal cells. This MCR was the third in t-AML. It contained miRNA-490 which was probably regulating fewer than a hundred genes, with a maximum context score for the FOS gene. Among several genes (table 6), CREB3L2 was overexpressed in BM-CD34+ cells. It is a DNA binding and basic leucine zipper dimerization (bZIP) transcription factor. It was reportedly fused with FUS in fibrosarcomas [59] via a t(7;16)(q34;p11) and with PPAR gamma in a subset of thyroid carcinoma via a t(3;7)(p25;q34) [60].

In our series of p-AML, a large 43 Mb MCR was situated between 7q31.3 and the telomere (table 6). Table 8 allowed us to divide this region into 5 smaller MCR that seemed to be different from those of t-AML. The only exception was the previously identified 7q33q34 MCR that was the only MCR common to t-AML and p-AML in the loss of 7q.

The most centromeric p-AML-specific deletion was a 2.2Mb MCR on 7q31.3. Among the 10 genes in the region, only WASL is reported to potentially play a role in the microthrombocytopenia, the characteristic sign of Wiskott-Aldrich syndrome [61].

The 7q34 MCR was the most frequent and the most specific in p-AML. It contains 5 genes (table 8) that are not obviously involved in malignancy and some (e.g. PARP12) are poorly known but all are more or less strongly expressed in CD33 myeloid cells.

They were located between 7q31.3 and 7q36.2. Obviously, there are too many genes in those 5 MCRs, but PTPRZ1, MLL3 and XRCC2 could be candidate leukemogenic genes.

+8q24.3

A gain of 170 Kb located on 8q24.3 was selected as a MCR from two cases in the present group of t-AML (Figure 1). This MCR was confirmed in other series (table 9), frequently in t-AML (8%) and less frequently in p-AML (2.1%). This finding is consistent with the +8q22qter MCR being the "drive" genes of trisomy 8 which can be observed in some t(8;21) AML [62]. This MCR was telomeric to the MYC and TRIB1 genes [63]. PSCA, implicated in prostate cancer and C8orf55, the "mesenchymal stem cell protein DSCD75" which plays a role in bone marrow cell interactions, could not be excluded. However JRK, which is moderately overexpressed in BM-CD34+ cells [6] encodes a putative DNA-binding protein [64] and exhibits homology with the CENP-B (centromere-binding protein B).

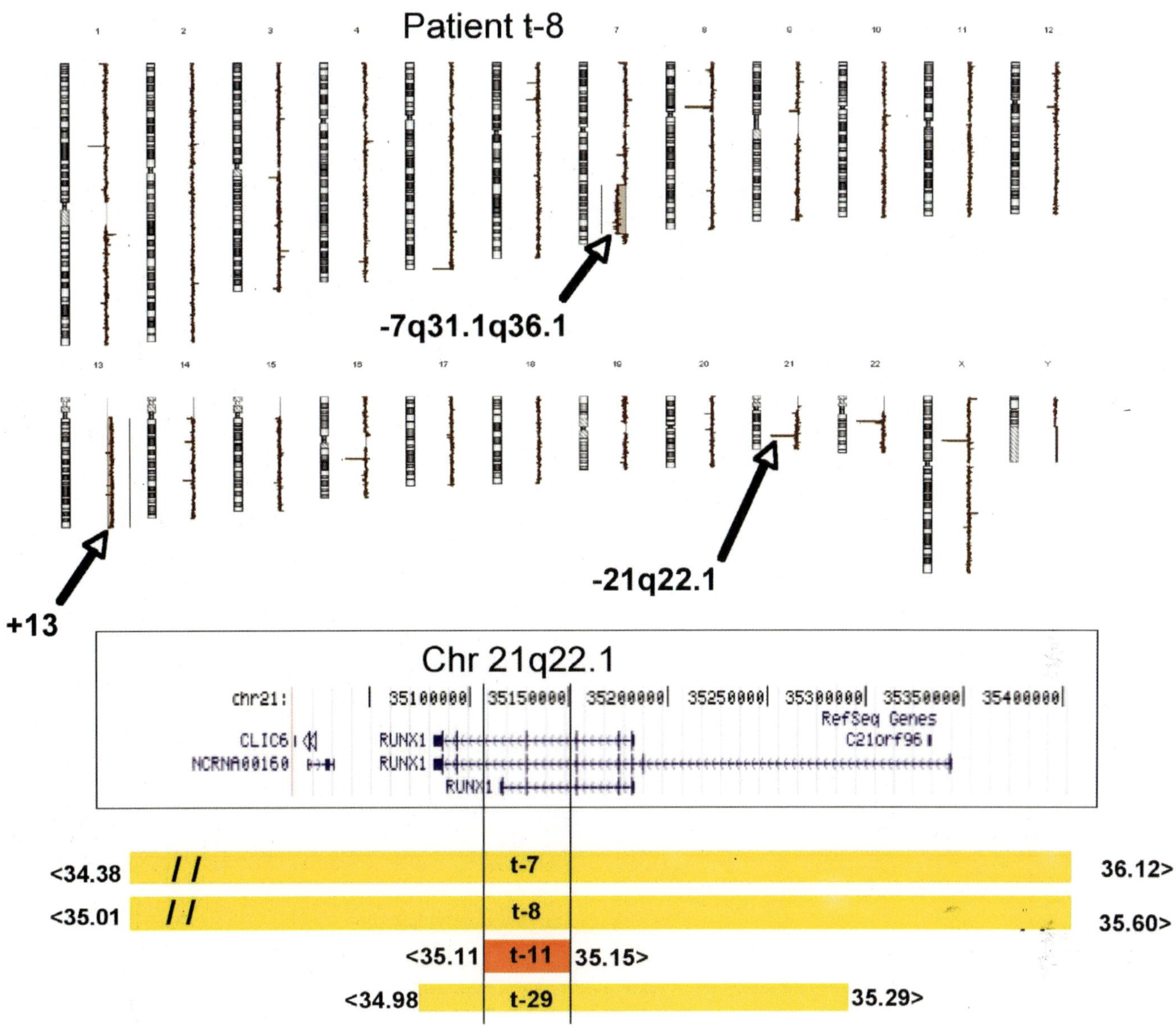

Figure 2. aCGH karyogram of patient t-8 and MCR delineation of RUNX1. A = A del (7q) and trisomy 13 are obvious. Cryptic deletions from 21q22.1 (corresponding to RUNX1) and from Xp11.4, that are smaller than 60kb, are nullosomic. On 22q11, the loss is a constitutive CNV of GGT1. B = A UCSC map (build 18) of the RUNX1 gene. C = The deletions of RUNX in four patients at the molecular level are labeled in orange and the smallest in red. The location of the breakpoints are indicated at the ends of the colored lines. Patient t-8 exhibits a homozygous 590 Kb deletion that encompassed the entire RUNX1 gene and could have occurred by an acquired isodisomy. Patient t-11 had the smallest deletion (40Kb) that was internal to RUNX1; t-29 had a deletion limited to RUNX1.

+11q24.2q24.3

Although no such result was found in our study, 5.6% of the p-AML in other series clearly showed gains or amplifications of this region that contains ETS1 and FLI1 genes. They are members of the ETS gene family that includes genes playing important roles in regulating hematopoiesis, proliferation, differentiation and apoptosis. Interestingly, these gains were found in cases presenting gains of the ETS2 and ERG genes (see below, the +21q22 paragraph).

−12p13

A 1.48Mb loss was defined as a MCR from three t-AML cases in the present report. The same area is recurrently lost in both types of AML (table 7, table 8). Among 17 genes, the 5′ part of ETV6 was lost. This ETS family transcription factor is a multi-partner gene with almost 28 different fusion genes via reciprocal translocations. It is implicated in multiple myeloid malignancies such as MDS and AML, but also in lymphoid malignancies and in fibrosarcomas [49]. CDKN1B encodes a cyclin-dependent kinase inhibitor. These two genes are considered as having tumor suppressor activity.

−17p13.2p13.1

Although no deletion of this region was found in our series, several reports claimed a loss of this MCR in 12% of t-AML and 3% of p-AML. This region, among several genes, exhibits loss of the TP53 tumor suppressor gene [49].

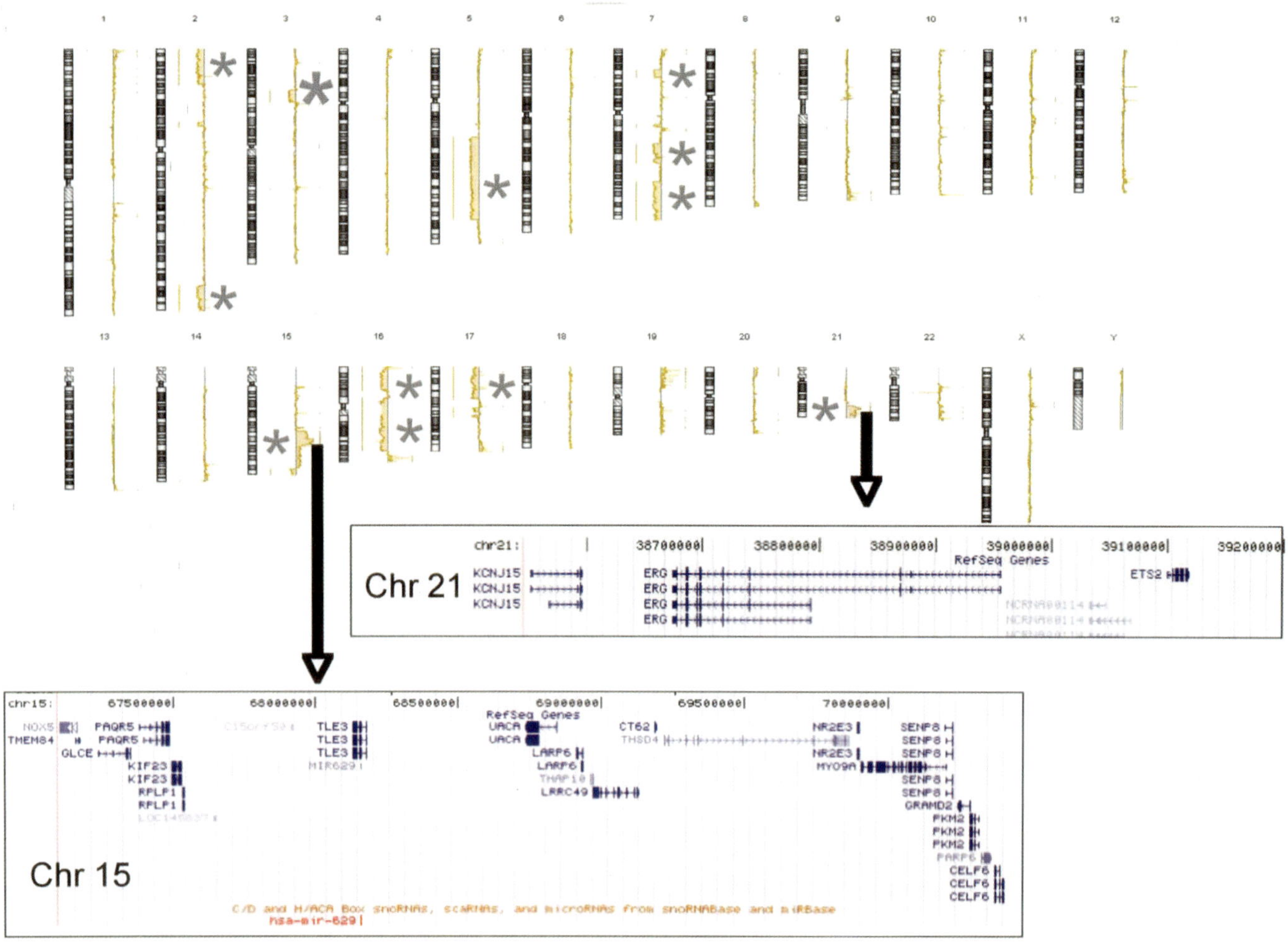

Figure 3. p-AML (case p24) with a complex karyotype. See the amplification of 15q23q24 and of 21q11.2q22.1 that are enlarged at the gene level. Multiple abnormalities (cf table 5) are asterisked.

−17q11.2

This MCR, that we found in a single case of t-AML (table 7), is the most frequent loss of the table 8 with 7.1% of in p-AML and 10% of in t-AML. This MCR contains the NF1 tumour suppressor gene NF1 which encodes neurofibromin, a GTPase-activating protein that negatively regulates RAS signaling by stimulating hydrolysis of Ras-GTP. Loss of NF1 can lead to a progressive myeloproliferative disorder in animal models [65] and in Juvenile myelomonocytic leukemia. Parkin [19] concluded that NF1 null states were present in 7% of AML. This important point confirmed that additional events were are required.

−18

Loss of different parts of chromosome 18 were highly recurrent in p-AML (table 8). In our series, we found a single p-AML with a 2.06 Mb deletion that had an equivalent MCR in table 8 which contains RAB27B and CCDC68 genes.

−21q22.12

This 40kb small MCR contains RUNX1 that was lost in 4 t-AML cases in the present series. Two patients had lost their two alleles either through double losses or deletion and D171N mutation. This mutation has been claimed to result in the proliferation of immature myeloid cells, an enhanced capacity for self-renewal, and the proliferation of primitive progenitors [66].

Patient t-29 had a normal karyotype [32] and a 310kb deletion that deleted most of the gene in a radiotherapy-induced leukemia [67].

Three deleted cases were exposed to multi-agent chemotherapy with alkylating agents. They exhibited a 7q-/-7 as previously reported [68] as well as patient t-12 that had a balanced abnormality involving RUNX1, only detected by classical karyotype. It has been suggested that the mutation of RUNX1 and gene losses localized on 7q could cooperate in leukemogenesis and predispose to leukemic transformation into t-AML following alkylating agents (figure 2). In table 8, seven other cases were observed in p-AML.

RUNX1, the subunit alpha of the Core Binding Factor (CBF), a heterodimeric transcription factor, plays a key role in the regulation of hematopoietic stem cell proliferation and differentiation. It is one of the most frequent targets of chromosome translocations via nearly forty different partners [49] in various forms of leukemia.

A germline mono-allelic mutation or deletion of RUNX1 [69] has been described in FPD (Familial Platelet Dysfunction) disease. A second mutation may appear at the AML stage, mostly with an M0 type in the FAB classification [70].

Point mutations of RUNXI have been described in radiation-induced MDS [67] or in therapy-induced transformation of myeloproliferative neoplasia [66].

Haploinsufficiency of RUNX1 leads to the loss of function of this gene (probably a tumor suppressor function). In the case of t-AML, the various point mutations are localized at the N-terminal, the DNA binding site [68].

+21q22

Distal 21q11.2qter polysomy was observed in three cases (table 6), two of which exhibited amplifications of this region in the context of a complex karyotype [21].

The first amplicon (table 5 and 6) from 14.29 to 17.97Mb harbored a cluster of miR-99a, miR-125b-2 and hsa-let-7c, each of which is predicted to regulate several hundred genes. Several of the genes in this amplicon (table 6) were overexpressed [35] in BM-CD34+ cells. SAMSN1, a hematopoietic adaptor was found to contain the SH3 and SAM domains 1, HSP13, BTG3 and NRIP1. This region was reported to be amplified by BAC aCGH in a series of patients with complex karyotypes [71] which showed that NRIP1 and SAMSN1 genes were up-regulated compared with their status in patients with normal karyotypes. The same area from LIP1 to miR-125b-2 is reported to be homozygously deleted in the Non-Small Cell Lung Cancer cell line Calu-6 [72].

The 1Mb-long second amplicon, observed in cases p-21 and p-24 was found to occur frequently in p-AML (table 9) and most of the cases also exhibited a gain of ETS1. It contained ERG and ETS2 genes. These two ETS transcription factor gene family members were overexpressed in BM-CD34+ cells. ERG can be fused with several genes in prostate cancer [73], in Ewing tumors [74] and in leukemias with a t(16;21)(p11;q22) and an FUS-ERG fusion [49]. It has been claimed that ERG is a megakaryocytic oncogene [75] together with ETS2 [76].

ERG and ETS2 were amplified in p-AML with complex karyotypes (figure 3) and ETS2 overexpression was highly correlated with the amplification, unlike ERG [71,77]. The preliminary results of a transcriptome study of case p-21 are in agreement with these findings. The RUNX1 region was not amplified in p-AML in our small sample.

Conclusion

High resolution cytogenomics obtained by aCGH and similar techniques already published allowed us to characterize numerous untargeted non random chromosome abnormalities. This work supports the hypothesis that they can be classified into several categories: abnormalities common to all AML (e.g. 8q24.3 gain or 17q11.2 deletion involving NF1); those more frequently found in t-AML (e.g. 7q21 or 7q33 deletions or even the specific gain of HOX genes); and those specifically found in p-AML (e.g. loss of the 139 to 152.8 Mb of 7q, 11q24 gain or 21q22 with amplifications of ERG and ETS2).

The genes involved in AML MCRs are often very well known in leukemogenesis but many others need to be explored.

Acknowledgments

The authors thank Lorna Saint Ange for editing, Lydie Da Costa for her friendly help, Didier Fauvet, Philippe Leopoldie, Caroline Dubois Gache, Bernard Clausse, Sebastien Forget for their invaluable assistance.

Author Contributions

Conceived and designed the experiments: NI PD AB. Performed the experiments: NI PD AB ST CR NA CP VL VS ALB JHB SdB. Analyzed the data: NI PD AB ST CR NA CP VL VS ALB JHB SdB. Contributed reagents/materials/analysis tools: NI PD AB ST CR NA CP VL VS ALB JHB SdB. Wrote the paper: NI PD AB.

References

1. Godley LA, Larson RA (2008) Therapy-related myeloid leukemia. Semin Oncol 35: 418–429.
2. Leone G, Pagano L, Ben-Yehuda D, Voso MT (2007) Therapy-related leukemia and myelodysplasia: susceptibility and incidence. Haematologica 92: 1389–1398.
3. Pedersen-Bjergaard J, Andersen MT, Andersen MK (2007) Genetic pathways in the pathogenesis of therapy-related myelodysplasia and acute myeloid leukemia. Hematology Am Soc Hematol Educ Program. pp 392–397.
4. Pedersen-Bjergaard J, Andersen MK, Andersen MT, Christiansen DH (2008) Genetics of therapy-related myelodysplasia and acute myeloid leukemia. Leukemia 22: 240–248.
5. Toujani S, Dessen P, Ithzar N, Danglot G, Richon C, et al. (2009) High resolution genome-wide analysis of chromosomal alterations in Burkitt's lymphoma. PLoS One 4: e7089.
6. Zhu J, Sanborn JZ, Benz S, Szeto C, Hsu F, et al. (2009) The UCSC Cancer Genomics Browser. Nat Methods 6: 239–240.
7. Iafrate AJ, Feuk L, Rivera MN, Listewnik ML, Donahoe PK, et al. (2004) Detection of large-scale variation in the human genome. Nat Genet 36: 949–951.
8. Redon R, Ishikawa S, Fitch KR, Feuk L, Perry GH, et al. (2006) Global variation in copy number in the human genome. Nature 444: 444–454.
9. Wong KK, deLeeuw RJ, Dosanjh NS, Kimm LR, Cheng Z, et al. (2007) A comprehensive analysis of common copy-number variations in the human genome. Am J Hum Genet 80: 91–104.
10. Skjelbred CF, Saebo M, Hjartaker A, Grotmol T, Hansteen IL, et al. (2007) Meat, vegetables and genetic polymorphisms and the risk of colorectal carcinomas and adenomas. BMC Cancer 7: 228.
11. Suzen HS, Guvenc G, Turanli M, Comert E, Duydu Y, et al. (2007) The role of GSTM1 and GSTT1 polymorphisms in head and neck cancer risk. Oncol Res 16: 423–429.
12. Sreeja L, Syamala V, Hariharan S, Syamala VS, Raveendran PB, et al. (2008) Glutathione S-transferase M1, T1 and P1 polymorphisms: susceptibility and outcome in lung cancer patients. J Exp Ther Oncol 7: 73–85.
13. Lin C-H, Li L-H, Ho S-F, Chuang T-P, Wu J-Y, et al. (2008) A large-scale survey of genetic copy number variations among Han Chinese residing in Taiwan. BMC Genetics 9: 92.
14. Schmetzer HM, Braun S, Wiesner D, Duell T, Gerhartz HH, et al. (2000) Gene rearrangements in bone marrow cells of patients with acute myelogenous leukemia. Acta Haematol 103: 125–134.
15. Roumier C, Eclache V, Imbert M, Davi F, MacIntyre E, et al. (2003) M0 AML, clinical and biologic features of the disease, including AML1 gene mutations: a report of 59 cases by the Groupe Francais d'Hematologie Cellulaire (GFHC) and the Groupe Francais de Cytogenetique Hematologique (GFCH). Blood 101: 1277–1283.
16. Dupret C, Asnafi V, Leboeuf D, Millien C, Ben Abdelali R, et al. (2005) IgH/TCR rearrangements are common in MLL translocated adult AML and suggest an early T/myeloid or B/myeloid maturation arrest, which correlates with the MLL partner. Leukemia 19: 2337–2338.
17. Schoch C, Haferlach T, Bursch S, Gerstner D, Schnittger S, et al. (2002) Loss of genetic material is more common than gain in acute myeloid leukemia with complex aberrant karyotype: a detailed analysis of 125 cases using conventional chromosome analysis and fluorescence in situ hybridization including 24-color FISH. Genes Chromosomes Cancer 35: 20–29.
18. Parkin B, Erba H, Ouillette P, Roulston D, Purkayastha A, et al. (2010) Acquired genomic copy number aberrations and survival in adult acute myelogenous leukemia. Blood.
19. Parkin B, Ouillette P, Wang Y, Liu Y, Wright W, et al. (2010) NF1 inactivation in adult acute myelogenous leukemia. Clin Cancer Res 16: 4135–4147.
20. Walter MJ, Payton JE, Ries RE, Shannon WD, Deshmukh H, et al. (2009) Acquired copy number alterations in adult acute myeloid leukemia genomes. Proc Natl Acad Sci U S A 106: 12950–12955.
21. Mrozek K (2008) Cytogenetic, molecular genetic, and clinical characteristics of acute myeloid leukemia with a complex karyotype. Semin Oncol 35: 365–377.
22. Peterson LF, Boyapati A, Ahn EY, Biggs JR, Okumura AJ, et al. (2007) Acute myeloid leukemia with the 8q22;21q22 translocation: secondary mutational events and alternative t(8;21) transcripts. Blood 110: 799–805.
23. Chen CZ, Li L, Lodish HF, Bartel DP (2004) MicroRNAs modulate hematopoietic lineage differentiation. Science 303: 83–86.
24. Karp X, Ambros V (2005) Developmental biology. Encountering microRNAs in cell fate signaling. Science 310: 1288–1289.
25. Calin GA, Croce CM (2006) MicroRNAs and chromosomal abnormalities in cancer cells. Oncogene 25: 6202–6210.

26. Garzon R, Fabbri M, Cimmino A, Calin GA, Croce CM (2006) MicroRNA expression and function in cancer. Trends Mol Med 12: 580–587.
27. Dixon-McIver A, East P, Mein CA, Cazier JB, Molloy G, et al. (2008) Distinctive patterns of microRNA expression associated with karyotype in acute myeloid leukaemia. PLoS One 3: e2141.
28. Paulsson K, Heidenblad M, Strombeck B, Staaf J, Jonsson G, et al. (2006) High-resolution genome-wide array-based comparative genome hybridization reveals cryptic chromosome changes in AML and MDS cases with trisomy 8 as the sole cytogenetic aberration. Leukemia 20: 840–846.
29. Rucker FG, Bullinger L, Schwaenen C, Lipka DB, Wessendorf S, et al. (2006) Disclosure of candidate genes in acute myeloid leukemia with complex karyotypes using microarray-based molecular characterization. J Clin Oncol 24: 3887–3894.
30. Suela J, Alvarez S, Cigudosa JC (2007) DNA profiling by arrayCGH in acute myeloid leukemia and myelodysplastic syndromes. Cytogenet Genome Res 118: 304–309.
31. Tyybakinoja A, Elonen E, Piippo K, Porkka K, Knuutila S (2007) Oligonucleotide array-CGH reveals cryptic gene copy number alterations in karyotypically normal acute myeloid leukemia. Leukemia 21: 571–574.
32. Akagi T, Ogawa S, Dugas M, Kawamata N, Yamamoto G, et al. (2009) Frequent genomic abnormalities in acute myeloid leukemia/myelodysplastic syndrome with normal karyotype. Haematologica 94: 213–223.
33. Akagi T, Shih LY, Kato M, Kawamata N, Yamamoto G, et al. (2009) Hidden abnormalities and novel classification of t(15;17) acute promyelocytic leukemia (APL) based on genomic alterations. Blood 113: 1741–1748.
34. Akagi T, Shih LY, Ogawa S, Gerss J, Moore SR, et al. (2009) Single nucleotide polymorphism genomic arrays analysis of t(8;21) acute myeloid leukemia cells. Haematologica 94: 1301–1306.
35. Su AI, Wiltshire T, Batalov S, Lapp H, Ching KA, et al. (2004) A gene atlas of the mouse and human protein-encoding transcriptomes. Proc Natl Acad Sci U S A 101: 6062–6067.
36. Monnier J, Samson M (2008) Cytokine properties of prokineticins. FEBS J 275: 4014–4021.
37. Grozdanov PN, Roy S, Kittur N, Meier UT (2009) SHQ1 is required prior to NAF1 for assembly of H/ACA small nucleolar and telomerase RNPs. RNA 15: 1188–1197.
38. Delhommeau F, Dupont S, Della Valle V, James C, Trannoy S, et al. (2009) Mutation in TET2 in myeloid cancers. N Engl J Med 360: 2289–2301.
39. Hu X, Stern HM, Ge L, O'Brien C, Haydu L, et al. (2009) Genetic alterations and oncogenic pathways associated with breast cancer subtypes. Mol Cancer Res 7: 511–522.
40. Stockwin LH, Vistica DT, Kenney S, Schrump DS, Butcher DO, et al. (2009) Gene expression profiling of alveolar soft-part sarcoma (ASPS). BMC Cancer 9: 22.
41. Evers C, Beier M, Poelitz A, Hildebrandt B, Servan K, et al. (2007) Molecular definition of chromosome arm 5q deletion end points and detection of hidden aberrations in patients with myelodysplastic syndromes and isolated del(5q) using oligonucleotide array CGH. Genes Chromosomes Cancer 46: 1119–1128.
42. Gao M, Liu Q, Zhang F, Han Z, Gu T, et al. (2009) Conserved expression of the PRELI domain containing 2 gene (Prelid2) during mid-later-gestation mouse embryogenesis. J Mol Histol 40: 227–233.
43. Tahvanainen J, Kallonen T, Lahteenmaki H, Heiskanen KM, Westermarck J, et al. (2009) PRELI is a mitochondrial regulator of human primary T-helper cell apoptosis, STAT6, and Th2-cell differentiation. Blood 113: 1268–1277.
44. Fiskus W, Wang Y, Sreekumar A, Buckley KM, Shi H, et al. (2009) Combined epigenetic therapy with the histone methyltransferase EZH2 inhibitor 3-deazaneplanocin A and the histone deacetylase inhibitor panobinostat against human AML cells. Blood 114: 2733–2743.
45. Fortier JM, Payton JE, Cahan P, Ley TJ, Walter MJ, et al. (2010) POU4F1 is associated with t(8;21) acute myeloid leukemia and contributes directly to its unique transcriptional signature. Leukemia 24: 950–957.
46. Niu C, Zhang J, Breslin P, Onciu M, Ma Z, et al. (2009) c-Myc is a target of RNA-binding motif protein 15 in the regulation of adult hematopoietic stem cell and megakaryocyte development. Blood 114: 2087–2096.
47. Staudt LM (2010) Oncogenic activation of NF-kappaB. Cold Spring Harb Perspect Biol 2: a000109.
48. Ferch U, Kloo B, Gewies A, Pfander V, Duwel M, et al. (2009) Inhibition of MALT1 protease activity is selectively toxic for activated B cell-like diffuse large B cell lymphoma cells. J Exp Med 206: 2313–2320.
49. Huret JL Atlas Genet Cytogenet Oncol Haematol.
50. Golub TR, Slonim DK, Tamayo P, Huard C, Gaasenbeek M, et al. (1999) Molecular classification of cancer: class discovery and class prediction by gene expression monitoring. Science 286: 531–537.
51. Thorsteinsdottir U, Mamo A, Kroon E, Jerome L, Bijl J, et al. (2002) Overexpression of the myeloid leukemia-associated Hoxa9 gene in bone marrow cells induces stem cell expansion. Blood 99: 121–129.
52. Eklund EA (2007) The role of HOX genes in malignant myeloid disease. Curr Opin Hematol 14: 85–89.
53. Sauvageau G, Lansdorp PM, Eaves CJ, Hogge DE, Dragowska WH, et al. (1994) Differential expression of homeobox genes in functionally distinct CD34+ subpopulations of human bone marrow cells. Proc Natl Acad Sci U S A 91: 12223–12227.
54. Kawagoe H, Humphries RK, Blair A, Sutherland HJ, Hogge DE (1999) Expression of HOX genes, HOX cofactors, and MLL in phenotypically and functionally defined subpopulations of leukemic and normal human hematopoietic cells. Leukemia 13: 687–698.
55. Quentmeier H, Dirks WG, Macleod RA, Reinhardt J, Zaborski M, et al. (2004) Expression of HOX genes in acute leukemia cell lines with and without MLL\ translocations. Leuk Lymphoma\ 45\: 567–574\.
56. Poliseno L, Salmena L, Riccardi L, Fornari A, Song MS, et al. (2010) Identification of the miR-106b~25 microRNA cluster as a proto-oncogenic PTEN-targeting intron that cooperates with its host gene MCM7 in transformation. Sci Signal 3: ra29.
57. Yamazaki T, Sasaki N, Nishi M, Yamazaki D, Ikeda A, et al. (2007) Augmentation of drug-induced cell death by ER protein BRI3BP. Biochem Biophys Res Commun 362: 971–975.
58. Murr R, Loizou JI, Yang YG, Cuenin C, Li H, et al. (2006) Histone acetylation by Trrap-Tip60 modulates loading of repair proteins and repair of DNA double-strand breaks. Nat Cell Biol 8: 91–99.
59. Panagopoulos I, Storlazzi CT, Fletcher CD, Fletcher JA, Nascimento A, et al. (2004) The chimeric FUS/CREB3l2 gene is specific for low-grade fibromyxoid sarcoma. Genes Chromosomes Cancer 40: 218–228.
60. Lui WO, Zeng L, Rehrmann V, Deshpande S, Tretiakova M, et al. (2008) CREB3L2-PPARgamma fusion mutation identifies a thyroid signaling pathway regulated by intramembrane proteolysis. Cancer Res 68: 7156–7164.
61. Sabri S, Foudi A, Boukour S, Franc B, Charrier S, et al. (2006) Deficiency in the Wiskott-Aldrich protein induces premature proplatelet formation and platelet production in the bone marrow compartment. Blood 108: 134–140.
62. Farra C, Awwad J, Valent A, Lozach F, Bernheim A (2004) Complex translocation (8;12;21): a new variant of t(8;21) in acute myeloid leukemia. Cancer Genet Cytogenet 155: 138–142.
63. Storlazzi CT, Fioretos T, Surace C, Lonoce A, Mastrorilli A, et al. (2006) MYC-containing double minutes in hematologic malignancies: evidence in favor of\ the episome model and exclusion of MYC as the target gene. Hum Mol Genet\ 15\: 933–942\.
64. Liu W, Seto J, Sibille E, Toth M (2003) The RNA binding domain of Jerky consists of tandemly arranged helix-turn-helix/homeodomain-like motifs and binds specific sets of mRNAs. Mol Cell Biol 23: 4083–4093.
65. Le DT, Kong N, Zhu Y, Lauchle JO, Aiyigari A, et al. (2004) Somatic inactivation of Nf1 in hematopoietic cells results in a progressive myeloproliferative disorder. Blood 103: 4243–4250.
66. Ding Y, Harada Y, Imagawa J, Kimura A, Harada H (2009) AML1/RUNX1 point mutation possibly promotes leukemic transformation in myeloproliferative neoplasms. Blood 114: 5201–5205.
67. Harada H, Harada Y, Tanaka H, Kimura A, Inaba T (2003) Implications of somatic mutations in the AML1 gene in radiation-associated and therapy-related myelodysplastic syndrome/acute myeloid leukemia. Blood 101: 673–680.
68. Christiansen DH, Andersen MK, Pedersen-Bjergaard J (2004) Mutations of AML1 are common in therapy-related myelodysplasia following therapy with alkylating agents and are significantly associated with deletion or loss of chromosome arm 7q and with subsequent leukemic transformation. Blood 104: 1474–1481.
69. Beri-Dexheimer M, Latger-Cannard V, Philippe C, Bonnet C, Chambon P, et al. (2008) Clinical phenotype of germline RUNX1 haploinsufficiency: from point mutations to large genomic deletions. Eur J Hum Genet 16: 1014–1018.
70. Preudhomme C, Renneville A, Bourdon V, Philippe N, Roche-Lestienne C, et al. (2009) High frequency of RUNX1 biallelic alteration in acute myeloid leukemia secondary to familial platelet disorder. Blood 113: 5583–5587.
71. Baldus CD, Bullinger L (2008) Gene expression with prognostic implications in cytogenetically normal acute myeloid leukemia. Semin Oncol 35: 356–364.
72. Yamada H, Yanagisawa K, Tokumaru S, Taguchi A, Nimura Y, et al. (2008) Detailed characterization of a homozygously deleted region corresponding to a candidate tumor suppressor locus at 21q11-21 in human lung cancer. Genes Chromosomes Cancer 47: 810–818.
73. Clark JP, Cooper CS (2009) ETS gene fusions in prostate cancer. Nat Rev Urol 6: 429–439.
74. Janknecht R (2005) EWS-ETS oncoproteins: the linchpins of Ewing tumors. Gene 363: 1–14.
75. Salek-Ardakani S, Smooha G, de Boer J, Sebire NJ, Morrow M, et al. (2009) ERG is a megakaryocytic oncogene. Cancer Res 69: 4665–4673.
76. Stankiewicz MJ, Crispino JD (2009) ETS2 and ERG promote megakaryopoiesis and synergize with alterations in GATA-1 to immortalize hematopoietic progenitor cells. Blood 113: 3337–3347.
77. Santoro A, Maggio A, Carbone P, Mirto S, Caronia F, et al. (1992) Amplification of ETS2 oncogene in acute nonlymphoblastic leukemia with t(6;21;18). Cancer Genet Cytogenet 58: 71–75.

2

Penicillamine Increases Free Copper and Enhances Oxidative Stress in the Brain of Toxic Milk Mice

Ding-Bang Chen[1,9], Li Feng[1,9], Xiao-Pu Lin[2], Wei Zhang[3], Fu-Rong Li[3], Xiu-Ling Liang[1], Xun-Hua Li[1]*

1 Department of Neurology, First Affiliated Hospital, Sun Yat-sen University, Guangzhou, China, **2** Nanfang Hospital, Southern Medical University, Guangzhou, China, **3** Laboratory Animal Centre, Sun Yat-sen University, Guangzhou, China

Abstract

Wilson disease (WD) is characterized by the accumulation of copper arising from a mutation in the ATP7B gene. Penicillamine (PA) makes 10–50% of the patients with neurologic symptoms neurologically worse at the early stage of administration. The aim of this study was to determine how the copper metabolism changes and whether the change impairs the brain of toxic milk (tx) mice, an animal model of WD, during the PA administration. The free copper and protein-bound copper concentrations in the serum, cortex and basal ganglia of tx mice with PA administration for 3 days, 10 days and 14 days, respectively, were investigated. The expression of copper transporters, ATP7A and CTR1,was analyzed by real-time quantitative PCR, immunofluorescence and Western blot. Then SOD, MDA and GSH/GSSG were detected to determine whether the oxidative stress changed correspondingly. The results revealed the elevated free copper concentrations in the serum and brain, and declined protein-bound copper concentrations in the brain of tx mice during PA administration. Meanwhile, transiently increased expression of ATP7A and CTR1 was observed generally in the brain parenchyma by immunofluorescence, real-time quantitative PCR and Western blot. Additionally, ATP7A and CTR1 were observed to locate mainly at Golgi apparatus and cellular membrane respectively. Intense staining of ATP7A in the choroid plexus was found in tx mice on the 3rd and 10th day of PA treatment, but rare staining of ATP7A and CTR1 in the blood-brain barrier (BBB). Decreased GSH/GSSG and increased MDA concentrations were also viewed in the cortex and basal ganglia. Our results suggested the elevated free copper concentrations in the brain might lead to the enhanced oxidative stress during PA administration. The increased free copper in the brain might come from the copper mobilized from brain parenchyma cells but not from the serum according to the ATP7A and CTR1 expression analysis.

Editor: Thomas Langmann, Center of Ophtalmology, Germany

Funding: The work was supported by grants from the National Natural Science Foundation of China(30671154,http://www.nsfc.gov.cn/Portal0/default106.htm). The funder had no role in study design, data collection and analysis, decision to publish, or preparation of the manuscript.

Competing Interests: The authors have declared that no competing interests exist.

* E-mail: lxunh001@yahoo.com.cn

9 These authors contributed equally to this work.

Introduction

Wilson disease (WD) is an autosomal recessive disease arising from a mutation in the ATP7B gene, which results in the failure of hepatocytes to excrete copper into bile, leading to the hepatic copper accumulation and cell injury. Eventually copper is released into the bloodstream and deposits in various other organs, notably the brain, kidneys, and cornea. Copper incorporation into the protein ceruloplasmin (Cp) is also impaired by dysfunction of ATP7B, leading to the reduced circulating holoceruloplasmin.

The treatment for WD patients involves reversing the positive copper balance. Chelators like penicillamine or trientine induce negative copper balance by cupriuresis [1]. The pivotal role of penicillamine in the initial treatment for WD patients with neurologic symptoms has been a matter of debate for the risk of neurological worsening for the past three decades. 10%–50% of patients neurologically worsened by PA and 50% of them never recovered to the level before treatment [2]. Trientine shares the propensity of penicillamine to deteriorate neurologic symptoms (about 25%) [3].

Previous study reported that free copper increased in the cerebrospinal fluid (CSF) and serum in WD patients with the neurologic manifestation during the penicillamine therapy [4]. Neurons were found an early and extensive death when treated with copper in vitro, which mirrored the concentration of the CSF of WD patients in previous report [5]. These findings indicated the increased free copper concentration in the brain might associate with the neurologic deterioration. The likely explanation for the drugs worsening the neurological symptoms was that a further elevation of copper level in the brain followed the mobilization of large stores of copper in the liver and/or the brain [4,6,7]. But there has been no direct evidence supporting the hypothesis yet.

Copper transport into cells is mediated by copper transporter1 (CTR1), which mediates copper uptake into mammalian cells, through the copper-stimulated endocytosis and degradation of CTR1 [8]. ATP7A and ATP7B are both copper transport proteins which participate in copper efflux out of cells,whereas ATP7A is the dominating copper transporter in neurons [9]. ATP7A moves towards the plasma membrane and removes excess copper in the presence of elevated extracellular copper concentrations [10]. Earlier studies reported the expression of the copper transpoter-s,ATP7A and CTR1, was higher in brain barriers than that in brain parenchyma by in situ brain perfusion technique with copper, and the copper transported into the brain was mainly achieved through the blood-brain barrier(BBB) [11,12].

In the serum copper is mainly carried by Cp, while the residue bound to albumin or small molecules. Free copper, which is commonly defined as the copper not covalently bound to Cp in the blood, is loosely bound to albumin and small molecules. Free copper, which is about 5–15% of serum copper in normal people, greatly expanded in WD patients and diffused out of the vascular compartment into extracellular fluids and tissues with toxic effects [13].The free copper concentration is assessed with the calculation of the serum non Cp-bound copper [1]. However, it was suggested copper transported into the brain through the blood-brain barrier (BBB) as free copper ions but not as albumin-bound copper [11]. The estimation of copper concentration by the traditional method didn't eliminate the role of albumin or other proteins which bound unnecessary copper and lessened the toxic effect.

The toxic milk (tx) mouse is a naturally occurring genetic and phenotypic model of WD derived from the wild-type (DL) mouse [14]. The mouse contains a methionine to valine substitution (M1356V) that renders the ATP7B protein dysfunctional and results in copper accumulation, which commences in the 3rd postnatal week, in a distribution resembling that observed in human WD cases. An increase of copper in the liver and the brain has been well characterized in tx mice [15]. In this study we investigated the concentrations of free copper and protein-bound copper in the serum and the brain tissue, separately, by a different method of ultrafiltration during PA treatment [16]. The expression of ATP7A and CTR1 was also detected to estimate the copper transporting activity in the brain. Furthermore we examined the possible neurotoxicity during the treatment. Superoxide dismutase (SOD) and reduced glutathione/oxidized glutathione (GSH/GSSG) ratio were measured as intracellular indicators of antioxidant responses, while the malondialdehyde (MDA) content as a lipid peroxidation index.

Results

Copper concentrations

The average serum free copper concentration detected by ultrafiltration method was about 8.9% of serum copper concentration, the sum of free copper and protein-bound copper, in control group of tx mice,while in DL mice it was 1.9%. The free copper concentrations in tx mice serum significantly elevated on the 3rd day after persistent PA administration ($P<0.05$), then declined progressively and below the level of control mice on the 14th day (Fig. 1). Obviously the free copper concentrations in DL mice were lower than tx mice and also lightly increased 3 days after PA administration ($P>0.05$). The protein-bound copper concentrations in tx mice serum were significantly lower than that in DL mice. In tx mice the mean protein-bound copper concentrations was nearly 200 ug/L and almost 2-fold increased on the 3rd day of PA treatment and kept the level up to the 14th day ($P<0.01$). In normal mice the copper bound to protein was slightly decreased during the PA treatment.

Figure 2 shows the free copper concentrations in the cortex and basal ganglia of tx mice were slightly higher than that of DL mice and also it shows the same tendency as that of the serum after administration, which significantly elevated ($P<0.05$)on the 3rd day and gradually lowered on the 10th and the 14th day. The free copper concentrations in DL mice were slightly decreased during the treatment. The protein-bound copper concentrations in the cortex and basal ganglia of the control tx mice were approximately 2-fold higher than that of DL mice,and gradually decreased along the administration compared with the control group ($P<0.01$). On the 14th day the protein-bound copper concentrations almost 25% decreased, while in DL mice the concentrations also slightly decreased during the administration.

Relative mRNA expression of ATP7A and CTR1

To make sure β-actin mRNA expression was unchanged during the PA treatment,the expression stability was analyzed by absolute standard curve method. The copies of β-actin did not change prominently in the cortex and basal ganglia of tx mice or DL mice during the PA treatment. Figure 3 showed the stable expression of β-actin mRNA in the basal ganglia of the mice.

Relative abundance values for ATP7A and CTR1 were compared between the mice with PA administration and the controls (Fig. 4). Compared to the controls, the mRNA expression of ATP7A 4-fold increased ($P<0.01$) on the 3rd day in tx mice cortex after PA treatment, and 6-fold ($P<0.01$) increased in the basal ganglia. But on the 10th day it decreased to the level before administration, and further, lowered down to approximately 0.4-fold ($P<0.05$) in the cortex and 0.5-fold ($P<0.05$) in the basal ganglia as high as the controls on the 14th day. In DL mice,ATP7A mRNA expression 1.7-fold increased ($P<0.05$) in the cortex and 1.8-fold ($P<0.05$) in the basal ganglia on the 3rd day, and 0.5- and 0.7-fold decreased ($P<0.05$) in the cortex and basal ganglia on the 10th day, respectively, while 0.4-fold decreased ($P<0.05$) in both locations on the 14th day.

CTR1 mRNA expression increased by 6.9-fold ($P<0.01$) in the cortex and 9.1-fold in the basal ganglia of tx mice on the 3rd day after administration, but on the 10th day, it decreased significantly. Compared to controls, CTR1 expression increased by 1.9-fold ($P<0.05$) in the cortex and by 2.1-fold ($P<0.05$) in the basal ganglia on the 10th day, while by 1.8- and 2.3-fold ($P<0.05$) on the 14th day in the cortex and basal ganglia, respectively. In DL mice, CTR1 expression increased by 2.5-fold ($P<0.05$) in the cortex and by 2.15-fold ($P<0.05$) in the basal ganglia on the 3rd day of administration as compared to controls. Then it dropped back to the level of the control in both locations on the 3rd and the 10th day.

Immunofluorescence of ATP7A and CTR1

Immunofluorescence staining of frozen brain sections with antibody to ATP7A was scarcely observed in all DL mice brain sections, but weak staining in the layer 5 pyramidal neurons in the cortex, that is, internal pyramidal layer neurons (data not shown). ATP7A antibody also stained the internal pyramidal layer neurons in the control tx mice. After PA administration, intense ATP7A staining was generally present in the brain on the 3rd and the 10th day, including the cortex, hippocampus, caudate putamen (CPu), thalamus and choroid plexus in lateral cerebral ventricles (Fig. 5), and the location with the most intense staining was the internal pyramidal layer neurons. On the 14th day, ATP7A staining generally declined in the brain sections.

Immunofluorescence staining of CTR1 showed the staining was seldom present in the brain tissues of DL mice with or without PA treatment (Data not shown). CTR1 staining in the brain sections of the control group of tx mice was also scarcely observed. On the 3rd day of administration, CTR1 staining was generally but not intensely detected in the tx brain tissues, including internal pyramidal layer cells in the cortex, hippocampus, Cpu and thalamus. On the 10th day, the CTR1 staining was still present in brain cells, but almost disappeared on the 14th day. CTR1 staining was not detected in the choroid plexus or the endyma cells in tx mice brain with or without PA treatment (Fig. 6).

Co-localization experiment showed the localization of ATP7A and CTR1 in brain cells during the PA treatment. We used

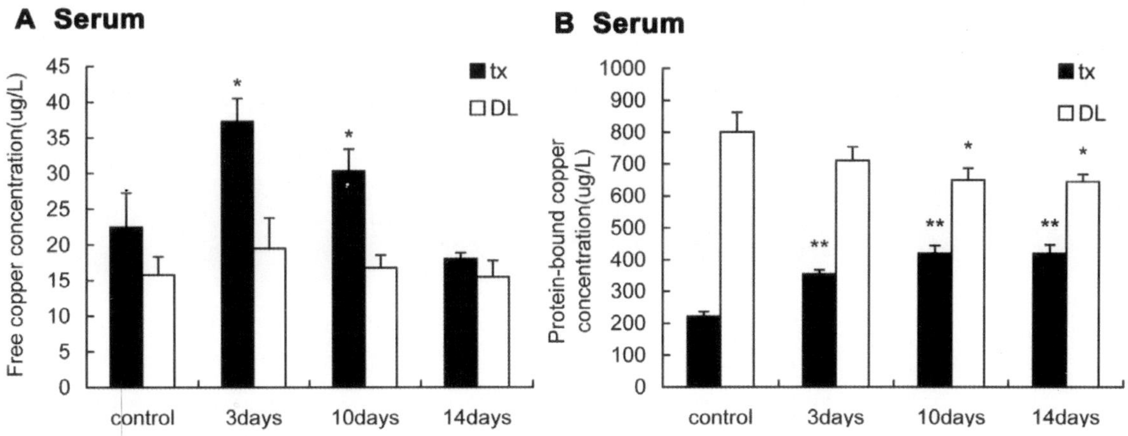

Figure 1. Detection of the free copper and protein-bound copper in the serum of tx and DL mice. Tx and DL mice were subjected to PA intragastric administration for 3 days, 10 days and 14 days, respectively. Mice without PA were controls. (A)The free copper concentrations in the tx mice serum increased on the 3rd day, and decreased on the 10th and the 14th day. The free copper concentrations didn't change significantly in DL mice. (B)The protein-bound copper concentrations in the serum 2-fold increased on the 3rd day compared to the controls and kept the level on the 10th and the 14th day, while slightly decreased along the administration in the serum of DL mice.(* $P<0.05$;** $P<0.01$).

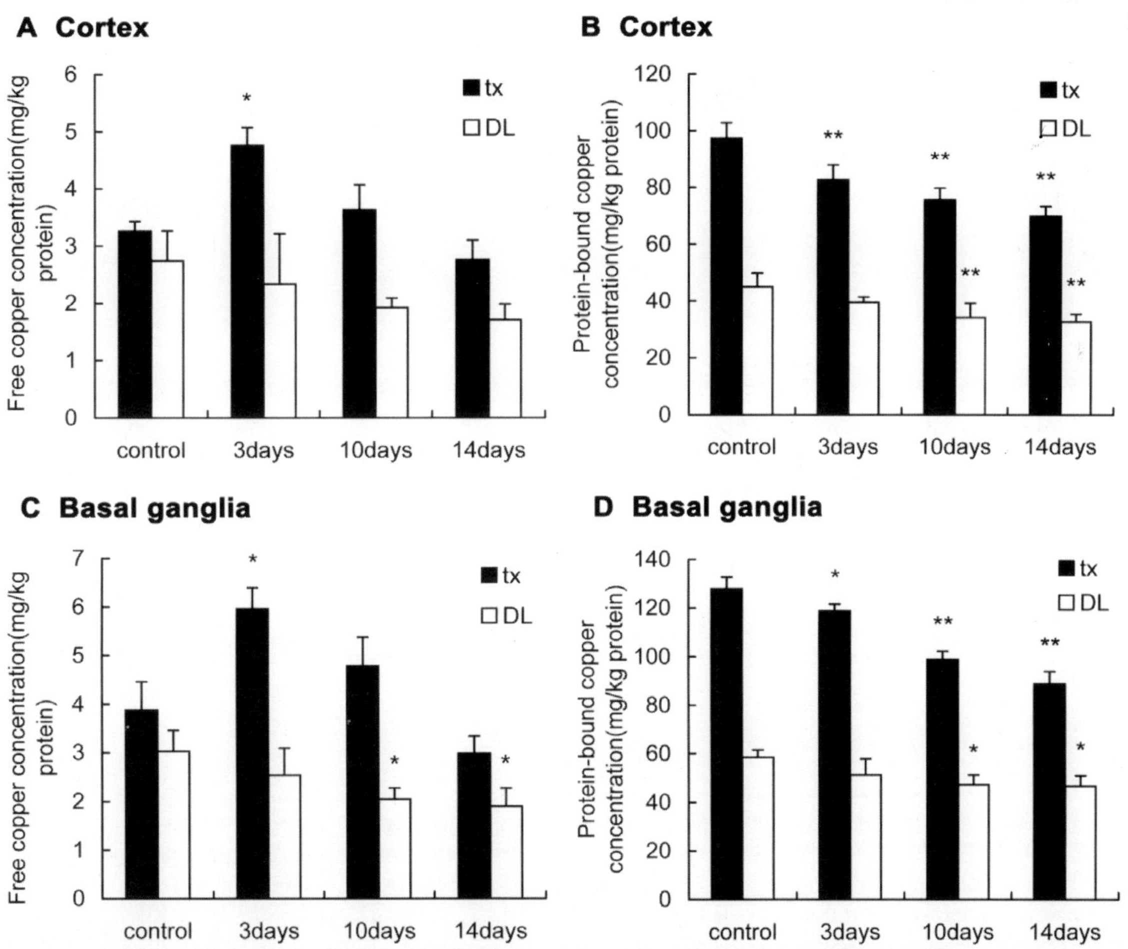

Figure 2. Detection of the free copper and protein-bound copper in the brain of tx and DL mice. (A)(C)The free copper concentrations in the cortex and basal ganglia of tx mice increased on the 3rd day and decreased on the 10th and 14th day,respectively. In DL mice the free copper decreased slightly along the administration. (B)(D) The protein-bound copper concentrations in the cortex and basal ganglia of tx and DL mice all decreased along the administration. The protein-bound copper concentrations in tx mice were about 2-fold higher than that of DL mice. (* $P<0.05$; ** $P<0.01$).

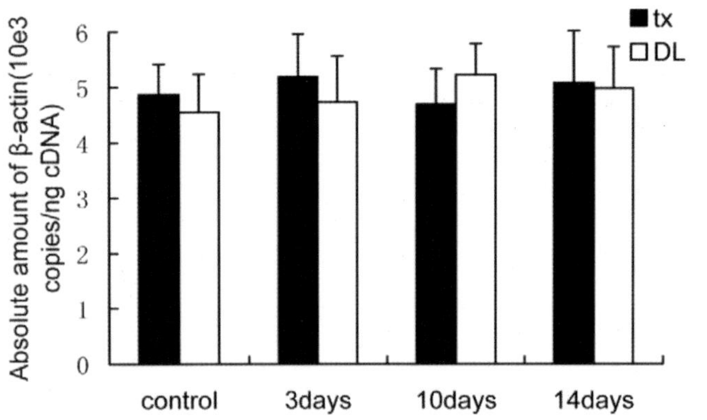

Figure 3. Absolute quantitation of β-actin in the cDNA from tissue. The copies of β-actin analyzed by absolute standard curve method did not change prominently in the basal ganglia of tx mice or DL mice during PA treatment.

GOLPH2/GOLM1, the golgi membrane protein 1, to label Golgi apparatus and viewed the co-localization of ATP7A and GOLPH2 under the oil immersion lens. Figure 7 showed that ATP7A mainly located at Golgi apparatus in the internal pyramidal layer of brain of tx mice during the PA treatment, while ATP7A staining seemed to exceed the scope of GOLPH2 staining on the 3rd day of the PA treatment. Meanwhile, we used NKCC1, the Na+/K+/2Cl− cotransporter located at cellular membrane, to label the cellular membrane. Figure 8 showed CTR1 co-located with NKCC1 in the internal pyramidal layer of cerebrum of tx mice, and it indicated that CTR1 located mainly at cellular membrane in tx mouse brain during the PA treatment.

In brain sections of tx mice intense ATP7A staining generally located in cells expressing CTR1. Figure 9 shows the co-localization in the Cpu of tx mice with 3 days PA administration. ATP7A expression in neurons was investigated using microtubulin-associated protein 2(MAP2), which was generally detected in neurons. This suggested that PA induced increased expressions of ATP7A and CTR1 in neurons. Previous study revealed that ATP7A and CTR1 achieved to transport copper into brain through BBB. The structure basis of BBB is composed of capillary endothelium and astrocytic endfeet, which ensheath the capillary

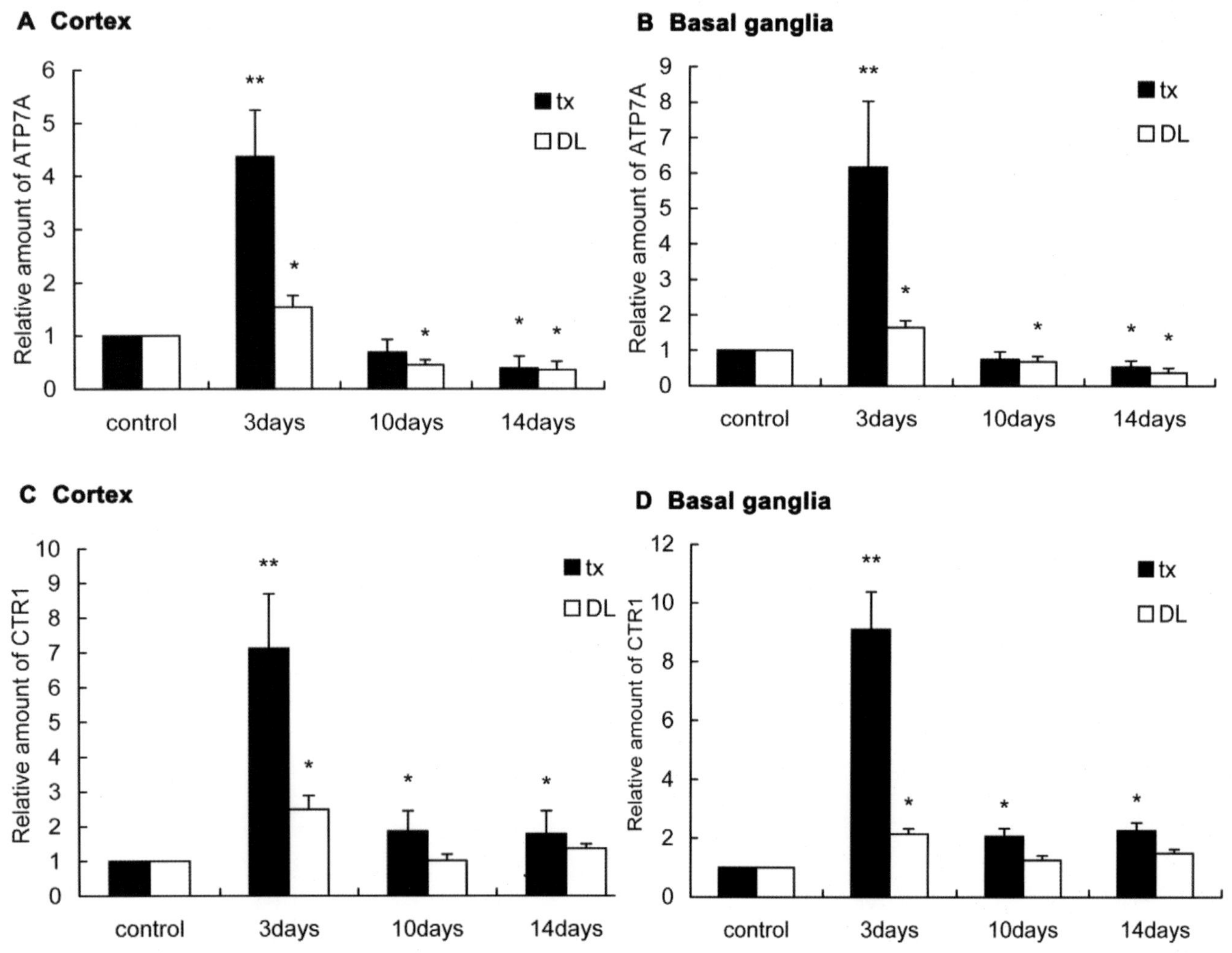

Figure 4. ATP7A and CTR1 mRNA expression in the brain of tx and DL mice. (A)(B)(C)(D)The ATP7A and CTR1 mRNA expression in the cortex and the basal ganglia increased significantly on the 3rd day, and declined close to the level of the control on the 10th and the 14th day. In DL mice mRNA expression of ATP7A and CTR1 also transiently increased on the 3rd day. In tx and DL controls, mRNA expression value was defined as 1.0. (* $P<0.05$, ** $P<0.01$).

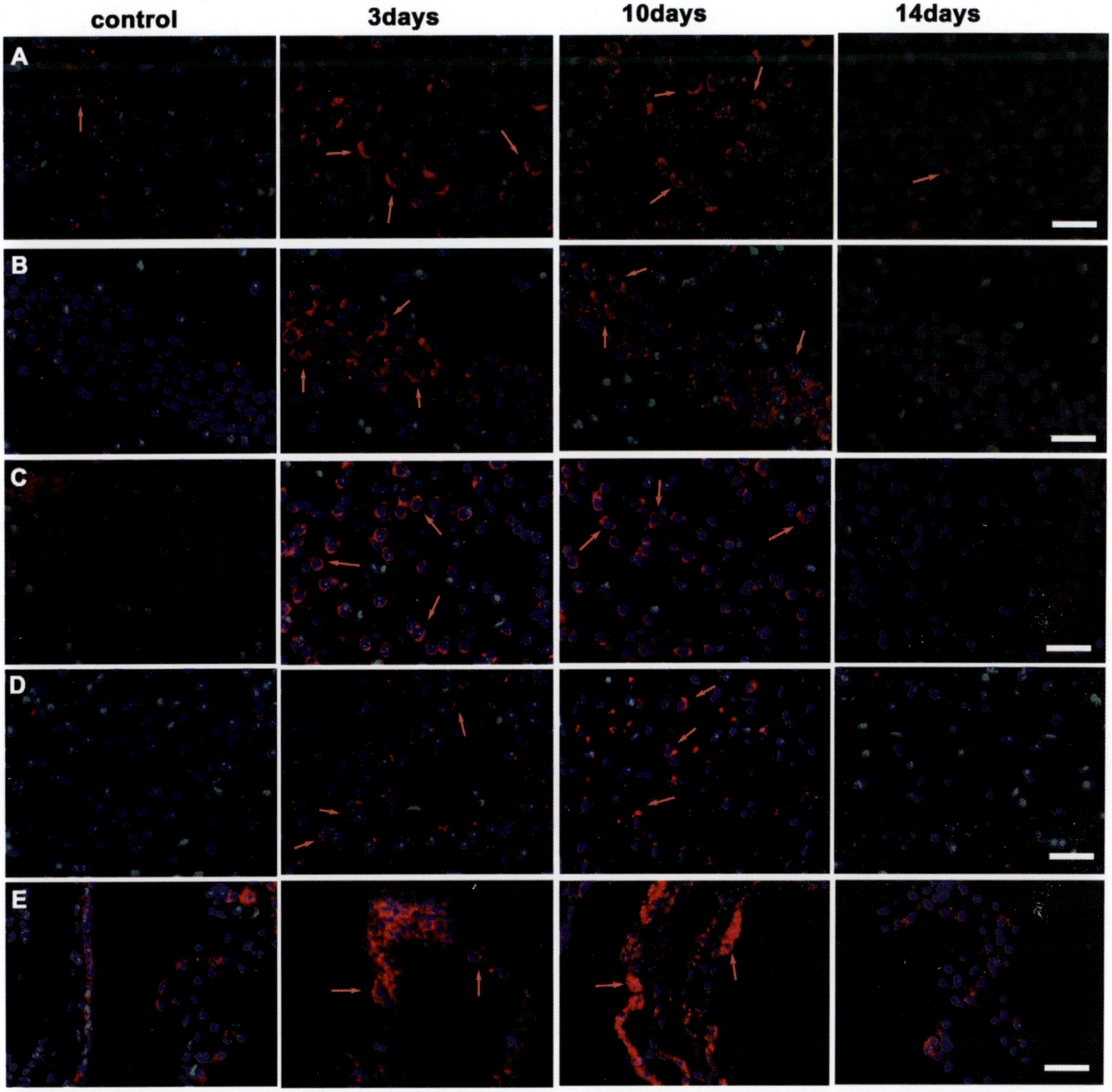

Figure 5. Detection of ATP7A by immunofluorescent staining (red) in the coronal brain slices of tx mice. Tx mice were subjected to PA administration for 3 days, 10days and 14days, respectively. (A) Internal pyramidal layer. ATP7A immunoreactivity staining was weak in internal pyramidal layer neurons in the control mice cortex, but increased significantly on the 3rd and the 10th day, then decreased on the 14th day. (B)hippocampus CA1 region, (C)caudate putamen(CPu), (D) central medial thalamic nucleus(CM),(E)choroid plexus in the lateral cerebral ventricles.ATP7A staining was weak in cells of hippocampus CA1 region, CPu, CM and choroid plexus in the control mice, and significantly increased on the 3rd day and the 10th day during PA administration, and declined on the 14th day. Scale bars = 30 um.

endothelium covering over 99% of the vascular endothelium. We used the cytoskeletal marker protein GFAP to identify astrocytes and astrocytic endfeet, and viewed little co-localization of ATP7A or CTR1 with GFAP as well as endothelial cells nucleus marked by DAPI in the basal lamina of BBB.

Western blot analysis for ATP7A and CTR1

To verify the changes of immunofluorescence staining of ATP7A and CTR1, the cortex and basal ganglia tissues of the mice with or without PA administration were examined with Western blot. The specificity of the anti-ATP7A and anti-CTR1 primary antibodies was confirmed by the protein bands with the size 170 kDa and 25 kDa, respectively. Compared with controls, the ATP7A expression 1.5-fold increased ($P<0.01$) in the cortex, and 2.6-fold ($P<0.01$) increased in the basal ganglia of tx mouse on the 3rd day after PA treatment (Figure 10). On the 10th day a 2.1-fold increased ATP7A expression was observed in the cortex as well as a more than 2.9-fold increase in basal ganglia. On the 14th

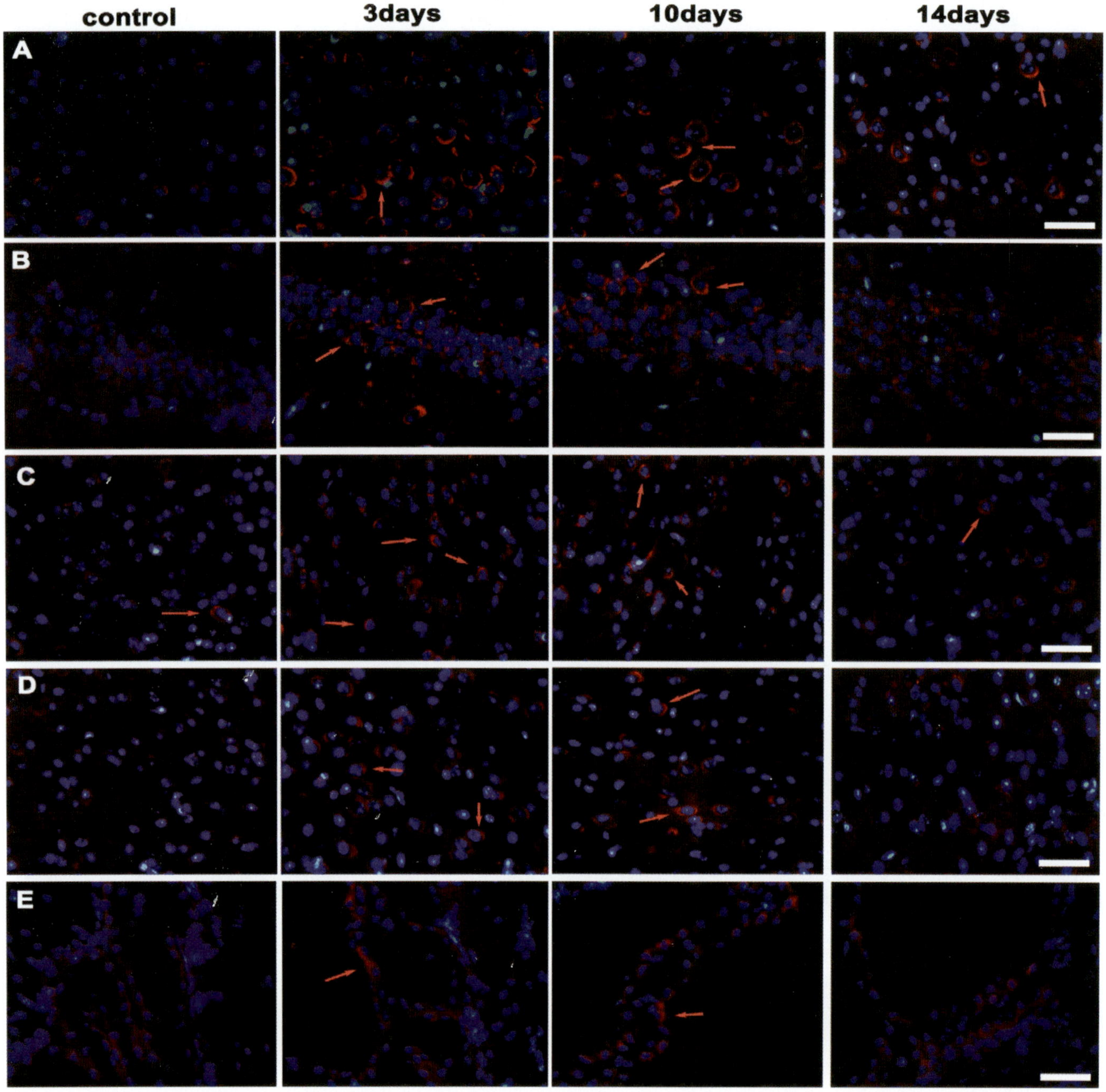

Figure 6. Detection of CTR1 by immunofluorescent staining (red) in the coronal brain slices of tx mice. (A) Internal pyramidal layer. There was almost no CTR1 immunoreactivity staining in the internal pyramidal layer neurons in control mice cortex. The staining presented on the 3rd and the 10th day, but declined on the 14th day during PA treatment. (B) hippocampus CA1 region, (C) caudate putamen (CPu), (D) central medial thalamic nucleus(CM). CTR1 staining was scarcely observed in cells of hippocampus CA1 region, CPu, and CM in the control mice, but presented on the 3rd and the 10th day during PA treatment, and declined on the 14th day. (E) choroid plexus in lateral cerebral ventricles. There was rare staining in the choroid plexus cells in tx mice with or without PA administration. Scale bars = 30 um.

day the ATP7A expression returned to the baseline in the control group. In DL mice ATP7A expression did not change in the cortex or basal ganglia during the PA administration.

CTR1 expression 2.2-fold ($P<0.01$) and 2.6-fold ($P<0.01$) increased on the 3rd day in tx mouse cortex and basal ganglia, respectively, while on the 10th day it 2.9-fold ($P<0.01$) and 3.1-fold ($P<0.01$) increased in tx mouse cortex and basal ganglia, respectively. CTR1 expression declined to the baseline on the 14th day in both regions above. In DL mice CTR1 expression did not change in the cortex and basal ganglia during the PA administration (Figure 11).

Oxidative-stress in the central nervous system

The activity of SOD in the cortex and the basal ganglia of tx and DL mice did not change during the two weeks PA administration. MDA was measured to estimate the lipid

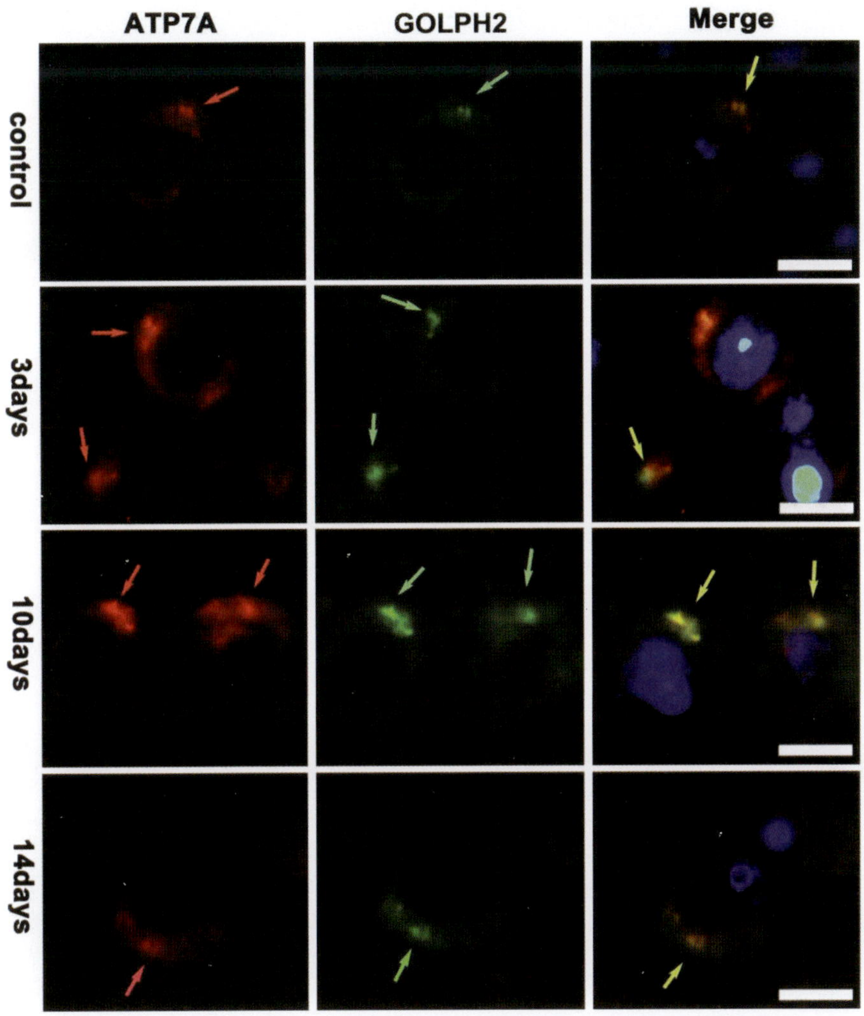

Figure 7. Co-localization of ATP7A and GOLPH2 in the internal pyramidal layer. The slices were from tx mice subjected to PA administration for 3 days, 10days and 14days, respectively. Golgi apparatus were labeled with GOLPH2. ATP7A(red) staining mainly co-located with GOLPH2(green) in the internal pyramidal layer of tx mice during the PA treatment, and the scope of ATP7A staining exceeded that of GOLPH2 on the 3rd day of the PA treatment. Scale bars = 10 um.

peroxidation in the brain. The result showed that the MDA concentrations in the cortex and the basal ganglia of tx mice increased on the 10th ($P<0.05$) and the 14th day ($P<0.01$) of the administration compared to controls. But it did not show any difference in DL mice. Analysis of GSH/GSSG ratios revealed that the GSH/GSSG declined gradually in the brains of tx mice after PA administration ($P<0.01$). It declined from the 3rd day of administration in the cortex and from the 10th day in the basal ganglia. It did not demonstrate the variation of GSH/GSSG ratios in DL mice during PA administration (Fig. 12).

Discussion

The neurological deterioration of WD patients during the chelator treatment has puzzled the neurologists for years. In a double blind study the spikes of the increased free copper levels in the serum associated in time with the WD patients' neurologic worsening [17]. But there are few researches on the change of copper in brain during the chelator treatment. In this study, we aimed to investigate the fluctuation of copper in the tx mice brain during PA treatment.

In our experiment the main content of serum copper in tx mice, which is the protein-bound copper, was significantly lower than DL mice. This was consistent with the reduced Cp due to the mutant ATP7B gene and verified this model. The transient increase of free copper in the serum of tx mice in the early days of PA administration was accordant with the previous report about WD patients [17]. Meanwhile, serum protein-bound copper also increased in tx mice during PA administration. This suggested that PA chelated a large amount of copper in the liver, followed by the increased copper in the serum. The mobilized copper mostly bound to the non-Cp proteins, such as albumin, which could be held-up by the ultrafiltration device and detected. When beyond the binding capability of serum proteins, the copper loosely bound to small molecules like amino acids or remained free, then filtrated through the membrane. In DL mice, the protein-bound copper was slightly decreased during the PA treatment, which might attributed to that PA reduced the copper potentially delivered to Cp by ATP7B in the liver.

In cells most of the copper is incorporated to the proteins including ceruloplasmin, cytochome oxidase, superoxide dismutase and metallothionein [18]. In our study most of the copper

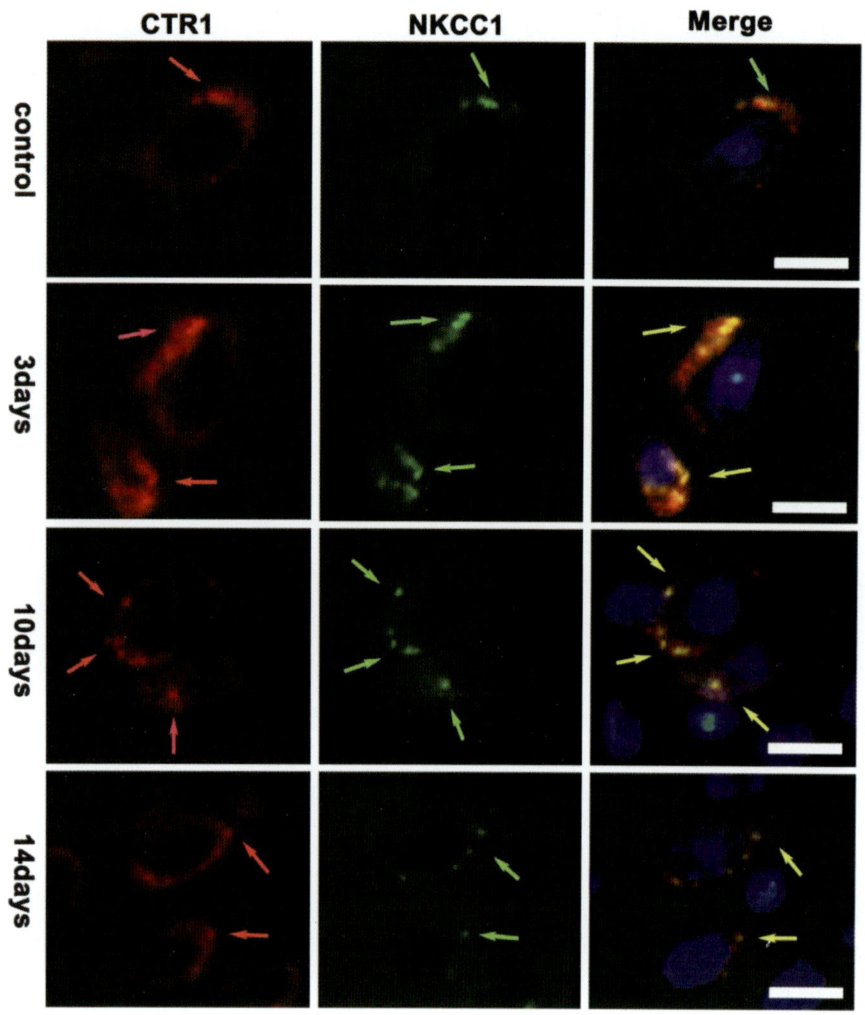

Figure 8. Co-localization of CTR1 and NKCC1 in the internal pyramidal layer. The slices were from tx mice subjected to PA administration for 3 days, 10days and 14days, respectively. Cellular membranes were labeled with NKCC1. CTR1(red) staining mainly co-located with NKCC1(green) in the internal pyramidal layer in cortex of tx mice during the PA treatment. Scale bars = 10 um.

bound to proteins in tissue were separated by the ultrafiltration device,and the residues, which were defined as free copper, included the copper ions and the copper binding with GSH, amino acid or other small molecules. These free copper elevated at the early stage of PA administration in the cortex and basal ganglia, whereas the protein-bound copper decreased gradually. It indicated PA removed copper from the brain at the early stage of treatment and induced the increase of free copper concentrations in tissue. Herein we provided the evidence of copper mobilized by PA in the brain, though it is still not sure whether the free copper came from the brain or the liver. What is interesting is that the protein-bound copper concentrations in the basal ganglia were approximately 25 mg/kg protein higher than those in the cortex. This may be one of the reasons for the very susceptibility of the basal ganglia in WD patients.

We further documented the transient increased mRNA expression of ATP7A and CTR1 after PA administration, and the immunofluorescence results demonstrated the same tendency as transcription, while the Western blot experiment further verified the transiently increased protein expression. It has been reported a decline in ATP7A expression in the cortex from the early postnatal period to adulthood in mice, and our data verified the feature that in the adult the ATP7A staining was the most intense in layer 5 pyramidal neurons of the cortex [19]. Our data showed enhanced ATP7A expression was ubiquitously observed in the brain of tx mice 3 days after PA treatment, and still the most intense in layer 5 pyramidal neurons. The experiment revealed that ATP7A primarily expressed in internal pyramidal layer neurons, and PA induced the increase of ATP7A expression generally in the brain of tx mice but not in DL mice. It is known that all the key regulators,including ATP7A and CTR1,mediating copper homeostasis in peripheral tissues are also present in the brain [9]. When copper elevated, ATP7A left the TGN and facilitated copper excretion. Copper also induced the mRNA expression and might regulate the transcription of ATP7A in a fish cell line [20]. In our study the increased ATP7A expression was in accordance with the concentrations of free copper,which suggested that the elevated expression of ATP7A may be induced by the increased copper in the brain on the early phages of PA treatment. Co-localization experiment revealed that ATP7A mainly located at Golgi apparatus during the PA treatment, while the scope of ATP7A immunostaining exceeded that of GOLPH2 staining in brain cells of tx mice on the 3rd day of the PA treatment. It indicated the alteration in subcellular localization of ATP7A during the PA

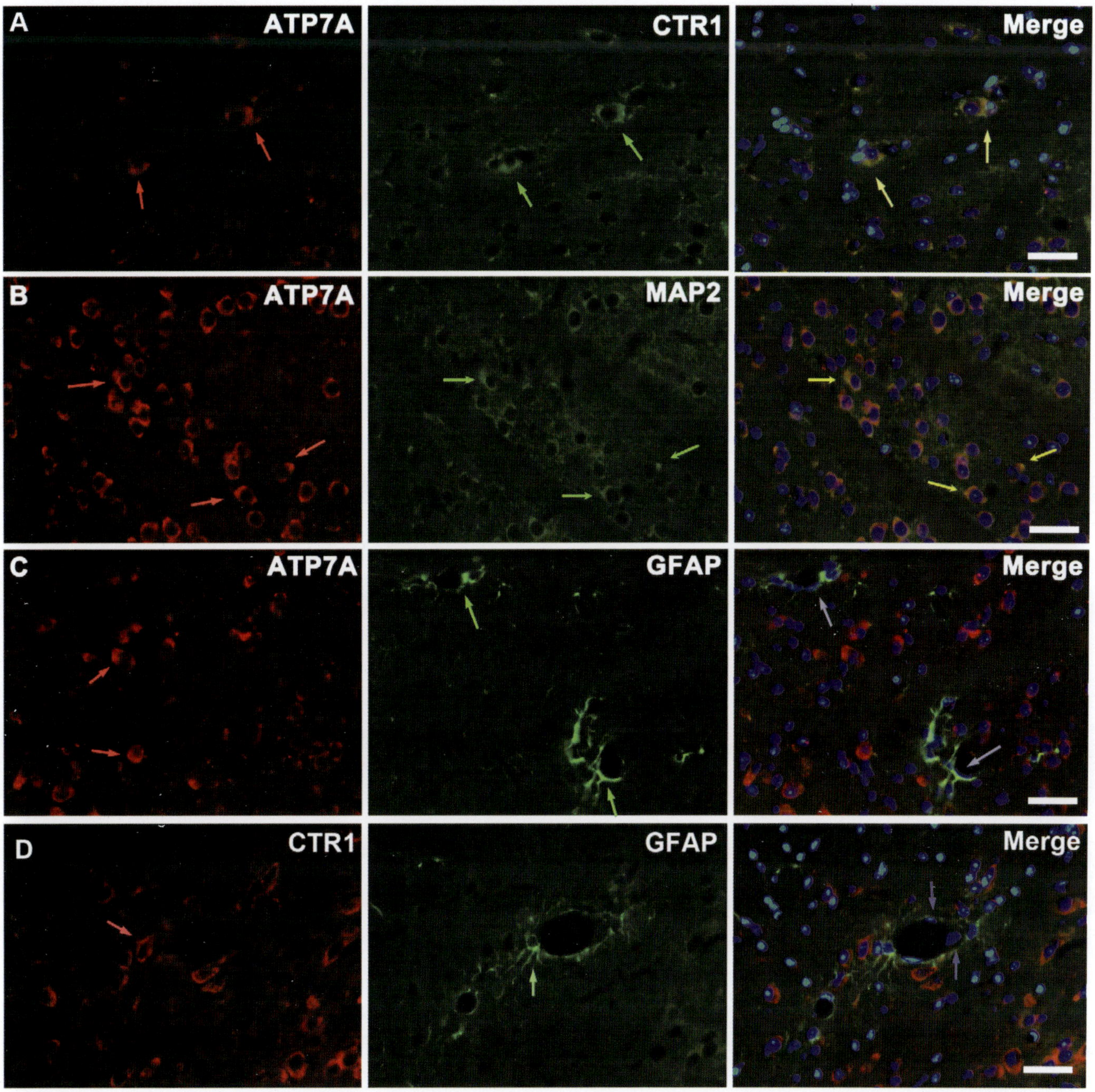

Figure 9. Immunofluorescent staining of ATP7A and CTR1 in neurons and astrocytes in the Cpu. The slices were from tx mice with 3 days PA administration. Neurons and astrocytes were labeled with MAP2 and GFAP, respectively. (A) ATP7A (red) immunoreactivity co-localization with CTR1 (green) in CPu (yellow arrows). (B)ATP7A (red) immunoreactivity co-localization with MAP2 (green) in CPu(yellow arrows). (C)ATP7A (red) immunoreactivity demonstrated little expression at BBB, which was formed by vascular endothelial cells (blue arrows) and astrocytic endfeet (green) ensheathing the endothelium. (D)CTR1 (red) immunoreactivity demonstrated little expression with vascular endothelial cells (blue arrows) and astrocytic endfeet (green). Scale bars = 30 um.

treatment,which might result from the trafficking of ATP7A from TGN to the vesicles induced by increased copper concentration.

The same tendency of the free copper concentrations in the serum and the brain tissues during PA administration brought about the question that whether the increased free copper in the brain came from the serum, or directly mobilized from the brain cells. The mechanism of copper transporting into the brain is still unclear. Previous data showed that the ATP7A and CTR1 expressed more profoundly in the brain barrier fractions (cerebral capillaries and choroid plexus) than in the brain parenchyma, and the copper transported into the brain primarily occured via the BBB as free ions [11,12]. Our data revealed most of the copper mobilized by PA in the serum was bound to proteins. If the free copper in the brain came from the serum, the copper transporters at BBB should be observed. In fact we found CTR1 and ATP7A hardly expressed in cells around BBB, which didn't support the

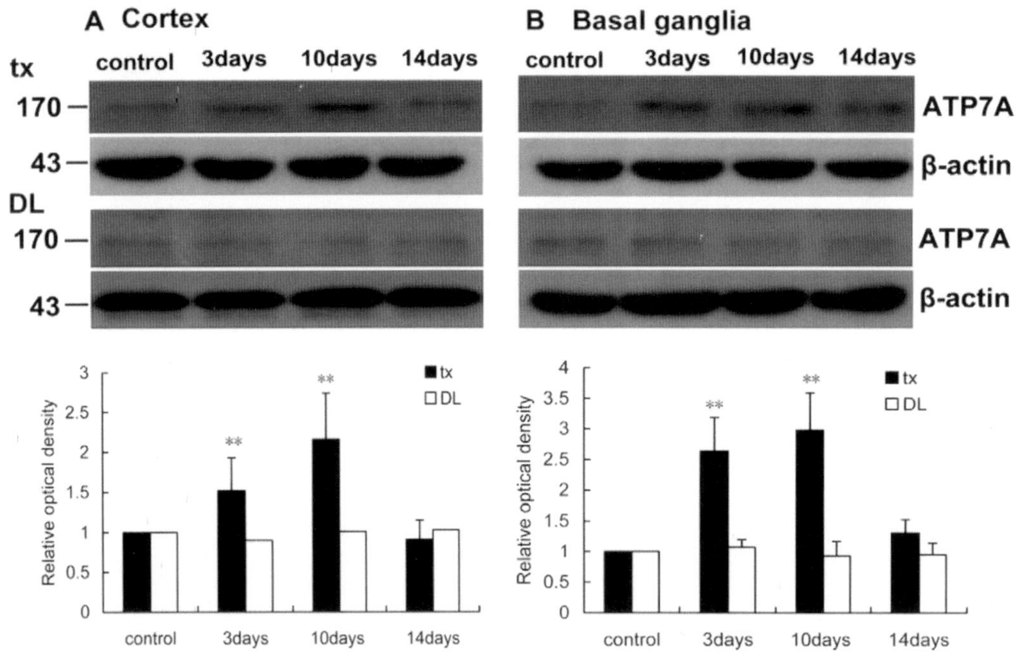

Figure 10. Western blot analysis of ATP7A in the cortex and basal ganglia of tx and DL mice. (A) ATP7A expression increased significantly ($P<0.01$) on the 3rd day and 10th day in tx mouse cortex during PA treatment, and declined closed to the level of the control on the 14th day. ATP7A expression did not change in DL mice during PA treatment. (B) ATP7A expression increased significantly ($P<0.01$) on the 3rd day and 10th day in tx mouse cortex, and declined closed to the level of the control on the 14th day, while it did not change in DL mice. Relative protein quantified as compared with tx or DL controls (normalized to 1.0). $^{**}p<0.01$ was considered significantly different from the control.

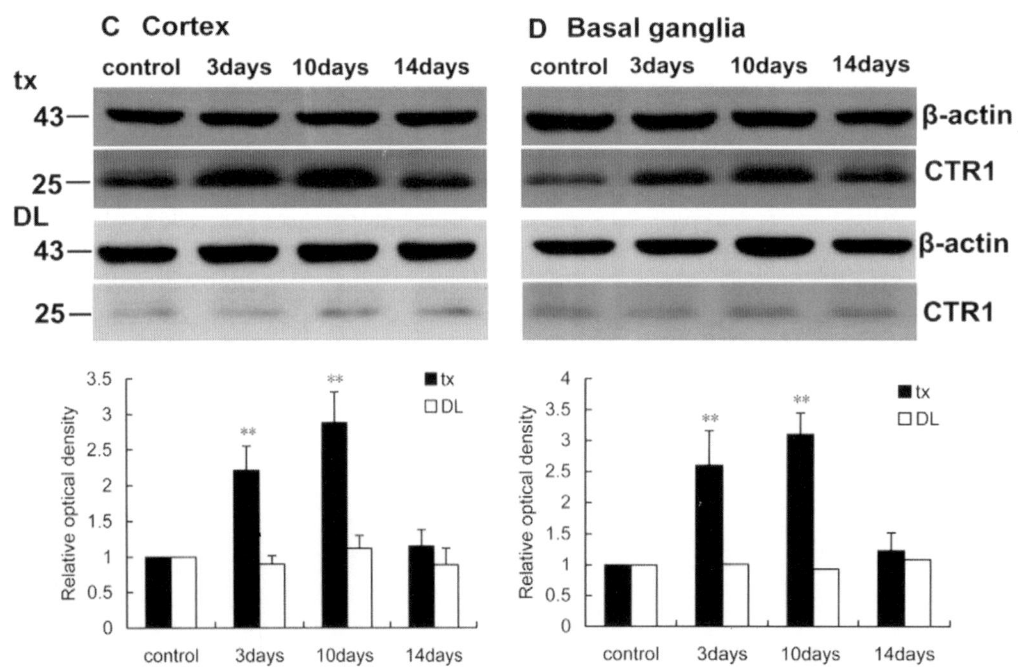

Figure 11. Western blot analysis of CTR1 in the cortex and basal ganglia of tx and DL mice. (A) CTR1 expression increased significantly ($P<0.01$) on the 3rd day and 10th day in tx mouse cortex, and declined closed to the level of the control on the 14th day. CTR1 expression did not change in DL mice during the PA treatment. (B) CTR1 expression increased significantly ($P<0.01$) on the 3rd day and 10th day in tx mouse cortex, and declined closed to the level of the control on the 14th day, while it did not change in DL mice. Relative protein quantified as compared with tx or DL controls (normalized to 1.0). $^{**}p<0.01$ was considered significantly different from the level of the control.

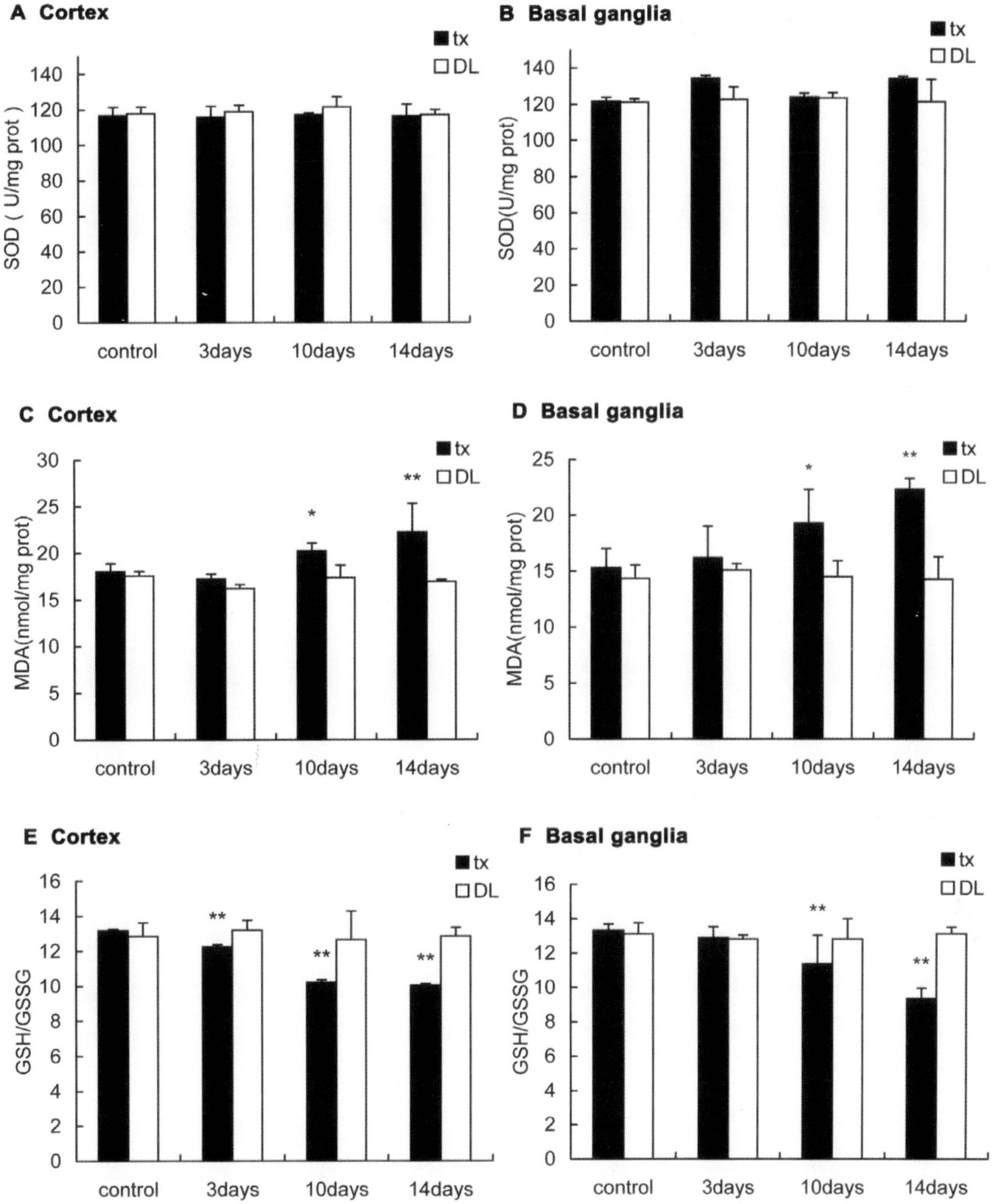

Figure 12. Oxidative-stress-related biomarkers assay in the cortex and the basal ganglia of the mice. (A)(B)SOD activity did not show change in tx or DL mice during the administration. (C)(D) MDA concentrations slightly increased during PA administration in the cortex and basal ganglia of tx mice but not in DL mice. (E)(F)GSH/GSSG ratios decreased gradually along the administration in the cortex and basal ganglia of tx mice, but not in DL mice. (* $P<0.05$; ** $P<0.01$).

hypothesis that the free copper originated from the serum. Compared with the weak signal before PA treatment, the ATP7A signal was abundant in the choroid plexus during two weeks treatment. It was likely that ATP7A played a role on regulating copper concentration in the brain and the CSF. The findings of in situ brain perfusion studies suggested copper was utilized and released into the CSF via the interstitial fluid and removed by the BCB from the CSF to blood [12]. Subsequently the increased expression of ATP7A might suggest that ATP7A exported the excess copper mobilized by PA from the brain cells, then the free copper increased in interstitial fluid which in turn led to the higher expression of ATP7A in the choroid plexus and secreted more copper into CSF.

CTR1 transcription didn't appear to change as a function of Cu status in mammal cells [21,22]. But in our work CTR1 staining and protein expression paralleled the transient increase of the mRNA expression with the increased signal in the cortex and the basal ganglia during the PA treatment, especially in layer 5 pyramidal neurons. CTR1 mostly located at the plasma membrane,where it functioned in uptake of copper. Its increased expression conflicted with the increasing of ATP7A, which played the opposite role of CTR1. This phenomenon may be explained by the following feedback mechanism. The brain cells of tx mice had been accommodated to the copper accumulation for long. However, the copper was quickly and indiscriminately chelated by PA, and the protein-bound copper, which performed the major physiologic function in the whole cells, decreased quickly during the PA treatment. Therefore, cells had to ingest the extracellular copper, reactively, to adjust the change and to meet the physiologic needs.

We suggested that the excessive oxidative stress might occur in the brain of tx mice after PA treatment. Copper induces oxidative stress by two mechanisms. First, it was suggested that reaction of Cu(I) with hydrogen peroxide and re-reduction of Cu(II) by superoxide via Fenton and Haber-Weiss chemistry yielded hydroxyl radicals [23,24,25]. Second, exposure to excessive copper significantly decreases the glutathione level which is the major water-soluble antioxidant in cells and directly reduces most of the ROS [26]. Copper-overloaded rats exhibited oxidative injuries with decreased GSH and increased MDA in the brain [27,28]. MDA also increased in the livers of rats with elevated copper [27]. In our study GSH/GSSG ratios decreased in the cortex and basal ganglia and this indicated declined reductive capacity and antioxidation during PA treatment. The increased MDA, the lipid peroxidation index, implied the increased oxidative stress and cellular damage. Though MDA and GSH/GSSG decreased, the SOD levels remained in our study. SOD protected cells from oxygen free radical by catalyzing the removal of O_2^-. Now the change of SOD activity induced by copper was not unanimous in different studies [28,29,30,31]. Different copper concentrations may result in different adjustment of the activity of SOD. Whether SOD is involved in the defence of copper-induced oxidative damaged is still controversial.

The tx mice did not demonstrate neurologic symptoms for lifetime. Nevertheless, in our study we found the evidence of increased free copper and increased oxidative biomarkers in the tx mice brain during PA administration. It suggested the neurotoxicity of PA administration in tx mice, even which didn't showed significant abnormalities of central nervous system. We presume two weeks administration may be too short to lead to prominent brain damage. Some of WD patients didn't demonstrate neurologic worsening during PA treatment, even suffered to obvious neuroligic symptoms. We suppose other factors, such as mutation styles, involved in the brain reacting to the chelator treatment.

In conclusion, the present study revealed the elevated free copper and declined protein-bound copper concentration in the cortex and basal ganglia of tx mice accompanied by general transiently increased of ATP7A and CTR1 in the brain during PA treatment. The scarce expression of ATP7A and CTR1 in the BBB and the increased ATP7A in choroid plexus suggested that the increased free copper in the brain might be mobilized from the brain parenchyma but not the serum. The declined oxidative biomarkers GSH/GSSG ratio and MDA concentrations indicated the oxidative stress raised by chelator treatment and this might be due to the increased free copper in the parenchyma. The increased free copper and oxidative stress partly explains the neurological deterioration of WD patients with PA treatment.

Materials and Methods

Ethic statement

All animal procedures were conducted in accordance with and approved by the animal ethics guidelines of the Institutional Animal Care and Use Committee of Sun Yat-sen University (ethics approval number20100603005). Strict attention was given to the care and use of animals according to Chinese Law. All efforts were made to minimize the number of animals used and their suffering.

Animals

Toxic milk mutant mice (tx mice) and control mice (DL mice) were kindly presented by professor Julian. Mercer(School of Life and Environmental Sciences,Deakin University, Australia) and arose in the Laboratory Animal Center of Sun Yat-sen University, Guangzhou, China. Mice were housed in a temperature-controlled, 12:12 light/dark room and were allowed free access to water and food. Pups of tx mice required fostering in order to survive and were routinely cross fostered within 5 days of birth to DL mice that had produced litters at the similar time. All mice used in this study were 16 weeks old (the peak time of copper deposition in tx mice).

Reagents and antibodies

The chemical was purchased from the following sources: D-Penicillamine (PA)(sigma), antibodies for immunofluorescence: goat anti-ATP7A antibody(goat anti-human), goat anti-NKCC1 antibody(Santa, USA), rabbit anti-CTR1 antibody(Novus biologicals, USA), rabbit anti-GOLPH2 antibody(Beijing Biosynthesis Biotechnology, China), mouse anti-microtubulin-associated protein 2(MAP2) antibody (Boster, China), mouse anti glial fibrillary acidic protein (GFAP) antibody (Cell signaling technology, USA). The following were used as secondary antibodies: Cy3-conjugated goat antirabbit immunoglobulin (Proteintech group, USA); Cy3-conjugated donkey antigoat immunoglobulin (Proteintech group, USA); and FITC-conjugated goat antimouse immunoglobulin (Proteintech group, USA), antibodies for Western blot: chicken anti-ATP7A antibody (Abcam,USA), rabbit anti-CTR1 antibody(Novus biologicals, USA), secondary antibodies: peroxidase anti-chicken IgG (Proteintech, USA), peroxidase-conjugated anti-rabbit IgG.

Experiment design

PA was dissolved in deionized water and given to mice (tx and DL mice) with intragastric administration at doses (200 mg/kg/d) in 2 divided dosages for 3 days, 10 days or 14 days respectively. Tx mice with PA were model intervention groups, and DL mice with PA were normal intervention groups ($n = 5$ for each time point in each index as following). Mice (tx and DL mice) given with deionized water through intragastric administration were taken as blank control groups.

Serum and tissue free and protein-bound copper concentration analysis

Animals ($n = 5$ for model intervention group and normal intervention group, $n = 3$ for both blank control groups, in each time point) euthanized by injection of chloral hydrate (350 mg/kg body). Blood samples were taken from the retrobulbar plexus. For serum preparation blood samples were centrifuged at room temperature for 10 mins. Animals were sacrificed by decapitation and cortex and basal ganglia samples were collected. Brain samples were homogenized in ten times the volumes of the buffer

(50 mM Tris buffer, PH 7.4), and centrifuged for 60 mins at 100000 g at 2°C [32]. The protein concentration of supernatant was quantitated by BCA protein assay kit (Thermo Scientific). The supernatant and serum samples were ultrafiltrated by the ultrafiltration centrifugal filter devices(Millipore, 3 kD) with low binding regenerated cellulose membrane. To retain albumin which binds much of the copper in blood except ceruloplasmin, and metallothionein which binds most of the copper in cells, we selected the type of 3 kD. The proteins larger than 3 kD molecular weight in the serum and homogenate of cortex and basal ganglia were held up by the ultrafiltration centrifugal filter devices (Millipore, 3 kD) in the concentrate. The copper being free ion and the copper binding with small molecules were in the filtrate (in this work we defined it as free copper). The filtrate and the concentrate were wet-ashed with the same volume of nitric acid. And copper concentrations were determined by air/acetylene flame atomic absorption spectrometry, using a Hitach Z5000 spectrophotometer.

Real-Time quantitative PCR

Animals were treated with PA or deionized water as described above (n = 5 for model intervention group and normal intervention group, n = 3 for both blank control groups, in each time point). Cortex and basal ganglia tissues were homogenated in Trizol reagent and total RNA was isolated. Two micrograms of RNA was used to synthesize single-strand cDNA by PrimeScript RT-PCR Kit (Takara, Japan).The resulting cDNA was used for Real-time PCR gene expression analysis of CTR1 and ATP7A. The specific primers for Atp7A(5′-AAACCTTGCGAGAAG-CAATTG, and 5′-GGGCA AAAGAGGTGTTTCCA),CTR1 (5′- TGATGATGATGCCTATGACCT, and 5′-G AAGA-TAGCCCGAGAGGGTC) and β-actin (5′-GACAGGATGGCA-GAAGGA GATTACT, and 5′-TGATCCACATCTGCTG-GAAGGT). Real time PCR was performed in triplicate on a DNA Engine Option (MJ Research) using a SYBR Green I kit (Takara, Japan).The following protocol was used for all genes: denaturation: 10 min-95°C;amplification and fluorescence acquisition (36 cycles): 15 s — 95°C, 10 s 60°C; 10 s — 72°C with a single fluorescence measurement; melting curve: from 40°C to 99°C, 0.1°C/s heating rate and continuous fluorescence measurement. Specificity of all products was verified by melting-curve analysis and by analysis on agarose gels. Abundance data for each gene is expressed as fold change. Samples were run in triplicate on each plate and the results were analyzed with the relative standard curve method. To make sure β-actin is a suitable reference gene,the expression stability was analyzed at the beginning of the experiment. A pair of specific primers for β-actin (TGCTGTC-CCTGTATGCCTCT,TCATCGTACTCC TGCTTGCT) was designed. The PCR product (676 bp) purified by E.Z.N.A®. Cycle-Pure Kit (Omega, USA) was determined by Beckman-coulter DU 800 spectrophotometer for the DNA concentration. Total DNA copies were calculated by a free software offered online by URI Genomics & Sequencing Center (http://www.uri.edu/research/gsc/resources/cndna.html), and purified PCR product was used as defined template of β-actin to perform a standard curve. The copies of β-actin in the cDNA from tissues was analyzed by absolute standard curve method.

Immunofluorescence of CTR1 and ATP7A

Animals were treated with PA or deionized water as described above (n = 5 for model intervention group and normal intervention group, n = 3 for both blank control groups, in each time point). Mice were anesthetized with chloral hydrate (350 mg/kg body) and perfused in the left ventricle with saline followed by 4% polyoxymethylene in 1×PBS, pH 7.4. The brain was extracted and post-fixed 6 h in 4% polyoxymethylene, then incubated overnight in 20% sucrose, then 30% sucrose and then embedded in Tissue-Tek Optimal Cutting Temperature compound(Sakura Fine Technical, Tokyo, Japan)at −20°C. Coronal section of 10 um were sliced and placed onto poly-L-lysine-coated slides. Slides were rehydrated in phosphate-buffered saline (PBS), and then permeabilized with 0.03% Triton X-100 in PBS for 15 min at room temperature. Slides were washed in PBS and blocked for 1 h at room temperature using 5% bovine serum albumin in PBS. Slides were then incubated overnight at 4°C with primary antibody (CTR1 at 1:100 or ATP7A at 1:300) in dilution buffer (1%BSA, in PBS). Unbound antibodies were removed by washing in PBS. After that the slides were incubated for 1 h in the dark with fluorescein isothiocyanate (FITC)-conjugated IgG, or Cyanine3 (Cy3) -conjugated donkey IgG. After a further wash in PBS, the slides were incubated with 4,6-diamidino-2-phenylindole (DAPI) at 500 ng/ml diluted in PBS for 15 minutes, and analyzed using an Olympus microscope.

Western blot analysis

Mice were sacrificed (n = 4 for model intervention group, n = 3 for normal intervention group) and tissues were prepared as previously described. Proteins (50 ug) were boiled in reducing buffer (final concentrations:16.7 mmol/L Tris-HCl, pH 6.8, 2% SDS, 0.83% b-mercaptoethanol,3.3% glycerol, and 0.016% bromophenol blue), electrophoresed in(8% for ATP7A, 10% for CTR1)SDS-PAGE gel (120 V) and transferred to Polyvinylidene fluoride membrane (Roch) using 100v for 90 min. Membranes were blocked with 5% skim milk for 1 h at room temperature, and incubated with the chicken anti-ATP7A antibody (1:1000, Abcam, USA) and the goat anti-CTR1 (1:1000, Novus biologicals, USA), respectively, in Tris-buffered saline containing 0.1% Tween-20 (TBST) at 4°C for 2 h. Membranes were then washed with TBST and incubated for 1 h at room temperature with peroxidase-conjugated anti-goat IgG or anti-chicken IgG (1:3000, Proteintech, USA) in TBST. Proteins were detected by chemiluminescence (Super ECL Plus Detection Reagent, Applygen, China). Densitometry was used to evaluate immunolabeled protein intensity. Pixel intensities were quantified using Multi Gauge software V2.2 (Fujifilm) and their levels were normalized against β-actin controls.

Oxidative-stress-related biomarkers assay

Sub-brain homogenate preparation. Animals were treated with PA or deionized water as described above (n = 5 for model intervention group and normal intervention group, n = 3 for both blank control groups, in each time point). The cortex and basal ganglia of the mice were homogenized in 0.1 mol/L PBS(PH7.3) at 4°C. The homogenate was centrifuged with 10000×g for 10 min at 4°C and the supernatant was collected for oxidative stress biochemical assay. The supernatant was subjected to the measurement of the protein contents. We used the BCA protein assay kit (Thermo Scientific) to quantify protein concentrations. Oxidative-stress-related biomarker levels were then normalized to milligram protein.

Assessment of SOD levels. The activity of superoxide dismutase (SOD) was measured by a modified nitrite method with a commercial-available kit (Nanjing Jiancheng Bioengineering Insititute, Jiangsu, China). Superoxide generated by hypoxanthine and xanthine oxidase was transformed to nitrite ion by hydroxylamine. Nitrite ion was measured by color densitometry at 550 nm using a coloring reagent. The least necessary amount of

SOD inhibited the rate of nitrite ion generation by 50% was defined as 1 U of SOD.

Assessment of MDA levels. For lipid peroxidation assay, we used a colorimetric microplate assay kit (Beyotime Institute of biotechnology, Zhejiang, China) to quantify the generation of malondialdehyde (MDA) according to the protocol. MDA was determined by measuring the red product, thiobarbituric acid(-TBA)-MDA, generated by TBA and MDA at 100°C for 15 min at 532 nm absorbance.

Assessment of GSH/GSSG ratio. The concentrations of total glutathione (T-GSH),reduced glutathione(GSH) and oxidized disulfide(GSSG) were measured by colorimetric microplate assay from the kits(Beyotime Institute of biotechnology, Zhejiang, China).The T-GSH level was determined by the method of 5,5-Dithio-bis(2-nitrobenzoic acid)(DNTB)-GSSG recycling assay. GSSG level was measured by measuring the 5-thio-2-nitrobenzoic acid (TNB) which was measured at 412 nm absorbance. The amount of reduced GSH was determined by subtracting the amount of GSSG from the total GSH. Then the GSH/GSSG ratios were calculated.

Statistics

Data presented in this work corresponded to the arithmetical mean±SEM. Statistical significance (one-way ANOVA, followed by post hoc Bonferroni) was performed using SPSS 13.0. Values were considered to differ significantly at the level of $p<0.05$.

Acknowledgments

The authors thank Ms Miao-Ying He (Laboratory Animal Center, Sun Yat-sen University, Guangzhou, China) for breeding the mice.

Author Contributions

Conceived and designed the experiments: XHL DBC. Performed the experiments: DBC LF XPL. Analyzed the data: DBC. Contributed reagents/materials/analysis tools: WZ FRL XLL. Wrote the paper: DBC LF XHL.

References

1. Roberts EA, Schilsky ML (2008) Diagnosis and treatment of Wilson disease: an update. Hepatology 47: 2089–2111.
2. Brewer GJ, Terry CA, Aisen AM, Hill GM (1987) Worsening of neurologic syndrome in patients with Wilson's disease with initial penicillamine therapy. Arch Neurol 44: 490–493.
3. Brewer GJ, Askari F, Lorincz MT, Carlson M, Schilsky M, et al. (2006) Treatment of Wilson disease with ammonium tetrathiomolybdate: IV. Comparison of tetrathiomolybdate and trientine in a double-blind study of treatment of the neurologic presentation of Wilson disease. Arch Neurol 63: 521–527.
4. Stuerenburg HJ (2000) CSF copper concentrations, blood-brain barrier function, and coeruloplasmin synthesis during the treatment of Wilson's disease. J Neural Transm 107: 321–329.
5. Reddy PV, Rao KV, Norenberg MD (2008) The mitochondrial permeability transition, and oxidative and nitrosative stress in the mechanism of copper toxicity in cultured neurons and astrocytes. Lab Invest 88: 816–830.
6. Britton RS (1996) Metal-induced hepatotoxicity. Semin Liver Dis 16: 3–12.
7. Porzio S, Iorio R, Vajro P, Pensati P, Vegnente A (1997) Penicillamine-related neurologic syndrome in a child affected by Wilson disease with hepatic presentation. Arch Neurol 54: 1166–1168.
8. Petris MJ, Smith K, Lee J, Thiele DJ (2003) Copper-stimulated endocytosis and degradation of the human copper transporter, hCtr1. J Biol Chem 278: 9639–9646.
9. Lutsenko S, Bhattacharjee A, Hubbard AL (2010) Copper handling machinery of the brain. Metallomics 2: 596–608.
10. Pase L, Voskoboinik I, Greenough M, Camakaris J (2004) Copper stimulates trafficking of a distinct pool of the Menkes copper ATPase (ATP7A) to the plasma membrane and diverts it into a rapid recycling pool. Biochem J 378: 1031–1037.
11. Choi BS, Zheng W (2009) Copper transport to the brain by the blood-brain barrier and blood-CSF barrier. Brain Res 1248: 14–21.
12. Monnot AD, Behl M, Ho S, Zheng W (2011) Regulation of brain copper homeostasis by the brain barrier systems: Effects of Fe-overload and Fe-deficiency. Toxicol Appl Pharmacol.
13. Brewer GJ (2010) Risks of copper and iron toxicity during aging in humans. Chem Res Toxicol 23: 319–326.
14. Rauch H (1983) Toxic milk, a new mutation affecting cooper metabolism in the mouse. J Hered 74: 141–144.
15. Allen KJ, Buck NE, Cheah DM, Gazeas S, Bhathal P, et al. (2006) Chronological changes in tissue copper, zinc and iron in the toxic milk mouse and effects of copper loading. Biometals 19: 555–564.
16. Bohrer D, Do Nascimento PC, Ramirez AG, Mendonca JK, De Carvalho LM, et al. (2004) Comparison of ultrafiltration and solid phase extraction for the separation of free and protein-bound serum copper for the Wilson's disease diagnosis. Clin Chim Acta 345: 113–121.
17. Brewer GJ, Askari F, Dick RB, Sitterly J, Fink JK, et al. (2009) Treatment of Wilson's disease with tetrathiomolybdate: V. Control of free copper by tetrathiomolybdate and a comparison with trientine. Transl Res 154: 70–77.
18. Tapiero H, Townsend DM, Tew KD (2003) Trace elements in human physiology and pathology. Copper. Biomed Pharmacother 57: 386–398.
19. Niciu MJ, Ma XM, El Meskini R, Ronnett GV, Mains RE, et al. (2006) Developmental changes in the expression of ATP7A during a critical period in postnatal neurodevelopment. Neuroscience 139: 947–964.
20. Minghetti M, Leaver MJ, Taggart JB, Casadei E, Auslander M, et al. (2011) Copper induces Cu-ATPase ATP7A mRNA in a fish cell line, SAF1. Comp Biochem Physiol C Toxicol Pharmacol 154: 93–99.
21. Lee J, Prohaska JR, Dagenais SL, Glover TW, Thiele DJ (2000) Isolation of a murine copper transporter gene, tissue specific expression and functional complementation of a yeast copper transport mutant. Gene 254: 87–96.
22. Tennant J, Stansfield M, Yamaji S, Srai SK, Sharp P (2002) Effects of copper on the expression of metal transporters in human intestinal Caco-2 cells. FEBS Lett 527: 239–244.
23. Halliwell B, Gutteridge JM (1984) Oxygen toxicity, oxygen radicals, transition metals and disease. Biochem J 219: 1–14.
24. Gaetke LM, Chow CK (2003) Copper toxicity, oxidative stress, and antioxidant nutrients. Toxicology 189: 147–163.
25. Jomova K, Vondrakova D, Lawson M, Valko M (2010) Metals, oxidative stress and neurodegenerative disorders. Mol Cell Biochem 345: 91–104.
26. Gaetke LM, Chow CK (2003) Copper toxicity, oxidative stress, and antioxidant nutrients. Toxicology 189: 147–163.
27. Sansinanea AS, Cerone SI, Streitenberger SA, Garcia C, Auza N (1998) [Oxidative effect of hepatic copper overload]. Acta Physiol Pharmacol Ther Latinoam 48: 25–31.
28. Ozcelik D, Uzun H (2009) Copper intoxication; antioxidant defenses and oxidative damage in rat brain. Biol Trace Elem Res 127: 45–52.
29. Zhang SS, Noordin MM, Rahman SO, Haron J (2000) Effects of copper overload on hepatic lipid peroxidation and antioxidant defense in rats. Vet Hum Toxicol 42: 261–264.
30. Ozcelik D, Ozaras R, Gurel Z, Uzun H, Aydin S (2003) Copper-mediated oxidative stress in rat liver. Biol Trace Elem Res 96: 209–215.
31. Cheng J, Ma H, Fan C, Zhang Z, Jia Z, et al. (2011) Effects of Different Copper Sources and Levels on Plasma Superoxide Dismutase, Lipid Peroxidation, and Copper Status of Lambs. Biol Trace Elem Res.
32. Sakurai H, Kamada H, Fukudome A, Kito M, Takeshima S, et al. (1992) Copper-metallothionein induction in the liver of LEC rats. Biochem Biophys Res Commun 185: 548–552.

3

Regulation of miR-146a by RelA/NFkB and p53 in STHdh^{Q111}/Hdh^{Q111} Cells, a Cell Model of Huntington's Disease

Jayeeta Ghose[1], Mithun Sinha[2], Eashita Das[1], Nihar R. Jana[3], Nitai P. Bhattacharyya[1]*

1 Crystallography and Molecular Biology Division, Saha Institute of Nuclear Physics, Kolkata, West Bengal, India, **2** Structural Genomics Division, Saha Institute of Nuclear Physics, Kolkata, West Bengal, India, **3** Division of Cellular and Molecular Neuroscience, National Brain Research Centre, Manesar, Haryana, India

Abstract

Huntington's disease (HD) is caused by the expansion of N-terminal polymorphic poly Q stretch of the protein huntingtin (HTT). Deregulated microRNAs and loss of function of transcription factors recruited to mutant HTT aggregates could cause characteristic transcriptional deregulation associated with HD. We observed earlier that expressions of miR-125b, miR-146a and miR-150 are decreased in STHdh^{Q111}/Hdh^{Q111} cells, a model for HD in comparison to those of wild type STHdh^{Q7}/Hdh^{Q7} cells. In the present manuscript, we show by luciferase reporter assays and real time PCR that decreased miR-146a expression in STHdh^{Q111}/Hdh^{Q111} cells is due to decreased expression and activity of p65 subunit of NFkB (RelA/NFkB). By reporter luciferase assay, RT-PCR and western blot analysis, we also show that both miR-150 and miR-125b target p53. This partially explains the up regulation of p53 observed in HD. Elevated p53 interacts with RelA/NFkB, reduces its expression and activity and decreases the expression of miR-146a, while knocking down p53 increases RelA/NFkB and miR-146a expressions. We also demonstrate that expression of p53 is increased and levels of RelA/NFkB, miR-146a, miR-150 and miR-125b are decreased in striatum of R6/2 mice, a mouse model of HD and in cell models of HD. In a cell model, this effect could be reversed by exogenous expression of chaperone like proteins HYPK and Hsp70. We conclude that (i) miR-125b and miR-150 target p53, which in turn regulates RelA/NFkB and miR-146a expressions; (ii) reduced miR-125b and miR-150 expressions, increased p53 level and decreased RelA/NFkB and miR-146a expressions originate from mutant HTT (iii) p53 directly or indirectly regulates the expression of miR-146a. Our observation of interplay between transcription factors and miRNAs using HD cell model provides an important platform upon which further work is to be done to establish if such regulation plays any role in HD pathogenesis.

Editor: Philipp J. Kahle, Hertie Institute for Clinical Brain Research and German Center for Neurodegenerative Diseases, Germany

Funding: This work was supported by the Institutional Grant to Saha Institute of Nuclear Physics for the Project 'Structural Proteomics and Genomics of Human Genetic Diseases' by the Department of Atomic Energy, Government of India. The funders had no role in study design, data collection and analysis, decision to publish, or preparation of the manuscript.

Competing Interests: The authors have declared that no competing interests exist.

* E-mail: nitaipada.bhattacharya@saha.ac.in

Introduction

Huntington's disease (HD) is an autosomal dominant neurodegenerative disorder caused by the expansion of polymorphic CAG repeats in exon1 of Huntingtin (*HTT*) gene. Among various molecular and cellular dysfunctions originated from mutations to *HTT* gene, which eventually lead to neuronal loss from striatal regions in HD patients, transcriptional deregulation is considered to be one of the important events [1,2]. Such deregulation of genes has been attributed, at least partially, to interactions and recruitments of several transcription factors to the mutant HTT aggregates [2,3]. Transcription factors (TFs) like TBP, CBP, p53, Sp1, NFkB and others are recruited to aggregates formed by mutant HTT, the hallmark of HD [4–9]. Functional consequence of such recruitment remains largely unknown. Recruitment of TFs to the aggregates may result in loss of functions of the TFs. This can explain the altered expressions of many genes in HD [2,3]. In the presence of mutated HTT exon1, repression of transcription from p53-responsive promoters is detected, indicating hypo function of p53 in HD [8]. However, the level of p53 is increased in various models of HD as well as in the affected tissue in HD patients possibly due to post transcriptional or post-translational modifications [4]. It has also been shown that p53 directly interacts with the promoter sequence of *HTT* gene that harbors multiple p53 response elements [10]. Increased expression of mutant HTT due to higher level of p53 in turn may increase the aggregates formed by mutant HTT. Direct evidence that p53 participates in the pathogenesis of HD is also available [11]. However, effects of recruitment and interaction of NFkB with mutant HTT in HD pathogenesis remains unclear. In a cell model of HD, it has been shown that NFkB activity is increased in the early stage when there are no visible aggregates of mutant HTT, while at a later stage when visible aggregates are formed, NFkB activity is reduced [12]. Similar decrease in NFkB activity after 72 hours of induction of mutant HTT was also observed in a cell model of HD, while in early stage of induction, NFkB activity was increased [13,14]. This dual role of mutant HTT on NFkB activity could be due to initial protective action of NFkB, which is suppressed at a later stage by the recruitment of NFkB into the aggregates. Alteration of NFkB activity may result in altered expression of NFkB regulated genes.

Micro RNA (miRNA) belongs to a class of small non-coding single stranded RNA, approximately 21 nucleotides long, and generally regulates gene expression negatively. Mature miRNA interacts mostly with 3′ untranslated regions (3′UTRs) of the genes in human and down regulates the expression of the targets either by degrading the mRNAs or by inhibiting their translation. In some cases, increased expression of target genes by miRNAs have also been reported [15]. Recent experiments show that at least in few specific cases, mature miRNA can alter the expression of genes even by binding to the coding regions as well as to the 5′ UTRs of its targets [16,17,18]. It thus provides further complex regulation of genes by miRNAs. It has been proposed on the basis of theoretical analysis that as many as 30% of genes in the human genome may be the targets of miRNAs [19]. However, latter estimates predict that as large as 90% of human genes are targets of miRNAs [20], although experimentally validated targets are limited. MiRNA genes are regulated in similar way as that of coding genes [21,22]. For example, p53 is known to increase as well as decrease the expression of several miRNAs [23–27]. Interestingly, p53 is one of the targets of miR-125b [28], which is itself negatively regulated by p53 [26]. RelA/NFkB regulates the expression of miR-146a [29]. The neuron-restrictive silencer factor (NRSF), also known as Repressor Element Silencing Transcription Factor (REST), another HTT interacting protein, regulates several miRNAs. Among them, miR-132, miR-124, miR-9 and miR-9* are down regulated in affected tissues of HD patients [30,31]. To investigate whether miRNA expressions are altered in HD, we recently identified changes in expressions of several miRNAs in STHdh^{Q111}/Hdh^{Q111} cells, a cell model of HD. We also characterized that miR-146a which is down regulated in the cell model targets TBP [32,33].

As RelA/NFkB regulates the expression of miR-146a [29], in the present manuscript, we first tested the hypothesis that down regulation of miR-146a could be due to decreased activity of NFkB in STHdh^{Q111}/Hdh^{Q111} cells. Further, we tested whether p53 is a target of miRNAs, which are down regulated in STHdh^{Q111}/Hdh^{Q111} cells [33]. We then focused on the regulation of miR-146a by both RelA/NFkB and p53. We observed that NFkB activity is compromised in STHdh^{Q111}/Hdh^{Q111} cells and exogenous expression of p65 sub-unit of NFkB i.e. RelA/NFkB increased the expression of mature miR-146a in STHdh^{Q111}/Hdh^{Q111} cells. In addition, we showed that increased level of p53 in ST$Hdh^{Q111}/$ Hdh^{Q111} cells could be due to decreased level of miR-150 and miR-125b. Besides, we also showed that exogenous p53 decreased the expression of RelA/NFkB and also reduced NFkB activity. Besides, p53 directly or indirectly regulated the expression of miR-146a. Further, results obtained with mutant HTT aggregates led us to postulate that in the presence of the aggregates there is an initial decrease in miR-125b and miR-150 expression. These down regulated miRNAs lead to increased p53 level. Elevated p53 then in turn, may decrease RelA/NFkB expression, NFkB activity and miR-146a expression.

Results

Regulation of miR-146a by RelA/NFkB in STHdh^{Q7}/Hdh^{Q7} and STHdh^{Q111}/Hdh^{Q111} cells

We have shown earlier that expressions of several miRNAs are altered in STHdh^{Q111}/Hdh^{Q111} cells in comparison with ST$Hdh^{Q7}/$ Hdh^{Q7} cells. Among the altered miRNAs, miR-146a is down regulated [33]. It is known that RelA/NFkB regulates the expression of miR-146a [29]. To investigate the possible role of RelA/NFkB in the observed down regulation of miR-146a in STHdh^{Q111}/Hdh^{Q111} cells, we first determined the steady state level (expression) of p65 sub-unit of NFkB i.e. RelA/NFkB in these cells. Western blot analysis revealed that the expression of RelA/NFkB (denoted by p65 in **Figure 1A**) was indeed decreased significantly ($n = 3$, $p = 0.018$) in STHdh^{Q111}/Hdh^{Q111} cells in comparison with that in STHdh^{Q7}/Hdh^{Q7} cells (**Figures 1A and 1B**). Using luciferase reporter assay with multiple NFkB responsive elements (denoted as NFkB-RE), we further observed that NFkB activity was also significantly ($n = 4$, $p = 0.0082$) compromised in STHdh^{Q111}/Hdh^{Q111} cells (**Figure 1C**). This was further confirmed by using gastrin promoter tagged reporter luciferase activity assay. It is known that RelA/NFkB regulates gastrin gene expression [34]. This result shown in **Figure 1D** confirms that NFkB activity is compromised in STHdh^{Q111}/Hdh^{Q111} cells ($n = 2$, $p = 0.034$).

Given that RelA/NFkB regulates miR-146a expression [29] and above observations that both RelA/NFkB steady state level and activity are compromised in STHdh^{Q111}/Hdh^{Q111} cells, we tested whether exogenous expression of p65 sub-unit of NFkB (RelA/NFkB) could rescue the expression of miR-146a in these cells. Transfection of RelA/NFkB (denoted by p65 in **Figure 2A**) in STHdh^{Q7}/Hdh^{Q7} and STHdh^{Q111}/Hdh^{Q111} cells increased the expression of the gene as determined by western blot analysis. In such condition, NFkB activity as revealed by reporter luciferase assay, was also increased significantly ($n = 4$, $p = 0.022$) as shown in **Figure 2B**. Mature miR-146a expression was increased in such condition in both STHdh^{Q7}/Hdh^{Q7} cells ($n = 3$, $p = 0.036$) and STHdh^{Q111}/Hdh^{Q111} cells ($n = 3$, $p = 0.045$) as shown in **Figure 2C**. Even though miR-146a expression increased in ST$Hdh^{Q111}/$ Hdh^{Q111} cells exogenously expressing RelA/NFkB in comparison to STHdh^{Q111}/Hdh^{Q111} cells with endogenous RelA/NFkB, it did not rescue up to the level observed in STHdh^{Q7}/Hdh^{Q7} cells. It is known that aspirin decreases NFkB activity [35]. We thus tested whether decreasing NFkB activity by aspirin could alter miR-146a expression. STHdh^{Q7}/Hdh^{Q7} cells treated with 2.0 mM aspirin for 24 hours decreased the basal NFkB activity significantly ($n = 2$, $p = 0.014$) (**Figure 2B**). In such condition, expression of miR-146a was significantly ($n = 2$, $p = 0.031$) reduced (**Figure 2D**). Taken together, we show that increasing the expression of RelA/NFkB in STHdh^{Q111}/Hdh^{Q111} cells increased miR-146a expression and reducing the expression of RelA/NFkB decreased miR-146a expression in STHdh^{Q7}/Hdh^{Q7} cells establishing that decreased RelA/NFkB expression could result in the decreased expression of miR-146a.

Over expression of p53 in STHdh^{Q111}/Hdh^{Q111} cells: role of miR-125b and miR-150

Expression of p53 is increased in STHdh^{Q111}/Hdh^{Q111} cells [32] as well as in various models of HD and post mortem HD brains. The exact mechanism for the increase of p53 protein in HD remains unknown. It has been shown by us that miR-125b is down regulated in STHdh^{Q111}/Hdh^{Q111} cells compared to the wild type cells [33]. Given that p53 is a validated target of miR-125b [28], we explored whether increased expression level of endogenous p53 in STHdh^{Q111}/Hdh^{Q111} cells could be due to decrease in the expression of miR-125b or any other miRNA down regulated in these cells [33]. We confirmed that the endogenous expression of p53 is increased in STHdh^{Q111}/Hdh^{Q111} cells (**Figures 3A and 3B**) compared to the wild type STHdh^{Q7}/Hdh^{Q7} cells. Luciferase activity of the reporter vector pmiR-Report with 150 bp (position 733–739) of the 3′-UTR of human p53 (p53-UTR1) containing miR-125b recognition site [28] was also significantly ($n = 3$, $p = 0.026$) increased in STHdh^{Q111}/Hdh^{Q111} cells compared to that observed in STHdh^{Q7}/Hdh^{Q7} cells (**Figure 3C**) indicating that down regulated miR-125b could target p53 and increase its

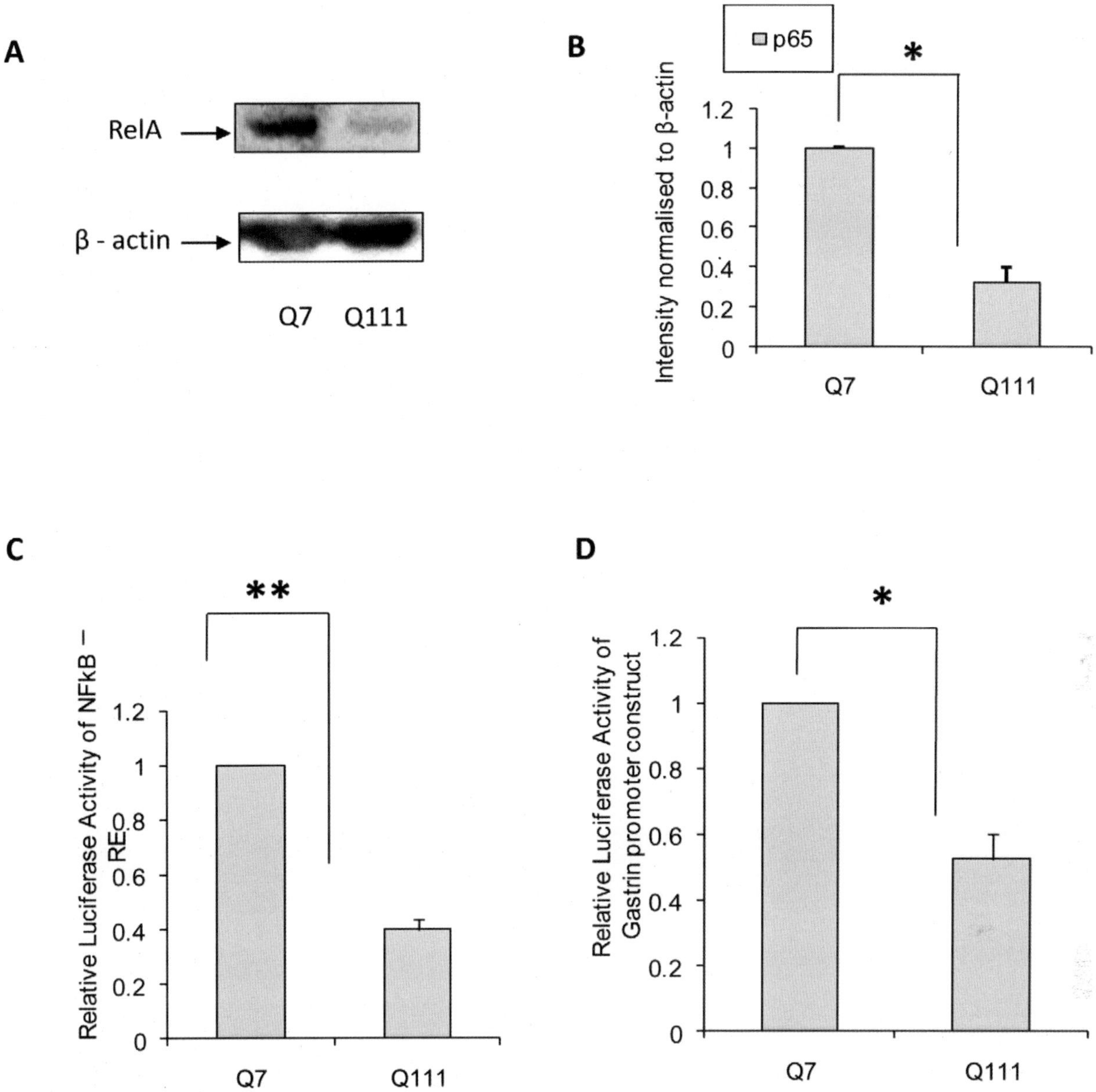

Figure 1. RelA/NFkB expression and activity in ST*Hdh*^{Q111}/*Hdh*^{Q111} and ST*Hdh*^{Q7}/*Hdh*^{Q7} cells. (**A**) Representative Western Blot showing decreased level of RelA/NFkB (denoted by p65 in the figure) in ST*Hdh*^{Q111}/*Hdh*^{Q111} cells compared to ST*Hdh*^{Q7}/*Hdh*^{Q7} cells; (**B**) Average integrated optical density (IOD) of p65 protein bands (RelA/NFkB) in *A*, normalized to β-actin level (n = 3, p = 0.018) in these cells; (**C**) Average luciferase activity using reporter luciferase with multiple NFkB response elements (denoted by NFkB-RE) in ST*Hdh*^{Q111}/*Hdh*^{Q111} cells compared to ST*Hdh*^{Q7}/*Hdh*^{Q7} cells. Normalization of protein level between ST*Hdh*^{Q7}/*Hdh*^{Q7} cells and ST*Hdh*^{Q111}/*Hdh*^{Q111} cells was done by taking the ratio of Relative Luciferase Units (RLU) of NFkB-RE and empty vector pGL3 in these cells. The normalized value obtained with ST*Hdh*^{Q7}/*Hdh*^{Q7} cells was taken as 1. Relative luciferase activity of NFkB-RE was found significantly lower (n = 4, p = 0.0082) in ST*Hdh*^{Q111}/*Hdh*^{Q111} cells compared to ST*Hdh*^{Q7}/*Hdh*^{Q7} cells; (**D**) Average reporter luciferase activity with Gastrin promoter (n = 2, p = 0.034) in ST*Hdh*^{Q7}/*Hdh*^{Q7} cells and ST*Hdh*^{Q111}/*Hdh*^{Q111} cells. Normalization of protein level between the cells was done by taking the ratio of Relative Luciferase Units (RLU) of Gastrin promoter construct and empty vector pGL3 in these cells. The normalized value obtained with ST*Hdh*^{Q7}/*Hdh*^{Q7} cells was taken as 1; Error bars represent standard deviation s of more than 2 experiments and each experiment was done in duplicate. "*" represents statistical significance; * $p \le 0.05$; ** $p < 0.01$.

expression. Further, over expression of pre-miR-125b that increased the expression of mature miR-125b significantly (data not shown) decreased reporter luciferase activity significantly in ST*Hdh*^{Q7}/*Hdh*^{Q7} cells (n = 3, p = 0.024) and ST*Hdh*^{Q111}/*Hdh*^{Q111} cells (n = 3, p = 0.0086) when co-expressed with p53-UTR1 (**Figure 3D**). In addition, exogenous expression of miR-125b decreased the endogenous expression of p53 (n = 3, p = 0.039), shown in **Figure 3E**. Taken together, these results confirmed the earlier observation that p53 is one of the targets of miR-125b [28]. Thus, the increased expression level of endogenous p53 in ST*Hdh*^{Q111}/*Hdh*^{Q111} cells could be due to decreased expression of endogenous miR-125b.

We searched mirbase [36] (http://www.mirbase.org/) and observed that human p53 could also be targeted by miR-150, which is decreased in ST*Hdh*^{Q111}/*Hdh*^{Q111} cells [33]. We cloned 136 bp (position 234–256) of the 3′-UTR of p53 (p53-UTR2)

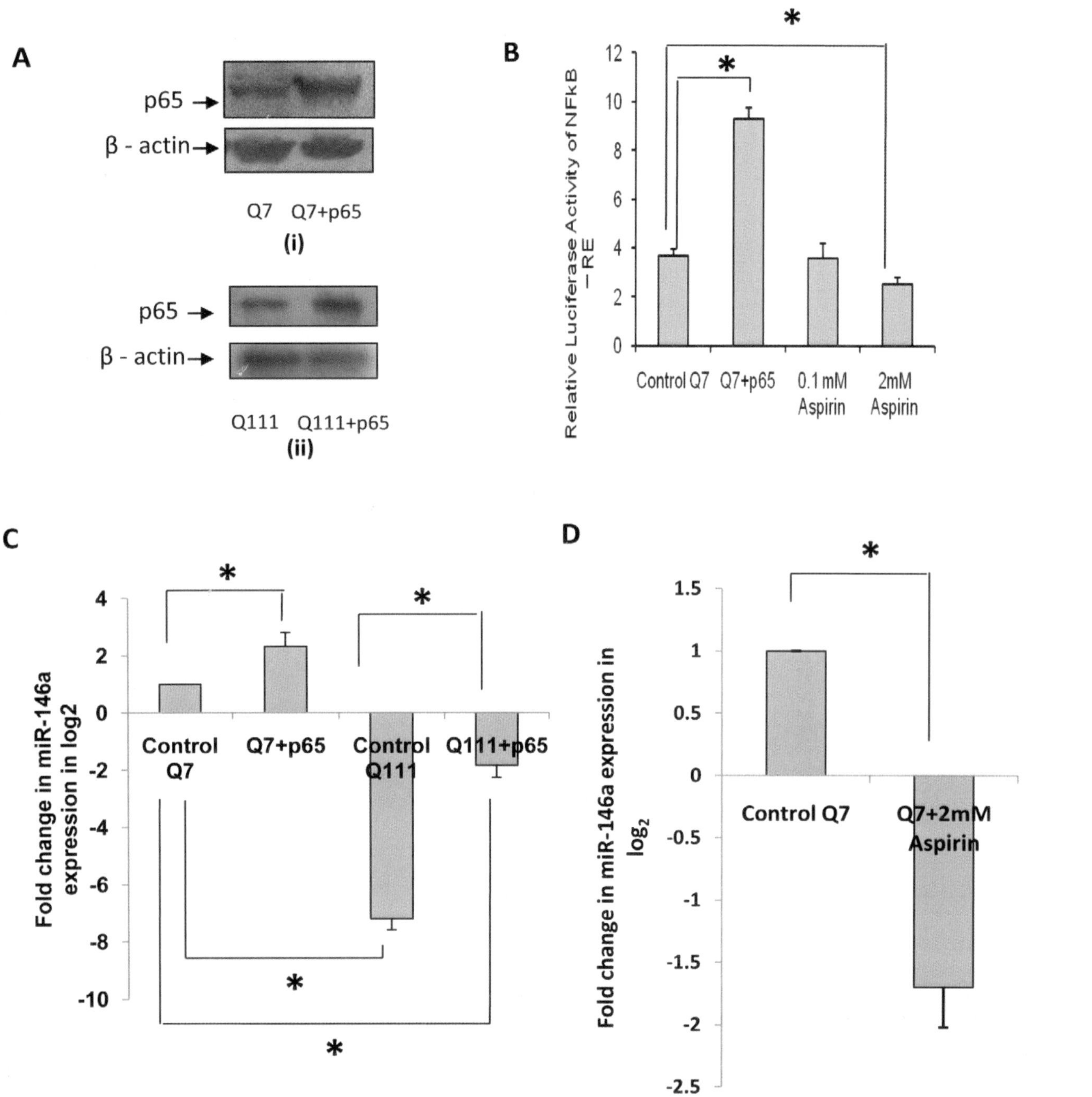

Figure 2. Regulation of miR-146a by RelA/NFkB in ST*Hdh*^{Q7}/*Hdh*^{Q7} and ST*Hdh*^{Q111}/*Hdh*^{Q111} cells. (**A**) Western Blot showing increased p65 protein (RelA/NFkB) level in (i) ST*Hdh*^{Q7}/*Hdh*^{Q7} cells expressing exogenous p65 subunit of NFkB (RelA/NFkB) compared to control ST*Hdh*^{Q7}/*Hdh*^{Q7} cells and in (ii) ST*Hdh*^{Q111}/*Hdh*^{Q111} cells expressing exogenous p65 subunit of NFkB (RelA/NFkB) compared to the control ST*Hdh*^{Q111}/*Hdh*^{Q111} cells; (**B**) Average luciferase activity of NFkB response element (NFkB-RE) in ST*Hdh*^{Q7}/*Hdh*^{Q7} cells and ST*Hdh*^{Q7}/*Hdh*^{Q7} cells expressing exogenous p65 subunit of NFkB (RelA/NFkB). Exogenous expression of p65 sub-unit of NFkB (RelA/NFkB) increased the luciferase activity significantly (n = 4, p = 0.022). Bars 3 and 4, from the left, represent changes in luciferase activity of NFkB-RE on treatment with 0.1 mM and 2 mM aspirin for 24 hours in ST*Hdh*^{Q7}/*Hdh*^{Q7} cells. Treatment with 2.0 mM aspirin reduced the luciferase activiy (n = 2, p = 0.014); (**C**) Fold increase in the expression of mature miR-146a detected by real time PCR using stem loop specific primers in p65 subunit of NFkB (RelA/NFkB) transfected ST*Hdh*^{Q7}/*Hdh*^{Q7} cells (n = 3, p = 0.036) and ST*Hdh*^{Q111}/*Hdh*^{Q111} cells (n = 3, p = 0.045). Expression of miR-17-5p was used as endogenous control. Expression of miR-146a was significantly higher in cells expressing p65 subunit of NFkB (RelA/NFkB); (**D**) Treatment with 2.0 mM aspirin decreased the expression of mature miR-146a in ST*Hdh*^{Q7}/*Hdh*^{Q7} cells (n = 2, p = 0.031). Error bars represent standard deviation s of more than 2 experiments and each experiment was done in duplicate. "*" represents statistical significance; * $p \leq 0.05$; ** $p < 0.01$.

containing the predicted recognition site of miR-150 in luciferase reporter vector as described above. We observed that the luciferase activity of the reporter with p53 3′-UTR containing the recognition site of miR-150, shown in **Figure S1 (A)**, was increased significantly (n = 3, p = 0.031) in ST*Hdh*^{Q111}/*Hdh*^{Q111} cells compared to that in ST*Hdh*^{Q7}/*Hdh*^{Q7}

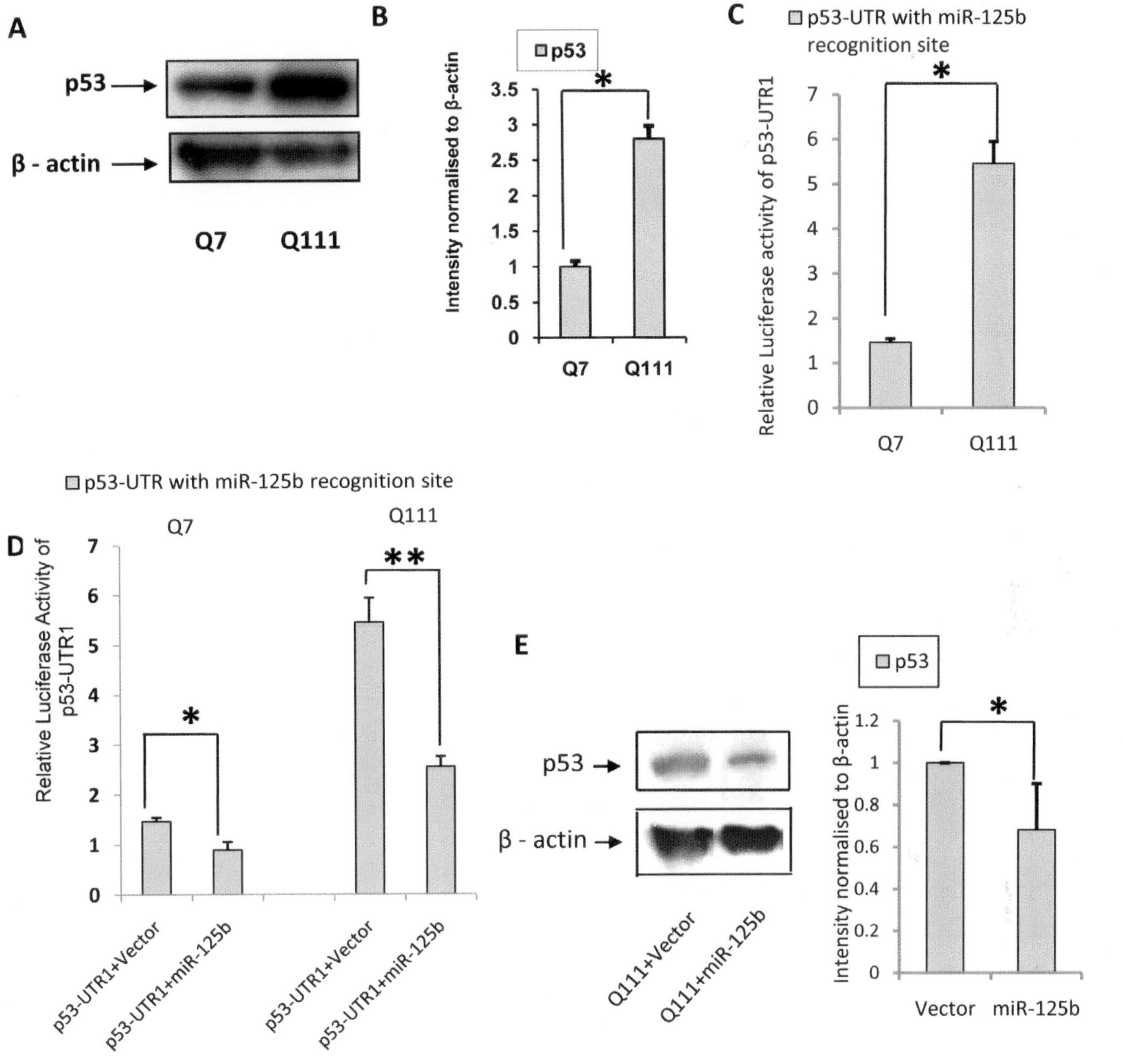

Figure 3. Endogenous expression of p53 in ST*Hdh*^{Q7}/*Hdh*^{Q7} and ST*Hdh*^{Q111}/*Hdh*^{Q111} cells: decreased miR-125b target p53. (A) Representative Western Blot showing increased p53 protein level in ST*Hdh*^{Q111}/*Hdh*^{Q111} cells compared to ST*Hdh*^{Q7}/*Hdh*^{Q7} cells; **(B)** Average integrated optical density (IOD) of p53 protein bands in *A*, normalized to β-actin level (n = 3, p = 0.024) in these cell lines. **(C)** Relative luciferase activity of cloned p53-3′UTR with miR-125b binding site (denoted by p53-UTR1) in ST*Hdh*^{Q111}/*Hdh*^{Q111} cells compared to ST*Hdh*^{Q7}/*Hdh*^{Q7} cells. Normalization of protein level between ST*Hdh*^{Q111}/*Hdh*^{Q111} cells and ST*Hdh*^{Q7}/*Hdh*^{Q7} cells was done by taking the ratio of RLU of cloned construct i.e. p53-UTR1 and empty vector pmiR. Relative luciferase activity of p53-UTR1 was found significantly higher (n = 3, p = 0.026) in ST*Hdh*^{Q111}/*Hdh*^{Q111} cells compared to ST*Hdh*^{Q7}/*Hdh*^{Q7} cells; **(D)** Reduced luciferase activity of p53-UTR1 co-transfected with pre-miR-125b in ST*Hdh*^{Q7}/*Hdh*^{Q7} cells (n = 3, p = 0.024) and ST*Hdh*^{Q111}/*Hdh*^{Q111} cells (n = 3, p = 0.0086) compared to those obtained in respective empty vector U61 tansfected cells; **(E)** Representative Western Blot showing reduction in p53 protein level in ST*Hdh*^{Q111}/*Hdh*^{Q111} cells 72 hours following transfection with pre-miR-125b compared to ST*Hdh*^{Q111}/*Hdh*^{Q111} cells transfected with empty vector U61, average IOD compared to β-actin (n = 3, p = 0.039) is shown in the adjacent bar diagram.

cells (**Figure 4A**). This result indicated that miR-150 could also target p53. We next cloned pre-miR-150 in pRNA-U61 vector. ST*Hdh*^{Q111}/*Hdh*^{Q111} cells transfected with this construct showed an increase in mature miR-150 levels as detected by Real Time PCR with stem loop specific primers. The result shown in **Figure 4B** was statistically significant (n = 3, p = 0.0056). Exogenous expression of cloned pre-miR-150 construct decreased the reporter luciferase activity of p53-UTR2 in both ST*Hdh*^{Q7}/*Hdh*^{Q7} (n = 3, p = 0.021) and ST*Hdh*^{Q111}/*Hdh*^{Q111} cells (n = 3, p = 0.040) as shown in **Figure 4C**. Moreover, over expression of pre-miR-150 decreased the endogenous expression of p53 in ST*Hdh*^{Q111}/*Hdh*^{Q111} cells (n = 3, p = 0.043) as shown by Western blot analysis (**Figure 4D**). These results indicate that p53 could be targeted by miR-150 as well.

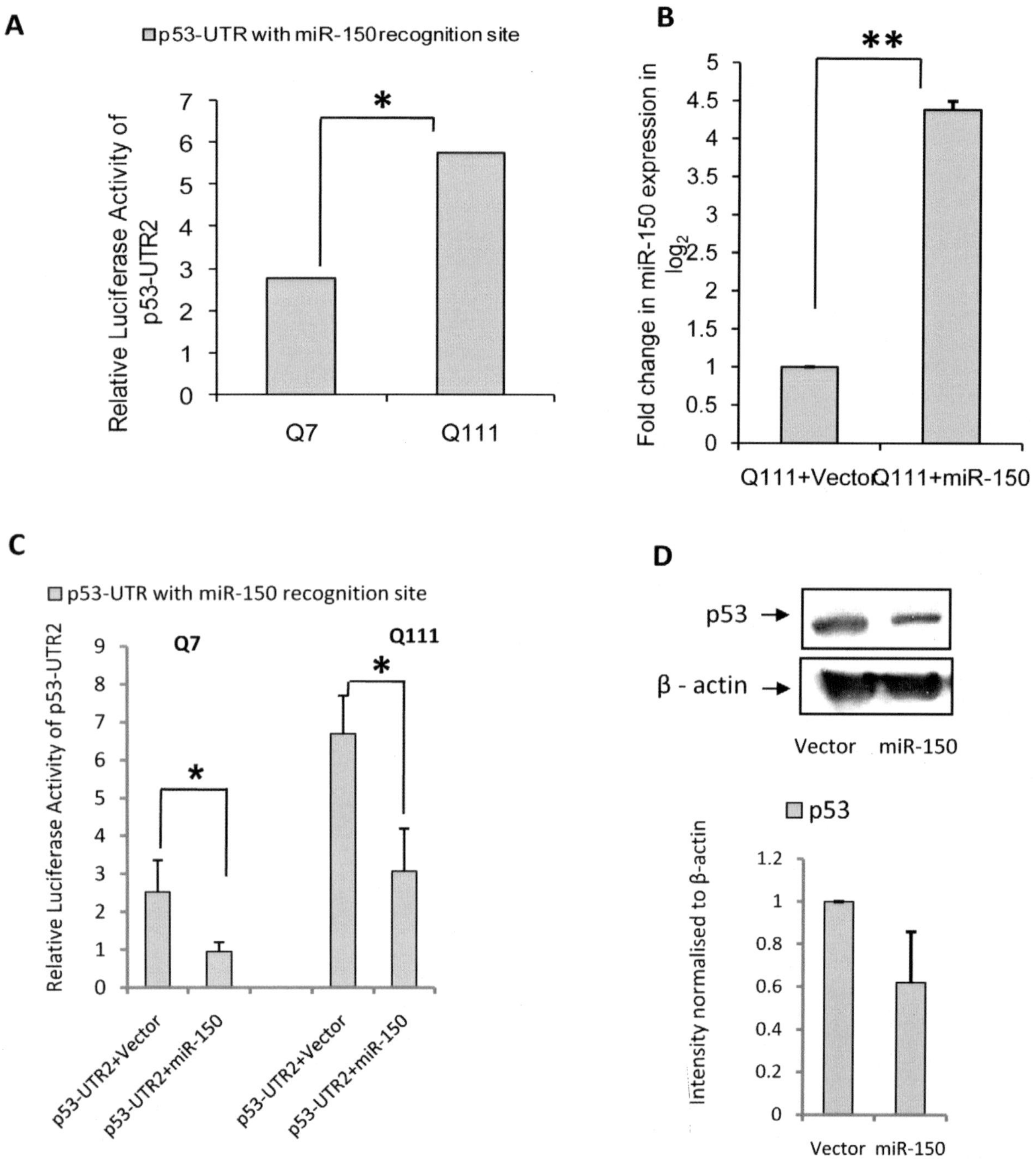

Figure 4. Reduced miR-150 also targets p53 in ST*Hdh*^{Q7}/*Hdh*^{Q7} and ST*Hdh*^{Q111}/*Hdh*^{Q111} cells. (**A**) Relative luciferase activity of cloned p53-3′UTR with miR-150 binding site (denoted by p53-UTR2) in ST*Hdh*^{Q111}/*Hdh*^{Q111} cells compared to ST*Hdh*^{Q7}/*Hdh*^{Q7} cells. Normalization of protein levels between the cells was done as described earlier. Relative luciferase activity of p53-UTR2 was found significantly higher (n = 3, p = 0.031) in ST*Hdh*^{Q111}/*Hdh*^{Q111} cells compared to ST*Hdh*^{Q7}/*Hdh*^{Q7} cells; (**B**) Fold increase (n = 3, p = 0.0056) in mature miR-150 expression detected by real time PCR using stem loop specific primers in ST*Hdh*^{Q111}/*Hdh*^{Q111} cells transfected with cloned pre-miR-150 compared to ST*Hdh*^{Q111}/*Hdh*^{Q111} cells transfected with empty vector U61, at 24 hours post transfection. Expression of miR-17-5p was used as endogenous control; (**C**) Reduced luciferase activity of p53-UTR2 co-transfected with pre-miR-150 in ST*Hdh*^{Q7}/*Hdh*^{Q7} cells (n = 3, p = 0.021) and ST*Hdh*^{Q111}/*Hdh*^{Q111} cells (n = 3, p = 0.04) compared to those obtained in respective empty vector U61 transfected cells; (**D**) Typical Western Blot showing reduction in p53 protein level in ST*Hdh*^{Q111}/*Hdh*^{Q111} cells 72 hours following transfection with pre-miR-150 compared to ST*Hdh*^{Q111}/*Hdh*^{Q111} cells transfected with empty vector U61. Average IOD compared to β-actin (n = 3, p = 0.043) is shown in the adjacent bar diagram.

As a negative control, we tested 213 bp (position 145–359 of the 3′ UTR) of p50 sub-unit of NFkB (also known as NFkB1) containing no predicted recognition sites for either miR-125b or miR-150 and did not observe any change in the luciferase activity significantly when the construct (p50-UTR) was co-transfected with cloned pre-miR-125b or pre-miR-150 in ST*Hdh*^{Q7}/*Hdh*^{Q7} cells (**Figure 5A**). This result showed that the decrease in the luciferase activity by exogenous expression of miR-150 was specific. Although endogenous p53 level was decreased by over expressing miR-125b or miR-150, there was no change in p53 level either in the presence of exogenous miR-19a or miR-146a (**Figure 5B and 5C**). Neither of these miRNAs has any predicted recognition site in the cloned 3′UTRs of p53 as revealed from miRbase. Taken together, these results show that p53 is specifically targeted by miR-125b and miR-150. Since the expressions of miR-125b and miR-150 were decreased in STHdh^{Q111}/Hdh^{Q111} cells compared to those obtained in STHdh^{Q7}/Hdh^{Q7} cells, we expressed these miRNAs in STHdh^{Q111}/Hdh^{Q111} cells and detected the endogenous expression of p53 as shown in **Figure 5D**. It is evident that exogenous expressions of both the miRNAs resulted in decreased expression of p53 in STHdh^{Q111}/Hdh^{Q111} cells. However, the level of expression did not reach exactly up to that of in STHdh^{Q7}/Hdh^{Q7} cells. Thus, decreased expressions of miR-125b and miR-150 in STHdh^{Q111}/Hdh^{Q111} cells could result in increased expression of p53.

Role of p53 in the expression of miR-146a in STHdh^{Q7}/Hdh^{Q7} and STHdh^{Q111}/Hdh^{Q111} cells

There are conflicting results regarding the functional interactions between RelA/NFkB and p53. Several reports show that p53 inhibits the transcriptional activity of RelA/NFkB [37–40] either by binding to the promoter sequences or by altering the interaction of NFkB with p53 and CBP. A different pathway has been identified where p53 enhances RelA/NFkB activity [41,42]. These observations prompted us to find whether increased expression of p53 in STHdh^{Q111}/Hdh^{Q111} cells had any influence on the down regulation of miR-146a. We exogenously expressed p53 in STHdh^{Q7}/Hdh^{Q7} cells and knocked down p53 in STHdh^{Q111}/Hdh^{Q111} cells and also in STHdh^{Q7}/Hdh^{Q7} cells using validated siRNA commercially available from Imgenex Corporation. Exogenous expression of p53 in STHdh^{Q7}/Hdh^{Q7} cells was confirmed by RT-PCR **Figure 6A (i)** as well as by western blot analysis **Figure 6A (ii)** while down regulation of the protein by siRNA in STHdh^{Q7}/Hdh^{Q7} cells was confirmed by western blot analysis as shown in **Figure 6B**. Detection of the expression of mature miR-146a in these cells revealed that in the presence of exogenous p53, miR-146a was down regulated significantly ($n = 3$, $p = 0.032$) while as expected, knocking down p53 up regulated the expression of the miRNA ($n = 3$, $p = 0.029$) as shown in **Figure 6C**.

To confirm further, we treated STHdh^{Q7}/Hdh^{Q7} cells with 5-Flurouracil (5-FU, 10 μg/ml for 12 h and 18 h), which is known to stabilize p53 protein [43]. In such condition, steady state level of p53 was increased (**Figure 7A**) and the expression of miR-146a was decreased significantly for both the time points as shown in **Figure 7B**. As we have shown above that miR-150 might target p53, we also expressed miR-150 in STHdh^{Q111}/Hdh^{Q111} cells and as expected, significant increase ($n = 3$, $p = 0.039$) in the expression of miR-146a was observed (**Figure 7C**), possibly due to down regulation of p53 by miR-150. Similar increase in miR-146a expression was observed when STHdh^{Q7}/Hdh^{Q7} cells were transfected with miR-150. However, when p53 was co-transfected with miR-150, no increase in the expression of miR-146a was observed. This result shows that decrease in p53 expression by miR-150 could be compensated here by the exogenous expression of p53 which does not have the 3′-UTR region bearing the target site of miR-150. Indeed miR-146a was down regulated when p53 was co-transfected with miR-150. However, the extent of decrease was less compared to when STHdh^{Q7}/Hdh^{Q7} cells were transfected with p53 alone as shown in **Figure 7D**. These results showed that in our experimental conditions, p53 directly or indirectly regulates the expression of miR-146a.

Regulation of p65 subunit of NFkB (RelA/NFkB) expression and activity by exogenous p53

It has been mentioned in the preceding section that there are conflicting results regarding the functional interactions between RelA/NFkB and p53. This conflicting result could arise from the dependence of cellular needs in different conditions of growth as well as for different types of cells. Depending on cellular needs, p53 may modulate NFkB activity differently. We tested whether p53 directly or indirectly regulates NFkB (RelA/NFkB) expression and activity. Exogenous expression of p53 significantly ($n = 3$, $p = 0.041$) reduced the steady state level of RelA/NFkB) in STHdh^{Q7}/Hdh^{Q7} cells (**Figure 8A**). Exogenous expression of p53 in STHdh^{Q7}/Hdh^{Q7} cells significantly decreased ($n = 3$, $p = 0.021$) the activity of NFkB whereas knocking down p53 by siRNA led to an increase in NFkB activity ($n = 3$, $p = 0.032$) in STHdh^{Q7}/Hdh^{Q7} cells. Reduction of p53 expression in STHdh^{Q111}/Hdh^{Q111} cells by expressing miR-150 that targets p53, significantly increased NFkB activity ($n = 4$, $p = 0.0482$) as detected by luciferase reporter assay (**Figure 8B**). Similar results were also obtained in HeLa cells expressing exogenous p53 and by knocking down p53 by siRNA (data not shown). Thus, in the presence of excess p53, RelA/NFkB expression and activity are reduced. This result showed that increased p53 in STHdh^{Q111}/Hdh^{Q111} cells might reduce NFkB activity. Besides, there are evidence of physical interaction between (RelA/NFkB) and p53 [37]. By co-immuno precipitation analysis, we confirmed such interaction in both STHdh^{Q7}/Hdh^{Q7} and STHdh^{Q111}/Hdh^{Q111} cells (**Figure 8C**). However, it remains unknown how p53 negatively regulates RelA/NFkB expression.

Poly Q aggregates cause alterations in the expressions of protein coding genes and miRNAs and removal of aggregates by chaperones rescue such changes

Formation of mutant HTT aggregates is the hallmark of HD and has been shown in several studies using cell [44] and animal models of HD as well as in the post mortem brains of HD patients. Recently, we have shown that HYPK, an interacting partner of HTT, possesses chaperone like activity and reduces mutant HTT aggregates and toxicity [45]. Besides, other chaperones including Hsp70 reduce mutant HTT aggregates [46]. Expression of DsRed tagged N-terminal HTT with 83Q coded by exon1 of *HTT* gene in STHdh^{Q7}/Hdh^{Q7} cells increased mutant HTT aggregates and in the presence of exogenous HYPK such aggregates are reduced (data not shown), similar to that which has been published earlier by us in other neuronal cells [44]. Expression of p53 was increased and RelA/NFkB expression was decreased (**Figure 9A**) in the presence of aggregates as revealed by RT-PCR. In such conditions, NFkB activity as determined by reporter luciferase assay was significantly ($n = 6$, $p = 0.0334$) decreased (**Figure 9B**). Expression of miR-146a was also significantly ($n = 4$, $p = 0.011$) decreased along with the expression of miR-125b and miR-150 as shown in **Figure 9C**, similar to that which has been shown in STHdh^{Q111}/Hdh^{Q111} cells [33]. HYPK-GFP and Hsp70-GFP were transfected into the cells which increased the level of HYPK and Hsp70 respectively as shown by Western blot analysis in **Figure 9D**.

Interestingly, when 83Q was co-transfected with HYPK-GFP or Hsp70-GFP in STHdh^{Q7}/Hdh^{Q7} cells, p53 expression was decreased and RelA/NFkB expression was recovered in comparison to that obtained in STHdh^{Q7}/Hdh^{Q7} cells expressing only mutant HTT exon1 (**Figure 10A and 10B**). NFkB activity was also significantly increased in such conditions in presence of HYPK-GFP ($n = 6$, $p = 0.031$) and Hsp70-GFP ($n = 6$, $p = 0.029$) in 83Q-DsRed transfected STHdh^{Q7}/Hdh^{Q7} cells (**Figure 10C**). Moreover, remov-

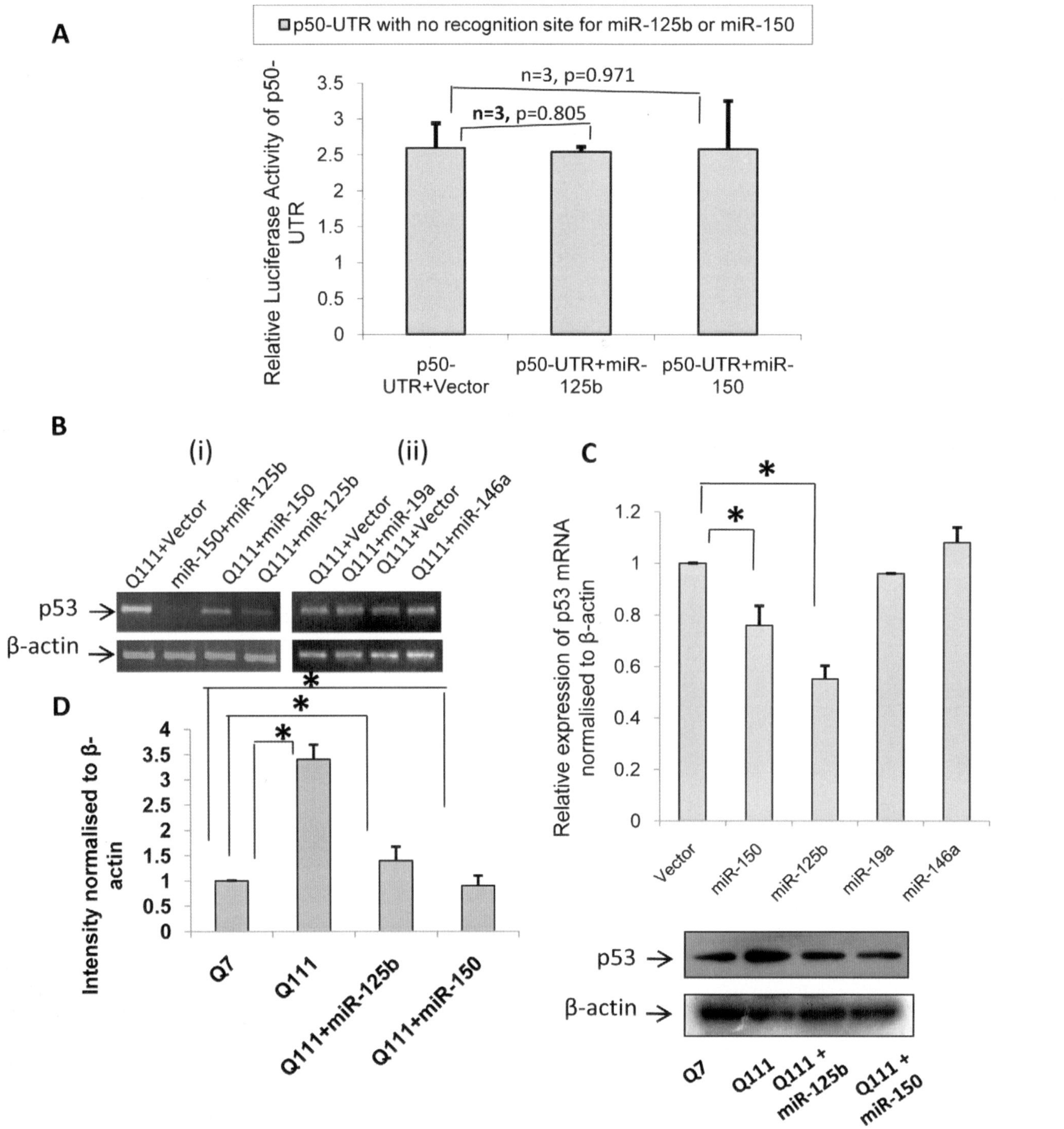

Figure 5. p53 is specifically targeted by miR-125b and miR-150 in HD cell model. (**A**) No change in relative luciferase activity of p50-3′UTR (bearing no predicted recognition site for miR-125b or miR-150) in cells co-transfected with pre- miR-125b and pre-miR-150 compared to cells co-transfected with empty vector U61; (**B**) RT-PCR showing (i) reduction in p53 mRNA in cells expressing exogenous pre-miR-150 and pre-miR-125b compared to cells expressing empty vector U61, (ii) no reduction in p53 mRNA in cells expressing exogenous pre-miR-19a and pre-miR-146a compared to cells expressing empty vector U61. (**C**) Average IOD showing relative expression of p53 mRNA in presence of over expressed miR-150 (n = 2, p = 0.021), miR-125b (n = 2, p = 0.029), miR-19a and miR-146a is given in the adjacent bar diagram (negative control). This indicates that p53 is specifically targeted by miR-125b and miR-150 in HD cell model. (**D**) Average IOD showing relative expression of p53 protein level in cell extracts prepared from ST*Hdh*^{Q7}/*Hdh*^{Q7}, ST*Hdh*^{Q111}/*Hdh*^{Q111} and in ST*Hdh*^{Q111}/*Hdh*^{Q111} cells transfected with miR-125b or miR-150. Immunoblot analysis show that the extent of p53 up regulation found in ST*Hdh*^{Q111}/*Hdh*^{Q111} cells when compared to ST*Hdh*^{Q7}/*Hdh*^{Q7} cells was reduced when ST*Hdh*^{Q111}/*Hdh*^{Q111} cells were transfected with miR-125b or miR-150.

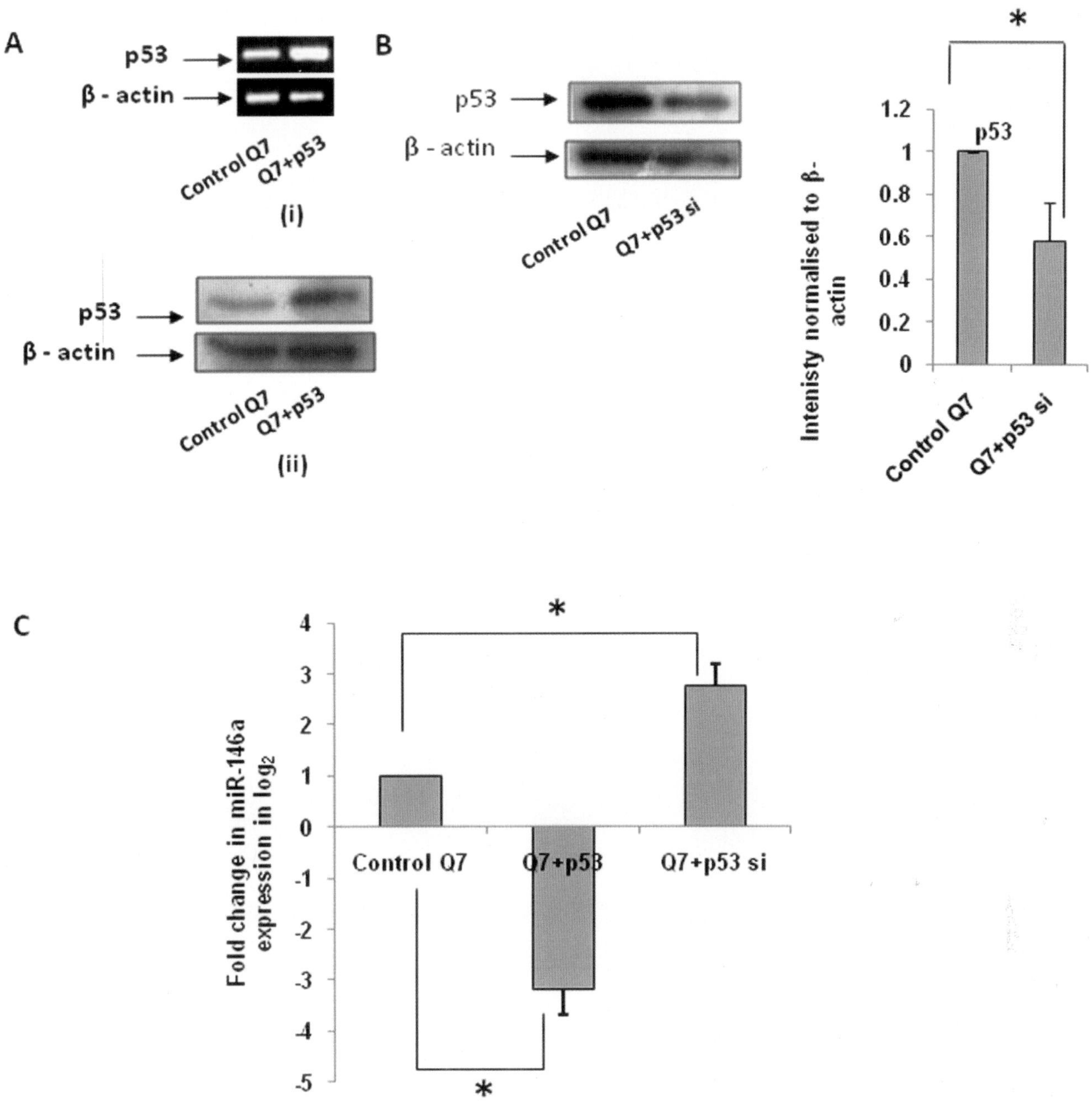

Figure 6. Role of p53 in the expression of miR-146a. (**A**) (i) RT-PCR showing p53 over expression upon transfection of exogenous p53-CFP in ST*Hdh*^{Q7}/*Hdh*^{Q7} cells compared to cells transfected with empty vector CFP and (ii) western blot showing p53 over expression at the protein level under similar conditions; (**B**) Representative Western Blot showing reduction in p53 protein level in ST*Hdh*^{Q7}/*Hdh*^{Q7} cells trasfected with pSuppressor plasmid containing p53 siRNA construct compared to ST*Hdh*^{Q7}/*Hdh*^{Q7} cells transfected with empty vector U61. Average IOD showing significant reduction in p53 protein level ($n = 3$, $p = 0.041$) compared to that of β-actin (control) is shown in the adjacent bar diagram; (**C**) Fold change in miR-146a expression in ST*Hdh*^{Q7}/*Hdh*^{Q7} cells in presence of over expressed p53 and reduced p53 levels respectively. miR-146a expression was significantly decreased ($n = 3$, $p = 0.032$) in ST*Hdh*^{Q7}/*Hdh*^{Q7} cells 72 hours post transfection with p53-CFP compared to empty vector CFP transfected cells and the expression was increased ($n = 3$, $p = 0.029$) in ST*Hdh*^{Q7}/*Hdh*^{Q7} cells compared to control ST*Hdh*^{Q7}/*Hdh*^{Q7} cells transfected with empty vector U61.

al of aggregates by HYPK and Hsp70 also rescued the expression of miR-146a, miR-125b and miR-150 (**Figure 10D**). It is to be noted that the ability to recover the expressions of miR-125b, miR-146a and miR-150 by Hsp70 was higher compared to that obtained with HYPK, reasons remaining unknown. This result shows that mutant HTT aggregates directly or indirectly increased p53 expression, reduced RelA/NFkB expression and activity and also reduced miR-146a, miR-125b and miR-150 expressions.

Expressions of p53, RelA/NFkB, miR-125b, miR-146a and miR-150 in striatal region of the brains of R6/2 mice

Transgenic mice (R6/2 strain), an animal model of HD [47] has been widely used by many investigators. Total RNA was isolated from paraffinised tissue sections of these R6/2 mice and their age-matched controls as described in the materials and methods section. cDNA was prepared using random hexamer to determine the expressions of p53 and RelA/NFkB in the striatal tissues.

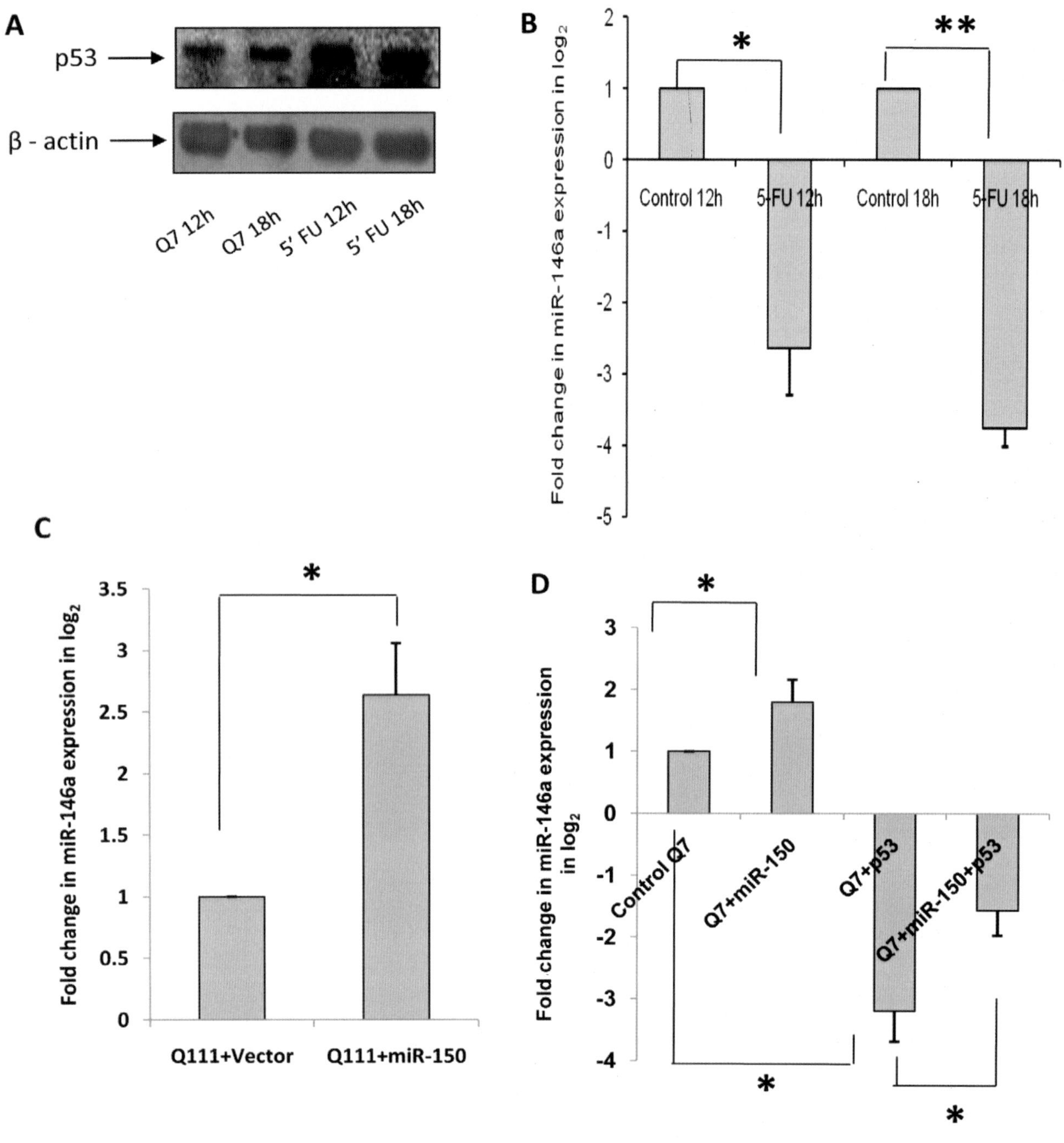

Figure 7. Stabilisation of p53 by 5-FU in ST*Hdh*^{Q7}/*Hdh*^{Q7} cells leads to decreased expression of miR-146a. (**A**) Typical Western Blot showing p53 stabilisation upon 5-FU treatment of ST*Hdh*^{Q7}/*Hdh*^{Q7} cells. ST*Hdh*^{Q7}/*Hdh*^{Q7} cells were treated with 10 μg/ml of 5-FU. Cells were harvested 12 hours and 18 hours successively post 5-FU treatment and immunoblotting with the cell extracts show an up regulation in p53 protein level in the treated cells compared to the untreated ones; (**B**) miR-146a expression was reduced significantly in ST*Hdh*^{Q7}/*Hdh*^{Q7} cells treated with 5-FU for 12 hours (n = 2, p = 0.038) and for 18 hours (n = 2, p = 0.0089) compared to the respective untreated cells; (**C**). Relative differences in miR-146a expression in presence of reduced p53 levels in ST*Hdh*^{Q111}/*Hdh*^{Q111} cells. miR-146a expression was increased significantly (n = 3, p = 0.039) in ST*Hdh*^{Q111}/*Hdh*^{Q111} cells 72 hours post transfection with pre-miR-150 compared to ST*Hdh*^{Q111}/*Hdh*^{Q111} cells transfected with empty vector U61. (**D**) Relative differences in miR-146a expression in endogenous ST*Hdh*^{Q7}/*Hdh*^{Q7} cells and in cells transfected respectively with pre-miR-150, p53 and pre-miR-150 and p53 alone. Mature miR-146a expression was increased significantly (n = 3, p = 0.03) in cells transfected with pre-miR-150 which has been shown to reduce p53. miR-146a expression was reduced in presence of p53 (n = 3, p = 0.032). However, the reduction was less in cells when p53 was co-transfected with pre-miR-150 (n = 3, p = 0.044).

Result obtained by RT-PCR revealed that expression of p53 was increased significantly (n = 3, p = 0.05), while the expression of RelA/NFkB was decreased significantly (n = 3, p = 0.04) compared to control (**Figure 11A**). As described above similar result was obtained in cell models of HD (**Figures 1A, 3A** and **9A**). Besides, cDNA prepared using stem-loop specific primers for mature miR-125b, miR-146a and miR-150 also revealed a decrease in the expressions of these miRNAs (n = 3, p<0.01), similar to that

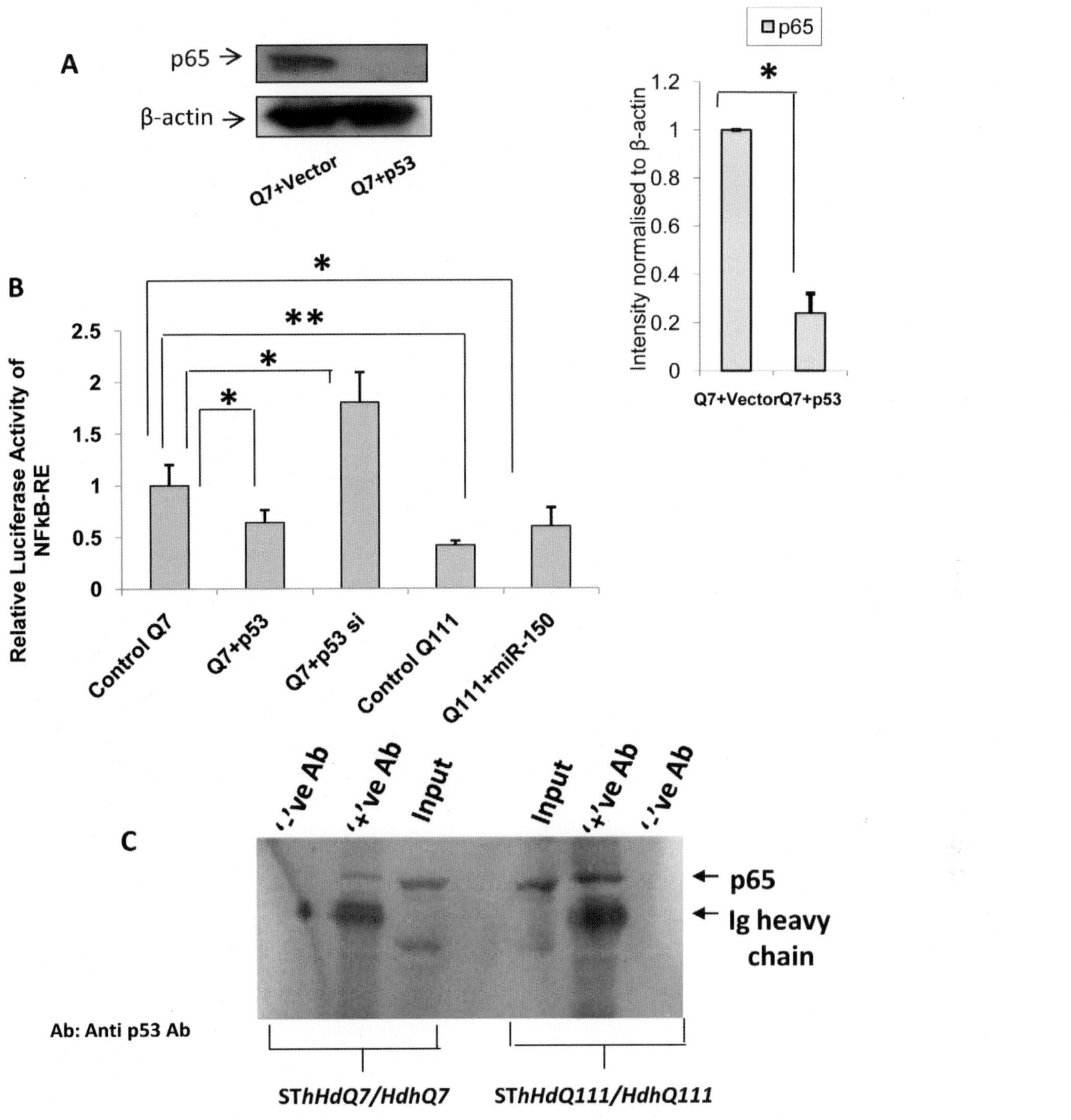

Figure 8. Regulation of RelA/NFkB expression and activity by p53. (**A**) Typical experiment by Western Blot showing decrease in NF-kB (p65) i.e. RelA/NFkB expression upon over expression of p53 in STHdh^{Q7}/Hdh^{Q7} cells. RelA/NFkB expression was decreased significantly ($n = 3$, $p = 0.0041$) in STHdh^{Q7}/Hdh^{Q7} cells 48 hours post transfection with p53-CFP compared to STHdh^{Q7}/Hdh^{Q7} cells transfected with empty vector CFP. Average IOD obtained by comparing with β-actin is shown in the adjacent bar diagram; (**B**) Decrease in luciferase activity ($n = 3$, $p = 0.0214$) of NFkB-RE in STHdh^{Q7}/Hdh^{Q7} cells 48 hours post transfection with p53-CFP compared to STHdh^{Q7}/Hdh^{Q7} cells transfected with empty vector CFP and increase in luciferase activity ($n = 3$, $p = 0.032$) of NFkB-RE in STHdh^{Q7}/Hdh^{Q7} cells 48 hours post transfection with p53 si compared to control STHdh^{Q7}/Hdh^{Q7} cells; increase in luciferase activity ($n = 4$, $p = 0.0482$) of NFkB-RE in STHdh^{Q111}/Hdh^{Q111} cells 48 hours post transfection with pre-miR-150 compared with that obtained in STHdh^{Q111}/Hdh^{Q111} cells transfected with empty vector U61. Relative luciferase activity of NFkB-RE obtained in control Q7 was taken as 1; (**C**) Co-immunoprecipitation analysis showing in vivo interaction of p53 with p65 sub-unit of NF-kB (RelA/NFkB) in wild type STHdh^{Q7}/Hdh^{Q7} cells and mutant STHdh^{Q111}/Hdh^{Q111} cells. Cell extracts prepared from STHdh^{Q7}/Hdh^{Q7} cells and STHdh^{Q111}/Hdh^{Q111} cells were immunoprecipitated by anti-p53 antibody coupled to agarose-protein G beads. Western blotting the p53 immunoprecipitated complex with anti-p65 antibody reveals such interaction as evident in lanes 2 and 6 denoted by '+' ve Ab.

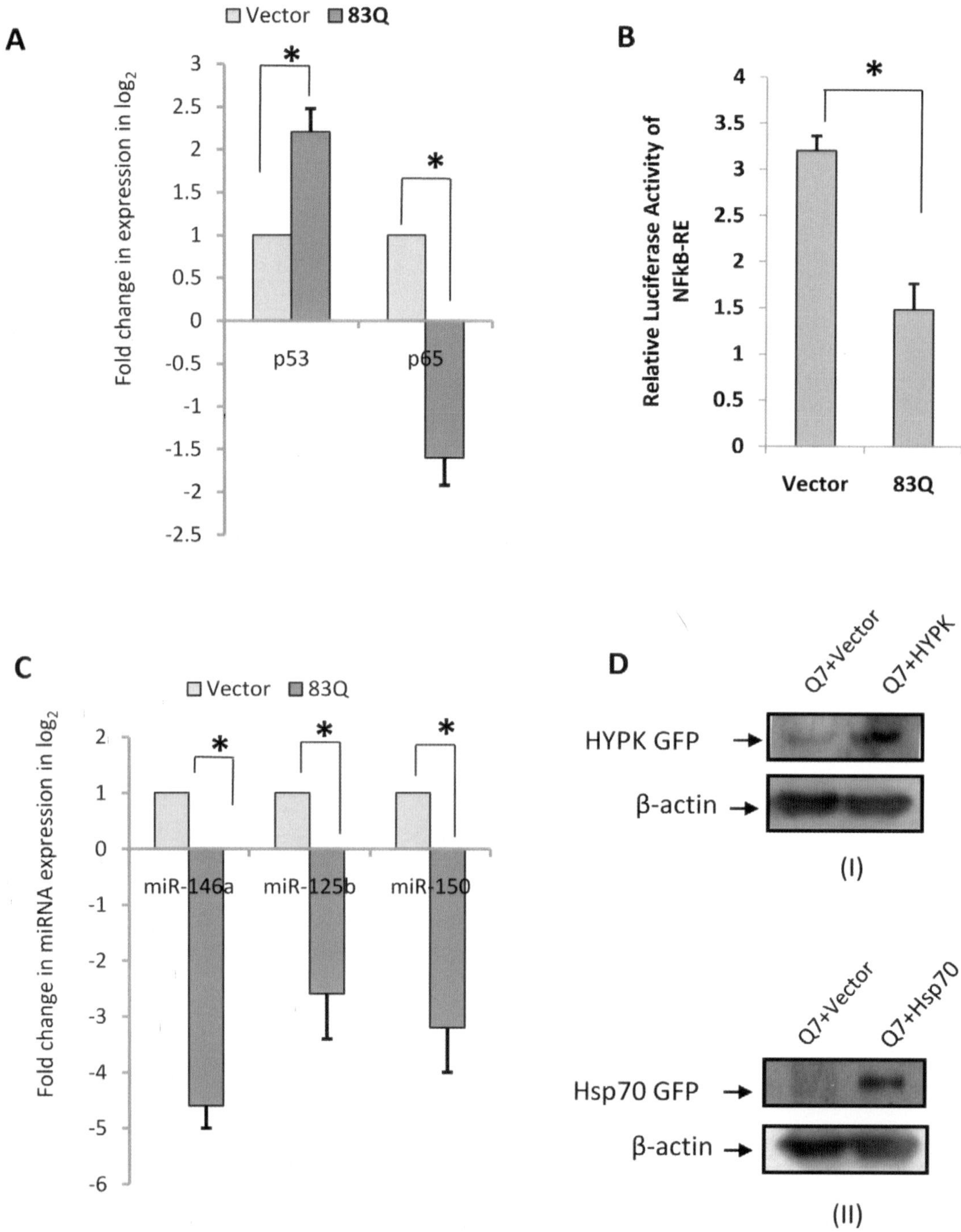

Figure 9. Poly Q aggregates alter the expressions of miR-125b, miR-150, p53, RelA/NFkB and miR-146a. (**A**) Increase in p53 expression ($n = 3$, $p = 0.028$) and decrease in RelA/NFkB expression ($n = 3$, $p = 0.031$) in 83Q DsRed transfected ST*Hdh*^{Q7}/*Hdh*^{Q7} cells compared to ST*Hdh*^{Q7}/*Hdh*^{Q7} cells transfected with empty vector DsRed. (**B**) Decrease in relative luciferase activity of NFkB-RE upon 83Q DsRed transfection in ST*Hdh*^{Q7}/*Hdh*^{Q7} cells. Average luciferase activity of NFkB-RE was significantly decreased ($n = 6$, $p = 0.0334$) in ST*Hdh*^{Q7}/*Hdh*^{Q7} cells 48 hours post transfection with 83Q DsRed compared to ST*Hdh*^{Q7}/*Hdh*^{Q7} cells transfected with empty vector DsRed. (**C**) Similarly, miR-146a expression ($n = 4$, $p = 0.011$), miR-125b expression ($n = 2$, $p = 0.048$) and miR-150 expressions ($n = 2$, $p = 0.039$) were decreased significantly in ST*Hdh*^{Q7}/*Hdh*^{Q7} cells 48 hours post transfection with 83Q DsRed compared to ST*Hdh*^{Q7}/*Hdh*^{Q7} cells 48 hours post transfection with empty vector DsRed. miR-17-5p was used as endogenous control to calculate fold change in each case; (**D**) Immunoblotting with cell extracts prepared from HYPK-GFP transfected ST*Hdh*^{Q7}/*Hdh*^{Q7} cells and Hsp70-GFP transfected ST*Hdh*^{Q7}/*Hdh*^{Q7} cells showed increase in the expression of HYPK (in panel I probed by anti-HYPK antibody) and Hsp70 (in panel II probed by anti-GFP antibody) respectively compared to those obtained in ST*Hdh*^{Q7}/*Hdh*^{Q7} cells transfected with empty vector GFP-C1.

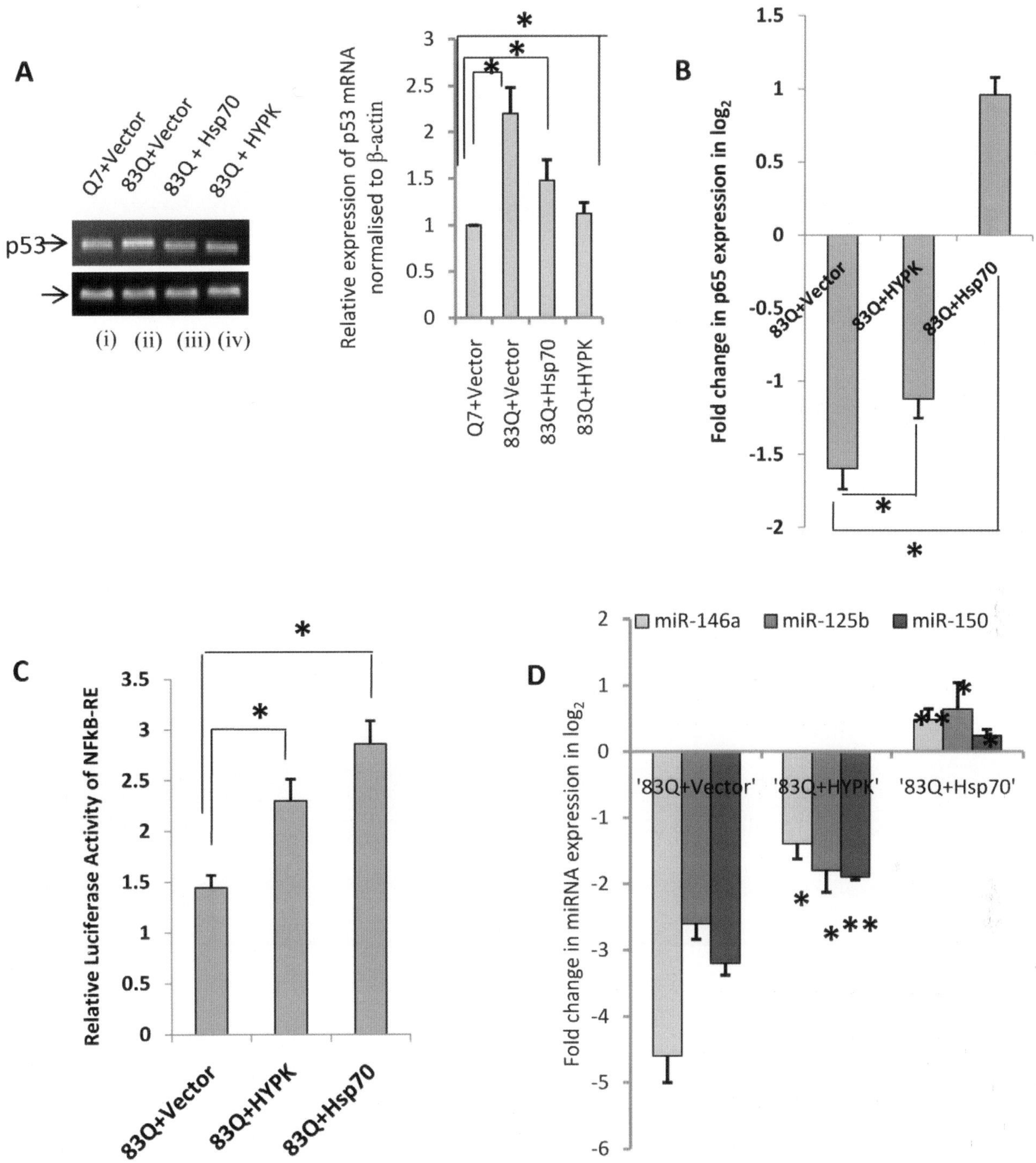

Figure 10. Removal of aggregates by chaperones rescue expression pattern of micoRNAs, p53 and RelA/NFkB. (**A**) RT-PCR showing increase in p53 expression in ST*Hdh*^{Q7}/*Hdh*^{Q7} cells co-transfected with 83Q DsRed and empty vector GFP-C1 (lane ii, n = 3, p = 0.028) and decrease in p53 expression in ST*Hdh*^{Q7}/*Hdh*^{Q7} cells co-transfected with 83Q DsRed and Hsp70-GFP (lane iii, n = 3, p = 0.025) and 83Q DsRed and HYPK-GFP (lane iv, n = 3, p = 0.019) compared to control ST*Hdh*^{Q7}/*Hdh*^{Q7} cells (lane i). Average IOD showing relative expression of p53 mRNA in each case is given in the adjacent bar diagram. (**B**) Changes in p65 (RelA/NFkB) expression in ST*Hdh*^{Q7}/*Hdh*^{Q7} cells co-transfected with 83Q DsRed and HYPK-GFP and 83Q DsRed and Hsp70-GFP compared to ST*Hdh*^{Q7}/*Hdh*^{Q7} cells co-transfected with 83Q DsRed and empty vector GFP-C1. The increase in RelA/NFkB expression was significant in the presence of HYPK-GFP (n = 6, p = 0.028) and also in the presence of Hsp70-GFP (n = 6, p = 0.022). (**C**) Revival of luciferase activity of NFkB-RE in presence of chaperones in 83Q DsRed transfected ST*Hdh*^{Q7}/*Hdh*^{Q7} cells. Luciferase activity of NFkB-RE in ST*Hdh*^{Q7}/*Hdh*^{Q7} cells co-transfected with 83Q DsRed and HYPK-GFP was significantly increased (n = 6, p = 0.031) when compared to that obtained in ST*Hdh*^{Q7}/*Hdh*^{Q7} cells transfected with 83Q DsRed and empty vector GFP-C1. Similar increase (n = 6, p = 0.029) in relative luciferase activity of NFkB-RE was observed in ST*Hdh*^{Q7}/*Hdh*^{Q7} cells 48 hours post transfection with 83Q DsRed and Hsp70-GFP; (**D**) Similarly, miR-146a expression (n = 3, p = 0.033), miR-125b expression and miR-150 expression were significantly increased in ST*Hdh*^{Q7}/*Hdh*^{Q7} cells 48 hours post transfection with 83Q DsRed and HYPK-GFP compared to ST*Hdh*^{Q7}/*Hdh*^{Q7} cells transfected with 83Q DsRed and empty vector GFP-C1. Such increase in miR-146a expression (n = 3, p = 0.0079), miR-125b expression and miR-150 expression were also observed with ST*Hdh*^{Q7}/*Hdh*^{Q7} cells 48 hours post transfection with 83Q DsRed and Hsp70-GFP. miR-17-5p was used as endogenous control to calculate fold change in each case.

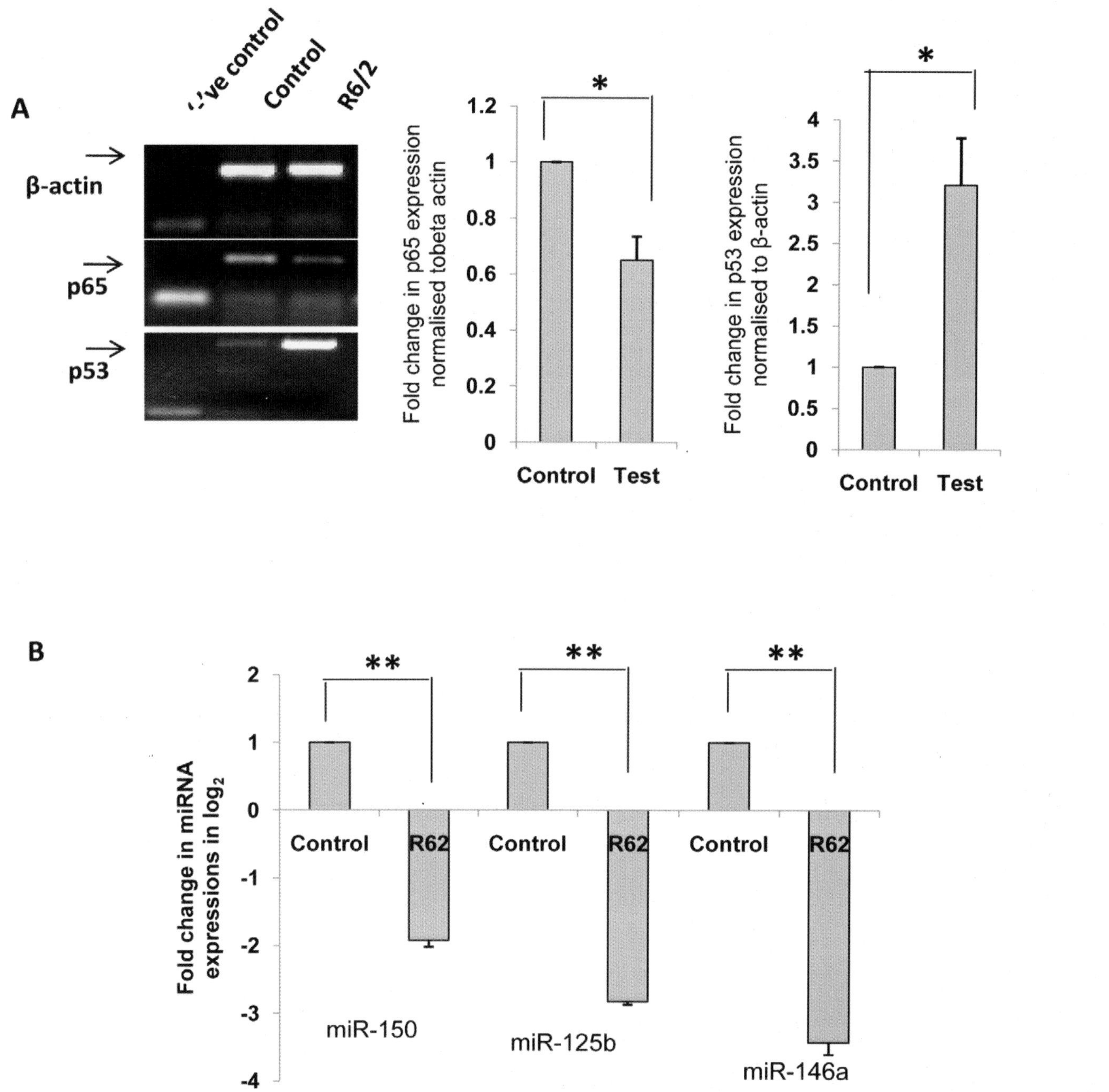

Figure 11. Expression pattern of p53, RelA/NFkB and microRNAs in striatal regions of the brains of R6/2 mice. (**A**) RT-PCR showing expression levels of β-actin, p65 sub-unit of NFkB (RelA/NFkB) and p53 in striatal regions of the brains of R6/2 mice and their age matched controls. Integrated optical density showing relative expression of p65 sub-unit of NFkB (RelA/NFkB) and p53 in the tissues normalized to β-actin are given in the adjacent bar diagrams. RelA/NFkB expression was found to be lesser (n = 3, p = 0.041) and p53 expression greater (n = 3, p = 0.05) in striatum of R6/2 mice when compared to their age matched controls. (**B**) Real time PCR analysis showing significant decrease in mature miR-150 expression (n = 3, p = 0.01), mature miR-125b expression (n = 3, p = 0.002) and mature miR-146a expression (n = 3, p = 0.008) in striatum of R6/2 mice.

obtained in $STHdh^{Q111}/Hdh^{Q111}$ cells [33]. This result shown in **Figure 11B** reveals that the alterations in the expressions of p53, RelA/NFkB, miR-125b, miR-146a and miR-150 might be involved in the pathogenesis of HD.

In order to see whether miR-146a, miR-125b and miR-150 were specifically down regulated than others in striatal region of the brains of R6/2 mice, we determined the expression levels of additional ten miRNAs in the mouse model and compared the results with that obtained earlier by us in HD cell model [33]. The results given in **Table S1** show that expressions of miR-100, miR-125b, miR-135a, miR-138, miR-150, miR-146a, miR-221 which were decreased in HD cell model [33] were also decreased in R6/2 mice and the expressions of miR-127-3p and miR-214 were increased in both $STHdh^{Q111}/Hdh^{Q111}$ cells [33] and the R6/2 mouse model. miR-145, miR-148a, miR-190 and miR-335 however showed different expression pattern in R6/2 mice and HD cell model [33]. Thus, out of the thirteen miRNAs whose expressions have been studied, expressions of eight miRNAs including miR-146a, miR-125b and miR-150 were decreased, expressions of two miRNAs (viz., miR-127 and miR-214) were increased and expressions of three miRNAs (viz., miR-145, miR-190 and miR-335) remained unchanged in R6/2 mice. Earlier observations by others showed miR-138, miR-218 and miR-222 to be down regulated in HD mouse models [30,48] which had also been confirmed by us in HD cell model [33].

We have already shown in the earlier section that Poly Q aggregates cause decrease in the expressions of miR-146a, miR-125b and miR-150 and removal of aggregates by chaperones rescue such changes. To address the specificity of such alteration of miR-146a, miR-125b and miR-150 in the presence of poly Q aggregates, mutated exon1 of HTT gene that translated to N-terminal HTT with 83 Q was exogenously expressed in four different cell lines viz., Neuro2A (mouse neuroblastoma cell line), ST*Hdh*^{Q7}/*Hdh*^{Q7} (mouse sriatal cells having two copies of full length HTT with 7Q), SH-SY5Y (human neuroblastoma cell line) and HeLa cells (human cells derived from cervical tumours) and the expression of twenty two miRNAs were studied in these cell models (**Table S1**). Similar cell models of HD had earlier been shown by us [44,45] and others. Of these twenty two miRNAs taken for study, eleven miRNAs were earlier found to be up regulated and eleven miRNAs were found to be down regulated by us in HD cell model [33]. Among the up regulated miRNAs in ST*Hdh*^{Q111}/*Hdh*^{Q111} cells, expressions of miR-214, miR-299 and miR-335 were also up regulated in three of the four cell models and expression of miR-199a was increased in two cell models. Expression of miR-148a, which was increased in ST*Hdh*^{Q111}/*Hdh*^{Q111} cells, was however decreased in all the four cell models. Among the down regulated miRNAs, expression of miR-146a was decreased in all the four cell models whereas expression of miR-125b and miR-150 were decreased in three of the four cell models excepting Neuro2A where expressions of those were up regulated. Expressions of miR-100 and miR-135b were also decreased in two of the four cell models. The results shown in **Table S1** suggests that although there is a heterogeneity in the expressions of miRNAs in different cell lines exogenously expressing mutated exon1 of HTT, miR-146a, miR-125b and miR-150 were preferentially decreased than others in the presence of poly Q aggregates.

A probable model showing the involvement of NFkB (RelA), p53 and miRNAs in the regulation of cell death in HD pathogenesis

The model shows that mutant HTT modulates the expressions of both p53 and RelA/NFkB, NFkB activity and decreases miR-146a, miR-125b and miR-150 expressions. In the presence of mutant HTT aggregates, miR-125b and miR-150 expressions decrease leading to an increased level of p53. The elevated p53 then in turn, further increases mutant HTT aggregates and decreases RelA/NFkB expression, NFkB activity and miR-146a expression.

Discussion

In this study, we present evidences to show that (i) in ST*Hdh*^{Q111}/*Hdh*^{Q111} cells decreased expression of miR-146a is mediated through decreased expression and activity of RelA/NFkB, (ii) increased expression of p53 in the same cells could be due to decreased expression of miR-125b and miR-150, (iii) p53 and RelA/NFkB regulate the expression of miR-146a and (iv) neuronal cells expressing N-terminal HTT with 83Q coded by exon1 exhibit decreased miR-125b and miR-150 expressions, increased p53 expression and reduced RelA/NFkB expression and activity and miR-146a expression. Such changes could be rescued by the expression of HYPK and Hsp70. Besides, we also show that expressions of miR-125b, miR-146a, miR-150 and RelA/NFkB were decreased while the expression of p53 was increased in striatal tissues of R6/2 mice models of HD.

Transcription factor RelA/NFkB is known to regulate the expression of miR-146a by binding to the upstream sequences [29]. RelA/NFkB dependent increase in the expression of miR-146a is shown earlier by several investigators in Alzheimer's disease (AD), viral infection, epilepsy and prion disease [49–52]. Increased expression of miR-146a results in the decreased expression of complement factor H (CFH) in AD and Herpes simplex virus type1 [49,50]. Even though elevated expression of miR-146a is reported in epilepsy and scrapie, no targets of the miRNA are reported. The reason for the difference in the expression of the miRNA in AD and HD remains unknown. Here, we show that the steady state level and activity of RelA/NFkB are reduced in ST*Hdh*^{Q111}/*Hdh*^{Q111} cells compared to those in ST*Hdh*^{Q7}/*Hdh*^{Q7} cells (**Figures 1A–1D**). Exogenous expression of RelA/NFkB restores NFkB activity as well as the expression of miR-146a (**Figures 2A, 2B and 2C**). Reducing the activity of NFkB by treatment with aspirin [35] also compromised miR-146a expression (**Figure 2D**). Taken together, the down regulation of miR-146a in ST*Hdh*^{Q111}/*Hdh*^{Q111} cells seen earlier [33] could be due to lower steady state level of RelA/NFkB in these cells. We then confirmed the earlier observation that the level of p53 is increased in ST*Hdh*^{Q111}/*Hdh*^{Q111} cells and also in other cell and animal models of HD [10,11,32]. However, the mechanism of such increased level of p53 was not known. Since p53 is a known target of miR-125b [28] and the expression of miR-125b is down regulated in ST*Hdh*^{Q111}/*Hdh*^{Q111} cells [33], we tested the hypothesis that increased expression of p53 in these cells could be due to decreased level of miR-125b. Increased reporter luciferase activity of human p53 3′-UTR (718 to 742) containing miR-125b recognition site viz., p53-UTR1 in ST*Hdh*^{Q111}/*Hdh*^{Q111} cells compared to that in ST*Hdh*^{Q7}/*Hdh*^{Q7} cells (**Figure 3C**) and decreased luciferase activity of the same in presence of exogenous miR-125b indicated that miR-125b could target p53 (**Figure 3D**). Using the prediction tool RNAhybrid [53] http://bibiserv.techfak.uni-bielefeld.de/rnahybrid/), we observed that mouse p53 (*Trp53*) could also be targeted by miR-125b at 3′-UTR position 413–435 as shown in **Figure S1 (B)**. Exogenous expression of miR-125b decreased the endogenous level of p53 in ST*Hdh*^{Q111}/*Hdh*^{Q111} cells (**Figure 3E**). These results confirmed that in ST*Hdh*^{Q111}/*Hdh*^{Q111} cells, increased p53 level could be mediated by decreased expression of miR-125b. Significant decrease of mature miR-150 was detected in ST*Hdh*^{Q111}/^{Q111} cells compared to that obtained in ST*Hdh*^{Q7}/*Hdh*^{Q7} cells [33] and also in neuronal cells expressing mutated exon1 of the *HTT* gene as well as in the post mortem brain of HD mice R6/2. We confirmed the prediction that human p53 could be a target of miR-150 at human p53 3′-UTR position 234–256. Mouse p53 (*Trp53*) could also be a target of miR-150 at 3′ UTR position 260–287 as shown in **Figure S1 (C)** using RNAhybrid [53]. Increased expression of luciferase reporter with predicted recognition site of miR-150 at the 3′-UTR of human p53 (p53-UTR2) in ST*Hdh*^{Q111}/*Hdh*^{Q111} cells in comparison to that in ST*Hdh*^{Q7}/*Hdh*^{Q7} cells was observed (**Figure 4A**). In the presence of exogenous miR-150, decreased expression of the same luciferase reporter in ST*Hdh*^{Q7}/*Hdh*^{Q7} cells (**Figure 4C**) and reduction of endogenous p53 in ST*Hdh*^{Q111}/*Hdh*^{Q111} cells (**Figure 4D**) were also observed. These results show that miR-150 also targets p53. However, 213 bp (145–359) of the 3′ UTR of NFkB1 (p50-UTR) containing no predicted binding site for either miR-125b or miR-150 showed no change in its luciferase activity (negative control) when the construct was co-transfected with cloned pre-miR-125b or pre-miR-150 (**Figure 5A**). Although endogenous p53 level was decreased by over expressing miR-125b and miR-150, there was no change in p53 level either in the presence of exogenous miR-19a or miR-146a (negative control), which bears no predicted recognition site in the 3′UTR of p53 (**Figure 5B**). Taken together, these results show that p53 is specifically targeted by miR-125b and miR-150. Report that expressions of miR-125b and miR-150 are decreased in ST*Hdh*^{Q111}/^{Q111} cells [**33**] and p53 is one of the targets of these two miRNAs provides an explanation for the increased expression of p53 in these cells. If this down regulation of miR-125b and miR-150 are confirmed along with increased p53 in the post mortem brains of HD, then it may explain the cause for elevated p53 and its role in HD pathogenesis as observed in other studies [4,10,11].

NFkB is known to resist apoptosis induction [54,55] while p53 in general, is a well-known inducer of apoptosis. Thus down regulation of RelA/NFkB and increased expression of p53 as observed in ST*Hdh*^{Q111}/*Hdh*^{Q111} cells, a cell model of HD, if replicated in HD patients could be one of the mechanisms of enhanced apoptosis observed in HD as reviewed by Imarisio et al., 2008 [1]. The differential pattern of expression of the two transcription factors NFkB and p53 in ST*Hdh*^{Q111}/*Hdh*^{Q111} cells, prompted us to search for any relationship that might exist between the expressions of these two transcription factors. We observed an inverse correlation between the levels of p53 and p65 sub-unit of NFkB (RelA/NFkB) in neuronal cells. Exogenous expression of p53 and stabilization of p53 by 5-FU treatment decreased the expression of RelA/NFkB and activity of NFkB. Reducing the expression of p53 either by siRNA or by expressing exogenous miR-150 increased NFkB activity as detected by the luciferase assay. It is unclear what exactly mediates such functional inverse relationship. CREB binding protein (CBP) is known to interact with both p53 and RelA/NFkB and depending on the preference either induces or prevents apoptosis. Sequestration of CBP to p53 may decrease NFkB activity [38]. Activated p53 is also known to induce NFkB DNA binding but at the same time suppresses its transcriptional activation [37]. This may provide an explanation for the decreased NFkB activity as observed in our studies. However, there is a report, which suggests for an activation of the transcription factor NFkB in response to apoptosis induced by p53 [41]. Besides, RelA/NFkB is also known to regulate p53 expression in tumor cells in response to hypoxia [56]. All these results show that p53 directly or indirectly regulates RelA/NFkB expression and activity of NFkB and thus the expression of miR-146a. The other possibility of direct interference of p53 on miR-146a expression could not be ruled out and requires further studies. Even though it is conceivable that p53 can modulate the activity of NFkB, how the expression of RelA/NFkB is compromised remains unknown.

Chaperones are known to protect mutant HTT aggregates possibly by preventing formation of aggregates. We have earlier shown that HYPK possesses chaperone like activity and reduces the aggregates formed by mutated N-terminal HTT coded by exon1 of the gene [45]. Exogenous expression of N-terminal HTT with 83Q increased the mutant HTT aggregates as have been observed by many authors including us [44]. In such condition, p53 expression was increased and RelA/NFkB expression was decreased (**Figure 9A**) similar to that obtained in endogenous ST*Hdh*^{Q111}/*Hdh*^{Q111} cells when compared with endogenous ST*Hdh*^{Q7}/*Hdh*^{Q7} cells. NFkB activity and expression of miR-146a, miR-125b and miR-150 were also reduced in such condition (**Figures 9B and 9C**). However, co-expression of HYPK together with mutant HTT exon1 reduced the aggregates, reduced p53 expression and recovered the activity of NFkB and miR-146a, miR-125b and miR-150 expressions (**Figures 10A–10D**). Similar results were also observed with Hsp70. Results obtained with ST*Hdh*^{Q111}/*Hdh*^{Q111} cells, a cell model of HD has been schematically represented in **Figure 12** to propose for a probable model showing the involvement of RelA/NFkB, p53 and miRNAs in the regulation of cell death in HD pathogenesis. The model shows that mutant HTT modulates the expression of p53 and p65 subunit of NFkB (RelA/NFkB), NFkB activity and miR-146a, miR-125b and miR-150 expressions. Since miR-125b and miR-150 target p53, we postulate that in the presence of mutant HTT aggregates there is an initial decrease in miR-125b and miR-150 expression. These down regulated miRNAs lead to increased p53 level as observed in presence of aggregates. The elevated p53 then in turn, further increases mutant HTT aggregates and decreases RelA/NFkB expression, NFkB activity and miR-146a expression.

In summary, we may conclude that in ST*Hdh*^{Q111}/*Hdh*^{Q111} cells, down regulation of miR-146a is mediated through RelA/NFkB. Increased p53 level in HD models could be mediated through down regulation of miR-125b and miR-150. p53 directly or indirectly regulates the expression of miR-146a. Identification of interplay between transcription factors and miRNAs regulating their targets remains one of the challenges in miRNA biology. Our investigation using HD cell lines provides important observations that miR-146a is regulated by p53 and RelA/NFkB and increased p53 could be mediated through down regulation of miR-125b and miR-150. It requires further studies to establish if such regulation plays any role in HD pathogenesis.

Materials and Methods

R6/2 mice

Ovarian transplanted hemizygote females carrying HD exon 1 gene with about 150 CAG repeats (strain name: B6CBA-Tg(Hdexon1)62Gpb/3J) were purchased from Jackson Laboratory and crossed with B6CBAF1/J males. The transgenic strain was maintained by crossing carrier males with CBA females. The genotyping was carried out using PCR as described previously by Mangirani et al., 1996 [47]. All animal experiments were performed according to the protocol approved by the Institutional Animal Ethics Committee of National Brain Research Centre, Manesar. Animals had free access to pelleted diet and water *ad libitum*. All efforts were made to minimize animal suffering. The transgenic mice along with their age-matched controls were anesthetized and then perfused with PBS containing 4% PFA in PBS, brain samples were collected and processed for paraffin embedding followed by cryosectioning with 20 μm thickness.

STHdh^{Q7}/Hdh^{Q7} and STHdh^{Q111}/Hdh^{Q111} cells

ST*Hdh*^{Q7}/*Hdh*^{Q7} cells express full-length wild type HTT with 7Q (homozygous) while ST*Hdh*^{Q111}/*Hdh*^{Q111} cells express full length mutated HTT with 111Q (homozygous) from the chromosomal region and is considered as a model for HD. These cell lines were established from wild type and homozygous mutant Hdh knock in embryonic mice respectively [32]. Dr. Marcy E. MacDonald of Massachusetts General Hospital, USA, kindly provided these cells to us. ST*Hdh*^{Q111}/*Hdh*^{Q111} cells exhibit dominant HD phenotypes and indicate a disruption of striatal cell homeostasis by the mutant HTT protein, via a mechanism that is different from its normal activity (ST*Hdh*^{Q7}/*Hdh*^{Q7} cells). This cell model of HD has been extensively used for identifying molecular alterations in HD [57–64].

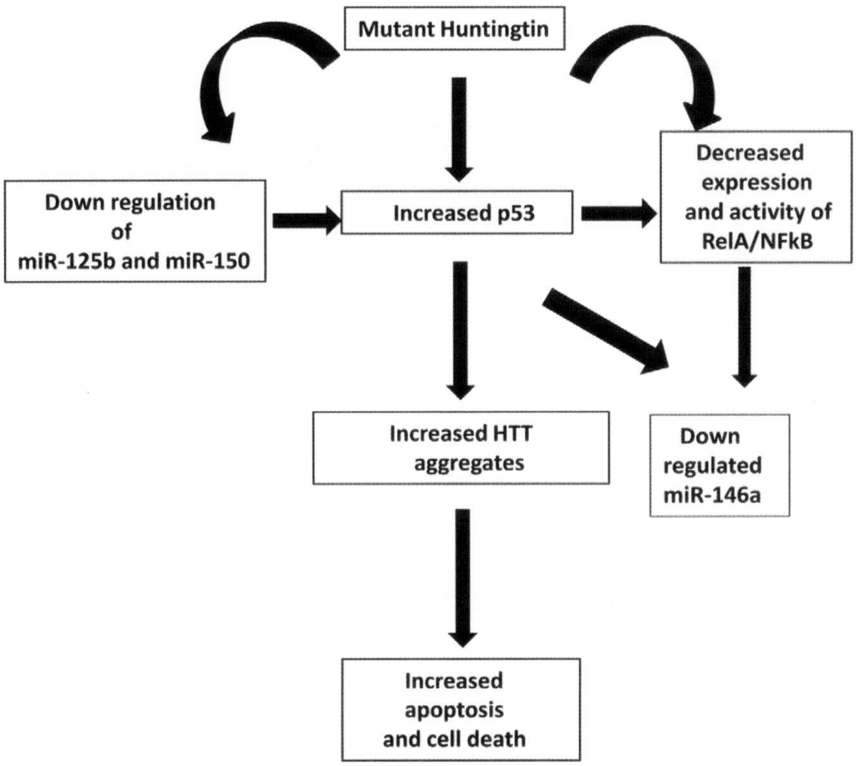

Figure 12. Proposed model for the involvement of RelA/NFkB, p53 and microRNAs in the regulation of cell death in HD pathogenesis. The model shows that mutant HTT modulates the expression of both p53 and p65 subunit of NFkB (RelA/NFkB) expression and activity and miR-146a, miR-125b and miR-150 expressions. Since miR-125b and miR-150 target p53, we postulate that in the presence of mutant HTT aggregates there is an initial decrease in miR-125b and miR-150 expression. These down regulated miRNAs lead to increased p53 level as observed in presence of aggregates. The elevated p53 then in turn, further increases mutant HTT aggregates and decreases NFkB/p65 expression (RelA/NFkB), NFkB activity and miR-146a expression.

Cell Culture

STHdh^{Q7}/Hdh^{Q7} and STHdh^{Q111}/Hdh^{Q111} cells, obtained from Dr. Marcy E. MacDonald, were cultured in DMEM (HiMedia, India) supplemented with 10% (v/v) heat inactivated FBS (Biowest, France), antibiotics penicillin/streptomycin PS 1% (v/v) and 400 µg/ml G418 (Invitrogen, USA) at 33°C in humidified condition and 5% CO_2. HeLa cells were cultured in MEM (HiMedia, India), 10% (v/v) FBS (Biowest, France), 1% (v/v) PS at 37°C in humidified condition and 5% CO_2. Growth conditions for HeLa cells [44] and growth conditions for Neuro2a cells [45] were similar to those which have already been published. Human derived neuroblastoma cells SH-SY5Y were cultured in DMEM (HiMedia, India), 10% (v/v) FBS (Biowest, France), 1% (v/v) PS at 37°C in humidified condition and 5% CO_2.

Antibodies and materials

Anti-p53 monoclonal antibody (1:200, Clone DO7, Imgenex, USA) was used for immuno-precipitation. Anti-p53 polyclonal (1:2000, Clone DO7, Imgenex, USA), anti-p65 monoclonal (1:1000, MAB3026, Chemicon, USA), anti-GFP monoclonal (1:4000, CATALOG No. 632375, Clontech, USA) and anti-β-actin monoclonal (1:10,000, A2228, Sigma Chemicals, USA) antibodies were used for immunoblot analysis. Anti-HYPK polyclonal was custom made by providing purified HYPK protein [45] to Imgenex Biotech Pvt. Ltd, India (1:1000, CP 40 07, Imgenex Biotech Pvt. Ltd, India). Anti-mouse IgG-HRP (1:8,000) and anti-rabbit IgG-HRP (1:6000) were purchased from GENEI, India and used as secondary antibodies. Aspirin was purchased from Central Drug House Laboratory Reagent, India and 5-Fluorouracil (5-FU) obtained from Sigma-Aldrich, USA was used.

DNA constructs

Precursor miRNA-125b (Chr11: 121970465–121970552, - strand) and precursor miRNA-150 (Chr19: 50004042–50004125, - strand) were amplified by PCR from human genomic DNA and respectively cloned into pU61 Hygro (Genescript, USA) vector using BamHI and HindIII (NEB, USA) sites. The primers used were miR-125b-U6-F: 5′-CGCGGATCCGTCTCAAGAAAGAAAACATTG-3′ and miR-125b-U6-R: 5′-CCCAAGCTTAAAAACACCAAATTT-CCAGGATGCAA-3′; miR_150_U6_F: 5′-CGCGGATCCCT-CCCCATGGCCCTGTCT-3′ and miR_150_U6_R: 5′-CCC-AAGCTTAAAAAGTCCCCAGGTCCCTGTCC-3′. Full-length human *p53* cDNA was obtained by PCR from human brain cDNA library and cloned into CFP vector using BamH1 and Sal1 sites. The primers used for cloning were p53_CFP_F: 5′-ACGCGTCGA-CGTGGAGCCGCAGTCAGATCCTA-3′ and p53_CFP_R: 5′-CGCGGATCCCAGTCTGAGTCAGGCCCTTC-3′. Full-length p65 subunit of NFkB (RelA), cloned into pLG3 vector was obtained as a kind gift from Dr. Susanta Roychoudhury, IICB, Kolkata. For knocking down p53, pSuppressorNeo p53 plasmid DNA containing p53 siRNA [65] construct (Imgenex, USA) was used.

For luciferase reporter assays, we cloned two fragments of the 3′ UTR of human p53 into pmiR-Report vector (Ambion, USA), one comprising of 150 bp (position 733–739) containing miR-125b recognition site and the other comprising of 136 bp (position

234–256) containing miR-150 recognition site. These regions were amplified by PCR from human genomic DNA and cloned in vector using the MluI and HindIII (NEB, USA) sites. The constructs were named p53-UTR1 and p53-UTR2 respectively. For NFkB1 (p50), 213 bp (position 145–359) of the 3′ UTR of NFkB1 containing no predicted recognition site for either miR-125b or miR-150 was cloned into the vector using SpeI and MluI (NEB) sites and was named p50-UTR. The following primers were used to generate the UTR constructs: p53-UTR1-F: 5′-CGACGCGTAAGGAAATCTCACCCCATCC-3′ and p53-UTR1-R: 5′-CCCAAGCTTAAGCGAGACCCAGTCTCAAA-3′; p53-UTR2-F: 5′-CGACGCGTGAGGAGGATGGGGAGTAGGA-3′ and p53-UTR2-R: 5′-CCCAAGCTTAAGTGGGCCCCTACCTAGAA-3′; p50-UTR-F: 5′-GGACTAGTTTGGCTTCCTTTCTTGGTTC-3′ and p50-UTR-R: 5′-CGACGCGTGGCGACCGTGATACCTTTAAT-3′. For functional assay of NFkB promoter, the plasmids NFkB luciferase, containing multiple copies of NFkB response elements (NFkB-RE) and Gastrin luciferase containing the promoter sequence of Gastrin cloned in pGL3 vector were obtained as a kind gift from Prof. Susanta Roychoudhury, IICB, Kolkata.

In order to induce poly Q mediated aggregation in ST*Hdh*^{Q7}/*Hdh*^{Q7} cells, Neuro2a cells, SH-SY5Y cells and HeLa cells, N-terminal HTT with 83Q coded by exon1 of the gene cloned into Ds Red-C1 vector was used. For removal of such aggregates with the help of chaperones in ST*Hdh*^{Q7}/*Hdh*^{Q7} cells, DNA constructs containing full-length Hsp70 cloned into EGFP-C1 vector and N terminal of HYPK also cloned into EGFP-C1 vectors were used. For control experiments, empty vectors DsRedC1 and pEGFPC1 (both from BD Biosciences, USA) were used.

RNA preparation

Total RNA was prepared from cultured cells using TriZol Reagent (Invitrogen, USA) according to manufacturer's protocol. RNA samples were quantitated using Biophotometer (Eppendorf, Germany).

RNA extraction from paraffin embedded tissue samples

RNA was isolated from tissue sections routinely processed by fixation and paraffin embedding that does not completely degrade RNAs. Further, it is suggested that RNA fragments of around 100 bases in length or more are still present even in organs fixed at later stages after removal and also in organs very rich in RNase such as the pancreas [66]. We isolated RNA from paraffin embedded tissue samples of R6/2 mice following the protocol described by Santa et al., 1998, Korbler et al., 2003 [67,68]. Using this method many investigators studied expressions of coding sequences of DNA like β-actin, Ikaros and Aliolos from paraffinised lymph node sections of patients with malignant disorders of the lymphopoietic system (Hodgkin's and non-Hodgkin's lymphoma) [68]. There have been previous reports of studies on miRNA expression patterns from total RNA isolated from formalin-fixed paraffin-embedded (FFPE) tissues and frozen cells [69,70,71].

In brief, isolation method for RNA from paraffin embedded tissues consists of the following steps: De-paraffinization: For RNA extraction from tissue sections obtained from R62 mice, two sections each of 20 μm thickness were taken per 1.5 ml eppendorf tube. The sections were deparaffinised by two rinses in xylene for 5 min each at room temperature followed by two centrifugations at room temperature for 10 min each at 10,000 g. Rehydration: After paraffin solubilization, a rehydration step was introduced where the supernatants from the previous step were carefully removed and the pellets were successively washed with 1 ml of absolute ethanol and 1 ml of 95% ethanol in DEPC water. After each step the tissue was collected by centrifugation at 10,000 g for 10 min. Protein digestion: After the final wash, alcohol was aspirated and the tissue pellets were air dried in a thermoblock at 37°C and re-suspended in 500 μl of digestion buffer (10 mM NaCl, 500 mM Tris, pH 7.6, 20 mM EDTA and 1% SDS). To obtain purified RNA, tissue proteins were removed by adding 500 μg/ml of the proteolytic enzyme proteinase K. The sections were then incubated at 45°C for 16 hours (overnight). Prior to RNA purification, proteinase K was inactivated at 100°C for 7 min in order to nullify its effects on PCR. RNA extraction: Total RNA was then extracted from these tissue sections by using Trizol reagent and following manufacturer's protocol. Concentrations of total RNA was measured and total RNA was used to measure expression levels of genes like β-actin (contol), p53 and RelA/NFkB (p65 sub-unit of NFkB) and microRNAs like miR-150, miR-125b, miR-146a and miR-17-5p after making the cDNA.

Quantitative real time for miRNAs and their analysis

For Real time quantitation of microRNA, 100 ng of total RNA was taken for cDNA preparation using mirna specific stem-loop primers (ABI), Mulv-Reverse transcriptase (Fermentas), RNase inhibitor (Fermentas) and dNTPs. cDNA was then subjected to the procedure as described in [33]. We earlier confirmed miR-17-5p expression to remain unaltered in various conditions and cells including HD cell model viz., ST*Hdh*^{Q7}/*Hdh*^{Q7} and ST*Hdh*^{Q111}/*Hdh*^{Q111} cells and thus it was used as an endogenous control in our laboratory [33]. Besides, miR-17-5p has also been found to be useful as a suitable endogenous control in other studies as well [72]. In the present work also the expression of miR-17-5p was found to remain unchanged in various conditions and cells used. Thus, miR-17-5p was used as endogenous control to calculate fold change in all RT-PCR studies. The fold changes were calculated in accordance with SDS software V 2.0.

Real time PCR for mRNAs analysis

For real time of mRNAs 1 μg of total RNA was subjected to DNase treatment (Sigma) followed by cDNA preparation using random hexamer primer (Fermentas), dNTPs and MuLv- Reverse transcriptase (Fermentas) following the procedure described in [33]. The primers used for RT-PCR were: p53_expression_F: 5′-TCCCCCTTGCCGTCCCAA-3′, p53_expression_R: 5′-CGTGCAAGTCACAGACTT-3′; RelA(mse)_expression_F: 5′-GGCCTCATCCACATG- AACTT-3′, RelA(mse)_expression_R: 5′-CACTGTCACCTGGAAGCAGA-3′; and Actin-β_F: 5′-TCCTGTGGCATCCACGA- AACT-3′, Actin-β_R: GAAGCATTTGCGGTGGAC. Yield of the PCR products was estimated from the integrated optical density (IOD) using Image Master VDS software (Amersham Bioscience, UK). Data show mRNA expression levels relative to those of *β-actin*; the former was then normalized to control expression levels for each experiment.

Luciferase assays

For reporter luciferase assay, ST*Hdh*^{Q7}/*Hdh*^{Q7} and ST*Hdh*^{Q111}/*Hdh*^{Q111} cells were plated the day before transfection at 5×10^4 cells per well in 24-well plates (Nunc, USA). The following day, 50 ng of p53-3′UTR in pmiR-Report luciferase vector was transfected into cells using Lipofectamine 2000 (Invitrogen) according to the manufacturer's instructions. 24 hours later, luciferase assays were performed (Sirius Luminometer, Berthold detection systems, USA) using Luciferase Reporter assay system (Promega) according to the manufacturer's protocol. 3 μg of total protein was taken for each assay. Transfection efficiency was normalized by co-transfecting cells with GFP-C1 and measuring the Fluoresence at 510 nm

(Fluoromax-3, Jobin Yvon Horiba, USA). The luciferase activity of cloned constructs in ST*Hdh*^{Q111}/*Hdh*^{Q111} and ST*Hdh*^{Q7}/*Hdh*^{Q7} cells were normalized to the activity of empty vector (pmiR-Report luciferase vector), to nullify difference in protein synthesis levels between the wild type ST*Hdh*^{Q7}/*Hdh*^{Q7} and ST*Hdh*^{Q111}/*Hdh*^{Q111} cells. The experiments were carried out in triplicate. For over expression studies, 200 ng of pmiR-Report with desired clone and 300 ng of cloned pre-miR-125b or pre- miR-150 were co-transfected and luciferase assay was done following the same procedure.

For functional assay of NFkB response element and Gastrin promoter construct, 1×10^5 ST*Hdh*^{Q7}/*Hdh*^{Q7} cells and 1.5×10^5 ST*Hdh*^{Q7}/*Hdh*^{Q7} and ST*Hdh*^{Q111}/*Hdh*^{Q111} cells were plated a day before transfection per well in 6-well plates. The following day, 1 µg of NFkB response element construct and Gastrin luciferase construct were separately transfected. 24 h or 48 h post transfection, cells were collected and luciferase assays were performed as discussed above. For inhibiting NFkB activity, cells were treated with 2 mM aspirin 24 hours prior to transfection. For over expression studies 1 µg of p53-CFP and 1 µg of empty vector (CFP) were separately co-transfected with NFkB response element construct in ST*Hdh*^{Q7}/*Hdh*^{Q7} cells and for knocking down p53, 1 µg of p53 siRNA construct was transfected in HeLa cells (data not shown) and ST*Hdh*^{Q7}/*Hdh*^{Q7} cells and 1 µg of miR-150 was transfected in ST*Hdh*^{Q111}/*Hdh*^{Q111} cells along with 1 µg of NFkB luciferase construct. Luciferase assay was performed in each case following the same procedure as discussed above.

Immunoblot analysis

Cells were washed with cold phosphate-buffered saline (PBS), scraped, pelleted by centrifugation and lysed on ice for 30 mins using RIPA lysis buffer (50 mM Tris-HCl pH 8, 1% NP40, 150 mM NaCl, 12 mM deoxycholic acid sodium salt, 0.1% SDS) with protease inhibitor cocktail (Thermo Scientific, USA). The supernatant collected after centrifugation (at 4°C for 15 min at 18,000 g) was estimated by Bradford assay (BioRad, Hercules, CA) according to manufacturer's protocol. The OD readings of the samples were measured at 595 nm in Biophotometer (Eppendorf). For immunoblots 30 or 60 µg of total protein, boiled in SDS PAGE sample buffer were run on 10% SDS-PAGE, transferred to PVDF membranes (Thermo Scientific, USA) and detected by immunoblottting with the indicated antibodies. Integrated optical density (IOD) of each band compared to individual loading control was measured using Image Master VDS software (Amersham Biosciences, UK).

Co-immunoprecipitation assay

For co-immunoprecipitation assay, cells washed in cold PBS were lysed in co-immunoprecipitation (co-IP) buffer (50 mM Tris, pH 8.0, 150 mM NaCl, 1% NP40 and complete protease inhibitor cocktail) for 1 hour at 4°C with gentle mixing on an eppendorf rotor. Cell lysates were then centrifuged at 16,000 g for 15 min at 4°C and 50 µg of supernatant (total soluble extract) was used as an input for immunoprecipitation. For each experiment, 200 µg of the supernatant in 200 µl co-IP buffer was pre-cleared with agarose-protein G beads (GENEI, Bangalore, India) at 4°C for 2 hours with gentle shaking and then centrifuged at 1000 g for 5 min at 4°C. The beads obtained were washed twice with co-IP buffer, boiled in SDS PAGE loading buffer and used as negative antibody. The supernatant obtained was incubated overnight with 1 µg of p53 antibody at 4°C with gentle shaking. Next day, agarose-protein G bead was added to it and kept shaking for 6 hours at 4°C. The beads were precipitated by centrifuging at 18,000 g for 15 min at 48C, washed thrice by co-immunoprecipitation buffer, boiled with SDS–PAGE loading buffer and run on 10% SDS–PAGE and analyzed by immunoblotting technique with anti-p65 antibody.

Statistical analysis

Statistical analysis was done with the help of Graphpad Software, QuickCalcs, (http://www.graphpad.com/quickcalcs/index.cfm). Student's t-test was performed between control and experimental values to determine their statistical significance.

Supporting Information

Figure S1 (A) hsa-miR-150 binds to the 3′UTR of human p53. The position (234–256) in human p53-3′UTR predicted by miRBase as the recognition site for hsa-miR-150. Texts in blue indicate the 'seed' region. **(B). mmu-miR-125b binds to the 3′UTR of mouse Trp53.** (I) The position (413–435) in mouse p53-3′UTR predicted by RNAhybrid as the recognition site for mmu-miR-125b. Texts in blue indicate the 'seed' region. Their predicted stable RNA-RNA duplex formed by the binding of miR-125b to the 3′UTR of mouse Trp53 is shown in panel (II). The RNA strand in green represents mmu-miR-125b and the RNA strand in brown represents 413–435 of the 3′UTR in the mouse Trp53 transcript. **(C). mmu-miR-150 binds to the 3′UTR of mouse Trp53.** (I) The position (260–287) in mouse p53-3′UTR predicted by RNAhybrid as the recognition site for mmu-miR-150. Texts in blue indicate the 'seed' region. Their predicted stable RNA-RNA duplex formed by the binding of miR-150 to the 3′UTR of mouse Trp53 is shown in panel (II). The RNA strand in green represents mmu-miR-150 and the RNA strand in brown represents 260–287 of the 3′UTR in the mouse Trp53 transcript.

Table S1 MicroRNA expression changes in 83Q DsRed transfected cells compared to controls. Expressions of several miRNAs were studied in striatal regions of the brains of R6/2 mice and in four different cell lines exogenously expressing N-terminal HTT with 83Q coded by the exon1 of HTT gene and the results thus obtained have been indicated in the table. miR-17-5p was taken as endogenous control and fold change greater than 1.5 was considered as deregulated. The results obtained were compared with those found in HD cell model [33]. Texts in bold show names of miRNAs which maintained similar trend in their individual expression pattern in at least four of the six different models used for comparison. miR-125b and miR-150 were down regulated by more than 1.5 fold in five of the models including R6/2 mice whereas miR-146a was down regulated in all the models. Other miRNAs which showed a consistent expression pattern across the models were miR-100, miR-214, miR-299, miR-335, miR-34a and miR-148a. However, miR-148a which was up regulated in HD cell model [33] had been shown to be down regulated in all other models. The remaining miRNAs which were deregulated in HD cell model [33] have however showed heterogeneity in their expression pattern across the various models. The results obtained indicate that despite differences in miRNA expressions in various models, miR-146a, miR-125b and miR-150 were preferentially down regulated than others in the presence of poly Q aggregates.

Acknowledgments

We thank Dr. Marcy E. MacDonald of Massachusetts General Hospital, USA for providing ST*Hdh*^{Q7}/*Hdh*^{Q7} and *STHdh*^{Q111}/*Hdh*^{Q111} cells. We also thank Dr. Susanta Roy Choudhury, Indian Institute of Chemical Biology, Kolkata, India for providing us with p65 sub-unit of NFkB cloned into pLG3 vector, NFkB response element construct and Gastrin luciferase constructs.

Author Contributions

Conceived and designed the experiments: JG MS NPB. Performed the experiments: JG MS ED. Analyzed the data: JG MS NPB. Contributed reagents/materials/analysis tools: NRJ. Wrote the paper: JG NPB.

References

1. Imarisio S, Carmichael J, Korolchuk V, Chen CW, Saiki S, et al. (2008) Huntington's disease: from pathology and genetics to potential therapies. Biochem J 412: 191–209.
2. Cha JH (2007) Transcriptional signatures in Huntington's disease. Prog Neurobiol 83: 228–48.
3. Sugars KL, Rubinsztein DC (2003) Transcriptional abnormalities in Huntington disease. Trends Genet 19: 233–238.
4. Bae BI, Xu H, Igarashi S, Fujimuro M, Agrawal N, et al. (2005) p53 mediates cellular dysfunction and behavioral abnormalities in Huntington's disease. Neuron 47: 29–41.
5. Dunah AW, Jeong H, Griffin A, Kim YM, Standaert DG, et al. (2002) Sp1 and TAFII130 transcriptional activity disrupted in early Huntington's disease. Science 296: 2238–2243.
6. Takano H, Gusella JF (2002) The predominantly HEAT-like motif structure of huntingtin and its association and coincident nuclear entry with dorsal, an NF-kB/Rel/dorsal family transcription factor. BMC Neuroscience 14: 3–15.
7. Nucifora FC, Jr., Sasaki M, Peters MF, Huang H, Cooper JK, et al. (2001) Interference by huntingtin and atrophin-1 with cbp-mediated transcription leading to cellular toxicity. Science 291: 2423–2428.
8. Steffan JS, Kazantsev A, Spasic-Boskovic O, Greenwald M, Zhu YZ, et al. (2000) The Huntington's disease protein interacts with p53 and CREB-binding protein and represses transcription. Proc Natl Acad Sci 97: 6763–6768.
9. Huang CC, Faber PW, Persichetti F, Mittal V, Vonsattel JP, et al. (1998) Amyloid formation by mutant huntingtin: threshold, progressivity and recruitment of normal polyglutamine proteins. Somat Cell Mol Genet 24: 217–233.
10. Feng Z, Jin S, Zupnick A, Hoh J, de Stanchina E, et al. (2006) p53 tumor suppressor protein regulates the levels of huntingtin gene expression. Oncogene 25: 1–7.
11. Ryan AB, Zeitlin SO, Scrable H (2006) Genetic interaction between expanded murine Hdh alleles and p53 reveal deleterious effects of p53 on Huntington's disease pathogenesis. Neurobiol Dis 24: 419–427.
12. Khoshnan A, Ko J, Watkin EE, Paige LA, Reinhart PH, et al. (2004) Activation of the IkappaB kinase complex and nuclear factor-kappaB contributes to mutant huntingtin neurotoxicity. J Neurosci 24: 7999–8008.
13. Goswami A, Dikshit P, Mishra A, Mulherkar S, Nukina N, et al. (2006) Oxidative stress promotes mutant huntingtin aggregation and mutant huntingtin-dependent cell death by mimicking proteasomal malfunction. Biochem Biophys Res Commun 342: 184–190.
14. Godavarthi SK, Narender D, Mishra A, Goswami A, Rao SN, et al. (2009) Induction of chemokines, MCP-1, and KC in the mutant huntingtin expressing neuronal cells because of proteasomal dysfunction. J Neurochem 108: 787–795.
15. Liu J (2008) Control of protein synthesis and mRNA degradation by microRNAs. Curr Opin Cell Biol 20: 214–221.
16. Ørom UA, Nielsen FC, Lund AH (2008) MicroRNA-10a binds the 5′ UTR of ribosomal protein mRNAs and enhances their translation. Mol Cell 30: 460–471.
17. Place RF, Li LC, Pookot D, Noonan EJ, Dahiya R (2008) MicroRNA-373 induces expression of genes with complementary promoter sequences. Proc Natl Acad Sci 105: 1608–1613.
18. Tay Y, Zhang J, Thomson AM, Lim B, Rigoutsos I (2008) MicroRNAs to Nanog, Oct4 and Sox2 coding regions modulate embryonic stem cell differentiation. Nature 455: 1124–1128.
19. Lewis BP, Burge CB, Bartel DP (2005) Conserved seed pairing, often flanked by adenosines, indicates that thousands of human genes are microRNA targets. Cell 120: 15–20.
20. Miranda KC, Huynh T, Tay Y, Ang YS, Tam WL, et al. (2006) A pattern-based method for the identification of MicroRNA binding sites and their corresponding heteroduplexes. Cell 126: 1203–1217.
21. Vo N, Klein ME, Varlamova O, Keller DM, Yamamoto T, et al. (2005) A cAMP-response element binding protein-induced microRNA regulates neuronal morphogenesis. Proc Natl Acad Sci 102: 16426–16431.
22. Hermeking H (2007) p53 enters the microRNA world. Cancer Cell 12: 414–418.
23. Chang TC, Wentzel EA, Kent OA, Ramachandran K, Mullendore M, et al. (2007) Transactivation of miR-34a by p53 broadly influences gene expression and promotes apoptosis. Mol Cell 26: 745–752.
24. He L, He X, Lim LP, de Stanchina E, Xuan Z, et al. (2007) A microRNA component of the p53 tumour suppressor network. Nature 447: 1130–1134.
25. Suzuki HI, Yamagata K, Sugimoto K, Iwamoto T, Kato S, et al. (2009) Modulation of microRNA processing by p53. Nature 460: 529–533.
26. Tarasov V, Jung P, Verdoodt B, Lodygin D, Epanchintsev A, et al. (2007) Differential regulation of microRNAs by p53 revealed by massively parallel sequencing: miR-34a is a p53 target that induces apoptosis and G1-arrest. Cell Cycle 6: 1586–1593.
27. Raver-Shapira N, Marciano E, Meiri E, Spector Y, Rosenfeld N, et al. (2007) Transcriptional activation of miR-34a contributes to p53-mediated apoptosis. Mol Cell 26: 731–743.
28. Le MTN, The C, Shyh-Chang N, Xie H, Zhou B, et al. (2009) MicroRNA-125b is a novel negative regulator of p53. Genes Dev 23: 862–876.
29. Taganov KD, Boldin MP, Chang KJ, Baltimore D (2006) NF-kappaB-dependent induction of microRNA miR-146, an inhibitor targeted to signaling proteins of innate immune responses. Proc Natl Acad Sci 103: 12481–12486.
30. Johnson R, Zuccato C, Belyaev ND, Guest DJ, Cattaneo E, et al. (2008) A microRNA-based gene dysregulation pathway in Huntington's disease. Neurobiol Dis 29: 438–445.
31. Packer AN, Xing Y, Harper SQ, Jones L, Davidson BL (2008) The bifunctional microRNA miR-9/miR-9* regulates REST and CoREST and is downregulated in Huntington's disease. J Neurosci 28: 14341–14346.
32. Trettel F, Rigamonti D, Hilditch-Maguire P, Wheeler VC, Sharp AH, et al. (2000) Dominant phenotypes produced by the HD mutation in STHdh(Q111) striatal cells. Hum Mol Genet 9: 2799–2809.
33. Sinha M, Ghose J, Das E, Bhattarcharyya NP (2010) Altered microRNAs in STHdh(Q111)/Hdh(Q111) cells: miR-146a targets TBP. Biochem Biophys Res Commun 396: 742–747.
34. Chakravorty M, Datta De D, Choudhury A, Roychoudhury S (2009) IL1B promoter polymorphism regulates the expression of gastric acid stimulating hormone gastrin. Int J Biochem Cell Biol 41: 1502–1510.
35. Kopp E, Ghosh S (1994) Inhibition of NF-kappa B by sodium salicylate and aspirin. Science 265: 956–959.
36. Griffiths-Jones S (2004) The MicroRNA Registry. Nucl Acids Res 32(Database Issue): D109–D11155.
37. Kawauchi K, Araki K, Tobiume K, Tanaka N (2008) Activated p53 induces NFkappaB DNA binding but suppresses its transcriptional activation. Biochem Biophys Res Commun 372: 137–141.
38. Wadgaonkar R, Phelps KM, Haque Z, Williams AJ, Silverman ES, et al. (1999) CREB-binding protein is a nuclear integrator of nuclear factor-κB and p53 signaling. J Biol Chem 274: 1879–1882.
39. Webster GA, Perkins ND (1999) Transcriptional cross talk between NF-kB and p53. Mol Cell Biol 19: 3485–3495.
40. Huang WC, Ju TK, Hung MC, Chen CC (2007) Phosphorylation of CBP by IKKalpha promotes cell growth by switching the binding preference of CBP from p53 to NF-kappaB. Mol Cell 26: 75–87.
41. Bohuslav J, Chen LF, Kwon H, Mu Y, Greene WC (2004) p53 induces NF-kappaB activation by an IkappaB kinase-independent mechanism involving phosphorylation of p65 by ribosomal S6 kinase 1. J Biol Chem 279: 26115–26125.
42. Ryan KM, Ernst MK, Rice NR, Vousden KH (2000) Role of NF-kappaB in p53-mediated programmed cell death. Nature 404: 892–897.
43. Xiao-Xin S, Mu-Shui D, Hua L (2007) 5-Fluorouracil Activation of p53 Involves an MDM2-Ribosomal Protein Interaction. J Biol Chem 282: 8052–8059.
44. Majumder P, Raychaudhuri S, Chattopadhyay B, Bhattacharyya NP (2007) Increased caspase-2, calpain activations and decreased mitochondrial complex II activity in cells expressing exogenous huntingtin exon 1 containing CAG repeat in the pathogenic range. Cell Mol Neurobiol 27: 1127–1145.
45. Raychaudhuri S, Sinha M, Mukhopadhyay D, Bhattacharyya NP (2008) HYPK, a Huntingtin interacting protein, reduces aggregates and apoptosis induced by N-terminal Huntingtin with 40 glutamines in Neuro2a cells and exhibits chaperone-like activity. Hum Mol Genet 17: 240–255.
46. Kaznacheeva AV, Guzhova IV, Margulis BA (2009) Protective Effect of Hsp70 Molecular Chaperone in Polyglutamine Diseases Is Realized by Sequestering of GAPDH. Biologicheskie Membrany 26: 314.
47. Mangarini L, Sathasivam K, Seller M, Cozens B, Harper A, et al. (1996) Exon 1 of the *HD* Gene with an Expanded CAG Repeat Is Sufficient to Cause a Progressive Neurological Phenotype in Transgenic Mice. Cell 87: 493–506.
48. Lee ST, Chu K, Im WS, Yoon HJ, Im JY, et al. (2010) Altered microRNA regulation in Huntington's disease models. Exp Neurol 227(1): 172–179.
49. Lukiw WJ, Zhao Y, Cui JG (2008) An NF-kB-sensitive Micro RNA-146a-mediated Inflammatory Circuit in Alzheimer's Disease and in Stressed Human Brain Cells. J of Biol Chem 283: 31315–31322.
50. Hill JM, Zhao Y, Clement C, Neumann DM, Lukiw WJ (2009) HSV-1 infection of human brain cells induces miRNA-146a and Alzheimer-type inflammatory Signalling. Neuroreport 20(16): 1500–1505.
51. Aronica E, Fluiter K, Iyer A, Zurolo E, Vreijiling J, et al. (2010) Expression pattern of miR-146a, an inflammation-associated microRNA, in experimental and human temporal lobe epilepsy. Eur J Neurosci 31(6): 1100–7.
52. Saba R, Goodman CD, Huzarewich LCH, Robertson C, Booth SA (2008) A miRNA signature of prion induced neurodegeneration. PLoS One 3(11): e3652.
53. Rehmsmeier M, Steffen P, Höchsmann M, Giegerich R (2004) Fast and effective prediction of microRNA/target duplexes. RNA 10: 1507–1517.

54. Beg AA, Baltimore D (1996) An essential role for NF-kappaB in preventing TNF-alpha-induced cell death. Science 274: 782–784.
55. Bertrand F, Atfi A, Cadoret A, L'Allemain G, Robin H, et al. (1998) A role for nuclear factor kappaB in the antiapoptotic function of insulin. J Biol Chem 273: 2931–2938.
56. Royds JA, Dower SK, Qwarnstrom EE, Lewis CE (1998) Response of tumour cells to hypoxia: role of p53 and NFkB. Mol Pathol 51: 55–61.
57. Gines S, Ivanova E, Seong IS, Saura CA, MacDonald ME (2003) Enhanced Akt signaling is an early pro-survival response that reflects N-methyl-D-aspartate receptor activation in Huntington's disease knock-in striatal cells. J Biol Chem 278: 50514–50522.
58. Gines S, Seong IS, Fossale E, Ivanova E, Trettel F, et al. (2003) Specific progressive cAMP reduction implicates energy deficit in presymptomatic Huntington's disease knock-in mice. Hum Mol Genet 12: 497–508.
59. Lee JM, Ivanova EV, Seong IS, Cashorali T, Kohane I, et al. (2007) Unbiased gene expression analysis implicates the huntingtin polyglutamine tract in extra-mitochondrial energy metabolism. PLoS Genet 3(8): e135.
60. Benn CL, SunT, Sadri-Vakili G, McFarland KN, DiRocco DP, et al. (2008) Huntingtin modulates transcription, occupies gene promoters in vivo, and binds directly to DNA in a polyglutamine-dependent manner. J Neurosci 28: 10720–10733.
61. Quintanilla RA, Jin YN, Fuenzalida K, Bronfman M, Johnson G (2008) Rosiglitazone treatment prevents mitochondrial dysfunction in mutant huntingtin-expressing cells: possible role of peroxisome proliferator-activated receptor-gamma (PPARgamma) in the pathogenesis of Huntington disease. J Biol Chem 283: 25628–25637.
62. Xifró X, García-Martínez JM, Del Toro D, Alberch J, Pérez-Navarro E (2008) Calcineurin is involved in the early activation of NMDA-mediated cell death in mutant huntingtin knock-in striatal cells. J Neurochem 105: 596–612.
63. Kong PJ, Kil MO, Lee H, Kim SS, Johnson GV, et al. (2009) Increased expression of Bim contributes to the potentiation of serum deprivation-induced apoptotic cell death in Huntington's disease knock-in striatal cell line. Neurol Res 31: 77–83.
64. Subramaniam S, Sixt KM, Barrow R, Snyder SH (2009) Rhes, a Striatal Specific Protein, Mediates Mutant-Huntingtin Cytotoxicity. Science 324: 1327–1330.
65. Kim H, Kokkotou E, Na X, Rhee SH, Moyer MP, et al. (2005) *Clostridium difficile* Toxin A–Induced Colonocyte Apoptosis Involves p53-Dependent p21(WAF1/CIP1) Induction via p38 Mitogen-Activated Protein Kinase. Gastroenterology 129: 1875–1888.
66. Stanta G, Schneider C (1991) RNA extracted from paraffin-embedded human tissues is amenable to analysis by PCR amplification. Biotechniques 11(3): 304–308.
67. Stanta G, Bonin S, Perin R (1998) RNA Extraction from Formalin-Fixed and Paraffin-Embedded Tissues. Methods in Molecular Biology 86: 23–26.
68. Korbler T, Grskovic M, Dominis M, Antica M (2003) A simple method for RNA isolation from formalin-fixed and paraffin-embedded lymphatic tisuues. Experimental and Molecular Pathology 74: 336–340.
69. Li J, Smyth P, Flavin R, Cahill S, Denning K, et al. (2007) Comparison of miRNA expression patterns using total RNA extracted from matched samples of formalin-fixed paraffin-embedded (FFPE) cells and snap frozen cells. BMC Biotechnol 29: 7–36.
70. Doleshal M, Magotra AA, Choudhury B, Cannon BD, Labourier E, et al. (2008) Evaluation and validation of total RNA extraction methods for microRNA expression analyses in formalin-fixed, paraffin-embedded tissues. J Mol Diagn 10(3): 203–211.
71. Liu A, Xu X (2011) MicroRNA Isolation from Formalin-Fixed, Paraffin-Embedded Tissues. Methods Mol Biol 724: 259–67.
72. Peltier HJ, Latham GJ (2008) Normalization of microRNA expression levels in quantitative RT-PCR assays: Identification of suitable reference RNA targets in normal and cancerous human solid tissues. RNA 14: 844–852.

Association of Coagulation Activation with Clinical Complications in Sickle Cell Disease

Kenneth I. Ataga[1]*, Julia E. Brittain[2], Payal Desai[1], Ryan May[3], Susan Jones[1], John Delaney[1¤], Dell Strayhorn[1], Alan Hinderliter[4], Nigel S. Key[1]

1 Division of Hematology/Oncology, University of North Carolina, Chapel Hill, North Carolina, United States of America, **2** Department of Biochemistry and Biophysics, University of North Carolina, Chapel Hill, North Carolina, United States of America, **3** Department of Biostatistics, University of North Carolina, Chapel Hill, North Carolina, United States of America, **4** Division of Cardiology, University of North Carolina, Chapel Hill, North Carolina, United States of America

Abstract

Background: The contribution of hypercoagulability to the pathophysiology of sickle cell disease (SCD) remains poorly defined. We sought to evaluate the association of markers of coagulation and platelet activation with specific clinical complications and laboratory variables in patients with SCD.

Design and Methods: Plasma markers of coagulation activation (D-dimer and TAT), platelet activation (soluble CD40 ligand), microparticle-associated tissue factor (MPTF) procoagulant activity and other laboratory variables were obtained in a cohort of patients with SCD. Tricuspid regurgitant jet velocity was determined by Doppler echocardiography and the presence/history of clinical complications was ascertained at the time of evaluation, combined with a detailed review of the medical records.

Results: No significant differences in the levels of D-dimer, TAT, soluble CD40 ligand, and MPTF procoagulant activity were observed between patients in the SS/SD/Sβ^0 thalassemia and SC/Sβ^+ thalassemia groups. Both TAT and D-dimer were significantly correlated with measures of hemolysis (lactate dehydrogenase, indirect bilirubin and hemoglobin) and soluble vascular cell adhesion molecule-1. In patients in the SS/SD/Sβ^0 thalassemia group, D-dimer was associated with a history of stroke ($p = 0.049$), TAT was associated with a history of retinopathy ($p = 0.0176$), and CD40 ligand was associated with the frequency of pain episodes ($p = 0.039$). In multivariate analyses, D-dimer was associated with reticulocyte count, lactate dehydrogenase, NT-proBNP and history of stroke; soluble CD40 ligand was associated with WBC count and platelet count; and MPTF procoagulant activity was associated with hemoglobin and history of acute chest syndrome.

Conclusions: This study supports the association of coagulation activation with hemolysis in SCD. The association of D-dimer with a history of stroke suggests that coagulation activation may contribute to the pathophysiology of stroke in clinically severe forms of SCD. More research is needed to evaluate the contribution of coagulation and platelet activation to clinical complications in SCD.

Editor: Dimas Tadeu Covas, University of Sao Paulo – USP, Brazil

Funding: This work was supported in part by NIH grants HL79915, HL091265, and HL094592. Support for this work was also provided by an award from the North Carolina State Sickle Cell Program. The funders had no role in the study design, data collection and analysis, decision to publish, or preparation of the manuscript.

Competing Interests: The authors have declared that no competing interests exist.

* E-mail: kataga@med.unc.edu

¤ Current address: Carolina School of Medicine, Greenville, North Carolina, United States of America

Introduction

Patients with sickle cell disease (SCD) have an increased risk of stroke, pulmonary hypertension, avascular necrosis of large joints, and pregnancy-related complications, all of which may be due, at least in part, to thrombotic vascular occlusion [1]. They also appear to have a higher risk of pulmonary embolism as well as pregnancy-related venous thromboembolism compared with race-matched controls without SCD [2,3]. In addition to these thrombotic complications, patients with SCD manifest alterations in platelet function, as well as changes in the procoagulant, anticoagulant and fibrinolytic systems in the direction of a procoagulant phenotype [4]. Furthermore, tissue factor (TF) antigen and TF procoagulant activity are reported to be elevated in the circulation of SCD patients when compared with normal controls [5–7]. As a result of these findings, SCD is frequently referred to as a "hypercoagulable state."

Despite the abundant laboratory evidence of hypercoagulability observed in these patients, it still remains uncertain whether the observed platelet activation, as well as increased thrombin and fibrin generation contributes to the vascular occlusive episodes that characterize SCD or are rather simple epiphenomena.

In the present study, we sought to evaluate the association of markers of coagulation and platelet activation with specific SCD-related clinical complications and laboratory variables in a cohort of patients followed at an adult sickle cell clinic. In addition, we evaluated the relationship between microparticle-associated tissue factor procoagulant activity, plasma markers of coagulation activation and platelet activation.

Methods

Patients and Study Design

The study subjects represent a cohort of patients followed at the Adult Sickle Cell Clinic at the University of North Carolina (UNC), Chapel Hill. The data were collected as part of an ongoing study to investigate the pathophysiology of pulmonary hypertension in SCD. Sixty four patients with SCD were included in the analyses that assessed the associations of plasma markers of coagulation and platelet activation with both SCD-related clinical complications and laboratory variables. Patients with SCD were assessed while in the non-crisis, "steady state" (no current acute painful episode or illness and none requiring medical intervention for at least 1 week); had not experienced an episode of acute chest syndrome in the 4 weeks preceding enrollment; and had no clinical evidence of congestive heart failure. None of the patients was on chronic red blood cell transfusion therapy. This study was approved by the Institutional Review Board at UNC, Chapel Hill and all subjects gave written informed consent to participate in accordance with the Declaration of Helsinki.

Blood Sample Collection and Preparation. The samples from the study group were obtained during research visits while in the non-crisis, "steady state." Blood samples were obtained via venipuncture using a 21-gauge needle and drawn into citrate-containing tubes. Plasma samples were prepared in a manner that minimized platelet activation as previously described [8]. The plasma samples were aliquoted and frozen immediately at −80°C for subsequent analysis.

Microparticle-Associated Tissue Factor (MPTF) Procoagulant Activity. Platelet-free plasma was obtained from citrated whole blood by centrifugation at 1,500 g for 15 minutes, followed by a clearing spin of 13,000 g for 2 minutes. Microparticles were isolated from platelet-free plasma by centrifugation at 21,000 g for 30 minutes. The pellet was re-suspended in HBSA (20 mM HEPES, pH 7.4, 150 mM NaCl, and 1 mg/ml bovine serum albumin) and re-centrifuged at 20,000 g for 30 minutes, before the final re-suspension in 250 μL HBSA, and MPTF procoagulant activity was measured as previously described using a chromogenic assay [9,10].

Plasma Markers of Thrombin Generation, Platelet Activation and Endothelial Activation

Quantification of D-dimer (DiaPharma, Westchester, OH), thrombin-antithrombin (TAT) complexes (Dade Behring, Marburg, Germany), soluble CD40 ligand (R&D systems, Minneapolis, MN) and human soluble vascular cell adhesion molecule-1 (soluble VCAM-1) (R&D systems, Minneapolis, MN) was accomplished using commercially available ELISA kits. Samples were assayed in duplicate and according to manufacturer's instructions. Measurements of N-terminal pro-brain natriuretic peptide (NT-proBNP) and other routine laboratory studies were performed by the McClendon Clinical Laboratory at UNC Hospitals.

Sickle Cell Disease-Related Clinical Complications

The presence or history of clinical complications in SCD patients was ascertained from a history at the time of evaluation, combined with a detailed review of the medical records. Acute pain episodes (or crises), acute chest syndrome, stroke and other SCD-related complications were defined using standard definitions [11–14]. Based on a modification of the definition from both the Cooperative Study of Sickle Cell Disease [11] and the Multicenter Study of Hydroxyurea [12], acute pain episodes referred to episodes that required a visit to a medical facility for acute sickling-related pain for which treatment with a parenterally administered analgesic was needed. Tricuspid regurgitant jet velocity was measured by Doppler echocardiography as previously described [15].

Statistical Analysis

Wilcoxon rank sum tests were used to compare distributions of continuous variables in two groups. Fisher's exact tests were used to compare categorical variables. Spearman rank correlations were used to identify associations between markers of coagulation activation and specified variables ($\alpha = 0.05$). Reported p-values are considered 'nominal' and are for individual tests, unadjusted for multiple comparisons because of the exploratory nature of this study. Multivariate analyses were performed using multiple regression to assess the associations between clinical and laboratory variables that were found to be associated with markers of coagulation and platelet activation (TAT, D-dimer, soluble CD40 ligand and MPTF procoagulant activity) in univariate analyses ($P<0{\cdot}15$). Backwards elimination using Akaike's Information Criterion (AIC) was used to select the best model. Statistical analyses were performed using R statistical software (www.r-project.org).

Results

Demographic and Laboratory Characteristics

Sixty four patients with SCD (SS: 47; SC: 7; $S\beta^0$ thalassemia: 4; $S\beta^+$ thalassemia: 5; and SD: 1) were evaluated. Due to the clinical heterogeneity of SCD, the patients were arbitrarily categorized into 2 groups based on presumed disease severity - SS/SD/$S\beta^0$ thalassemia and SC/$S\beta^+$ thalassemia. The demographic and baseline laboratory characteristics of all the study subjects are shown in Table 1. As expected, patients in the SS/SD/$S\beta^0$ thalassemia group had significantly lower hemoglobin values (8.9 g/dL vs. 10.65 g/dL, $p<0.0001$), but higher platelet counts (412×10^9/L vs. 320.5×10^9/L; $p=0.0058$), reticulocyte counts (6.6% vs. 3.25%; $p=0.0011$), total bilirubin (2.2 mg/dL vs. 0.95 mg/dL; $p<0.0001$), indirect bilirubin (2.11 mg/dL vs. 0.86 mg/dL; $p<0.0001$) and lactate dehydrogenase (894 U/L vs. 641 U/L; $p=0.0011$) than patients in the SC/$S\beta^+$ thalassemia group. No significant differences were observed in the WBC count or in the level of soluble VCAM-1 when patients in both groups were compared.

Correlation of Markers of Coagulation and Platelet Activation with Laboratory Variables

No significant differences in the levels of D-dimer (1424 ng/mL; interquartile range [IQR], 745–2536 ng/mL vs. 1533.4 ng/mL; IQR, 591–2006 ng/mL, $p=0.47$), TAT (5.63 ng/L; IQR, 3.62–8.9 ng/L vs. 4.86 ng/L; IQR, 3.91–6.19 ng/L, $p=0.59$), soluble CD40 ligand (0.453 ng/mL; IQR, 0.339–0.60 ng/mL vs. 0.409 ng/mL; IQR, 0.201–0.60 ng/mL, $p=0.24$), and MPTF procoagulant activity (0.145 pg/mL, IQR 0.094–0.265 pg/mL, vs. 0.115 pg/mL, IQR 0.056–0.173 pg/mL, $p=0.17$) were observed when patients in the SS/SD/$S\beta^0$ thalassemia group were compared with patients in the SC/$S\beta^+$ thalassemia group. We observed a significant correlation between TAT and D-dimer ($r=0.66$; $p<0.0001$) (Figure 1). However, no correlations were observed between TAT and soluble CD40 ligand ($r=0.016$, $p=0.91$) or between TAT and MPTF procoagulant activity ($r=0.064$, $p=0.63$). Similarly, no correlations were observed between D-dimer and soluble CD40 ligand ($r=-0.17$; $p=0.19$)

Table 1. Baseline Clinical and Laboratory Characteristics of Study Subjects.

Variable	SS/SD/Sβ^0 thalassemia (N = 52)	SC/Sβ^+ thalassemia (N = 12)	p value
Age	37.5 (26.75, 46.25)	49 (30.25, 59.0)	0.068
*Gender: Female	29	7	1.0
*Hydroxyurea therapy (Yes)	34	4	0.054
White Blood Cell ($\times 10^9$/L)	9.1 (7.7, 11.0)	8.65 (4.7, 9.9)	0.28
Hemoglobin (g/dL)	8.9 (8.0, 9.6)	10.65 (9.9, 11.3)	$<$0.0001
Platelet Count ($\times 10^9$/L)	412 (325, 539)	320.5 (245, 386)	0.0058
Reticulocyte Count (%)	6.6 (4.5, 9.4)	3.25 (1.9, 5.0)	0.0011
Lactate Dehydrogenase (U/L)	894 (700, 1380)	641 (560, 681)	0.0011
Total Bilirubin (mg/dL)	2.2 (1.1, 3.4)	0.95 (0.65, 1.08)	$<$0.0001
Indirect Biliribin (mg/dL)	2.11 (1.01, 3.21)	0.86 (0.56, 0.98)	$<$0.0001
Soluble vascular cell adhesion molecule-1 (ng/mL)	1952 (1110, 3188)	1707 (1240, 2544)	0.45
*History of stroke (Yes)	4	1	1.0
*History of avascular necrosis (Yes)	26	5	0.76
*History of leg ulcer (Yes)	12	0	0.10
*Use of hydroxyurea (Yes)	34	4	0.06
*History of retinopathy (Yes)	14	7	0.09
*Pain crisis $\geq$3 in previous year	15	1	0.15
*History of acute chest syndrome (Yes)	48	7	0.0086
*History of priapism (Yes)	7	0	0.29

Data are presented as medians and interquartile ranges (25th and 75th percentiles).
*The results of a Fishers Exact Test.

or between D-dimer and MPTF procoagulant activity ($r = 0.11$, $p = 0.40$).

The plasma markers of coagulation activation, TAT and D-dimer, were associated with laboratory measures of hemolysis (Table 2). There was a correlation between TAT and lactate dehydrogenase ($r = 0.57$, $p < 0.0001$) (Figure 2), with borderline correlations between TAT and total bilirubin ($r = 0.25$; $p = 0.054$), indirect bilirubin ($r = 0.26$, $p = 0.051$), and hemoglobin ($r = -0.24$; $p = 0.071$). TAT was also correlated with the absolute monocyte count ($r = 0.27$; $p = 0.035$) and NT-proBNP ($r = 0.35$; $p = 0.005$). Similarly, D-dimer was correlated with lactate dehydrogenase ($r = 0.56$; $p < 0.0001$) (Figure 3), indirect bilirubin ($r = 0.26$; $p = 0.048$), hemoglobin ($r = -0.32$; $p = 0.012$), NT proBNP ($r = 0.42$; $p < 0.0001$), with borderline correlations with absolute monocyte count ($r = 0.23$; $p = 0.074$). Both TAT ($r = 0.37$; $p = 0.004$) and D-dimer ($r = 0.49$; $p < 0.0001$) (Figure 4) were also correlated with soluble VCAM-1.

Soluble CD40 ligand was correlated with WBC count ($r = 0.30$; $p = 0.018$) and platelet count ($r = 0.40$; $p = 0.0014$), but was not correlated with lactate dehydrogenase, total bilirubin, indirect bilirubin or hemoglobin (Table 3). No correlations were observed between MPTF procoagulant activity and measures of hemolysis or other measured laboratory variables.

When the analyses were limited to only patients in the SS/SD/Sβ^0 thalassemia group, there was a significant correlation between TAT and lactate dehydrogenase ($r = 0.62$, $p < 0.0001$), indirect bilirubin ($r = 0.296$, $p = 0.044$), and NT-proBNP ($r = 0.32$, $p = 0.026$), with borderline correlation with total bilirubin ($r = 0.28$, $p = 0.053$) and absolute monocyte count ($r = 0.25$, $p = 0.089$). Similarly, we observed significant correlations between D-dimer and lactate dehydrogenase ($r = 0.60$, $p < 0.0001$), hemoglobin ($r = -0.29$, $p = 0.039$), fetal hemoglobin ($r = -0.31$, $p = 0.035$), and NT-proBNP ($r = 0.49$, $p < 0.0001$), with borderline correlations with platelet count ($r = -0.28$, $p = 0.053$), total bilirubin ($r = 0.24$, $p = 0.093$) and indirect bilirubin ($r = 0.26$, $p = 0.07$). Soluble CD40 ligand was correlated

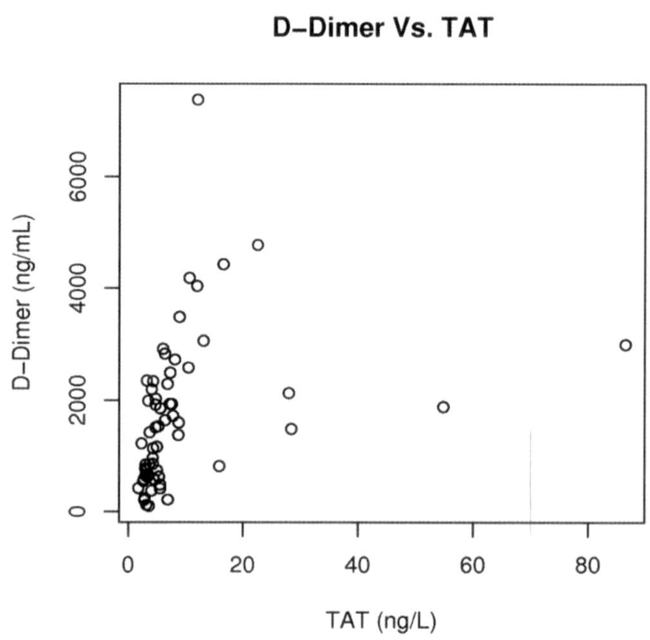

Figure 1. TAT is correlated with D-dimer in sickle cell disease. Plasma TAT is significantly correlated with plasma D-dimer in our study cohort ($r = 0.66$; $p < 0.0001$).

Table 2. Correlation of Markers of Coagulation Activation with Laboratory Variables.

Biomarker	Laboratory Variable	Number of Patients	r value	95% Confidence Interval	p value
TAT	White blood cell count	60	0.038	−0.242–0.31	0.77
	Absolute neutrophil count	60	−0.078	−0.338–0.19	0.55
	Absolute monocyte count	60	0.273	0.018–0.494	0.035
	Hemoglobin	60	−0.235	−0.457–0.005	0.071
	Platelet count	60	−0.154	−0.401–0.096	0.24
	Reticulocyte count	59	0.195	−0.041–0.412	0.14
	Hemoglobin F	57	−0.165	−0.416–0.112	0.22
	Lactate dehydrogenase	60	0.57	0.376–0.717	<0.0001
	Total bilirubin	61	0.248	0.026–0.45	0.054
	Direct bilirubin	58	0.015	−0.251–0.272	0.91
	Indirect bilirubin	58	0.258	0.028–0.456	0.051
	NT-proBNP	61	0.354	0.129–0.541	0.005
D-dimer	White blood count	61	−0.027	−0.287–0.234	0.83
	Absolute neutrophil count	61	−0.112	−0.381–0.16	0.39
	Absolute monocyte count	61	0.231	−0.038–0.486	0.074
	Hemoglobin	61	−0.318	−0.528–0.074	0.013
	Platelet count	61	−0.193	−0.45–0.078	0.14
	Reticulocyte count	60	0.197	−0.055–0.425	0.13
	Hemoglobin F	58	−0.148	−0.4–0.122	0.27
	Lactate dehydrogenase	61	0.559	0.372–0.697	<0.0001
	Total bilirubin	62	0.236	0.015–0.436	0.065
	Direct bilirubin	59	0.113	−0.188–0.387	0.39
	Indirect bilirubin	59	0.258	0.028–0.466	0.048
	NT-proBNP	62	0.417	0.192–0.6	<0.0001

TAT – Thrombin-antithrombin complexes.
NT-proBNP – N-terminal pro-brain natriuretic peptide.

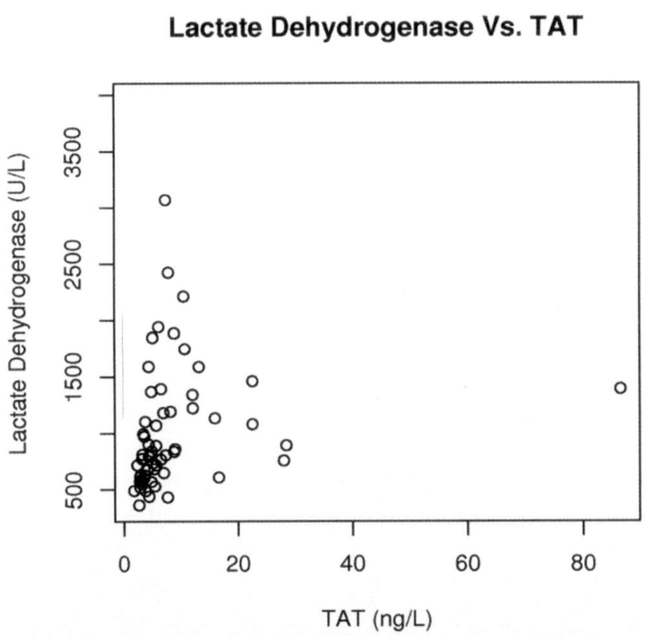

Figure 2. TAT is correlated with lactate dehydrogenase in sickle cell disease. TAT is correlated with lactate dehydrogenase in our study cohort (r = 0.57, p<0.0001).

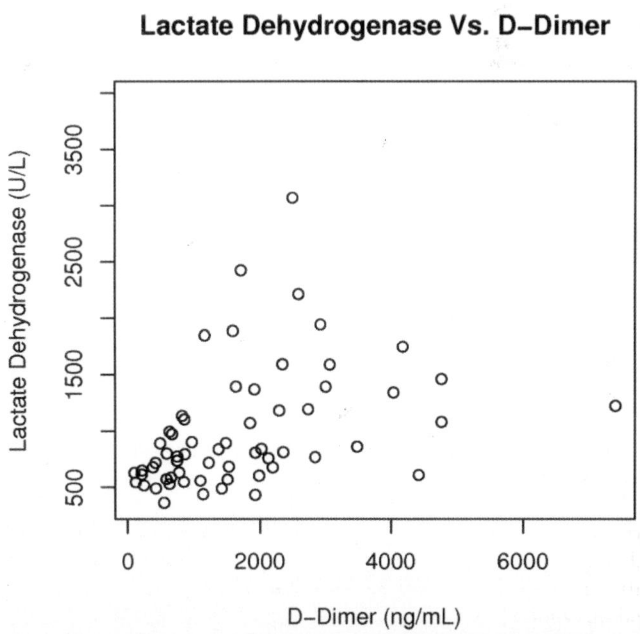

Figure 3. D-dimer is correlated with lactate dehydrogenase in sickle cell disease. D-dimer is correlated with lactate dehydrogenase in our study cohort (r = 0.56; p<0.0001).

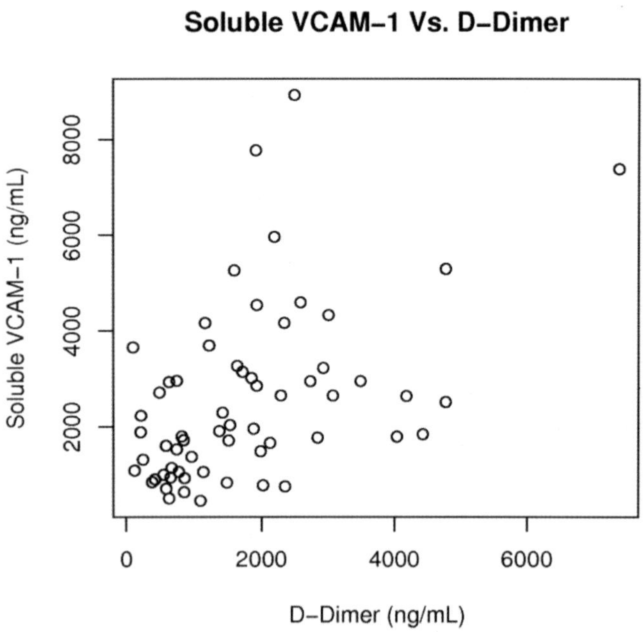

Figure 4. D-dimer is correlated with soluble VCAM-1 in sickle cell disease. D-dimer is correlated with soluble VCAM-1 in our study cohort ($r=0.49$; $p<0.0001$).

with platelet count ($r=0.41$, $p=0.003$), but not correlated with lactate dehydrogenase, total bilirubin, indirect bilirubin or hemoglobin. MPTF procoagulant activity was correlated with hemoglobin ($r=0.31$, $p=0.034$), but not correlated with measures of hemolysis or other measured laboratory variables.

Association of Measures of Coagulation and Platelet Activation with Clinical Complications. The level of TAT was significantly higher in patients with a history of retinopathy compared to those without this complication (6.05 ng/L; IQR, 4.91, 10.98 ng/L vs. 4.52 ng/L; IQR, 3.22, 7.33 ng/L, $p=0.023$) (Table 4). In addition, the level of TAT was lower in patients on hydroxyurea therapy compared to those not on such therapy (4.39 ng/L; IQR, 3.25, 8.77 ng/L vs. 6.5 ng/L; IQR, 5.08, 8.76 ng/L, $p=0.044$). D-dimer appeared to be associated with a history of stroke (3003.1 ng/mL [FEU]; IQR, 1513, 3067 ng/mL [FEU] vs. 1399.5 ng/mL [FEU]; 648.8, 2217 ng/mL [FEU], $p=0.062$), although the difference was not statistically significant. When those patients with a measurable tricuspid regurgitant jet velocity were evaluated ($N=43$), there was no correlation between D-dimer and tricuspid regurgitant jet velocity ($r=0.25$, $p=0.10$). There was an association between MPTF procoagulant activity and a history of acute chest syndrome (0.1445 pg/mL; IQR, 0.11, 0.268 pg/mL vs. 0.07 pg/mL; IQR, 0, 0.149 pg/mL, $p=0.045$) (Table 5). Finally, soluble CD40 ligand appeared to be associated with the frequency of pain episodes (<3 episodes vs. ≥3 episodes in the past year: 0.406 ng/mL; IQR, 0.428, 0.677 ng/mL vs.

Table 3. Correlation of Microparticle-Associated Tissue factor Procoagulant Activity and Platelet Activation with Laboratory Variables.

Biomarker	Laboratory Variable	Number of Patients	r value	95% Confidence Interval	p value
MPTF	White blood cell count	59	−0.177	−0.443–0.106	0.18
	Absolute neutrophil count	59	−0.144	−0.413–0.146	0.28
	Absolute monocyte count	59	−0.134	−0.404–0.144	0.31
	Hemoglobin	59	0.15	−0.123–0.409	0.26
	Platelet count	59	−0.159	−0.398–0.091	0.23
	Reticulocyte count	58	−0.063	−0.325–0.208	0.64
	Hemoglobin F	56	0.211	−0.047–0.444	0.12
	Lactate dehydrogenase	59	0.011	−0.255–0.271	0.94
	Total bilirubin	60	0.019	−0.248–0.281	0.89
	Direct bilirubin	57	−0.045	−0.308–0.233	0.74
	Indirect bilirubin	57	0.024	−0.258–0.293	0.86
	NT-proBNP	60	−0.1	−0.352–0.166	0.45
CD40 ligand	White blood count	61	0.303	0.065–0.518	0.018
	Absolute neutrophil count	61	0.215	−0.031–0.448	0.096
	Absolute monocyte count	61	0.079	−0.187–0. 339	0.55
	Hemoglobin	61	−0.096	−0.372–0.182	0.46
	Platelet count	61	0.4	0.168–0.595	0.0014
	Reticulocyte count	60	0.098	−0.17–0.359	0.46
	Hemoglobin F	58	0.023	−0.252–0.299	0.86
	Lactate dehydrogenase	61	−0.08	−0.355–0.197	0.54
	Total bilirubin	62	−0.048	−0.287–0.194	0.71
	Direct bilirubin	59	−0.104	−0.328–0.123	0.43
	Indirect bilirubin	59	−0.015	−0.261–0.238	0.91
	NT-proBNP	62	0.104	−0.172–0.359	0.42

MPTF PCA – Microparticle-associated tissue factor procoagulant activity.
NT-proBNP – N-terminal pro-brain natriuretic peptide.

0.498 ng/mL; IQR, 0.292, 0.579 ng/mL, p = 0.058), although the difference was not statistically significant.

When the analyses were limited to patients in the SS/SD/Sβ^0 thalassemia group, we observed associations between D-dimer and a history of stroke (3035.2 ng/mL [FEU]; IQR 2559, 3494 vs. 1269.6 ng/mL [FEU]; IQR 688.4, 2347, p = 0.049), TAT and history of retinopathy (7.145 ng/L; IQR 5.225, 12.01vs. 4.465 ng/L; IQR 3.215, 7.332, p = 0.018), and soluble CD40 ligand and frequency of pain episodes (<3 episodes vs. ≥3 episodes in the past year: 0.398 ng/mL; IQR 0.308, 0.568 ng/mL vs. 0.543 ng/mL; IQR 0.434, 0.730 ng/mL, p = 0.039), but the previously observed association between MPTF procoagulant activity and acute chest syndrome was no longer significant (0.148 pg/mL; IQR 0.115, 0.274 pg/mL vs. 0.094 pg/mL; IQR 0.047, 0.155 pg/mL, p = 0.32). There appeared to be a correlation between tricuspid regurgitant jet velocity and D-dimer (r = 0.3, p = 0.067), although this was not statistically significant.

Multivariate Analyses

Clinical and laboratory variables were selected for use in the multivariate model via a backwards elimination procedure using AIC as the fit criterion. The clinical variables were history of stroke, retinopathy, avascular necrosis, history of leg ulcers, and history of acute chest syndrome. The laboratory variables were lactate dehydrogenase, hemoglobin, reticulocyte count, white blood cell count, absolute neutrophil count, platelet count, total bilirubin, direct bilirubin, and NT-proBNP (Table 6). In this multivariate model, D-Dimer was associated with reticulocyte count (estimate: 92.56, p = 0.04), lactate dehydrogenase (estimate: 1.22, p = 0.0002), NT-proBNP (estimate: 0.44, p<0.0001) and history of stroke (estimate: 984.01, p = 0.051). This means that for continuous variables such as lactate dehydrogenase, we expect an increase in D-dimer by 1.22 units for every 1 unit increase in lactate dehydrogenase. For binary responses such as history of stroke, the estimated value of 984.01 indicates that having a history of stroke is predicted to result in an increase in D-dimer of 984.01 ng/mL [FEU] compared to no history of stroke. Soluble CD40 ligand was associated with WBC count (estimate: 0.04, p = 0.05), and platelet count (estimate: 0.001, p = 0.0016). Finally, MPTF procoagulant activity was associated with hemoglobin (estimate: 0.024, p = 0.023), and history of acute chest syndrome (estimate: 0.103, p = 0.029).

Discussion

Although SCD is characterized by hypercoagulability [1,4], the contribution of coagulation and platelet activation to disease pathophysiology remains poorly defined. Plasma levels of TAT, prothrombin fragment 1.2 and D-dimer are increased in patients with SCD during the non-crisis, "steady state" and are further increased during acute pain episodes [16]. D-dimer levels are reported to correlate with the frequency of pain episodes measured during the following year [16] as well as the interval for development of pain episodes, suggesting that coagulation activation may contribute to vaso-occlusion in SCD. Platelets are also activated in SCD during the non-crisis, "steady state," with further activation during acute pain episodes [7,16]. In addition, platelet activation, marked by activated fibrinogen receptor, has been reported to correlate with echocardiography-derived tricuspid jet regurgitant velocity suggesting an association with pulmonary hypertension in SCD [17].

In our present cross-sectional study, we observed no differences in markers of coagulation and platelet activation when patients in the SS/SD/Sβ^0 thalassemia group were compared to patients in the SC/Sβ^+ thalassemia group. Patients with sickle cell anemia (HbSS) have previously been reported to have higher plasma levels of markers of coagulation activation compared to patients with HbSC disease [18]. The reason for the absence of a difference between the groups in our study is uncertain, but may be related to the arbitrary grouping of the various genotypes based on the

Table 4. Association of Markers of Coagulation Activation with Clinical Variables.

Biomarker	Clinical Variable	N	Yes (Median, IQR)	N	No (Median, IQR)	p value
TAT (ng/L)	History of stroke	5	13.1 (4.83, 22.55)	55	5.09 (3.62, 7.73)	0.25
	Avascular necrosis	31	5.33 (3.66, 8.30)	30	5.35 (3.70, 9.90)	0.66
	History of leg ulcer	12	5.52 (3.73, 8.73)	48	4.95 (3.36, 6.42)	0.45
	Use of hydroxyurea	36	4.39 (3.25, 8.77)	25	6.5 (5.08, 8.76)	0.044
	History of retinopathy	20	6.05 (4.91, 10.98)	39	4.52 (3.22, 7.33)	0.023
	Pain crisis ≥3 in previous year	15	5.62 (4.26, 12.31)	40	5.38 (3.73, 7.92)	0.70
	History of acute chest syndrome	53	5.42 (3.75, 8.81)	8	4.84 (3.56, 7.13)	0.47
	History of priapism	6	4.81 (3.69, 9.13)	20	5.25 (4.03, 10.98)	0.84
D-dimer (ng/mL [FEU])	History of stroke	5	3003.1 (1513, 3067)	56	1399.5 (648.8, 2217)	0.062
	Avascular necrosis	31	1487 (760.3, 2023)	31	1883.7 (643.4, 2414)	0.72
	History of leg ulcer	12	1269.6 (716.4, 2023)	49	1513.3 (669.7, 2350)	0.77
	Use of hydroxyurea	37	1095.9 (589.4, 2023)	25	1719.4 (1164, 2490)	0.14
	History of retinopathy	20	1626.4 (827.2, 2878)	40	1300.2 (648.8, 2168)	0.41
	Pain crisis ≥3 in previous year	16	1235.5 (562.1, 2076)	40	1587.7 (768.5, 2408)	0.41
	History of acute chest syndrome	54	1500.2 (752.3, 2347)	8	1331.8 (467.1, 1953)	0.39
	History of priapism	6	688.5 (600.2, 2123)	20	1325.6 (580.6, 2339)	0.79

TAT – Thrombin-antithrombin complexes.
N – Number of patients.

Table 5. Association of Microparticle-Associated Tissue factor Procoagulant Activity and Platelet Activation with Clinical Variables.

Biomarker	Clinical Variable	N	Yes (Median, IQR)	N	No (Median, IQR)	p value
MPTF PCA (pg/mL)	History of stroke	4	0.208 (0.17, 0.23)	55	0.14 (0.087, 0.246)	0.46
	Avascular necrosis	30	0.15 (0.117, 0.215)	30	0.135 (0.051, 0.278)	0.54
	History of leg ulcer	12	0.136 (0.072, 0.26)	47	0.143 (0.091, 0.225)	0.89
	Use of hydroxyurea	35	0.144 (0.115, 0.246)	25	0.14 (0.065, 0.215)	0.52
	History of retinopathy	20	0.136 (0.081, 0.174)	38	0.143 (0.089, 0.262)	0.42
	Pain crisis ≥3 in previous year	14	0.144 (0.117, 0.294)	40	0.141 (0.069, 0.219)	0.42
	History of acute chest syndrome	52	0.145 (0.11, 0.268)	8	0.07 (0, 0.149)	0.045
	History of priapism	6	0.218 (0.144, 0.271)	19	0.14 (0.105, 0.225)	0.48
CD40 ligand (ng/mL)	History of stroke	5	0.487 (0.409, 0.543)	56	0.444 (0.309, 0.619)	0.76
	Avascular necrosis	31	0.454 (0.354, 0.627)	31	0.424 (0.308, 0.544)	0.39
	History of leg ulcer	12	0.468 (0.404, 0.552)	49	0.43 (0.302, 0.624)	0.53
	Use of hydroxyurea	37	0.429 (0.308, 0.624)	25	0.447 (0.378, 0.575)	0.92
	History of retinopathy	20	0.398 (0.282, 0.628)	40	0.462 (0.373, 0.597)	0.28
	Pain crisis ≥3 in previous year	16	0.498 (0.428, 0.677)	40	0.406 (0.292, 0.579)	0.058
	History of acute chest syndrome	54	0.453 (0.334, 0.615)	8	0.36 (0.214, 0.474)	0.19
	History of priapism	6	0.43 (0.401, 0.516)	20	0.416 (0.285, 0.667)	0.84

MPTF PCA – Microparticle-associated tissue factor procoagulant activity.
N – Number of patients.

Table 6. Multivariate Analysis.

	Covariate	Number of patients	Estimate	p value
TAT	Intercept	52	3.14	0.099
	Lactate dehydrogenase		0.003	0.082
	History of stroke		4.59	0.13
	History of retinopathy		2.94	0.093
D-dimer	Intercept	53	51.2	0.89
	Reticulocyte count		92.56	0.042
	Lactate dehydrogenase		1.22	0.0002
	Indirect bilirubin		−112.8	0.19
	NT-proBNP		0.438	<0.0001
	History of stroke		984.01	0.051
	History of avascular necrosis		−437.39	0.10
	History of leg ulcer		−566.43	0.10
	History of retinopathy		521.84	0.073
CD40 ligand	Intercept	51	0.032	0.79
	White blood cell count		0.044	0.049
	Absolute neutrophil count		−0.044	0.15
	Platelet count		0.001	0.0016
	Indirect bilirubin		−0.031	0.062
MPTF PCA	Intercept	53	−0.14	0.21
	Hemoglobin		0.024	0.023
	NT-proBNP		0.000	0.16
	History of retinopathy		−0.054	0.13
	History of acute chest syndrome		0.103	0.029

TAT – Thrombin-antithrombin complexes.
MPTF PCA – Microparticle-associated tissue factor procoagulant activity.
NT-proBNP – N-terminal pro-brain natriuretic peptide.

presumed severity of disease. Furthermore, as patients with more "severe" genotypes are more likely to be treated with hydroxyurea, it is possible that the lack of a difference may be due to a decrease in disease severity following hydroxyurea therapy. This presumption is supported by our finding of an association between TAT and hydroxyurea use on univariate analysis. In addition, hydroxyurea has previously been reported to decrease D-dimer levels in patients with SCD [19], suggesting that this drug may decrease the coagulation activation observed in SCD.

As expected, we observed significant correlations between TAT and D-dimer. This is consistent with previous reports in SCD [16]. Similar to previous publications by our group and others [15,20], our finding of correlations between both TAT and D-dimer with measures of hemolysis extends and confirms the contribution of hemolysis to coagulation activation in SCD. Heme, an inflammatory mediator and a product of hemolysis, has been shown to induce TF expression on the surface of both macrovascular and microvascular endothelial cells in a concentration-dependent manner [21]. In addition, heme produces an upregulation of the expression of TF mRNA, TF protein, and TF procoagulant activity in endothelial cells in a time-dependent manner, effects that may be mediated, at least in part, by the transcription factor, NFkappaB. Thus, heme-induced endothelial TF expression may provide a pathophysiologic link between hemolysis and the coagulation activation in SCD. Unlike a previous report that suggested an association between hemolysis and platelet activation [17], no correlation was observed between soluble CD40 ligand and measures of hemolysis in our study. Surprisingly, no correlations were observed between the measured plasma markers of coagulation activation (TAT and D-dimer) with either soluble CD40 ligand or MPTF procoagulant activity in our study. As CD40 ligand is known to induce the expression of TF in SCD [7], the reason for the lack of association between the plasma markers of coagulation activation and soluble CD40 ligand is uncertain. Furthermore, although MPTF procoagulant activity has previously been reported to correlate with plasma markers of coagulation activation in SCD [22], a recent report showed that while whole blood TF procoagulant activity was correlated with TAT, D-dimer, as well as markers of hemolysis, inflammation and endothelial activation, no such correlations were observed between MPTF procoagulant activity and any of these markers [23]. As a result, the contribution of MPTF procoagulant activity to coagulation activation in SCD remains uncertain.

The correlation of both TAT and D-dimer with soluble VCAM-1 suggests a relationship between activation of the coagulation system and endothelial activation in SCD. Furthermore, the correlation of TAT (and possibly D-dimer) with the absolute monocyte count suggests that monocytes may play a role in the coagulation activation in SCD. Monocytes are activated [24], abnormally express TF [5] and are a source of TF-positive microparticles [22] in SCD. There is increasing evidence of a crosstalk between coagulation activation and inflammation [25]. SCD is often referred to as a chronic inflammatory disease [26,27] and circulating endothelial cells in SCD patients are reported to express TF [28]. While the observed association between plasma markers of coagulation activation and measures of inflammation in our study does not prove causality, the inflammatory state in SCD may indeed contribute to hypercoagulability in SCD. Studies in transgenic SCD mice demonstrate that the induction of ischemia-reperfusion injury by exposure of the mild sickle-cell phenotype, NY1DD mice, to a hypoxic environment followed by a return to ambient air resulted in increased TF expression in the pulmonary veins [29].

The association between D-dimer and a history of stroke suggests that coagulation activation may contribute to the pathogenesis of stroke in SCD. Although the pathophysiology of stroke in SCD is complex, large vessel arterial obstruction with superimposed thrombosis is commonly observed in patients with thrombotic stroke [30]. Despite the absence of a significant association between coagulation activation and echocardiography-derived tricuspid regurgitant jet velocity in our study, autopsy series show the presence of in situ thrombosis in the pulmonary vasculature of patients with SCD-related pulmonary hypertension [31]. A recent study evaluating the relative role played by cells and plasma in the hypercoagulability observed in β thalassemia patients showed evidence of hypercoagulability based on thromboelastometry evaluation, but thrombin generation determined in platelet-poor plasma was not significantly different from healthy individuals [32]. With the known contribution of red blood cells and other cellular elements to hypercoagulability in SCD, this finding suggests that much like in β thalassemia, evaluation of whole blood may be required to accurately demonstrate associations between coagulation activation and clinical complications in SCD. The absence of an association between coagulation activation and echocardiography-derived tricuspid regurgitant jet velocity in our study may also reflect the small number of patients with catheterization-proven pulmonary hypertension in our cohort. Indeed, a recent multicenter study found no evidence of pulmonary hypertension following right heart catheterization in 72 of 96 patients with elevated tricuspid regurgitant jet velocities on echocardiography, suggesting that Doppler echocardiography may overestimate the prevalence of this condition [33].

The association between soluble CD40 ligand and the frequency of pain episodes in the past year in the SS/SD/Sβ^0 thalassemia group suggests that platelet activation may contribute to the pathogenesis of acute pain episodes in SCD. This finding is consistent with a previous report showing a correlation between platelet procoagulant activity assessed by annexin V binding and the frequency of pain episodes measured during the following year [16]. Platelet-derived CD40 ligand has been shown to induce tissue factor expression, endothelial cell expression of ICAM-1 and B-cell proliferation in SCD [7] and as such may play a role in disease pathophysiology.

Our study has several limitations. The patients were recruited from a specialty clinic at a tertiary care medical center, and may not represent all patients with SCD. The study population is relatively small, while the number of comparisons made is relatively large. We have reported only nominal p-values for each statistical test, with no adjustment made for multiple comparisons, reflecting the exploratory nature of this study. As with all cross-sectional studies, this analysis demonstrates associations, but cannot prove causation.

In summary, our study supports and extends the association of coagulation activation with hemolysis in SCD. TAT was associated with D-dimer, but these markers of coagulation activation were not associated with soluble CD40 ligand or MPTF procoagulant activity. We also show that D-dimer is associated with a history of stroke in patients with clinically severe forms of SCD. More research is needed to evaluate the pathophysiology of coagulation and platelet activation and their contribution to clinical complications in SCD.

Acknowledgments

The authors thank Ms. Melissa Caughey, MPH for help with the echocardiographic studies.

Author Contributions

Conceived and designed the experiments: KIA JEB. Performed the experiments: JEB JD. Analyzed the data: KIA RM. Contributed reagents/materials/analysis tools: JEB AH NSK. Wrote the paper: KIA JEB PD RM SJ JD DS AH NSK.

References

1. Ataga KI, Key NS (2007) Hypercoagulability in sickle cell disease: new approaches to an old problem. Hematology Am Soc Hematol Educ Program. pp 91–96.
2. Stein PD, Beemath A, Meyers FA, Skaf E, Olson RE (2006) Deep venous thrombosis and pulmonary embolism in hospitalized patients with sickle cell disease. Am J Med 119: 897.e7–e11.
3. James AH, Jamison MG, Brancazio LR, Myers ER (2006) Venous thromboembolism during pregnancy and the postpartum period: incidence, risk factors and mortality. Am J Obst Gynecol 194: 1311–1315.
4. Francis RB (1991) Platelets, coagulation, and fibrinolysis in sickle cell disease: their possible role in vascular occlusion. Blood Coagul Fibrinolysis 2: 341–353.
5. Key NS, Slungaard A, Dandelet L, Nelson SC, Moertel C, et al. (1998) Whole blood tissue factor procoagulant activity is elevated in patients with sickle cell disease. Blood 91: 4216–4223.
6. Mohan JS, Lip GYH, Wright J, Bareford D, Blann AD (2005) Plasma levels of tissue factor and soluble E-selectin in sickle cell disease: relationship to genotype and to inflammation. Blood Coagul Fibrinolysis 16: 209–214.
7. Lee SP, Ataga KI, Orringer EP, Parise LV (2006) Biologically active CD40 ligand is elevated in sickle cell disease: potential role for platelet-mediated inflammation. Arterioscler Thromb Vasc 26: 1626–1631.
8. Brittain JE, Hulkower B, Jones SK, Strayhorn D, De Castro L, et al. (2010) Placenta growth factor in sickle cell disease: association with hemolysis and inflammation. Blood 115: 2014–2020.
9. Manly DA, Wang J, Glover SL, Kasthuri R, Liebman HA, et al. (2009) Increased microparticle tissue factor activity in cancer patients with Venous Thromboembolism. Thromb Res 125: 511–512.
10. Khorana AA, Francis CW, Menzies KE, Wang JG, Hyrien O, et al. (2008) Plasma tissue factor may be predictive of venous thromboembolism in pancreatic cancer. J Thromb Haemost 6: 1983–1985.
11. Platt OS, Thorington BD, Brambilla DJ, Milner PF, Rosse WF, et al. (1991) Pain in sickle cell disease. Rates and risk factors. N Engl J Med 325: 11–16.
12. Charache S, Terrin ML, Moore RD, Dover GJ, Barton FB, et al. (1995) Effect of hydroxyurea on the frequency of painful crises in sickle cell anemia. Investigators of the Multicenter Study of Hydroxyurea in Sickle Cell Anemia. N Engl J Med 332: 1317–1322.
13. Vichinsky EP, Neumayr LD, Earles AN, Williams R, Lennette ET, et al. (2000) Causes and outcomes of the acute chest syndrome in sickle cell disease. National Acute Chest Syndrome Study Group. N Engl J Med 342: 1855–1865.
14. Ohene-Frempong K, Weiner SJ, Sleeper LA, Miller ST, Embury S, et al. (1998) Cerebrovascular accidents in sickle cell disease: rates and risk factors. Blood 91: 288–294.
15. Ataga KI, Moore CG, Hillery CA, Jones S, Whinna HC, et al. (2008) Coagulation activation and inflammation in sickle cell disease-association pulmonary hypertension. Haematologica 93: 20–26.
16. Tomer A, Harker LA, Kasey S, Eckman JR (2001) Thrombogenesis in sickle cell disease. J Lab Clin Med 137: 398–407.
17. Villagra J, Shiva S, Hunter LA, Machado RF, Gladwin MT, et al. (2007) Platelet activation in patients with sickle disease, hemolysis-associated pulmonary hypertension and nitric oxide scavenging by cell-free hemoglobin. Blood 110: 2166–72.
18. Westerman MP, Green D, Gilman-Sachs A, Beaman K, Freels S, et al. Antiphospholipid antibodies, proteins C and S, and coagulation changes in sickle cell disease. J Lab Clin Med 134: 352–62.
19. Orringer EP, Jones S, Strayhorn D, Hoffman E, Parker J, et al. (1996) The Effect of Hydroxyurea (HU) Administration on Circulating D-Dimer Levels in Patients with Sickle Cell Anemia. Blood 88: 496a.
20. van Beers EJ, Spronk HM, Ten Cate H, Duits AJ, Brandjes DP, et al. (2008) No association of the hypercoagulable state with sickle cell disease related pulmonary hypertension. Haematologica 93: e42–44.
21. Setty BN, Betal SG, Zhang J, Stuart MJ (2008) Heme induces endothelial tissue factor expression: potential role in hemostatic activation in patients with hemolytic anemia. J Thromb Haemost 6: 2202–2209.
22. Shet AS, Aras O, Gupta K, Hass MJ, Rausch DJ, et al. (2003) Sickle blood contains tissue factor-positive microparticles derived from endothelial cells and monocytes. Blood 102: 2678–2683.
23. Setty Y, Key NS, Rao AK, Krishnan S, Gayen-Betal S, et al. (2010) Tissue factor procoagulant activity and coagulation activation in sickle cell disease: Relationship with biomarkers of hemolysis and inflammation. Blood 116: 4210A.
24. Belcher JD, Marker PH, Weber JP, Hebbel RP, Vercellotti GM (2000) Activated monocytes in sickle cell disease: potential role in the activation of vascular endothelium and vaso-occlusion. Blood 96: 2451–2459.
25. Levi M, ten Cate H, van der Poll T (2002) Endothelium: Interface between coagulation and inflammation. Crit Care Med 30: S220–224.
26. Platt OS (2000) Sickle cell anemia as an inflammatory disease. J Clin Invest 106: 337–338.
27. Hebbel RP, Osarogiagbon R, Kaul D (2004) The endothelial biology of sickle cell disease: inflammation and a chronic vasculopathy. Microcirculation 11: 129–51.
28. Solovey A, Gui L, Key NS, Hebbel RP (1998) Tissue factor expression by endothelial cells in sickle cell anemia. J Clin Invest 101: 1899–1904.
29. Solovey A, Kollander R, Shet A, Milbauer LC, Choong S, et al. (2004) Endothelial cell expression of tissue factor in sickle mice is augmented by hypoxia/reoxygenation and inhibited by lovastatin. Blood 104: 840–846.
30. Prengler M, Pavlakis SG, Prohovnik I, Adams RJ (2002) Sickle cell disease: the neurological complications. Ann Neurol 51: 543–552.
31. Adedeji MO, Cespedes J, Allen K, Subramony C, Hughson MD (2001) Pulmonary thrombotic arteriopathy in patients with sickle cell disease. Arch Pathol Lab Med 125: 1436–1441.
32. Tripodi A, Cappellini MD, Chantarangkul V, Padovan L, Fasulo MR, et al. (2009) Hypercoagulability in splenectomized thalassemic patients detected by whole-blood thromboelastometry, but not by thrombin generation in platelet-poor plasma. Haematologica 94: 1520–1527.
33. Parent F, Bachir D, Inamo J, Lionnet F, Driss F, et al. (2011) A hemodynamic study of pulmonary hypertension in sickle cell disease. N Engl J Med 365: 44–53.

5

A Genome-Wide Association Study of Total Bilirubin and Cholelithiasis Risk in Sickle Cell Anemia

Jacqueline N. Milton[1], Paola Sebastiani[1], Nadia Solovieff[1], Stephen W. Hartley[1], Pallav Bhatnagar[4], Dan E. Arking[4], Daniel A. Dworkis[2], James F. Casella[5], Emily Barron-Casella[5], Christopher J. Bean[6], W. Craig Hooper[6], Michael R. DeBaun[7], Melanie E. Garrett[8], Karen Soldano[8], Marilyn J. Telen[8], Allison Ashley-Koch[8], Mark T. Gladwin[9], Clinton T. Baldwin[2], Martin H. Steinberg[2], Elizabeth S. Klings[2,3]*

1 Department of Biostatistics, Boston University School of Public Health, Boston, Massachusetts, United States of America, **2** Department of Medicine, Boston University School of Medicine, Boston, Massachusetts, United States of America, **3** The Pulmonary Center, Boston University School of Medicine, Boston, Massachusetts, United States of America, **4** McKusick-Nathans Institute of Genetic Medicine, Johns Hopkins University School of Medicine, Baltimore, Maryland, United States of America, **5** Department of Pediatrics, Division of Pediatric Hematology, Johns Hopkins University School of Medicine, Baltimore, Maryland, United States of America, **6** Clinical and Molecular Hemostasis Laboratory Branch, Division of Blood Disorders, National Center on Birth Defects and Developmental Disabilities, Centers for Disease Control and Prevention, Atlanta, Georgia, United States of America, **7** Vanderbilt School of Medicine, Nashville, Tennessee, United States of America, **8** Department of Medicine, Duke University Medical Center, Durham, North Carolina, United States of America, **9** Division of Pulmonary, Allergy and Critical Care Medicine and the Vascular Medicine Institute, University of Pittsburgh, Pittsburgh, Pennsylvania, United States of America

Abstract

Serum bilirubin levels have been associated with polymorphisms in the *UGT1A1* promoter in normal populations and in patients with hemolytic anemias, including sickle cell anemia. When hemolysis occurs circulating heme increases, leading to elevated bilirubin levels and an increased incidence of cholelithiasis. We performed the first genome-wide association study (GWAS) of bilirubin levels and cholelithiasis risk in a discovery cohort of 1,117 sickle cell anemia patients. We found 15 single nucleotide polymorphisms (SNPs) associated with total bilirubin levels at the genome-wide significance level (p value $<5\times10^{-8}$). SNPs in *UGT1A1, UGT1A3, UGT1A6, UGT1A8* and *UGT1A10*, different isoforms within the *UGT1A* locus, were identified (most significant rs887829, $p=9.08\times10^{-25}$). All of these associations were validated in 4 independent sets of sickle cell anemia patients. We tested the association of the 15 SNPs with cholelithiasis in the discovery cohort and found a significant association (most significant p value 1.15×10^{-4}). These results confirm that the *UGT1A* region is the major regulator of bilirubin metabolism in African Americans with sickle cell anemia, similar to what is observed in other ethnicities.

Editor: Ana Paula Arez, Instituto de Higiene e Medicina Tropical, Portugal

Funding: This study was funded by National Institutes of Health/National Heart, Lung and Blood Institute grant # 1RC2HL101212. The funders had no role in study design, data collection and analysis, decision to publish, or preparation of the manuscript.

Competing Interests: The authors have declared that no competing interests exist.

* E-mail: klingon@bu.edu

Introduction

Cholelithiasis is the most common gastrointestinal disease to require hospitalization worldwide [1]. Most gallstones are primarily comprised of cholesterol; however, in certain patient risk groups, bile pigment stones are extremely common and represent a significant cause of morbidity. These stones are associated with increased serum unconjugated bilirubin levels, which occur in a number of conditions including hemolytic anemia. In other patient groups, ineffective erythropoiesis, ileal diseases, or gastrointestinal resections producing increased colonic spillage of bile salts, predispose to bile pigment stones [2].

Patients with sickle cell disease (SCD), particularly those with sickle cell anemia (homozygosity for *HBB* glu6val), are at risk for bile pigment cholelithiasis due to the association of this disease with hemolysis which produces an unconjugated hyperbilirubinemia [3]. Cholelithiasis occurs in up to 70% of these patients, resulting from the precipitation of polymerized calcium bilirubinate within the gallbladder lumen when the ion product of calcium and unconjugated bilirubin exceeds its solubility. Up to 50% of these patients undergo cholecystectomy at some point during their lifetimes, suggesting increased associated morbidity, creating a need for hospitalization, and potential mortality from infectious or other complications related to this process(1).

Cholelithiasis risk, for both cholesterol and bile pigment stones, is thought to be partially mediated by genes impacting bilirubin metabolism [4,5,6]. Genome-wide association studies (GWAS) of three large Caucasian cohorts have identified single nucleotide polymorphisms (SNPs) in *UGT1A1* that are responsible for 18% of clinical variability of serum bilirubin [7]. Sequencing of the *UGT1A1* gene in patients with Gilbert's syndrome, associated with unconjugated hyperbilirubinemia, revealed that an important modulator of enzyme activity is the length of TA repeats in the promoter region; the greater the number of repeats being associated with the highest serum bilirubin levels and cholelithiasis risk [8,9].

Genome-wide studies examining hyperbilirubinemia and cholelithiasis risk have not been performed in persons of African descent with sickle cell anemia. However, sequencing of *UGT1A1* has been undertaken in SCD cohorts in Guadeloupe, Portugal, Jamaica, India and the United States; genotyping of 324 SCD children from the Cooperative Study of Sickle Cell Disease (CSSCD) revealed that the common (TA)6 and (TA)7 alleles were present in 75% [10–15]. The (TA)7/(TA)7 genotype was associated with increased serum bilirubin levels and cholelithiasis risk compared with the (TA)6/(TA)7 and (TA)6/(TA)6 genotypes across cohorts with suggestions that those with a (TA)8 allele are at highest risk, suggesting a similar pattern of inheritance as observed in Caucasians [10–15]. Treatment with hydroxyurea, known to decrease the hemolytic rate in sickle cell anemia patients, was unable to decrease bilirubin levels to normal levels in those with the (TA)7/(TA)7 genotype suggesting that this genetic defect may represent a new pharmacologic target for these patients [14].

One of the reasons for the focus on *UGT1A1* in genetic studies relates to its known importance in bilirubin metabolism [8,9]. Upon release into the plasma, heme is metabolized to bilirubin via the actions of heme oxygenase-1. Bilirubin is poorly water soluble and in order for excretion to occur, disruption of its hydrogen bonds via a process termed glucuronidation, or conjugation, is essential. Glucuronidation of bilirubin is mediated by a family of enzymes termed the uridine-diphosphoglucuronate glucuronosyltransferases (UGT). Of these, *UGT1A1* is the most important regulator of this process clinically and is one of the isoforms of the *UGT1A* gene complex comprised of 9 transcriptional units. Unconjugated or indirect bilirubin is responsible for all of the toxic effects of hyperbilirubinemia, supporting the clinical importance of this class of enzymes. Additionally, as alluded to previously, genetic studies of other patient populations characterized by hyperbilirubinemia, Gilbert's syndrome and cystic fibrosis, have demonstrated an association between genetic variants within dinucleotide repeats in the promoter of *UGT1A1* and bile pigment stone formation [7].

We conducted a GWAS of serum total bilirubin in the largest number of African American sickle cell anemia patients studied to date to determine if genetic variants played a role in the increased risk of cholelithiasis observed in this population. Our analysis shows that *UGT1A1* is the major regulator of bilirubin levels in African Americans with sickle cell anemia, and that genetically mediated differences in bilirubin conjugation play an important role in cholelithiasis risk in these patients.

Materials and Methods

Ethics Statement

All studies were approved by the Institutional Review Board of Boston Medical Center, Duke University, University of Pittsburgh, Johns Hopkins University, Washington University and the University of North Carolina at Chapel Hill. Additionally, IRB approval was acquired from all of the sites participating in the Walk-PHaSST, Multicenter Study of Hydroxyurea Use and SITT trials for subject enrollment. All patients signed informed written consent for participation in these studies.

Study Subjects

The discovery set consisted of 1,117 African American subjects from the CSSCD [16,17]. The replication cohorts were comprised of 195 subjects from the Multicenter Study of Hydroxyurea (MSH), 522 subjects from the Pulmonary Hypertension and Sickle Cell Disease with Sildenafil Therapy (Walk-PHaSST) study (NCT00492531) [18], 530 subjects from the Outcome Modifying Genes study (referred to subsequently as "Duke") that enrolled patients from Duke University Medical Center, the University of

Table 1. Patient Characteristics in CSSCD, MSH and Walk-PHaSST cohorts.

Clinical Variable	CSSCD			MSH			Walk-PHaSST		
	Overall (N = 1117)	Men (N = 533)	Women (N = 584)	Overall (N = 195)	Men (N = 96)	Women (N = 99)	Overall (N = 522)	Men (N = 241)	Women (N = 281)
Log Total Bilirubin (mg/dL)*	1.13(0.5)	1.19(0.5)	1.13(0.5)	1.09(0.6)	1.15(0.6)	1.04(0.6)	3.67(0.7)	3.81(0.7)	3.55(0.7)
Reticulocyte (%)	12.09(5.9)	11.79(5.6)	12.09(5.9)	15.06(8.1)	14.13(7.8)	15.90(8.3)	8.61(5.5)	8.99(5.6)	8.28(5.5)
AST (units/dL)	50.52(32.2)	48.68(34.5)	50.52(32.2)	41.45(19.3)	42.03(19.1)	40.91(19.6)	46.27(34.9)	51.55(41.4)	41.77(27.4)
ALT (units/dL)	22.14(22.6)	22.25(24.7)	22.14(22.6)	24.14(15.8)	24.81(15.6)	23.52(16.1)	28.33(22.4)	30.23(23.3)	26.61(21.5)
Hemoglobin (g/dL)	8.43(8.5)	8.49(1.3)	8.43(8.5)	8.56(1.4)	9.01(1.4)	8.14(1.3)	9.37(2.0)	9.63(2.1)	9.14(1.8)
LDH (mg/dL)	421.1(91.1)	438.1(88.4)	421.1(91.1)	NA	NA	NA	454.43(292.6)	493.05(316.4)	421.92(267.2)
Age (years)	16.41(11.5)	15.29(11.1)	16.41(11.5)	28.61(6.2)	28.61(6.2)	30.28(8.4)	36.69(13.2)	34.87(13.1)	38.25(13.2)

*Walk-PHaSST bilirubin measurement is in SI units.
Summary statistics of patient characteristics in the CSSCD, MSH, and WALK-PHaSSTstudies. For each study, the first column reports statistics (mean and standard deviation) for all patients included in the analysis and the second and third columns report statistics stratified by gender.

Table 2. Patient Characteristics of the Duke and SITT cohorts.

Clinical Variable	Duke			SITT		
	Overall (N = 530)	Men (N = 242)	Women (N = 288)	Overall (N = 905)	Men (N = 480)	Women (N = 425)
Log Total Bilirubin (mg/dL)*	0.83 (0.7)	0.89 (0.8)	0.78 (0.7)	1.12(0.6)	1.16(0.6)	1.08(0.6)
Reticulocyte (%)	10.35 (6.0)	10.22 (6.0)	10.45 (6.1)	11.89(5.5)	12.01(5.6)	11.75(5.4)
AST (units/dL)	46.56 (34.6)	47.69 (29.2)	45.61 (38.5)	NA	NA	NA
ALT (units/dL)	30.93 (28.2)	32.41 (28.7)	29.69 (27.8)	NA	NA	NA
Hemoglobin (g/dL)	8.75 (1.8)	9.20 (2.1)	8.40 (1.6)	8.12(1.1)	8.01(1.1)	8.26(1.1)
LDH (mg/dL)	NA	NA	NA	NA	NA	NA
Age (years)	33.67 (11.9)	32.34 (11.0)	34.79 (12.6)	8.96(2.4)	9.07(2.5)	8.84(2.4)

Summary statistics of patient characteristics in the DUKE and SITT studies. For each study, the first column reports statistics (mean and standard deviation) for all patients included in the analysis and the second and third columns report statistics stratified by gender.

North Carolina Chapel Hill, Emory University, East Carolina University Comprehensive Sickle Cell Centers, and the Carolinas Health Center, and 905 samples from the SITT silent cerebral infarct trial (NCT00072761). The timing of each of these studies impacted hydroxyurea use. None of the patients from the CSSCD discovery set were treated with hydroxyurea as recruitment for this study concluded in 1998. To eliminate potential confounding effects of hydroxyurea, in the MSH, pre-hydroxyurea levels of total bilirubin were utilized [19].

Genotyping

The DNA from the CSSCD, MSH, and Walk-PHaSST samples were genotyped at Boston University using the Illumina Human610-Quad SNP array, with approximately 600,000 SNPs and the Illumina HumanCNV370-duo bead chip (MSH). The Duke samples were also genotyped using the Human610-Quad SNP array, whereas the SITT cohort was genotyped in two stages. In stage 1, a subset of 573 recruited samples was genotyped at the Center for Inherited Disease Research (CIDR) using Illumina HumanHap650Y array. The genotype data for the remaining 509 samples were generated at the Center for Disease Control (CDC) in collaboration with Washington University using Illumina Infinium HumanOmni1-Quad array. To infer un-typed SNPs and fill-in missing data across Omni1M and HumanHap650Y platforms, imputation was performed by using Hidden Markov model implemented in MaCH software [20]. All samples genotyped at Boston University were processed according the manufacturer's protocol and BeadStudio Software was used to make genotype calls utilizing the Illumina pre-defined clusters. Samples with less than a 95% call rate were removed and SNPs with a call rate <97.5% were re-clustered. After re-clustering, SNPs with call rates >97.5%, cluster separation score >.25, excess heterozygosity between −.10 and .10, and minor allele frequency >5% were retained in the analysis. We used the genome-wide identity by descent analysis in PLINK to discover unknown relatedness. Pairs with identity by descent measurements greater

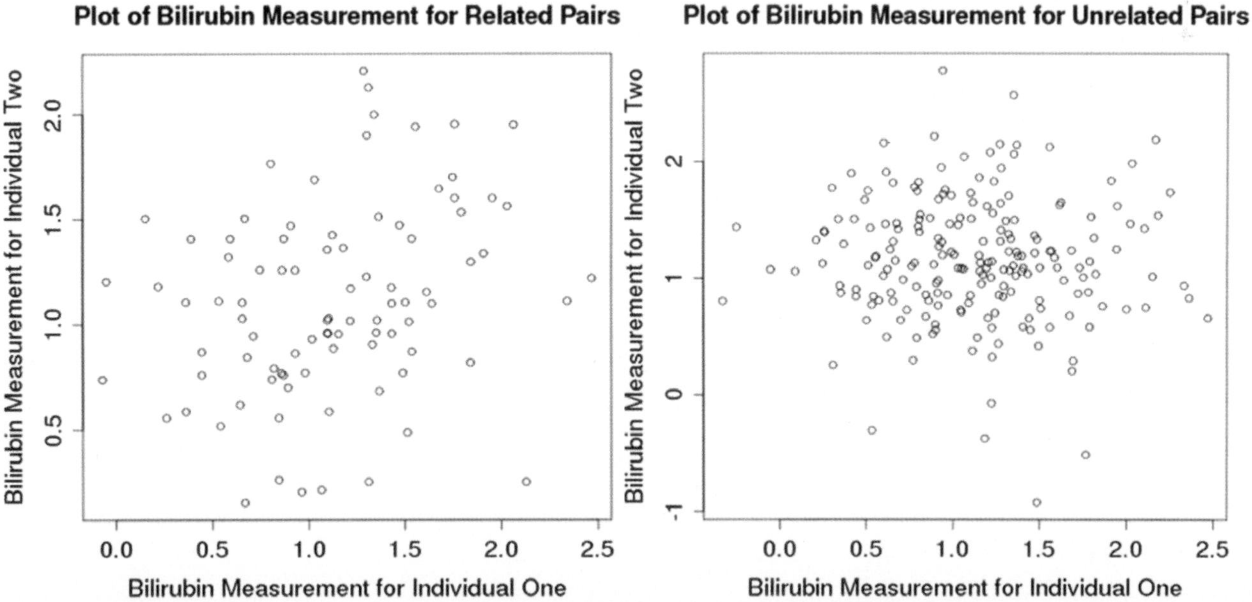

Figure 1. Plot of serum bilirubin among 90 sibling pairs in the CSSCD (A) and 200 pairs of unrelated individuals randomly selected from the CSSCD (B). In each scatter plot, the x- and y-axes show levels of total bilirubin. The correlation coefficient in the 90 sibling pairs was 0.27, while the average correlation coefficient of bilirubin levels in the pairs of unrelated individuals was −0.002.

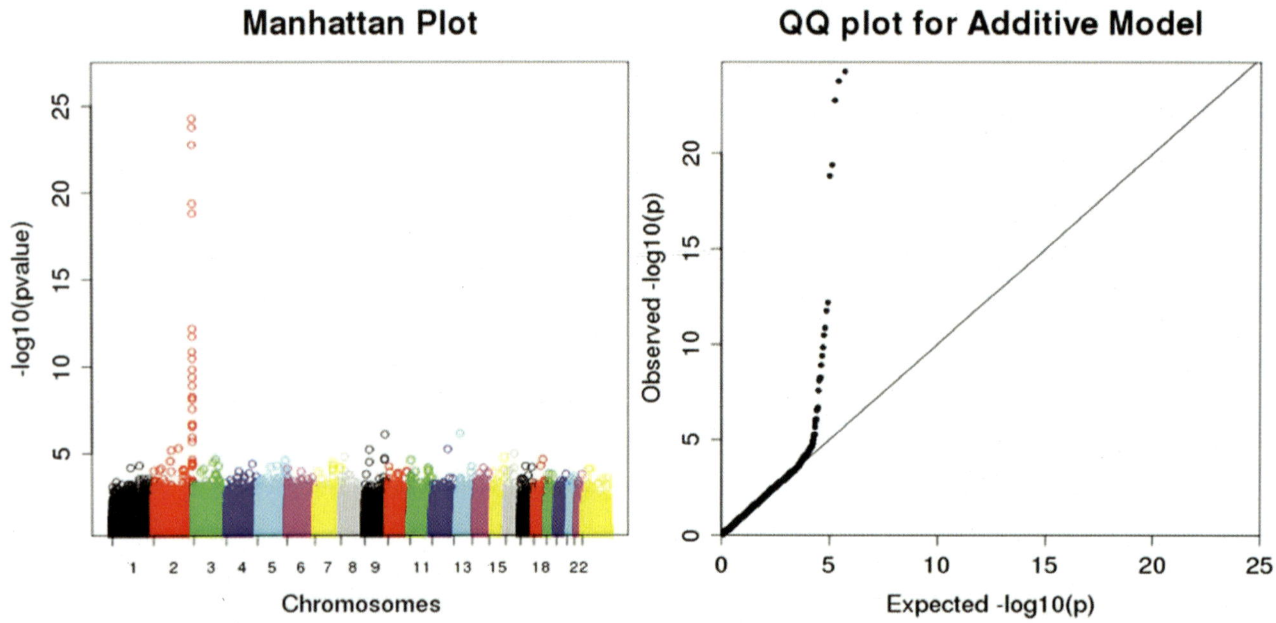

Figure 2. Summary of the GWAS data from the CSSCD Cohort. The Manhattan plot (A) displays the –log10(p value) of the associations tested in the CSSCD cohort using the additive model. Color bands represent chromosomes, and SNPs are ordered by their physical position within each chromosome. The large spike in chromosome 2 corresponds to the *UGT1A1, UGT1A3, UGT1A8* and *UGT1A10* regions. The QQ-plot (B) displays the observed (y-axis) versus expected (x-axis) –log10 (p-value). From the QQ plot, there is minimal to no inflation in the test statistic.

than .2 were deemed to be related subjects. Related subjects within individual or different studies were removed. We also removed samples with inconsistent gender findings defined by heterozygosity of the X chromosome and gender recorded in the database. Quality control parameters for the DUKE and SITT samples were comparable. In SITT, a 98% cutoff was used for both the sample and SNP call rates in the combined dataset (n = 1082), and resulted the exclusion of 6 individuals and 1,260 SNPs from the study. Seventy seven samples were identified as first-degree relatives (pairs with identity by descent measurements > 0.4), and 1 individual from each pair was removed. Twenty six individuals were identified as genetic outliers using EIGENSTRAT (>6 standard deviations on any of the top ten principal components) and removed. Additionally, 68 samples were also dropped from the study, due to missing phenotype data, leaving 905 samples for subsequent analysis.

Phenotype

Serum total and direct bilirubin, lactate dehydrogenase (LDH), hemoglobin concentrations, and reticulocyte counts were measured using automated chemical and hematologic analyzers at the individual medical centers participating in these studies.

For the CSSCD patients, longitudinal bilirubin measurements were collected from phases 1, 2, and 3 of the study [16]. Only steady state measurements were used (4 months removed from blood transfusion). The longitudinal measurements of 3,250 study patients were analyzed using a Bayesian hierarchical mixed model that included a random effect per patient to account for the repeated measurements, as well as random intercept and age effects that were allowed to vary with the clinics. The random intercept and age effects were used to remove the between-site systematic differences. Markov Chain Monte Carlo method in Openbugs was used to estimate the predicted total bilirubin values, and log-transformed median predicted values were used as the phenotype for the GWAS. The details of the analysis are available as (Information S1). For MSH, Duke, Walk-PHaSST and SITT patients, the log transformed baseline total bilirubin was used.

CSSCD subjects were assessed for gallstones by cholecystogram, plain film report, and abdominal ultrasound. A combination of questionnaires and medical records were utilized to determine a history of cholelithiasis or cholecystectomy. The cholelithiasis phenotype was dichotomized into: a) those who had gallstones (or history of), a history of cholecystectomy, a nonfunctional gallbladder; or b) none of these conditions. Of the 1,062 CSSCD patients with gallstone information, 348 had gallstones, or a nonfunctional gallbladder, cholecystectomy or a history of one of these events.

Heritability of Total Bilirubin

To further examine heritability of serum bilirubin in the CSSCD population, we examined the correlation of serum bilirubin in 90 sibling pairs. As a comparison, we randomly selected serum bilirubin values for 200 unrelated pairs 1,000 times to get an average of the estimated correlation among unrelated individuals.

Description of GWAS and Secondary Genetic Association Analyses

The association between total bilirubin levels and each SNP that passed quality control was tested using multiple linear regression, adjusting for age and gender using the additive and genotypic model in PLINK software. Age and gender were both included as covariates, as both were found to have a significant association with total bilirubin levels ($p<0.0001$ for both covariates). The minor allele was the coded allele in the additive model. To control for population stratification, a separate GWAS was performed on the discovery set adjusting for age, gender and the top ten principal components calculated using EIGENSOFT [21].

Haploview was employed to generate LD heatmaps using genotype data from the CSSCD. The SNPs that reached genome-

Table 3. Single Nucleotide Polymorphisms Associated with Total Bilirubin Levels.

Variant Information							CSSCD		MSH		WALK-PHaSST		Duke		SITT	
SNP	Chr	BP	Coded Allele	Noncoded Allele	MAF	Genes	*B*	pvalue	β	pvalue	β	pvalue	β	pvalue	β	pvalue
rs7586110	2	234255266	C	A	0.2632	UGT1A6–UGT1A10*	0.11	2.63E−08	0.07	.03347	.20	.000107	0.21	2.20E−05	0.24	8.65E−14
rs10168155	2	234261575	A	G	0.3735	UGT1A6–UGT1A10*	0.11	5.72E−09	NA	NA	0.18	0.000164	0.26	4.44E−09	0.24	3.52E−16
rs10168416	2	234261826	G	C	0.2402	UGT1A6–UGT1A10*	0.12	5.55E−09	NA	NA	0.21	4.46E−05	0.21	4.03E−05	0.26	1.16E−13
rs6759892	2	234266408	C	A	0.3766	UGT1A6–UGT1A10*	0.10	7.71E−09	0.08	.0045	.18	.000112	0.26	4.44E−09	0.24	7.31E−17
rs1105880	2	234266704	G	A	0.3628	UGT1A6–UGT1A10*	0.11	1.20E−09	NA	NA	0.18	0.000121	0.27	1.84E−09	0.26	3.13E−18
rs2070959	2	234266930	G	A	0.2468	DNAJB3,UGT1A3–UGT1A10ψ	0.13	4.05E−10	0.07	.05408	0.21	5.56E−05	0.22	1.62E−05	0.26	1.24E−15
rs1105879	2	234266941	C	A	0.3024	UGT1A6–UGT1A10*	0.13	1.39E−11	0.07	.02737	0.18	.000189	0.24	1.10E−06	0.28	7.68E−20
rs17863787	2	234275833	C	A	0.2498	UGT1A6–UGT1A10*	0.14	3.34E−11	NA	NA	0.28	1.22E−08	0.22	8.75E−06	0.28	4.93E−18
rs3755319	2	234332321	A	C	0.2913	UGT1A1–UGT1A10 ψ	−0.14	1.82E−12	NA	NA	−0.26	5.59E−08	−0.29	5.07E−09	−0.28	2.21E−18
rs887829	2	234333309	A	G	0.4532	UGT1A1–UGT1A10 ψ	0.19	5.27E−25	NA	NA	0.37	1.56E−18	0.33	2.30E−14	0.41	3.16E−46
rs6742078	2	234337378	A	C	0.433	UGT1A1–UGT1A10 ψ	0.18	1.71E−23	NA	NA	0.36	3.67E−17	0.33	3.18E−14	0.38	1.43E−43
rs4148324	2	234337461	C	A	0.4459	UGT1A1–UGT1A10 ψ	0.16	1.56E−19	NA	NA	0.35	4.89E−16	0.33	4.58E−14	0.37	2.55E−38
rs3771341	2	234337978	A	G	0.3998	UGT1A1–UGT1A10 ψ	0.17	4.17E−20	NA	NA	0.35	1.53E−15	0.28	2.08E−10	0.39	1.26E−37
rs4148325	2	234338048	A	G	0.4525	UGT1A1–UGT1A10 ψ	0.18	1.66E−24	NA	NA	0.37	2.13E−18	0.33	2.36E−14	0.40	2.11E−47
rs4148326	2	234338201	A	G	0.3874	UGT1A1–UGT1A10 ψ	−0.13	6.57E−13	NA	NA	−0.28	7.17E−11	−0.27	3.80E−09	−0.31	5.44E−26

Genome wide significant SNPs in the CSSCD study and their replicates in the independent cohorts. The table reports the SNP identifier from dbSNP, chromosome, physical coordinates (hg18), the coded allele in PLINK (also minor allele) and the non-coded allele, the minor allele frequency (MAF) from the CSSCD cohort, the gene clusters where the SNP is located, and regression coefficientt and p-value in each study. Additive models of association were used in all studies. NA in the MSH means the SNP was unavailable in the 370 Illumina array.

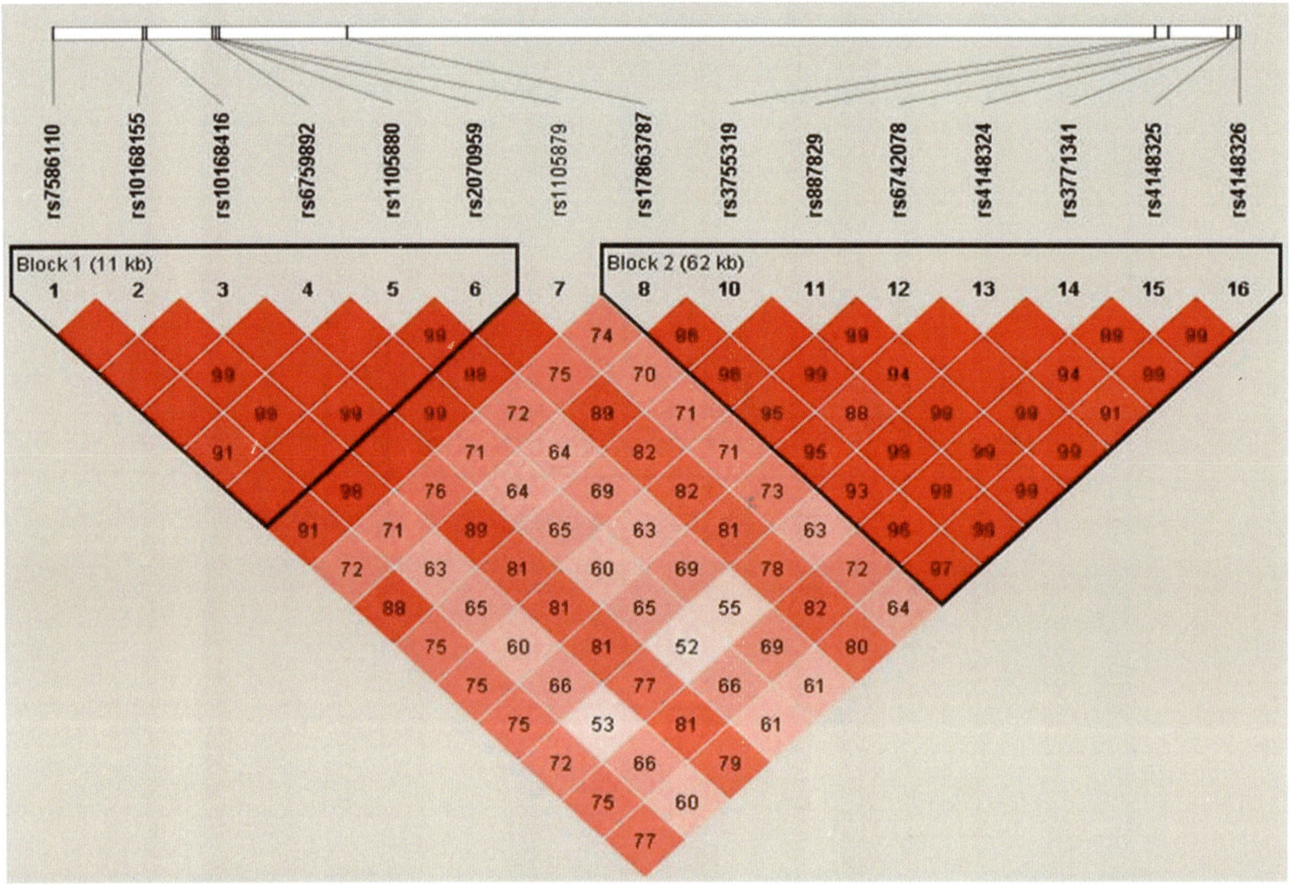

Figure 3. LD Structure in the CSSCD Cohort. LD plots for regions in genes *UGT1A1, UGT1A3, UGT1A4, UGT1A5, UGT1A6, UGT1A7, UGT1A8, UGT1A9* and *UGT1A10* on chromosome 2 in the CSSCD subjects. The LD plot was generated using Haploview 4.2. Each diamond represents the D' value between two SNPs. The LD color scheme is: white D'<1 and LOD<2, blue D' = 1 and LOD<2; shades of pinkish-red D'<1 and LOD≥2 and bright red D' = 1 and LOD≥2.

Table 4. Single Nucleotide Polymorphisms Associated with Cholelithiasis.

SNP	Chr	BP	Coded Allele	Non-Coded Allele	MAF	OR	P value
rs7586110	2	234255266	C	A	0.2632	1.366	0.05779
rs10168155	2	234261575	A	G	0.373	1.393	0.02858
rs10168416	2	234261826	G	C	0.2402	1.417	0.03765
rs6759892	2	234266408	C	A	0.3763	1.415	0.02134
rs1105880	2	234266704	G	A	0.3628	1.408	0.02277
rs2070959	2	234266930	G	A	0.2468	1.4	0.04248
rs1105879	2	234266941	C	A	0.303	1.356	0.05056
rs17863787	2	234275833	C	A	0.2498	1.324	0.09915
rs3755319	2	234332321	A	C	0.2913	0.561	0.001284
rs887829	2	234333309	A	G	0.4532	1.715	0.00032
rs6742078	2	234337378	A	C	0.433	1.635	0.001044
rs4148324	2	234337461	C	A	0.4459	1.654	0.000878
rs3771341	2	234337978	A	G	0.3998	1.661	0.00087
rs4148325	2	234338048	A	G	0.4525	1.757	0.000175
rs4148326	2	234338201	A	G	0.3874	0.524	0.000115

Results of SNP association analysis with cholelithiasis in the CSSCD study using the additive model. The minor allele is the coded allele, and the OR is the odds for cholelithiasis in carriers of one extra copy of the coded allele.

Table 5. Association Analysis with LDH, Reticulocyte Counts and Hemoglobin Concentration.

SNP	LDH		Reticulocytes		Hemoglobin	
	β	pval	β	pval	β	pval
rs7586110	−0.01206	0.235	0.01255	0.4964	0.02221	0.6891
rs10168155	−0.00587	0.5304	−0.0032	0.8501	0.04552	0.3687
rs10168416	−0.0042	0.6886	0.01099	0.563	0.02353	0.6808
rs6759892	−0.00604	0.5171	0.001128	0.9466	0.04249	0.4034
rs1105880	0.000316	0.9729	7.16E−05	0.9966	0.04007	0.4277
rs2070959	−0.00319	0.7579	0.01636	0.3834	0.003175	0.9552
rs1105879	−0.00135	0.8891	0.02488	0.1554	0.0182	0.7298
rs17863787	0.00116	0.9146	0.006013	0.7586	0.004455	0.9399
rs3755319	−0.00043	0.9653	0.006524	0.7188	0.01732	0.7509
rs887829	−0.00528	0.558	−0.01726	0.2922	0.06559	0.1825
rs6742078	−0.00786	0.3855	−0.01868	0.2558	0.05936	0.2303
rs4148324	−0.00463	0.6104	−0.02468	0.1339	0.06086	0.2193
rs3771341	−0.00911	0.3252	−0.01876	0.2654	0.07966	0.1158
rs4148325	−0.00799	0.3732	−0.02165	0.1877	0.06967	0.1576
rs4148326	0.003204	0.7309	0.01245	0.462	0.02886	0.5721

Results of SNP association analysis with other hemolytic phenotypes including hemoglobin, LDH and reticulocyte count in the CSSCD Study.

wide significance in the CSSCD sample were analyzed for association in the other cohorts. In SITT, the genetic associations were performed after adjustments for the same covariates (age, gender and top ten principal components). To account for the uncertainty of imputed data, the estimated allele dosage was analyzed using ProABEL under a linear regression framework [22]. Duke only controlled for age and gender, because previous analyses had indicated there was not appreciable population stratification in that data set. In a secondary analysis, SNPs that achieved genome-wide significance from the additive model were tested for association with the cholelithiasis in the CSSCD cohort. This association was tested using an additive multiple logistic regression model, adjusting for age. The same SNPs were also tested for association with LDH, reticulocyte counts and hemoglobin concentration, using the same Bayesian hierarchical model.

Results

Patient Characteristics and Heritability of Total Bilirubin Levels

Patient characteristics for each cohort are shown in Tables 1 and 2. The CSSCD cohort was younger than the MSH, Duke, and Walk-PHaSST cohorts. Each of the cohorts were equally divided between males and females. Examination of the serum bilirubin levels amongst 90 sibling pairs revealed a positive correlation ($r = 0.270$, $p = 0.009$), consistent with heritability of bilirubin levels (Figure 1A). In contrast, there was no correlation amongst 1,000 randomly selected pairs ($r = -.002$ average p value $= 0.502$, Figure 1B).

Association Between *UGT* SNPs and Serum Bilirubin Levels

After our quality control procedures, 569,615 SNPs were analyzed in the GWAS of serum bilirubin in the CSSCD. Figure 2A shows the Manhattan plot, with the results of the GWAS for the additive model and the large spike of significant associations in chromosome 2. The QQ plot (Figure 2B) shows no inflation (lambda factor, $\lambda = 1.01$) suggesting that there is no confounding by population stratification. To confirm this, we repeated the analysis after adjustment for the top ten principal components and the magnitude and significance of the top SNPs did not change. Fifteen SNPs reached genome-wide significance for both the genotypic and additive models and we report only the results from the additive model (Table 3). These genes are located on a contiguous part of chromosome 2 of the *UGT1* region. The linkage disequilibrium (LD) structure of these SNPs in Figure 3 shows two blocks in LD, although all 15 SNPs are in very strong LD (D'>0.53) (the LD structure of these SNPs can be show in terms of r^2 in Information S1). To determine if these 15 SNPs were part of one or multiple independent signals, another GWAS was performed adjusting for age, sex and our top SNP, rs887829. None of the fourteen SNPs showed a significant association with serum bilirubin after this adjusted analysis (complete results can be seen in Information S1), thus suggesting that these 15 SNPs are a part of the same signal. A complete list of the SNPs with a p value less than 5×10^{-05} consistent with genome-wide significance can be found in Information S1. An increase in the number of minor alleles in all SNPs except rs4148326 and rs3755319 was associated with an increase in log total bilirubin (effect sizes ranging from 0.108 to 0.1838), so that the less common alleles are the risk alleles; however, the other two SNPs showed effect estimates in the opposite direction (effect sizes ranging from −.13 to −.14), so that the minor alleles are associated with lower levels of serum bilirubin. Only four of the SNPs that reached genome-wide significance in the CSSCD population were available for genotyping on the 370K array used for the MSH samples, while all of them were genotyped in the Duke, Walk-PHaSST and SITT cohorts. All of the SNPs were significantly associated with bilirubin levels and had a regression coefficient in the same direction in both the discovery and replication sets (Table 3).

SNPs Associated with Bilirubin Levels are also Associated with Cholelithiasis

Table 4 shows the association between the 15 genome-wide significant SNPs and the odds for cholelithiasis. Twelve of the 15 SNPs were significantly associated with cholelithiasis ($p < .05$) and all of them had associated odds ratios for cholelithiasis in a direction consistent with that observed in the analysis of total bilirubin: An increase in the number of risk alleles for all SNPs except rs4148326 and rs3755319 was associated with an increased odds for cholelithiasis (odds ratios ranging from 1.324 to 1.757). The other two SNPs showed effect estimates in the opposite direction (odds ratios of .524 and .561). We also tested whether these 15 SNPs were significantly associated with LDH levels, hemoglobin concentration and reticulocyte count to see if there was an association with markers of hemolysis. None of the SNPs showed an association with LDH, hemoglobin concentration or reticulocyte count (Table 5).

Discussion

Intravascular hemolysis in sickle cell anemia patients produces increased circulating heme levels and has been associated with clinical complications including cholestatic jaundice and cholelithiasis [10,23–25,26–28] Unconjugated hyperbilirubinemia is a risk factor for the development of bile pigment stones in sickle cell disease and other hemolytic anemias [12,29–41]. Typically, bilirubin is formed from metabolism of heme, which is derived principally from erythrocytic hemoglobin. Heme is oxidatively metabolized by heme oxygenase-1 into biliverdin, which is subsequently reduced enzymatically by biliverdin reductase to bilirubin. Upon formation, bilirubin is water insoluble, due to the presence of internal hydrogen bonding that creates a contorted molecule structure, inhibiting solubility. This form of bilirubin, termed unconjugated or indirect bilirubin, is responsible for all of the toxic effects of bilirubin observed clinically. To permit excretion, bilirubin complexes with albumin and is transported via the bloodstream to the liver, where it undergoes glucuronidation by the UGT family of enzymes; *UGT1A1* is the only one with clinical relevance in humans [42]. *UGT1A* is a gene complex composed of 9 transcriptional units encoding an isoform of the *UGT* gene [30,31]. The most common genetic cause of impaired bilirubin glucuronidation occurs in Gilbert's syndrome, which follows an autosomal recessive inheritance pattern and most commonly affects Caucasians of European descent [43,44]. Clinically, these patients have a mild indirect hyperbilirubinemia, which worsens during periods of stress or febrile illnesses [45]. Genetic studies of these patients have identified a dinucleotide repeat polymorphism $(TA)_{5-8}$ in the TATA box of the *UGT1A1* gene promoter that is associated with reduced *UGT* expression and produces hyperbilirubinemia [30–31,37,46–47]. This polymorphism has also been observed in small cohorts of sickle cell anemia patients suggesting a common pathogenic link between ethnically divergent etiologies of indirect hyperbilirubinemia [5,10–15,33]. In the current study, genome-wide genetic screening of a large cohort of sickle cell anemia patients not only confirmed these findings but also supported their biological relevance.

In addition to defects in bilirubin metabolism, genetic alterations in the glucuronidation pathway have been linked to abnormalities in the hepatic metabolism of certain medications, pre-disposition to cardiovascular disease and certain types of malignancy suggesting a clinical level of importance beyond cholelithiasis [35,42,48–53]. How this relates to the pathogenesis of sickle cell anemia is not entirely clear clinically, but may be worthy of future study.

In genetic studies of primarily Caucasian cohorts, cholelithiasis and serum bilirubin levels are heritable traits. Family-based studies show that the *UGT* locus accounted for a significant proportion of the variation observed in both of these variables [18,54–56]. Our study is the first to use GWAS to examine an African American population with sickle cell anemia, a condition where hemolysis predisposes patients to hyperbilirubinemia, to determine the heritability of serum bilirubin levels. Fifteen SNPs in *UGT1A1, UGT1A3, UGT1A4, UGT1A5, UGT1A6, UGT1A7, UGT1A8* and *UGT1A9* reached genome-wide significance for association with total bilirubin levels in the CSSCD cohort; 13 of these were also associated with the presence or history of cholelithiasis. These findings were confirmed in 4 other cohorts totaling 3,269 patients, unusual for a rare disease such as sickle cell anemia, and representing a greater number of patients than all of the previous studies of this population combined.

SNPs we identified in the current study have been linked to hyperbilirubinemia in other populations. SNP rs887829, the most significant SNP associated with bilirubin levels identified in the CSSCD, Duke and Walk-PHaSST cohorts, was previously observed in associated with total bilirubin levels in a GWAS of 4,300 Sardinians [57]. This study also reported a significant association with bilirubin and the *SLCO1B3* locus; however, we were unable to replicate these results in our study due to unavailability or low MAF of the markers in our array. In a study performed by Cheng et al. examining genetic variants associated with serum bilirubin in 619 healthy African Americans revealed that the top SNP was rs887829 ($p = 1.77 \times 10^{-22}$) [58]. This suggests that this variant is not unique to African Americans with sickle cell disease. It has been theorized that this SNP may confer protection against malaria which may explain its penetrance amongst African populations. SNP rs887829 is located in the promoter region of *UGT1A1*, 221 bp upstream from the $(TA)_n$ repeat sequence. Horsfall et al. found a strong association was found between rs887829 and the $(TA)_7$ and $(TA)_8$ repeat sequence suggesting that this may be a marker for the (TA)7/(TA)7 or 8 genotypes [34]. This proximity to the promoter element and strong level of association suggest that rs887829 is a marker for the $(TA)_n$ repeats and that additional sequencing of this gene would be redundant [58]. SNP rs6742078, identified in the current study, was associated with total bilirubin in a meta-analysis previously performed by Johnson et al., including the Framingham Heart Study, Rotterdam Study and Age, Gene, Environment and Susceptibility-Reykjavik study cohorts [33]. In addition, SNPs rs3755319, rs7586110, and rs6759892 were also found to be significantly associated with total bilirubin in a cohort of 4,300 Sardinians [57]. SNP rs887829 was found to be associated with cholelithiasis in a study published by Buch et al., in which a cohort of 2,606 German cholelithiasis patients was compared with 1,121 South American controls (OR = 1.73, p value .003) [11].

There was no association between LDH, hemoglobin concentration or reticulocyte count, markers of hemolysis, and the SNPs identified in the present study. A potential explanation for this is the weak association between bilirubin levels and hemolytic rate. While the "gold standard" for hemolysis is the red cell lifespan, this is rarely performed and surrogate blood biomarkers such as reticulocyte count, LDH, bilirubin and haptoglobin levels are used clinically to estimate the degree of hemolysis. None of these measures are specific for hemolysis. An elevated serum bilirubin level in sickle cell anemia reflects multiple pathophysiologic processes that include liver disease in addition to hemolysis and therefore may lack the phenotypic specificity required for genetic association studies of hemolysis. Another possible reason for this finding is that the genes associated with bilirubin levels are all involved in bilirubin catabolism and not production suggesting that they are not reflective of the processes leading to bilirubin formation.

In summary, SNPs in *UGT1A1* are most tightly associated with bilirubin levels in African Americans with sickle cell anemia. This study in conjunction with those conducted in other populations at risk for unconjugated hyperbilirubinemia and other cohorts of sickle cell anemia patients support the concept that genetically mediated differences in bilirubin conjugation play an important role in the cholelithiasis risk. It is possible that targeting this pathway pharmacologically may offer new therapeutic options for these patients.

Supporting Information

Information S1 Description of the Bayesian hierarchical model used to create the phenotype in the CSSCD cohort. Supplementary Figure 1 contains information on the LD structure of the UGT1A region in the CSCCD cohort. Supplementary Table 1 contains information on the analysis of the association between bilirubin and after adjusting for our most significant SNP. Figure 1: LD Structure in CSSCD Cohort. LD plots for regions in genes *UGT1A1, UGT1A3, UGT1A4, UGT1A5, UGT1A6, UGT1A7, UGT1A8, UGT1A9* and *UGT1A10* on chromosome 2 in the CSSCD subjects. The LD plot was generated using Haploview 4.2. Each diamond represents the r^2 value between two SNPs. The LD color scheme is: white $r^2 = 0$,

$0<r^2<1$ grey (the darker the shade of grey, the higher the r^2 value), black $r^2 = 1$.

Author Contributions

Conceived and designed the experiments: PS MHS CTB ESK. Performed the experiments: JNM PS CTB NS DAD KS MEG WCH CJB. Analyzed the data: JNM NS PS CTB MHS ESK AEAK MJT MEG KS SWH PB. Contributed reagents/materials/analysis tools: MJT MRD JFC EBC CTB MHS MTG DEA. Wrote the paper: JNM PS ESK. Edited manuscript: PS MHS MTG MJT AEAK JFC MRD ESK DEA.

References

1. Adam S, Jonassaint J, Kruger H, Kail M, Orringer EP, et al. (2008) Surgical and obstetric outcomes in adults with sickle cell disease. Am J Med, 121, 916–921.
2. Au WY, Cheung WC, Chan GC, Ha SY, Khong PL, et al. (2003) Risk factors for hyperbilirubinemia and gallstones in Chinese patients with beta thalassemia syndrome. Haematologica, 88, 220–222.
3. Au WY, Cheung WC, Hu WH, Chan GC, Ha SY, et al. (2005) Hyperbilirubinemia and cholelithiasis in Chinese patients with hemoglobin H disease. Ann. Hematol, 84, 671–674.
4. Strassburg CP, Manns MP, Tukey RH (1998) Expression of the UDP-glucuronosyltransferase 1A locus in human colon. Identification and characterization of the novel extrahepatic UGT1A8. J. Biol. Chem., 273, 8719–8726.
5. Vasavda N, Menzel S, Kondaveeti S, Maytham E, Awogbade M, et al. (2007) The linear effects of alpha-thalassaemia, the UGT1A1 and HMOX1 polymorphisms on cholelithiasis in sickle cell disease. Br. J. Haematol., 138, 263–270.
6. Vogel A, Kneip S, Barut A, Ehmer U, Tukey RH, et al. (2001) Genetic link of hepatocellular carcinoma with polymorphisms of the UDP-glucuronosyltransferase UGT1A7 gene. Gastroenterology, 121, 1136–1144.
7. Benjamin EJ, Dupuis J, Larson MG, Lunetta KL, Booth SL, et al. (2007) Genome-wide association with select biomarker traits in the Framingham heart study. BMC Med. Genet, 8 Suppl 1, S11.
8. Bosma PJ, Chowdhury JR, Bakker C, Gantla S, de Boer A, et al. (1995) The genetic basis of the reduced expression of bilirubin UDP-glucuronosyltransferase 1 in Gilbert's syndrome. N. Engl. J. Med., 333, 1171–1175.
9. Bosma PJ, van der Meer IM, Bakker CT, Hofman A, Paul-Abrahamse M, et al. (2003) UGT1A1*28 allele and coronary heart disease: The Rotterdam study. Clin. Chem., 49, 1180–1181.
10. Chaar V, Keclard L, Diara JP, Leturdu C, Elion J, et al. (2005) Association of UGT1A1 polymorphism with prevalence and age at onset of cholelithiasis in sickle cell anemia. Haematologica, 90, 188–199.
11. Passon RG, Howard TA, Zimmerman SA, Schultz WH, Ware RE (2001) Influence of bilirubin uridine diphosphate-glucuronosyltransferase 1A promoter polymorphisms on serum bilirubin levels and cholelithiasis in children with sickle cell anemia. J. Pediatr. Hematol. Oncol., 23, 448–451.
12. Haverfield EV, McKenzie CA, Forrester T, Bouzekri N, Harding R, et al. (2005) UGT1A1 variation and gallstone formation in sickle cell disease. Blood, 105, 968–972.
13. Carpenter SL, Lieff S, Howard TA, Eggleston B, Ware RE (2008) UGT1A1 promoter polymorphisms and the development of hyperbilirubenemia and gallbladder disease in children with sickle cell anemia. Am J Hematol; 83(10): 800–803.
14. Italia KY, Jijina FF, Jain D, Merchant R, Nadkarni AH, et al. (2010) The effect of UGT1A1 promoter polymorphism on bilirubin response to hydroxyurea therapy in hemaglobinopathies. Clin Biochem, 43(16–17): 1329–1332.
15. Martins R, Morais A, Dias A, Soares I, Rolao C, et al. (2008) Early modification of sickle cell disease clinical course by UDP-glucuronosyltransferase 1A1 gene promoter polymorphism. J Hum Genet, 53(6): 524–528.
16. Went MS, Wethers D, Smith J, Steinberg MH (1992) Laboratory profile of sickle cell disease: a cross-sectional analysis. The Cooperative Study of Sickle Cell Disease. Journal of Clinical Epidemiology, 45, 893–90.
17. Sebastiani P, Solovieff N, Hartley SW, Milton JN, Riva A, et al. (2010) Genetic modifiers of the severity of sickle cell anemia identified through a genome-wide association study. Am. J. Hematol., 85, 29–35.
18. Machado RF, Barst RJ, Yovetich NA, Hassell KL, Kato GJ, et al. (2011) Hospitalization for pain in patients with sickle cell disease with sildenafil for elevated TRV and low exercise capacity. Blood, 118, 855–864.
19. Steinberg MH, Barton F, Castro O, Pegelow CH, Ballas SK, et al. (2003) Effect of hydroxyurea on mortality and morbidity in adult sickle cell anemia: Risks and benefits up to 9 years of treatment. JAMA, 289, 1645–1651.
20. Li Y, Willer CJ, Ding J, Scheet P, Abecasis GR (2010) MaCH: Using sequence and genotype data to estimate haplotypes and unobserved genotypes. Genetic Epidemiology, 34, 816–34.
21. Price AL, Patterson NJ, Plenge RM, Weinblatt ME, Shadick NA, et al. (2006) Principal components analysis corrects for stratification in genome-wide association studies. Nature Genetics, 38, 904–909.
22. Aulchenko YS, Struchalin MV, van Duijn CM (2010) ProbABEL package for genome-wide association analysis of imputed data. BMC Bioinformatics, 11, 134.
23. Buch S, Schafmayer C, Volzke H, Seeger M, Miquel JF, et al. (2010) Loci from a genome-wide analysis of bilirubin levels are associated with gallstone risk and composition. Gastroenterology, 139, 1942–1951.e2.
24. Cecchin E, Innocenti F, D'Andrea M, Corona G, De Mattia E, et al. (2009) Predictive role of the UGT1A1, UGT1A7, and UGT1A9 genetic variants and their haplotypes on the outcome of metastatic colorectal cancer patients treated with fluorouracil, leucovorin, and irinotecan. J. Clin. Oncol., 27, 2457–2465.
25. Chaar V, Keclard L, Etienne-Julan M, Diara JP, Elion J, et al. (2006) UGT1A1 polymorphism outweighs the modest effect of deletional (–3.7 kb) alpha-thalassemia on cholelithogenesis in sickle cell anemia. Am. J. Hematol., 81, 377–379.
26. Reiter CD, Wang X, Tanus-Santos JE, Hogg N, Cannon RO, et al. (2002) Cell-free hemoglobin limits nitric oxide bioavailability in sickle-cell disease. NatMed, 8, 1383–1389.
27. Taylor JG 6th, Nolan VG, Mendelsohn L, Kato GJ, Gladwin MT, et al. (2008) Chronic hyper-hemolysis in sickle cell anemia: Association of vascular complications and mortality with less frequent vasoocclusive pain. PLoS One, 3, e2095.
28. Van Erpecum KJ (2011) Pathogenesis of cholesterol and pigment gallstones: An update. Clin. Res. Hepatol. Gastroenterol., 35, 281–7.
29. Clementi M, Di Gianatonio E, Fabris L, Forbosco P, Strazzabosco M, et al. (2007) Inheritance of hyperbilirubinemia: Evidence for a major autosomal recessive gene. Dig Liver Dis, 39, 351–355.
30. Galanello R, Piras S, Barella S, Leoni GB, Cipollina MD, et al. (2001) Cholelithiasis and Gilbert's syndrome in homozygous beta-thalassaemia. Br. J. Haematol., 115, 926–928.
31. Gaston M RW (1982) The cooperative study of sickle cell disease: Review of study design and objectives. Am J Pediatr Hematol Oncol, 4, 197–201.
32. Haider MZ, Ashebu S, Aduh P, Adekile AD (1998) Influence of alpha-thalassemia on cholelithiasis in SS patients with elevated Hb F. Acta Haematol., 100, 147–150.
33. Heeney MM, Howard TA, Zimmerman SA, Ware RE (2003) UGT1A promoter polymorphisms influence bilirubin response to hydroxyurea therapy in sickle cell anemia. J. Lab. Clin. Med., 141, 279–282.
34. Horsfall LJ, Zeitlyn D, Tarekegn A, Bekele E, Thomas MG, et al. (2011) Prevalence of clinically relevant UGT1A alleles and haplotypes in African populations. Annals of Human Genetics, 236–246.
35. Hunt SC, Kronenberg F, Eckfeldt JH, Hopkins PN, Myers RH, et al. (2001) Association of plasma bilirubin with coronary heart disease and segregation of bilirubin as a major gene trait: The NHLBI family heart study. Atherosclerosis, 154, 747–754.
36. Johnson AD, Kavousi M, Smith AV, Chen MH, Dehghan A, et al. (2009) Genome-wide association meta-analysis for total serum bilirubin levels. Hum. Mol. Genet., 18, 2700–2710.
37. Kama NA, Atli M, Doganay M, Kologlu M, Reis E, et al. (2001) Practical recommendations for the prediction and management of common bile duct stones in patients with gallstones. Surg. Endosc., 15, 942–945.
38. Kang TW, Kim HJ, Ju H, Kim JH, Jeon YJ, et al. (2010) Genome-wide association of serum bilirubin levels in Korean population. Hum. Mol. Genet., 19, 3672–3678.
39. Kato GJ, Gladwin MT, Steinberg MH (2007) Deconstructing sickle cell disease: Reappraisal of the role of hemolysis in the development of clinical subphenotypes. Blood Rev., 21, 37–47.
40. Kato GJ, McGowan V, Machado RF, Little JA, Taylor J, et al. (2006) Lactate dehydrogenase as a biomarker of hemolysis-associated nitric oxide resistance, priapism, leg ulceration, pulmonary hypertension, and death in patients with sickle cell disease. Blood, 107, 2279–2285.
41. Kohle C, Mohrle B, Munzel PA, Schwab M, Wernet D, et al. (2003) Frequent co-occurrence of the TATA box mutation associated with Gilbert's syndrome (UGT1A1*28) with other polymorphisms of the UDP-glucuronosyltransferase-1 locus (UGT1A6*2 and UGT1A7*3) in Caucasians and Egyptians. Biochem. Pharmacol., 65, 1521–1527.
42. Perera MA, Innocenti F, Ratain MJ (2008) Pharmacogenetic testing for uridine diphosphate glucuronosyltransferase 1A1 polymorphisms: Are we there yet? Pharmacotherapy, 28, 755–768.
43. Persico M, Persico E, Bakker CT, Rigato I, Amoroso A, et al. (2001) Hepatic uptake of organic anions affects the plasma bilirubin level in subjects with Gilbert's syndrome mutations in UGT1A1. Hepatology, 33, 627–632.
44. Teng HC, Huang MJ, Tang KS, Yang SS, et al. (2007) Combined UGT1A1 and UGT1A7 variant alleles are associated with increased risk of Gilbert's syndrome in Taiwanese adults. Clin. Genet., 72, 321–328.
45. Krawczyk M, Wang DQ, Portincasa P, Lammert F (2011) Dissecting the genetic heterogeneity of gallbladder stone formation. Semin Liver Dis, 31, 157–172.

46. Kronenberg F, Coon H, Gutin A, Abkevich V, Samuels ME, et al. (2002) A genome scan for loci influencing anti-atherogenic serum bilirubin levels. Eur J Hum Genet, 10, 539–546.
47. Rantner B, Kollerits B, Anderwald-Stadler M, Klein-Weigel P, Gruber I, et al. (2008) Association between the UGT1A1 TA-repeat polymorphism and bilirubin concentration in patients with intermittent claudication: Results from the CAVASIC study. Clin. Chem., 54, 851–857.
48. Lammert F, Matern S (2005) The genetic background of cholesterol gallstone formation: An inventory of human lithogenic genes. Curr. Drug Targets. Immune. Endocr. Metabol. Disord., 5, 163–170.
49. Lammert F, Sauerbruch T (2005) Mechanisms of disease: The genetic epidemiology of gallbladder stones. Nat. Clin. Pract. Gastroenterol. Hepatol., 2, 423–433.
50. Lin JP, O'Donnell CJ, Schwaiger JP, Cupples LA, Lingenhel A, et al. (2006) Association between the UGT1A1*28 allele, bilirubin levels, and coronary heart disease in the Framingham heart study. Circulation, 114, 1476–1481.
51. Lingenhel A, Kollerits B, Schwaiger JP, Hunt SC, Gress R, et al. (2008) Serum bilirubin levels, UGT1A1 polymorphisms and risk for coronary artery disease. Exp. Gerontol., 43, 1102–1107.
52. Portincasa P, Moschetta A, Palasciano G (2006) Cholesterol gallstone disease. Lancet, 368, 230–239.
53. Schwertner HA, Vitek L (2008) Gilbert syndrome, UGT1A1*28 allele, and cardiovascular disease risk: Possible protective effects and therapeutic applications of bilirubin. Atherosclerosis, 198, 1–11.
54. Liu J, Yang XM, Liu G, Chang LS, Zhang LR, et al. (2009) Association between genetic polymorphism of UGT1A7 and susceptibility of bladder cancer. Zhonghua Yi Xue Za Zhi, 89, 3122–3125.
55. McDonagh AF (2010) Controversies in bilirubin biochemistry and their clinical relevance. Semin Fetal Neonatal Med, 15, 141–147.
56. Ockenga J, Vogel A, Teich N, Keim V, Manns MP, et al. (2003) UDP glucuronosyltransferase (UGT1A7) gene polymorphisms increase the risk of chronic pancreatitis and pancreatic cancer. Gastroenterology, 124, 1802–1808.
57. Sanna S, Busonero F, Maschio A, McArdle PF, Usala G, et al. (2009) Common variants in the SLCO1B3 locus are associated with bilirubin levels and unconjugated hyperbilirubinemia. Hum. Mol. Genet., 18, 2711–2718.
58. Chen G, Ramos E, Adeyemo A, Shriner D, Zhou J, et al. (2011) GWAS for serum bilirubin in African Americans. European Journal of Human Genetics, 1–6.

6

Isofagomine *In Vivo* Effects in a Neuronopathic Gaucher Disease Mouse

Ying Sun[1,3], Huimin Ran[1,3], Benjamin Liou[1,3], Brian Quinn[1,3], Matt Zamzow[1,3], Wujuan Zhang[2,3], Jacek Bielawski[4], Kazuyuki Kitatani[4,5], Kenneth D. R. Setchell[2,3], Yusuf A. Hannun[4], Gregory A. Grabowski[1,3]*

1 The Division of Human Genetics, University of Cincinnati College of Medicine, Cincinnati, Ohio, United States of America, **2** The Division of Pathology and Laboratory Medicine, Cincinnati Children's Hospital Medical Center, University of Cincinnati College of Medicine, Cincinnati, Ohio, United States of America, **3** The Department of Pediatrics, University of Cincinnati College of Medicine, Cincinnati, Ohio, United States of America, **4** The Department of Biochemistry and Molecular Biology, Medical University of South Carolina, Charleston, South Carolina, United States of America, **5** The Department of Clinical Laboratory, Tottori University Hospital, Tottori University, Yonago, Japan

Abstract

The pharmacological chaperone, isofagomine (IFG), enhances acid β-glucosidase (GCase) function by altering folding, trafficking, and activity in wild-type and Gaucher disease fibroblasts. The *in vivo* effects of IFG on GCase activity, its substrate levels, and phenotype were evaluated using a neuronopathic Gaucher disease mouse model, 4L;C* (V394L/V394L + saposin C-/-) that has CNS accumulation of glucosylceramide (GC) and glucosylsphingosine (GS) as well as progressive neurological deterioration. IFG administration to 4L;C* mice at 20 or 600 mg/kg/day resulted in life span extensions of 10 or 20 days, respectively, and increases in GCase activity and protein levels in the brain and visceral tissues. Cerebral cortical GC and GS levels showed no significant reductions with IFG treatment. Increases of GC or GS levels were detected in the visceral tissues of IFG treated (600 mg/kg/day) mice. The attenuations of brain proinflammatory responses in the treated mice were evidenced by reductions in astrogliosis and microglial cell activation, and decreased p38 phosphorylation and TNFα levels. Terminally, axonal degeneration was present in the brain and spinal cord from untreated and treated 4L;C* mice. These data demonstrate that IFG exerts *in vivo* effects by enhancing V394L GCase protein and activity levels, and in mediating suppression of proinflammation, which led to delayed onset of neurological disease and extension of the life span of 4L;C* mice. However, this was not correlated with a reduction in the accumulation of lipid substrates.

Editor: Raphael Schiffmann, Baylor Research Institute, United States of America

Funding: This work was supported by grants to GAG (R01 NS/DK36681 and R21 HD059823) and YAH (CA087584), and to KK, the Japan Society for the Promotion of Science (Grant-in-Aid for Young Scientists-Start-up, 21890144). The funders had no role in study design, data collection and analysis, decision to publish, or preparation of the manuscript.

Competing Interests: The authors have declared that no competing interests exist.

* E-mail: Greg.Grabowski@cchmc.org

Introduction

Gaucher disease is caused by mutations in *GBA1* that encodes acid β-glucosidase (glucocerebrosidase, GCase, EC3.2.1.45). The resultant defective GCase leads to accumulation of the substrates, glucosylceramide (GC) and glucosylsphingosine (GS) [1]. The disease has three clinical variants: Type 1 is primarily a visceral and nonneuropathic disease whereas types 2 and 3 are a continuum of neuronopathic and visceral diseases ranging from acute (type 2, infantile) to subacute (type 3) progressive CNS degenerative diseases [1,2].

Enzyme therapy with regular infusions of mannose-terminated recombinant human enzymes (imiglucerase, Genzyme; velaglucerase alfa, Shire) has become the standard-of-care for significantly involved type 1 patients [3]. The effects on liver, spleen, hematologic parameters, and bone are dose dependent [4,5]. Children show excellent responses in growth and bone disease to enzyme therapy [6]. Alternatively, reductions in GC levels can be achieved by partial inhibition of GC synthase, an essential enzyme in the biosynthesis of complex glycosphingolipids [7], i.e. substrate reduction therapy (SRT). SRT with N-butyldeoxynojirimycin (miglustat) shows improvement in some Gaucher disease parameters [8]. Eliglustat Tartrate {(1R,2R)-Octanoic acid [2-(2′,3′-dihydro-benzo [1,4] dioxin-6′-yl)-2-hydroxy-1-pyrrolidin-1-methyl-ethyl]-amide-L-tartaric acid salt}, an analog of 1-phenyl-2-decanoylamino-3-morpholino-1-propanol (PDMP), is a novel potent inhibitor (IC_{50}~24 nM) of GC synthase. This compound significantly reduces GC accumulation in visceral tissues and cells in the Gaucher disease mouse model [9,10]. In addition, phase 2 studies in humans show therapeutic effects that mimic those of higher dose enzyme therapy [11]. However, the compound does not reach significant levels in the brain since it is a pGP substrate. [9].

Directly modulating mutant enzyme activity by small molecules was proposed as an attractive alternative approach to treat Gaucher disease using pharmacological chaperones [12,13]. Competitive inhibitors specific for such enzymes could stabilize mutant enzyme proteins in endoplasm reticulum, assist the enzyme trafficking to lysosome, and restoring the activity [13,14]. IFG, a potent inhibitor of GCase, is an effective *in vitro* pharmacological chaperone that can enhance selected mutant GCases in fibroblasts [14,15]. IFG treatment of human patient fibroblasts facilitates mutant enzyme trafficking to lysosome and enhances protein and activity levels for the mutant GCases N370S, V394L, and L444P [14,15,16].

Here, IFG was evaluated *in vivo* in a neuronopathic GCase deficient mouse model [17] for its effect on mutant GCase activity, substrate levels, and phenotypic improvement.

Results

Treatment of 4L;C* mice with IFG

The *in vivo* effects of IFG were tested using 4L;C* mice that develop neurological signs, including a duck-like waddling gait at ~30 days, and then die from progressive CNS disease by ~48 days. Three to five days prior birth, IFG was added to the drinking water of pregnant dames in a dose calculated to provide ~20 mg/kg/d based on measured water intake (see methods). At postnatal day 7 (P7), one cohort was maintained on 20 mg/kg/d IFG and a second cohort on 600 mg/kg/d (Fig. 1A). The body weights (BW) of the mice were recorded from P7 to terminal stage. The 4L;C* mice receiving 20 mg/kg/d IFG showed normal increases of BW to ~35 days and then declined to ~70% of WT levels at terminal stage (Fig. 2A). The trend of BW change was similar to that observed with untreated 4L;C* mice. These treated 4L;C* mice developed the characteristic duck-walk gait at 40-44 days and their life span was 54 days on average or about 6–10 days longer than untreated mice (Fig. 2B). The 4L;C* mice receiving 600 mg/kg/d showed slow decreases in BW after 50 days (Fig. 2A). They did not develop duck-walking, but showed spastic-like gait starting 47–50 days (Fig. 1B). The average life span was 63 days or about 15–18 days longer than controls, or ~34% increase in lifespan (Fig. 2B). The untreated and 20 mg/kg/d IFG treated 4L;C+/− mice showed comparable BW attainments to WT and exhibited a normal phenotype during the entire study period. In comparison, 4L;C+/− mice treated with 600 mg/kg/d IFG showed slightly lower body weight (data not shown). The untreated 4L;C* mice are infertile and male 4L;C* mice treated with 20 or 600 mg/kg/d IFG produced only a single litter.

Additional regimes of IFG treatment were tested. The 4L;C* mice were treated with IFG in a 3-day-on/4-day-off trial. These mice received IFG starting 3-days prior birth at 20 mg/kg/d as above. Then, IFG was stopped from P3 to P7 (4-days off) and then it was given at 20 mg/kg/d for the next 3 days (3-day on). The cycle was continued until the end stage. The mice on this 3-day-on/4-day-off schedule showed no differences of phenotype, onset of signs, or life span (55 days) compared to the mice receiving 20 mg/kg/d of uninterrupted treatment. If IFG treatment was started on postnatal day 25 at 600 mg/kg/d, there was less of an

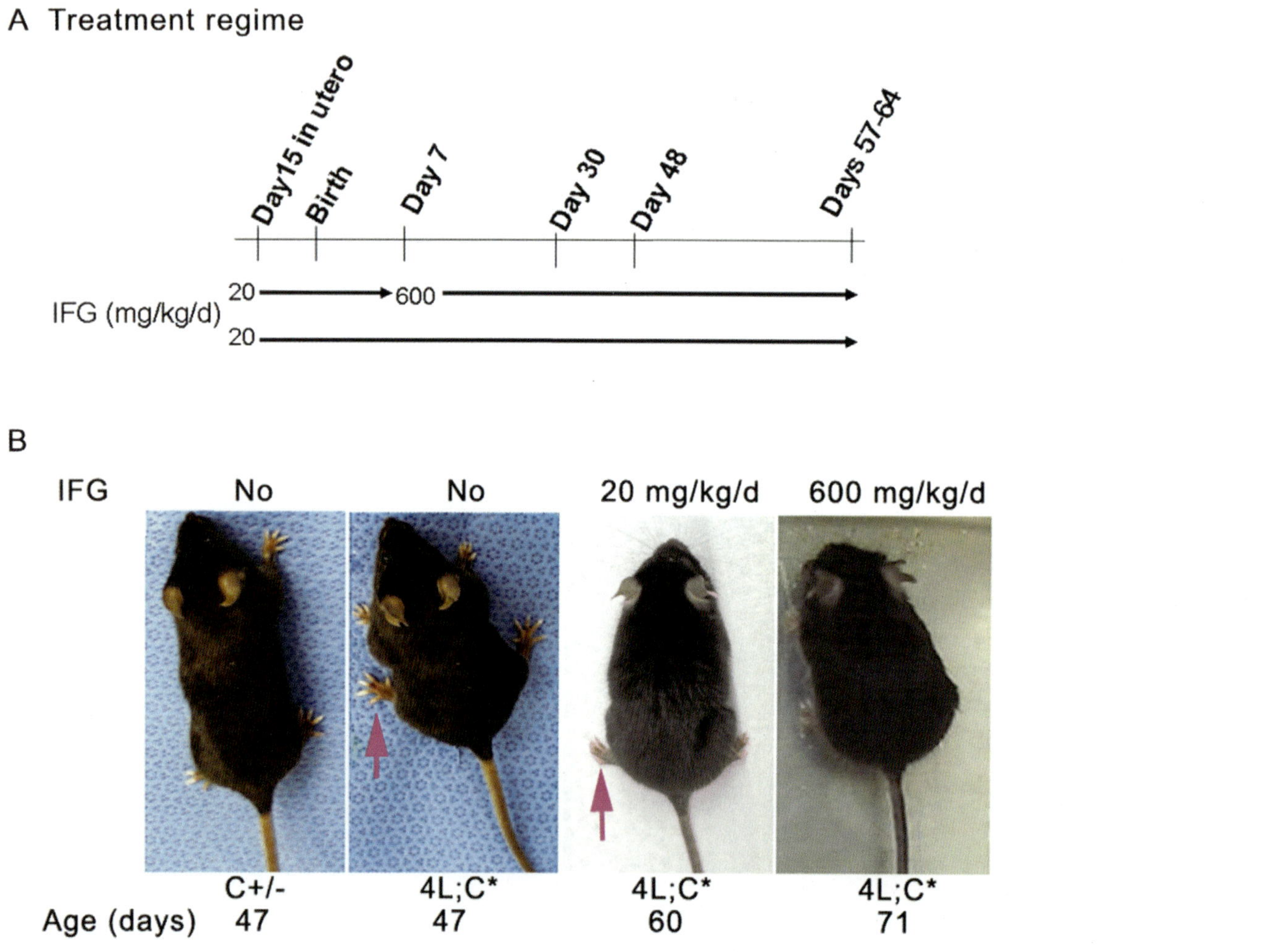

Figure 1. Treatment and phenotypes. (A) IFG treatment regime. IFG was given to pregnant females 3 to 5 days prior birth at 20 mg/kg/d. The first cohort was continued on 20 mg/kg/d for entire course. The dose for the second cohort was increased to 600 mg/kg/d at postnatal 7days. (B) Phenotypes of IFG treated 4L;C* mice. The mice with 20 mg/kg/d IFG showed delayed duck-walk gait (arrow) as seen in the untreated 4L;C* mice. The mice on 600 mg/kg/d IFG showed spastic walk.

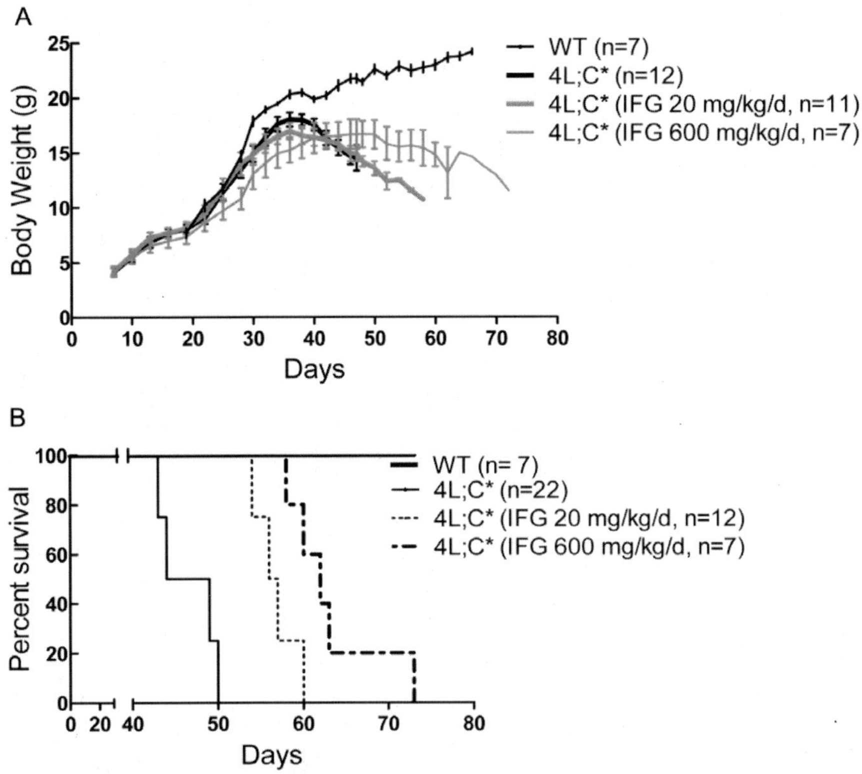

Figure 2. Life span and body weight. (A) Both treated and untreated 4L;C* mice had normal growth of their body weight till 35 days. The body weight of untreated 4L;C* mice started to decline at ~35 days. The mice on 20 mg/kg/d IFG showed decrease of body weight at ~35 days. The body weight of 4L;C* mice treated by 600 mg/kg/d IFG started decreasing at ~48 days. Their body weight grew slower than untreated 4L;C* mice. (B) The mice in both cohorts had significantly extended life span to average 54 days ($p = 0.0002$) by 20 mg/kg/d or 63 days ($P < 0.0001$) by 600 mg/kg/d IFG treatment relative to the untreated mice (~48 days). The Kaplan-Meier survival curves were analyzed using the Mantel-Cox Test.

effect on the life span of 4L;C* mice (54 days) compared to starting the same dose prior to birth (63 days). In 5 litters in which IFG (600 mg/kg/d) was begun at 3–5 days prior birth, all such pups died on postnatal days 1 to 3. The pups in one litter survived when this treatment started 2 days prior to birth. The results indicate that earlier treatment started had better efficacy, but that non-toxic doses were needed before the greater benefit of higher doses could be observed; 600 mg/kg/d extended the life span compared 20 mg/kg/d, and the administration of 600 mg/kg/d prior to birth is toxic to the pups.

IFG enhanced GCase activity and protein

The mutant GCase activity and protein levels in the tissues were analyzed in 4L;C* mice (Fig. 3). In the liver, IFG administration enhanced the mutant GCase activity by 3-fold at 20 mg/kg/d and by 6-fold at 600 mg/kg/d compared to that in untreated 4L;C mice. The 6-fold increase of V394L GCase activity corresponded to ~25% of WT levels, and was similar to the maximal effect observed in cultured skin fibroblasts from V394L/V394L or 4L;C* mice (data not shown). On 600 mg/kg/d, the mutant GCase activity was increased to a lesser extent in midbrain (1.4-fold) and spleen (1.9-fold). Lung mutant GCase activity was increased by 3.3-fold or 1.3-fold in the mice treated with IFG at 600 or 20 mg/kg/d, respectively. Immunoblot analyses using a specific anti-mouse GCase antibody showed that IFG increased GCase protein levels in the liver to WT levels (600 mg/kg/d) and to 21% of WT levels (20 mg/kg/d). In liver, these respective increases in GCase protein were about 28- or 5-fold compared to untreated 4L;C* (Fig. 3B). The results indicated a discrepancy between the activity and protein increases, and indicate that the IFG *in vivo* effect on activity was either inefficient or inhibitory. Also, tissue specific effects were observed with the liver enzyme having a greater response to IFG than that in the brain, spleen and lung. Whether this is due to enzyme differences in the various tissues or, more likely, IFG tissue distribution is unknown.

Substrate levels in IFG treated mice

GC and GS levels in 4L;C* tissues were determined by LC/MS. The tissues were collected from IFG treated (20 and 600 mg/kg/d) 4L;C*, untreated 4L;C* and WT mice at 14, 28, 44 days, and at terminal stages. Compared to untreated 4L;C*, GC and GS levels in various tissues were either unchanged or increased (Fig. 4 and Fig. 5). The longer treatments with 600 mg/kg/d led to GC and/or GS increases in visceral tissues (Fig. 4B and Fig. 5). The cerebral cortical levels were not significantly different in treated mice (Fig. 4A). At terminal stages, GC and GS levels in 600 mg/kg/d IFG treated brains were increased over baseline (Fig. 4A).

Cerebral cortical lactosylceramide (LacCer) and lactosylsphingosine (LacSph) levels in 4L;C* mice were not reduced by IFG treatment (Fig. 6). In general, LacCer and LacSph levels were either increased or unchanged in 600 mg/kg/d IFG treated mice compared to either untreated or to 20 mg/kg/d treated mice. Ceramide levels in 4L;C cortex and liver were at WT levels and were not altered by IFG treatment (data not shown). These data indicated that GC and GS levels were not substantially reduced in IFG treated 4L;C* mice. High dose (600 mg/kg/d) IFG caused accumulation of GC or GS in selected visceral tissues.

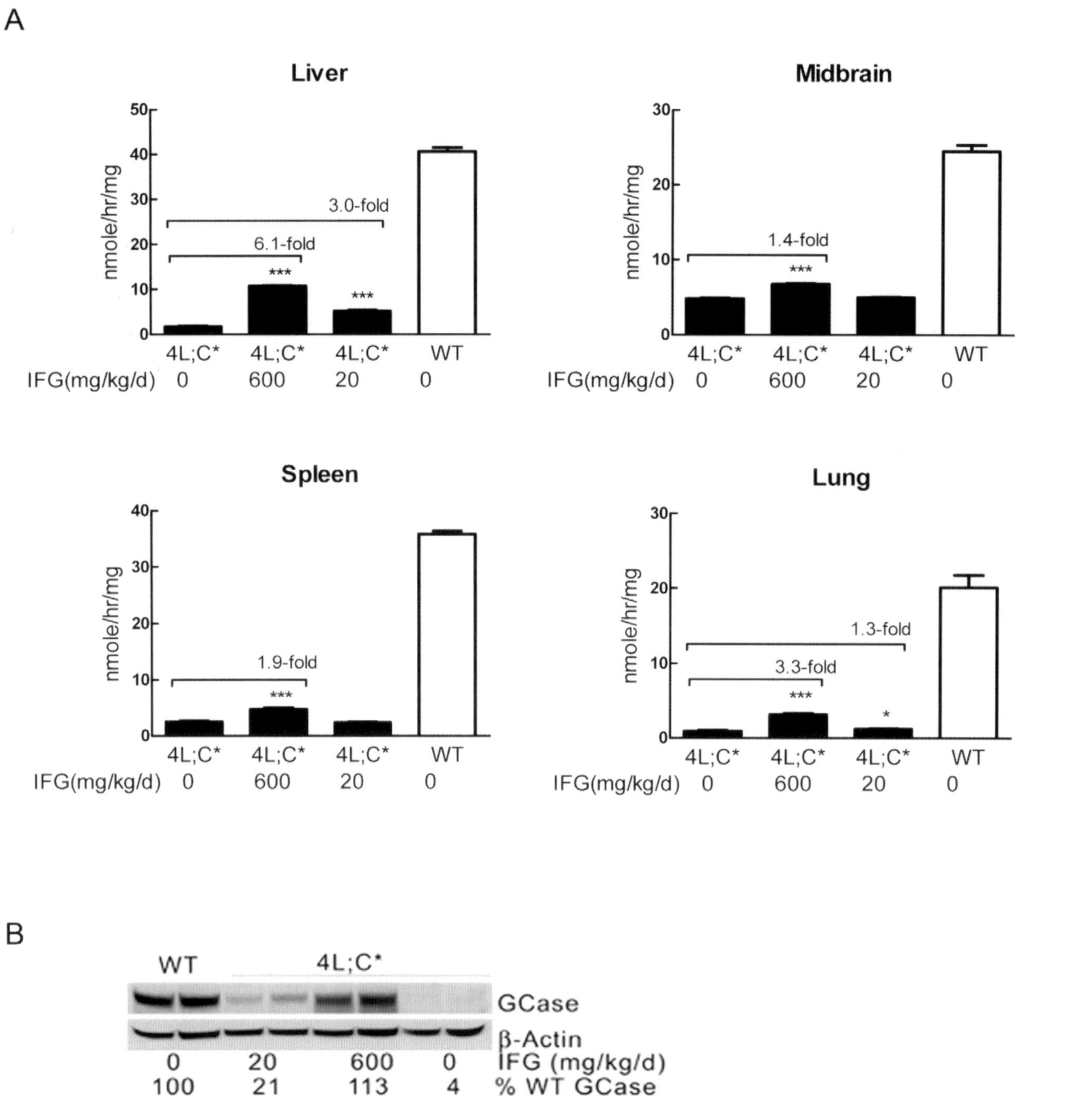

Figure 3. GCase activity and protein. (A) GCase activity was significantly increased in the treated 4L;C* liver by 3-fold in 20 mg/kg/d or 6-fold in 600 mg/kg/d IFG treatment groups, respectively. In the midbrain GCase was significantly increased by 1.4-fold in 4L;C* mice treated with 600 mg/kg/d IFG, but not changed with 20 mg/kg/d IFG compared to the untreated group. The GCase activity in the 4L;C* spleen was enhanced by 600 mg/kg/d IFG, whereas both 20 mg and 600 mg/kg/d IFG increased GCase activity in the lung. (B) GCase protein was increased in the liver of IFG (20 or 600 mg/kg/d) treated 4L;C* mice. GCase protein were determined by immunoblot analyses using anti-mouse GCase antibody and normalized to β-actin signal in the same sample. The levels were presented as percentage relative to GCase in WT mice. All the tissues used in GCase activity and protein analyses were from 28 days old mice. The data represent the mean±S.E. for three mice assayed in triplicate and analyzed by Student's t-test. ***, $p<0.001$.

IFG suppressed proinflammation

Proinflammation is a pathologic response in 4L;C* brain as demonstrated by microglial cell activation and astrogliosis [17]. IFG (20 or 600 mg/kg/d) treated 4L;C* showed decreased CD68 staining of microglial cells at 44 days, indicating suppression of microglial cell activation (Fig. 7A). With the disease progressing to the terminal stages, the CD68 positive microglial cells increased in both dosage groups (Fig. 7A). GFAP signals were increased, indicating astrogliosis. In the 20 mg/kg/d IFG treated 4L;C* brain stem, GFAP signals were weak at 44 days and increased by 57 days, i.e., terminal stage (Fig. 7B). Immunoblot analyses of GFAP of 44 day midbrain samples showed the reduction of GFAP level in IFG treated mice (Fig. 7C). High dose IFG (600 mg/kg/d) was more effective in

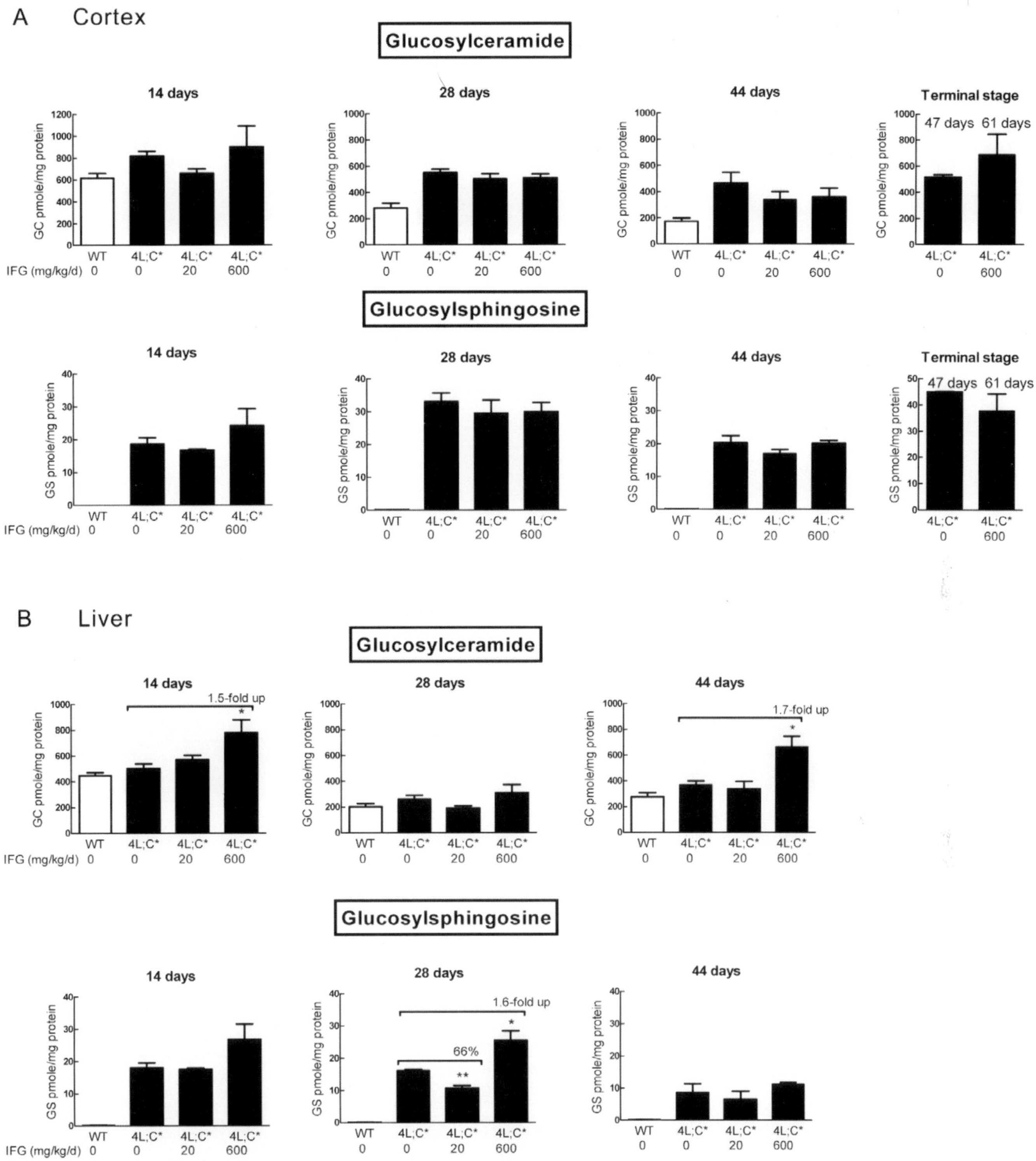

Figure 4. Analyses of GC and GS levels in the cortex and liver by LC/MS. (A) Cortex GC and GS levels in IFG treated 4L;C* did not show significant reduction relative to the untreated mice. GC and GS levels remained accumulated at terminal stage in 600 mg/kg/d IFG treated 4L;C* brain. (B) Increased liver GC were detected in 600 mg/kg/d IFG treated 4L;C* mice at 14 and 44 days relative to untreated 4L;C* liver. GS level decreased in 20 mg/kg/d IFG treated 4L;C* liver at 28 days. GS level in 600 mg/kg/d IFG treated 28 day liver were higher than untreated 4L;C* liver. The data represent the mean±S.E. and analyzed by Student's t-test. *, $p<0.05$ ($n=3$ mice). The GC and GS levels were normalized by protein level in the tissues lysate.

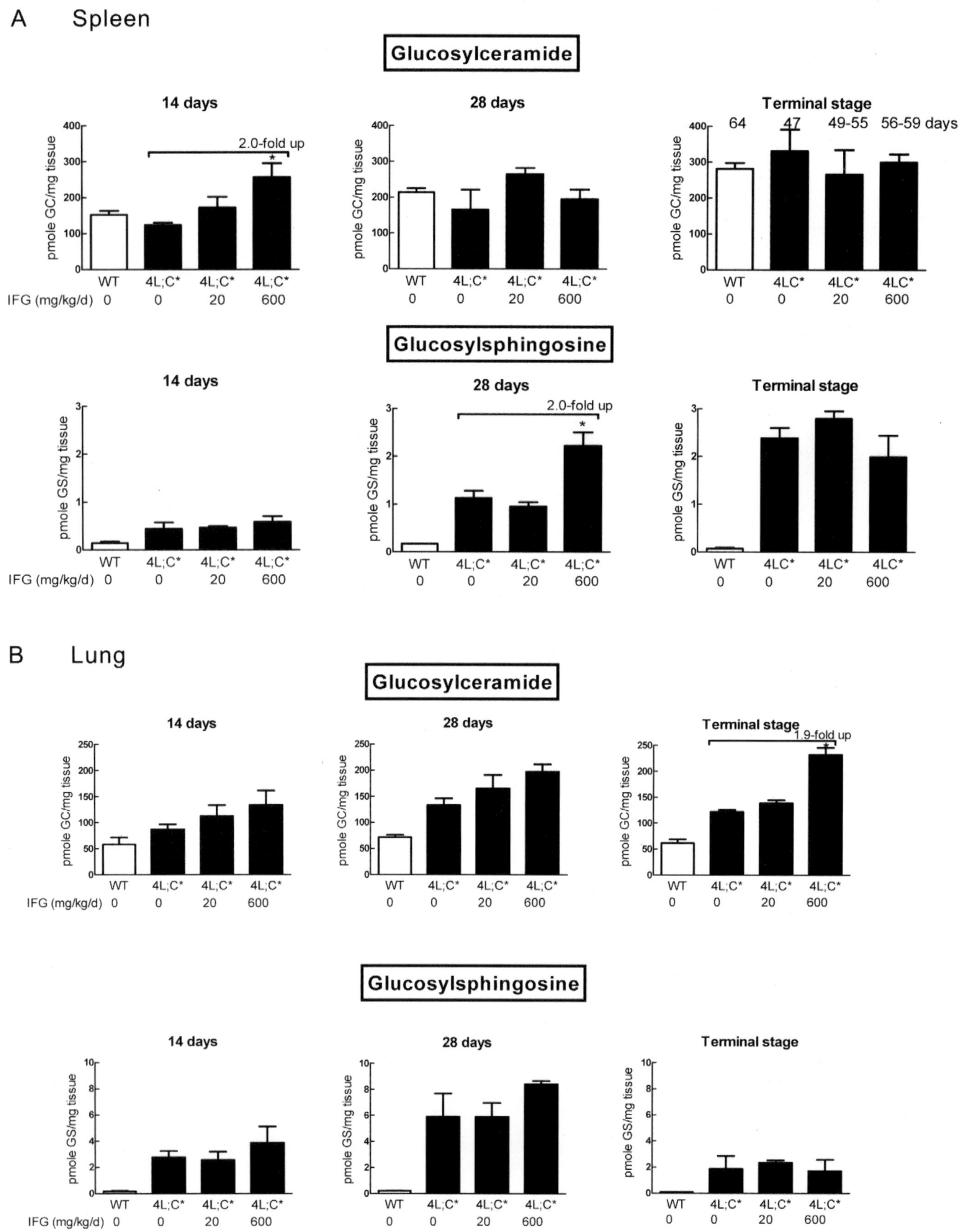

Figure 5. Analyses of GC and GS levels in the spleen and lung by LC/MS. (A) Spleen GC level in 4L;C* mice was not different from that in the WT. GS level was accumulated in 4L;C* spleen. By 600 mg/kg/d IFG treatment, GC or GS were increased by 2-fold in 4L;C* spleen at 14 day or 28 day,

respectively. (B) GC and GS were accumulated in 4L;C* lung. IFG treatment did not reduce the substrate level in 4L;C* lung. Increased GC level was in 600 mg/kg/d IFG treated lung at terminal stage (Age was same as spleen in Fig. 5A). The data represent the mean±S.E. and analyzed by Student's t-test. *, $p<0.05$ ($n=3$ mice). The GC and GS levels were normalized by tissue weight.

reducing GFAP signal levels than the lower dose in age matched samples.

p38 is involved in mediating inflammatory cytokine expression [18,19]. By immunoblotting with anti-Phosphorylated/active-p38 antibody, decreased phospho-p38 levels were detected in IFG treated 4L;C* midbrain, and the effect was dose dependent (Fig. 7D). The mRNA levels of p38α, β, γ, and δ were not significantly altered in the treated and untreated 4L;C* relative to WT, as determined by qRT-PCR analyses (data not shown). TNFα and IL6 are up-regulated during inflammation. By qRT-PCR analyses, increased TNFα and IL-6 mRNA levels were found in untreated 4L;C* midbrains (Fig. 7E) and brain stems (data not shown). TNFα levels were reduced by ~50% in IFG treated mice at 44 days and remained at decreased levels until the terminal stage (51 or 57 days). IL-6 mRNA levels remained elevated during IFG treatment with either dose at 44 days and at terminal stages. These results suggest that IFG attenuates the proinflammatory responses of microglial cells and astrocytes in 4L;C* brain.

Histology

The 4L;C* mice display axonal degeneration in the brainstem and spinal cord [17]. Axonal degeneration was found by H&E staining of brain stem and spinal cord sections from the 4L;C* mice untreated or treated with either 20 or 600 mg/kg/d IFG (Fig. 8A). Ultrastructural studies showed axonal inclusions in both treated and untreated 4L;C* mouse brain stems (Fig. 8B), midbrain and spinal cord (data not shown). These findings show that IFG treatment did not fundamentally change the brain pathology in 4L;C* mice.

Discussion

Pharmacological chaperones are a class of small molecules that enhance enzyme stability and can assist in trafficking of mutant enzymes from endoplasmic reticulum to normal destination such as the lysosome for GCase. IFG is a specific reversible GCase inhibitor (K_i ~20 nM) of WT GCase [20]. The binding of IFG to the active site of GCase locks the enzyme in its substrate-bound conformation and thermodynamically stabilizes the enzyme [21]. IFG binding affinity for GCase is greater (K_i ~<12 nM) at the neutral pH of the ER and lesser (K_i ~>50 nM) at the acidic lysosomal pH (Liou and Grabowski observations). Importantly, IFG enhances mutant activity in fibroblast having the N370S [15,20] and the L444P GCase in lymphoid lines and fibroblasts [16] (Liou and Grabowski unpublished). Using partially purified N370S GCase, IFG stabilizes the enzyme to thermal denaturation [21] (Liou and Grabowski unpublished). These findings suggest the potential for IFG as a therapeutic mutant enzyme enhancer that either improves enzyme stability or trafficking to the lysosome or both. The latter would facilitate dissociation of the GCase-IFG complex in the lysosome and allowing the GCase to bind its natural substrates. The finding that GCase in IFG treated cells have enhanced activity after dilution of the inhibitor implies that the free GCase retains an enhanced conformation for some time

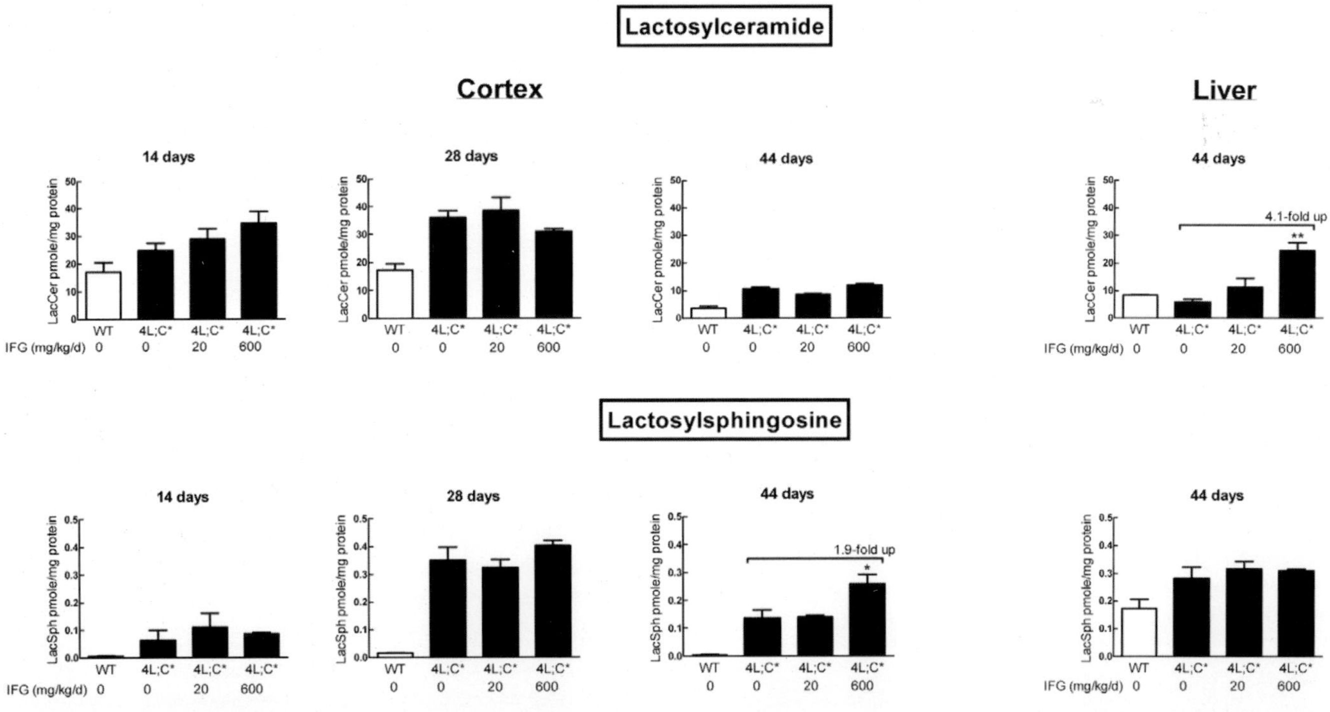

Figure 6. Analyses of lactosylceramide and lactosylsphingosine levels by LC/MS. Lactosylceramide (LacCer) level was not decreased in IFG treated 4L;C* cortex relative to the untreated mice. Increased lactosylsphingosine (LacSph) was detected in 600 mg/kg/d IFG treated cortex at 44 days. In the liver, LacSph level was not altered, but LacCer was increased in 600 mg/kg/d IFG treated mice at 44 days. The data represent the mean±S.E. and analyzed by Student's t-test. **, $p<0.01$; *, $p<0.05$ ($n=3$ mice). The GSL levels were normalized by protein level in the tissues lysate.

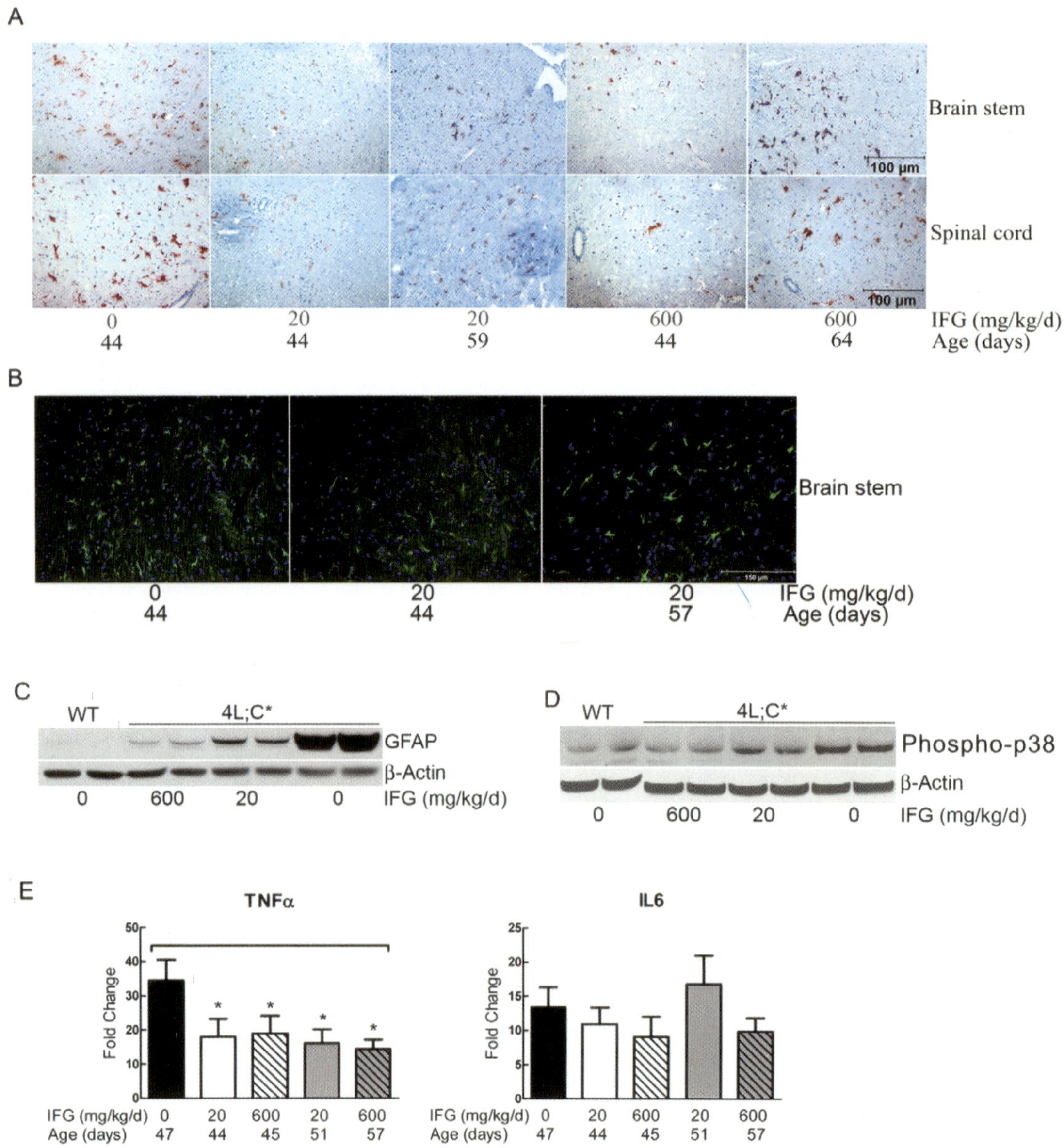

Figure 7. Proinflammation. (A) The brain stem and spinal cord sections were stained with anti-CD68 antibody, a macrophage-like marker. Positive CD68 signals (brown) on microglial cells demonstrated proinflammation. IFG (20 or 600 mg/kg/d) treated 4L;C* showed decreases of proinflammation at 44 days and increases of proinflammation at 59 or 64 days (terminal stage). (B) Enhanced GFAP staining (green) was in untreated 44 days old 4L;C* brain stem. IFG (20 mg/kg/d) treated 4L;C* showed decreases of GFAP signal at 44 days. GFAP signal were increased at terminal stage at 57 days. (C) GFAP protein in 44 days midbrain tissues was determined by immunoblot. Compared to untreated 4L;C*, GFAP levels were decreased in 20 mg/kg/d IFG and further reduced in 600 mg/kg/d IFG treated midbrain. (D) Phospho-p38 in 44 days midbrain tissues was analyzed by immunoblot. Increased Phospho-p38 was in untreated 4L;C* midbrain relative to WT. Phospho-p38 level was decreased in 20 mg/kg/d IFG treated midbrain and nearly to WT level in 600 mg/kg/d IFG treated mice. (E) TNFα and IL-6 mRNA in midbrain was determined by qRT-PCR. TNFα and IL-6 mRNA levels were increased by 35- and 13-fold in the untreated 4L;C* midbrain, respectively. In IFG (20 or 600 mg/kg/d) treated midbrain, TNFα mRNA were reduced at 44 or 45 days and at terminal stage (51 or 57 days). IL-6 mRNA level was not altered by IFG treatment. The data represent the mean±S.E. and analyzed by Student's t-test (n = 3 mice, assayed in duplicate).

after dissociation. Importantly, orally administered IFG distributes to visceral organs and the brain [16], suggesting an improved delivery compared to enzyme therapy that has little or no delivery to lungs, bone marrow, lymphoid tissues, and brain [22]. However, with these promising *in vitro* assay results, *in vivo* demonstration of improved substrate clearance and therapeutic efficiency remained to be shown.

In this study, a neuronopathic GCase-based mouse model having the V394L mutation was evaluated for IFG's *in vivo* effect on enzyme activity and substrate levels in CNS and visceral organs. This model was generated by crossing V394L homozygous to saposin C null mice. V394L homozygous mutant mice have residual enzyme activity of 4–10% of WT levels that is sufficient to maintain substrate flux and not present major GC or GS accumulation or cause a significant abnormal phenotype [23,24]. Since saposin C deficiency reduces GCase stability to proteolysis [25], the 4L;C* mice have decreased 4L GCase and develop a major neurological phenotype associated with

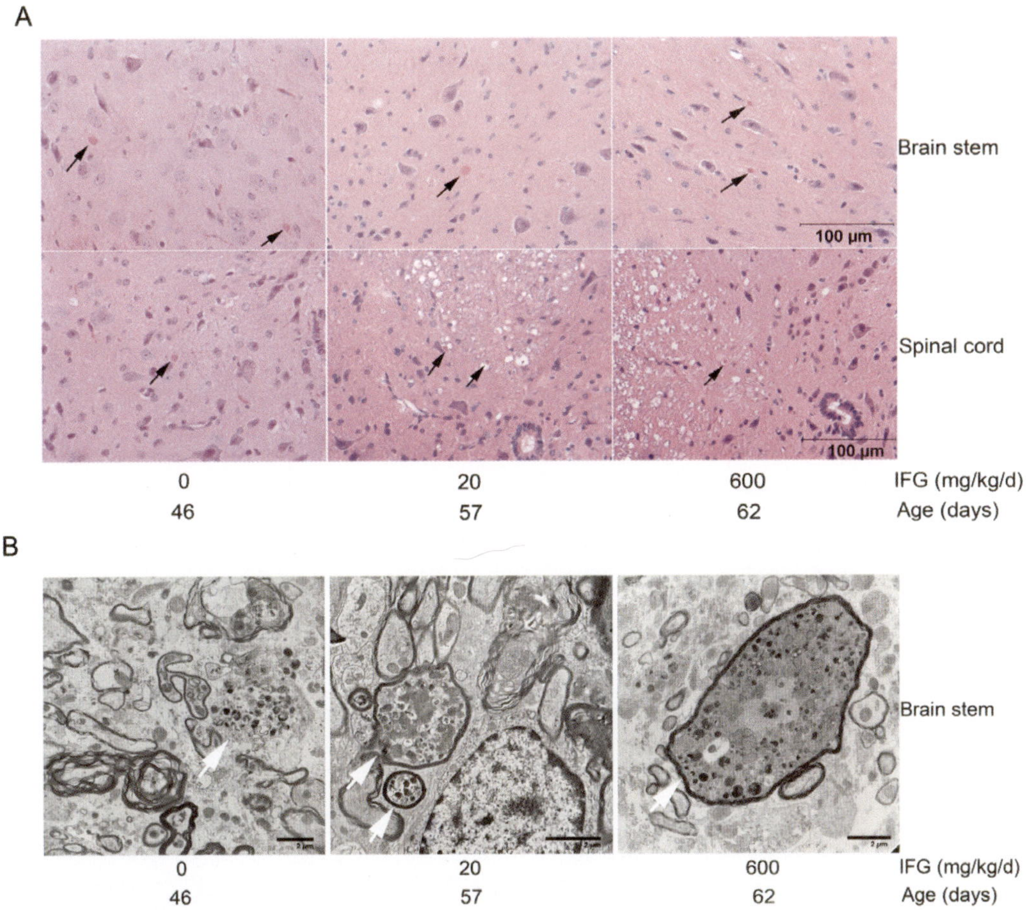

Figure 8. Histopathology. (A) H&E stained brain stem and spinal cord sections showed axonal degeneration (arrow) in untreated 4L;C* and 4L;C* mice treated by 20 or 600 mg/kg/d IFG. The tissues were collected at terminal stage. (B) Electron microscopy of brain stem. Axonal inclusions (arrow) in brain stem were present in untreated 4L;C* (left panel) at 43 days, 20 mg/kg/d IFG treated 4L;C* mice at 55 days (middle panel) and 600 mg/kg/d IFG treated 4L;C* mice at 62 days (right panel).

accumulation of GS and GC in the brain [17]. Importantly, the saposin C-/- mice do not show proinflammation until after 6 months of age in the visceral or brain. In addition, the saposin C-/- mice do not develop any phenotype or pathology until after 10 months of age. In saposin C-/- mouse model, absence of saposin C reduced GCase protein by ~50% of WT levels and led to activity reductions, but GC and GS levels are not increased in the brain and visceral tissues [26]. The phenotype of 4L;C* mouse model mimics some neuronopathic variants of human Gaucher disease. Here, IFG treatment of 4L;C* mice enhanced the V394L GCase protein and activity levels up to 25% of WT levels in the livers and about 2-fold in the brain. This was not accompanied by significant reductions in the accumulated substrates, GC and GS. Indeed, substrate levels increased under high dose IFG (600 mg/kg/d) treatment. This inhibitory effect of IFG and the mutant GCase was clearly toxic/lethal to developing pups as was evident when pregnant dames were administered this dose. Lower doses (20 mg/kg/d) did not have such toxic effect. To overcome such inhibitory effects, an on/off regimen had been suggested [16]. Here, no differences were found on the phenotype onset or life span between the on/off and continuous treatments. Lacking significant reduction of substrate levels by IFG in this model could be attributed to inhibitory effect on GCase from locally excessive IFG, and/or absence of saposin C's protection.

Despite the lack of IFG effect on the GC and GS levels, the treatment extended 4L;C*'s lifespan by >25%. Importantly, the pathological microglial infiltration in the untreated mice was delayed in the treated mice until the terminal stage. Thus, IFG treatment slowed disease progression, but did not change the ultimate disease outcome. Intriguingly, in the IFG treated mice, proinflammation was suppressed in the middle stage of treatment (44 days). However, the effect was lost in the terminal state and this was not different from the end stage in untreated mice. Such effects on the anti-proinflammatory responses were dose dependent, suggesting specific effect of IFG. Proinflammatory responses have been associated with neurodegeneration of other lysosomal storages diseases [27], and anti-inflammatory treatments attenuated the phenotype and extending lifespan [28,29,30]. The molecular targets for IFG to have such anti-proinflammatory effects are unknown. TNFα and IL-6 are the proinflammation cytokines that are dependent on p38 signaling for their production [18], which has implications in neurodegenerative diseases [31,32]. IL-6 protein and mRNA levels remained elevated during IFG treatment. However, the reductions of brain TNFα and phosporylation of p38 with IFG treatment suggests that these pathways are involved in the IFG mediated proinflammatory attenuation. In cell lines, ceramide generated from GC through the salvage pathway by enhancing GCase activity can reduce p38-mediated decreases in IL-6 levels, which would be anti-inflammatory [19]. In the brain, the total levels of GC and ceramide were not affected by IFG, and, therefore, the IL-6 pathway does not appear functional in this *in vivo* system. However, p38 phosphorylation was significantly reduced suggesting some connection. One intriguing possibility is that while the total levels of GC and ceramide remained the same, their subcellular distribution may have been different. Based on chaperone function, we could speculate that levels of GC and ceramide may have been partly corrected in the target organelle (e.g. lysosome) but not in other compartments.

Alternatively, off-target effects of IFG might be evoked. IFG is an iminosugar that is a member of the class of inhibitors for glycosidases and glycosyltransferases. Iminosugars have therapeutic applications in the diseases associated with the metabolism of glycoconjugates to treat tumor metastasis, influenza virus infection, and lysosomal storage diseases [33,34]. Single oral dose of 600 mg/kg to the rat achieves IFG concentration of 1.7 μM in the brain [16]. The continuous dosing of IFG (20 and 600 mg/kg/d) used here could have achieved much higher concentration in the brain than the K_i for GCase (20 nM). At such high concentrations, IFG could inhibit other glycosidase involved in inflammatory pathways, e.g. chitinase [35].

This study revealed the importance of *in vivo* analyses of the effects of pharmacological small molecules on mutant enzyme's function. Clearly, the ultimate effects on substrate reductions are essential for GCase or other lysosomal enzymes. Thus, *ex vivo* results of increasing GCase activity and protein by chaperones are insufficient to conclude that *in vivo* substrate degradation will occur and need to be interpreted cautiously when evaluating additional new compounds.

Materials and Methods

Materials

The following were from commercial sources: NuPAGE 4–12% Bis-Tris gel, NuPAGE MES SDS running buffer (Invitrogen, Carlsband, CA). 4-methyl-umbelliferyl-β-D-glucopyranoside (4MU-Glc; Biosynth AG, Switzerland). Sodium taurocholate (Calbiochem, La Jolla, CA). M-PER Mammalian Protein Extraction Reagent and BCA protein Assay reagent (Pierce, Rockford, IL). Hybond^{TM}-ECL^{TM} nitrocellulose membrane and ECL detection reagent (Amersham Biosciences, Piscataway, NJ). Anti-fade/DAPI, Methyl green, ABC Vectastain and Alkaline phosphatase kit II (Black) (Vector Laboratory, Burlingame, CA). Rat anti-mouse CD68 monoclonal antibodies (Serotec, Oxford, UK). Mouse anti-GFAP monoclonal antibody (Sigma, St. Louis, MO). Rabbit anti-active p38 polyclonal antibody (Promega, Madison, WI). IFG tartrate was provided by Amicus Therapeutics (Cranbury, NJ).

Animal care and drug treatment

4L;C* mice generation was as described [17]. Briefly, 4L;C* (V394L/V394L, saposin C-/-) mice were obtained from cross breeding saposin C+/-, V394L/V394L male and female mice. The strain background of 4L;C* was C57BL/6J/129SvEV. *In utero* IFG treatment was accomplished by providing the pregnant dames drinking water containing the requisite amount of IFG for 3–5 days prior to birth. In addition, mothers were kept on IFG during the weaning period so that the pups had continuous exposure to IFG via breast milk. Following weaning the mice were administrated IFG in drinking water under various specified regimens. Average daily water intake for each mouse is ~5 ml. At postnatal day 7, cohorts were treated with IFG either 600 or 20 mg/kg/d. Body weight, cage activity, and neurological phenotypes of the mice were monitored daily. The mice were maintained in microisolators in accordance with institutional guidelines under Institutional Animal Care and Use Committee (IACUC) approval at Cincinnati Children's Hospital Research Foundation (CCHRF). IACUC at CCHRF approved the study described in this manuscript with Animal Use Protocol number 8D10085. Other dosing schemes were as indicated in the text.

Histology and immunohistochemistry

After being anesthetized, the mice were perfused with saline followed by 4% paraformaldehyde prior tissues dissection. The tissues fixed in 10% formalin were processed for paraffin sections and stained with hematoxylin and eosin (H&E). Paraffin sections of brain and spinal cords were stained with mouse anti-GFAP as an astrocyte marker. Biotinylated goat anti-mouse IgG and streptavidin conjugated fluorescent 480 (green) were applied to the sections. DAPI (blue) in antifade was used for cell nuclei staining. Tissues fixed in 4% paraformaldehyde were processed for frozen blocks. Frozen sections were stained with rat anti-CD68 monoclonal antibody [36]. Methyl green was used for cell nuclei staining. Karnovsky's fixative was used for ultrastructural studies.

Glycosphingolipid analyses

Glycosphingolipids (GSLs) in the brain and liver lysates were extracted and analyzed by LC/MS at the Lipidomic Core at the Medical University of South Carolina [37]. GC and galactosylceramide in brain were separated for the LC/MS analyses. GC and GS levels in the tissue were normalized to protein content in the lysate.

GSLs in spleen and lung tissue (5 mg) were extracted [36], and GC and GS analyses were carried out at CCHRF by ESI-LC-MS/MS using a Waters Quattro Micro API triple quadrupole mass spectrometer (Milford, MA) interfaced with Acquity UPLC system. Nitrogen was used as nebulizer and argon was used as collision gas. The source temperature was maintained at 120°C, and the desolvation temperature was kept at 450°C. The drying gas (N_2) was maintained at ca. 800 L/h whereas the cone flow gas was off. The multiplier was set at an absolute value of 650. Online chromatographic separation was achieved using a Supelcosil-LC-18-DB column (33×3.0 mm i.d. 3.0 μm). Gradient elution with methanol and water charged with ammonium acetate and formic acid were employed.

Optimized parameters for GC and GS were determined with individual standard compounds (Avanti Polar lipids, Inc.). For quantification of GCs, the ESI-MS/MS was operated in the multiple reaction monitoring (MRM) mode for monitoring transition pair of the individual protonated precursor ions and their common product ion m/z 264. GS was monitored by mass transition m/z 462.3>282.4. Calibration curves were built for C16, C18 and C24:1 GC using C12 GC as the internal standard. Quantification of GCs with various fatty acid chain lengths was realized by using the curve of each GC species with closest number of chain length. The quantification of GS was based on the curve using C8 GS as internal standard. The linear response for GCs and GS was in the range of 50 pg–25 ng. The extracted spleen and lung samples were suspended in methanol containing internal standard and injected into the LC/MS. The GC and GS levels in the spleen and lung were normalized to tissue weight.

Analyses of GCase activity

Tissues were collected from saline perfused mice, homogenized in 0.25% Na taurocholate and 0.25% Triton X-100 and their GCase activities were determined fluorometrically [24,38]. Assay mixtures were incubated in the presence of CBE for 60 min (37°C) to correct for the presence of non-lysosomal GCase and β-glucosidases that cleave 4MU-Glc. WT mice tissues were run in parallel as control. Data were analyzed by Student's t-test.

Immunoblots

Mouse liver GCase protein detection by immunoblot was as described [36]. The amounts of GCase protein were quantitated with ImageQuant software and normalized to β-actin in the same samples. Midbrain tissues were homogenized in M-PER Mammalian Protein Extraction Reagent and subjected to electrophoresis on NuPAGE 4-12% Bis-Tris gel. The protein was transferred to Hybond^{TM}-ECL^{TM} nitrocellulose membrane. GFAP protein in the samples was reacted with anti-GFAP antibody [39]. Anti-active p38 polyclonal antibody was used to detect Phosphorylated p38 (Phospho-p38) in the samples resolved on 10% Bis-Tris gel [19]. The signals were detected with ECL detection reagent (GE Healthcare, Piscataway, NJ) according to manufacturer's instructions.

qRT-PCR

RNAs in midbrain or brain stem tissues were extracted using TOTALLY RNA kit (Ambion Inc.) and purified with RNeasy Mini kit (Qiagen). Reverse transcription of total RNA (1 µg) for each sample was carried out using RT^2 First Strand Kit (SA Biosciences). Quantitative RT-PCR (qRT-PCR) was performed on ABI Prism 7000 sequence detection system. The primers for mouse TNFα, IL6, and GAPDH were from SA Biosciences. In PCR mixtures, cDNA aliquots were analyzed using 400 nM of each primer and RT^2 Real-Time SYBR Green/ROX PCR master mix (SA Biosciences). PCR amplifications were run in duplicate as follows: 2 min at 50°C and 10 min at 95°C, followed by 40 cycles of 15 s at 95°C and 1 min at 60°C. Relative quantification of TNFα or IL6 referenced to internal control, GAPDH, was analyzed by ΔΔCt Analysis. The fold changes of each gene were normalized by WT samples. Three mice from each group were used and the experiments were repeated twice.

Acknowledgments

The authors thank Venette Inskeep, Juying Xu, Spence Perry, Sean Gray and Didi Zhu for their technical assistance, Lisa McMillin, Meredith Farmer and Sabina Sylvest for skilled tissue preparation, Chris Woods for the photograph preparation and Michelle Cooley for her clerical expertise.

Author Contributions

Conceived and designed the experiments: YS GAG. Performed the experiments: HR BL BQ MZ WZ JB KK YS. Analyzed the data: YS WZ KK KDRS YAH GAG. Contributed reagents/materials/analysis tools: KDRS YAH. Wrote the paper: YS KDRS YAH GAG.

References

1. Grabowski GA, Petsko GA, Kolodny EH (2010) Gaucher disease. In: Valle D, Beaudet A, Vogelstein B, Kinzler KW, Antonarakis SE et al, eds. The Online Metabolic and Molecular Bases of Inherited Diseases. New York: The McGraw-Hill Companies, Inc.
2. Gupta N, Oppenheim IM, Kauvar EF, Tayebi N, Sidransky E (2010) Type 2 Gaucher disease: Phenotypic variation and genotypic heterogeneity. Blood Cells Mol Dis.
3. Weinreb NJ, Charrow J, Andersson HC, Kaplan P, Kolodny EH, et al. (2002) Effectiveness of enzyme replacement therapy in 1028 patients with type 1 Gaucher disease after 2 to 5 years of treatment: a report from the Gaucher Registry. Am J Med 113: 112–119.
4. Wenstrup RJ, Kacena KA, Kaplan P, Pastores GM, Prakash-Cheng A, et al. (2007) Effect of enzyme replacement therapy with imiglucerase on BMD in type 1 Gaucher disease. J Bone Miner Res 22: 119–126.
5. Grabowski GA, Kacena K, Cole JA, Hollak CE, Zhang L, et al. (2009) Dose-response relationships for enzyme replacement therapy with imiglucerase/alglucerase in patients with Gaucher disease type 1. Genet Med 11: 92–100.
6. Burrow TA, Cohen MB, Bokulic R, Deutsch G, Choudhary A, et al. (2007) Gaucher disease: progressive mesenteric and mediastinal lymphadenopathy despite enzyme therapy. J Pediatr 150: 202–206.
7. Radin NS (1994) Rationales for cancer chemotherapy with PDMP, a specific inhibitor of glucosylceramide synthase. Mol Chem Neuropathol 21: 111–127.
8. Weinreb NJ, Barranger JA, Charrow J, Grabowski GA, Mankin HJ, et al. (2005) Guidance on the use of miglustat for treating patients with type 1 Gaucher disease. Am J Hematol 80: 223–229.
9. McEachern KA, Fung J, Komarnitsky S, Siegel CS, Chuang WL, et al. (2007) A specific and potent inhibitor of glucosylceramide synthase for substrate inhibition therapy of Gaucher disease. Mol Genet Metab 91: 259–267.
10. Marshall J, McEachern KA, Chuang WL, Hutto E, Siegel CS, et al. (2010) Improved management of lysosomal glucosylceramide levels in a mouse model of type 1 Gaucher disease using enzyme and substrate reduction therapy. J Inherit Metab Dis 33: 281–289.
11. Lukina E, Watman N, Arreguin EA, Banikazemi M, Dragosky M, et al. (2010) A phase 2 study of eliglustat tartrate (Genz-112638), an oral substrate reduction therapy for Gaucher disease type 1. Blood 116: 893–899.
12. Fan JQ (2008) A counterintuitive approach to treat enzyme deficiencies: use of enzyme inhibitors for restoring mutant enzyme activity. Biol Chem 389: 1–11.
13. Sawkar AR, Cheng WC, Beutler E, Wong CH, Balch WE, et al. (2002) Chemical chaperones increase the cellular activity of N370S beta -glucosidase: a therapeutic strategy for Gaucher disease. Proc Natl Acad Sci U S A 99: 15428–15433.
14. Mu TW, Fowler DM, Kelly JW (2008) Partial restoration of mutant enzyme homeostasis in three distinct lysosomal storage disease cell lines by altering calcium homeostasis. PLoS Biol 6: e26.
15. Steet RA, Chung S, Wustman B, Powe A, Do H, et al. (2006) The iminosugar isofagomine increases the activity of N370S mutant acid beta-glucosidase in Gaucher fibroblasts by several mechanisms. Proc Natl Acad Sci U S A 103: 13813–13818.
16. Khanna R, Benjamin ER, Pellegrino L, Schilling A, Rigat BA, et al. (2010) The pharmacological chaperone isofagomine increases the activity of the Gaucher disease L444P mutant form of beta-glucosidase. FEBS J.
17. Sun Y, Liou B, Ran H, Skelton MR, Williams MT, et al. (2010) Neuronopathic Gaucher disease in the mouse: viable combined selective saposin C deficiency and mutant glucocerebrosidase (V394L) mice with glucosylsphingosine and glucosylceramide accumulation and progressive neurological deficits. Hum Mol Genet 19: 1088–1097.
18. Zhang J, Shen B, Lin A (2007) Novel strategies for inhibition of the p38 MAPK pathway. Trends Pharmacol Sci 28: 286–295.
19. Kitatani K, Sheldon K, Anelli V, Jenkins RW, Sun Y, et al. (2009) Acid beta-glucosidase 1 counteracts p38delta-dependent induction of interleukin-6: possible role for ceramide as an anti-inflammatory lipid. J Biol Chem 284: 12979–12988.
20. Lieberman RL, Wustman BA, Huertas P, Powe AC, Jr., Pine CW, et al. (2007) Structure of acid beta-glucosidase with pharmacological chaperone provides insight into Gaucher disease. Nat Chem Biol 3: 101–107.
21. Lieberman RL, D'Aquino JA, Ringe D, Petsko GA (2009) Effects of pH and iminosugar pharmacological chaperones on lysosomal glycosidase structure and stability. Biochemistry 48: 4816–4827.
22. Xu YH, Sun Y, Barnes S, Grabowski GA (2010) Comparative therapeutic effects of velaglucerase alfa and imiglucerase in a Gaucher disease mouse model. PLoS One 5: e10750.
23. Xu YH, Reboulet R, Quinn B, Huelsken J, Witte D, et al. (2008) Dependence of reversibility and progression of mouse neuronopathic Gaucher disease on acid beta-glucosidase residual activity levels. Mol Genet Metab.
24. Xu YH, Quinn B, Witte D, Grabowski GA (2003) Viable mouse models of acid beta-glucosidase deficiency: the defect in Gaucher disease. Am J Pathol 163: 2093–2101.
25. Sun Y, Qi X, Grabowski GA (2003) Saposin C is required for normal resistance of acid beta-glucosidase to proteolytic degradation. J Biol Chem 278: 31918–31923.
26. Sun Y, Ran H, Zamzow M, Kitatani K, Skelton MR, et al. (2010) Specific saposin C deficiency: CNS impairment and acid beta-glucosidase effects in the mouse. Hum Mol Genet 19: 634–647.
27. Jeyakumar M, Thomas R, Elliot-Smith E, Smith DA, van der Spoel AC, et al. (2003) Central nervous system inflammation is a hallmark of pathogenesis in mouse models of GM1 and GM2 gangliosidosis. Brain 126: 974–987.
28. Jeyakumar M, Smith DA, Williams IM, Borja MC, Neville DC, et al. (2004) NSAIDs increase survival in the Sandhoff disease mouse: synergy with N-butyldeoxynojirimycin. Ann Neurol 56: 642–649.
29. Smith D, Wallom KL, Williams IM, Jeyakumar M, Platt FM (2009) Beneficial effects of anti-inflammatory therapy in a mouse model of Niemann-Pick disease type C1. Neurobiol Dis 36: 242–251.

30. Luzi P, Abraham RM, Rafi MA, Curtis M, Hooper DC, et al. (2009) Effects of treatments on inflammatory and apoptotic markers in the CNS of mice with globoid cell leukodystrophy. Brain Res 1300: 146–158.
31. Munoz L, Ralay Ranaivo H, Roy SM, Hu W, Craft JM, et al. (2007) A novel p38 alpha MAPK inhibitor suppresses brain proinflammatory cytokine up-regulation and attenuates synaptic dysfunction and behavioral deficits in an Alzheimer's disease mouse model. J Neuroinflammation 4: 21.
32. Klegeris A, Pelech S, Giasson BI, Maguire J, Zhang H, et al. (2008) Alpha-synuclein activates stress signaling protein kinases in THP-1 cells and microglia. Neurobiol Aging 29: 739–752.
33. Butters TD, Dwek RA, Platt FM (2005) Imino sugar inhibitors for treating the lysosomal glycosphingolipidoses. Glycobiology 15: 43R–52R.
34. Nishimura Y (2009) Gem-diamine 1-N-iminosugars as versatile glycomimetics: synthesis, biological activity and therapeutic potential. J Antibiot (Tokyo) 62: 407–423.
35. Zhu Z, Zheng T, Homer RJ, Kim YK, Chen NY, et al. (2004) Acidic mammalian chitinase in asthmatic Th2 inflammation and IL-13 pathway activation. Science 304: 1678–1682.
36. Sun Y, Quinn B, Witte DP, Grabowski GA (2005) Gaucher disease mouse models: point mutations at the acid {beta}-glucosidase locus combined with low-level prosaposin expression lead to disease variants. J Lipid Res 46: 2102–2113.
37. Kitatani K, Sheldon K, Rajagopalan V, Anelli V, Jenkins RW, et al. (2009) Involvement of acid beta-glucosidase 1 in the salvage pathway of ceramide formation. J Biol Chem 284: 12972–12978.
38. Xu YH, Ponce E, Sun Y, Leonova T, Bove K, et al. (1996) Turnover and distribution of intravenously administered mannose-terminated human acid beta-glucosidase in murine and human tissues. Pediatr Res 39: 313–322.
39. Sun Y, Witte DP, Ran H, Zamzow M, Barnes S, et al. (2008) Neurological deficits and glycosphingolipid accumulation in saposin B deficient mice. Hum Mol Genet 17: 2345–2356.

7

Urinary Copper Elevation in a Mouse Model of Wilson's Disease Is a Regulated Process to Specifically Decrease the Hepatic Copper Load

Lawrence W. Gray[1], Fangyu Peng[2], Shannon A. Molloy[3], Venkata S. Pendyala[1], Abigael Muchenditsi[1], Otto Muzik[4], Jaekwon Lee[5], Jack H. Kaplan[3], Svetlana Lutsenko[1]*

1 Department of Physiology, Johns Hopkins University, School of Medicine, Baltimore, Maryland, United States of America, **2** Department of Radiology, University of Texas Southwestern Medical Center, Dallas, Texas, United States of America, **3** Department of Biochemistry and Molecular Genetics, University of Illinois at Chicago, Chicago, Illinois, United States of America, **4** Carman and Ann Adams Department of Pediatrics and Department of Radiology, Wayne State University, School of Medicine, Detroit, Michigan, United States of America, **5** Redox Biology Center, Department of Biochemistry, University of Nebraska, Lincoln, Nebraska, United States of America

Abstract

Body copper homeostasis is regulated by the liver, which removes excess copper via bile. In Wilson's disease (WD), this function is disrupted due to inactivation of the copper transporter ATP7B resulting in hepatic copper overload. High urinary copper is a diagnostic feature of WD linked to liver malfunction; the mechanism behind urinary copper elevation is not fully understood. Using Positron Emission Tomography-Computed Tomography (PET-CT) imaging of live *Atp7b*$^{-/-}$ mice at different stages of disease, a longitudinal metal analysis, and characterization of copper-binding molecules, we show that urinary copper elevation is a specific regulatory process mediated by distinct molecules. PET-CT and atomic absorption spectroscopy directly demonstrate an age-dependent decrease in the capacity of *Atp7b*$^{-/-}$ livers to accumulate copper, concomitant with an increase in urinary copper. This reciprocal relationship is specific for copper, indicating that cell necrosis is not the primary cause for the initial phase of metal elevation in the urine. Instead, the urinary copper increase is associated with the down-regulation of the copper-transporter Ctr1 in the liver and appearance of a 2 kDa Small Copper Carrier, SCC, in the urine. SCC is also elevated in the urine of the liver-specific *Ctr1*$^{-/-}$ knockouts, which have normal ATP7B function, suggesting that SCC is a normal metabolite carrying copper in the serum. In agreement with this hypothesis, partially purified SCC-Cu competes with free copper for uptake by Ctr1. Thus, hepatic down-regulation of Ctr1 allows switching to an SCC-mediated removal of copper via kidney when liver function is impaired. These results demonstrate that the body regulates copper export through more than one mechanism; better understanding of urinary copper excretion may contribute to an improved diagnosis and monitoring of WD.

Editor: Paul Cobine, Auburn University, United States of America

Funding: This work was supported by the National Institutes of Health grants 5F31DK084730 to LWG, 5R01DK079209 to JL, and 5P01GM067166 to SL and JHK. The mass-spectrometry work was done at the Metal Ion Core (Oregon Health and Science University), supported by NIH instrumentation grant S10-RR025512. The funders had no role in study design, data collection and analysis, decision to publish, or preparation of the manuscript.

Competing Interests: The authors have declared that no competing interests exist.

* E-mail: lutsenko@jhmi.edu

Introduction

Copper is an essential trace element that is required for catalytic activity of key metabolic enzymes involved in oxidative stress response, respiration, blood clotting, and many other physiologic processes. Deficit of copper in the diet is associated with cardiac hypertrophy and neurologic abnormalities, whereas genetically induced copper insufficiency (in Menkes disease or as a result of genetic manipulations in animals) is lethal [1]. Although copper is essential for normal growth and development, excessive copper is toxic. This toxicity is best illustrated by Wilson's disease (WD), a potentially lethal human disease caused by inactivating mutations in the copper transporter ATP7B and massive copper accumulation in the liver [2]. Normally, in humans and other mammals, liver is the main organ that maintains copper homeostasis. In hepatocytes, ATP7B transports excess copper into vesicles for subsequent excretion into the bile [3]. In a healthy organism, this is the primary route of copper removal and little copper is found in the urine.

In WD, the copper excretion pattern changes dramatically. Inactivation of ATP7B impairs copper export into the bile. Copper content of the liver becomes greatly elevated causing, with time, significant pathologic changes in liver morphology and function [2]. Patients with WD also have high urinary copper (208 to 466 μg per day), which serves as an important diagnostic marker for the disease [4,5]. The origin of high copper in WD urine is not obvious because most of the incoming copper is thought to be trapped in the liver. Disease-induced cell necrosis may result in the release of copper from damaged hepatocytes into the bloodstream. However, experiments directly testing this hypothesis are lacking. Furthermore, elevated copper in the urine is observed in several other conditions (hepatitis, cancer, pregnancy) [6–8], when ATP7B function is presumed normal, suggesting existence of a secondary mechanism for copper excretion. A better mechanistic understanding of copper elevation in the urine would facilitate early diagnosis of WD and the treatment monitoring. Consequently, we utilized the *Atp7b*$^{-/-}$ mice, an established model for WD, to investigate the basis of urinary copper elevation.

Atp7b$^{-/-}$ mice, like WD patients, accumulate copper first in the liver and later in other tissues and have a marked liver pathology [9]. Without intervention of chelation therapy, the disease in these animals progresses through three major stages. At Stage I (up to 6–8 weeks after birth), copper accumulates rapidly in the liver and induces changes in cell cycle machinery and lipid metabolism; however no major histological changes are apparent [10]. At Stage II (12–20 weeks), there are numerous metabolic changes, and liver shows clear signs of inflammation, necrosis, and bile ducts proliferation. In animals older than 30 weeks (Stage III), there is a significant recovery of liver morphology and function [11] along with copper sequestration in highly concentrated deposits, appearance of regenerating nodules and continuing bile ducts proliferation [11]. In the present study, we used *Atp7b*$^{-/-}$ mice to show that the loss of ATP7B-mediated copper export also results in activation of a specific secondary export pathway that diminishes copper load in the liver. This pathway involves time-dependent down-regulation of the copper uptake transporter *Ctr1* in the liver and upregulation of a distinct small copper carrier(s), SCC, in the urine.

Results

Copper in the urine of Atp7b$^{-/-}$ mice increases with age but does not directly follow liver pathology

In *Atp7b*$^{-/-}$ mice, the liver morphology and function are most impaired at Stage II of the disease (12–20 weeks of age), and both parameters are improved in older animals [11]. Consequently, we tested whether the urinary copper follows liver pathology in *Atp7b*$^{-/-}$ mice by measuring copper concentration and total copper output in the urine of animals of various ages. In wild-type mice, urinary copper output and copper concentration were largely unchanged with some decrease in the total copper output observed in animals older than 14 weeks. In contrast, the amount of copper excreted in the urine of *Atp7b*$^{-/-}$ mice increased with age (Figure 1). A marked increase in copper concentration was detected between 7 and 20 weeks; a statistically significant change in both concentration and total copper output was most pronounced at 14–20 weeks (Figure 1). This increase coincides with marked pathologic changes in the liver [11]. In animals older than 20 weeks (when copper levels in the liver decreases and liver morphology and function are partially restored) the amount of copper in the urine remained high and the total output was similar to that at 14–20 weeks. Thus, inactivation of *Atp7b* produces age-dependent elevation of copper export through the kidney, which cannot be fully explained by liver necrosis.

Upregulation of copper export is followed by changes in renal function

We also noticed that although total copper output was high in *Atp7b*$^{-/-}$ mice older than 20 weeks (Figure 1B), the urinary concentration of copper of these animals was significantly lower compared to younger animals (Figure 1A). To gain a better insight into variations of urinary copper concentration, we measured food and water intake as well as total urine volume (Figure 2). Compared to age-matched controls, food (Figure 2B) and water intake (Figure 2A) did not differ significantly for *Atp7b*$^{-/-}$ animals before 20 weeks; however, after 20 weeks both water intake (Figure 2A) and urine volume (Figure 2C) increased dramatically,

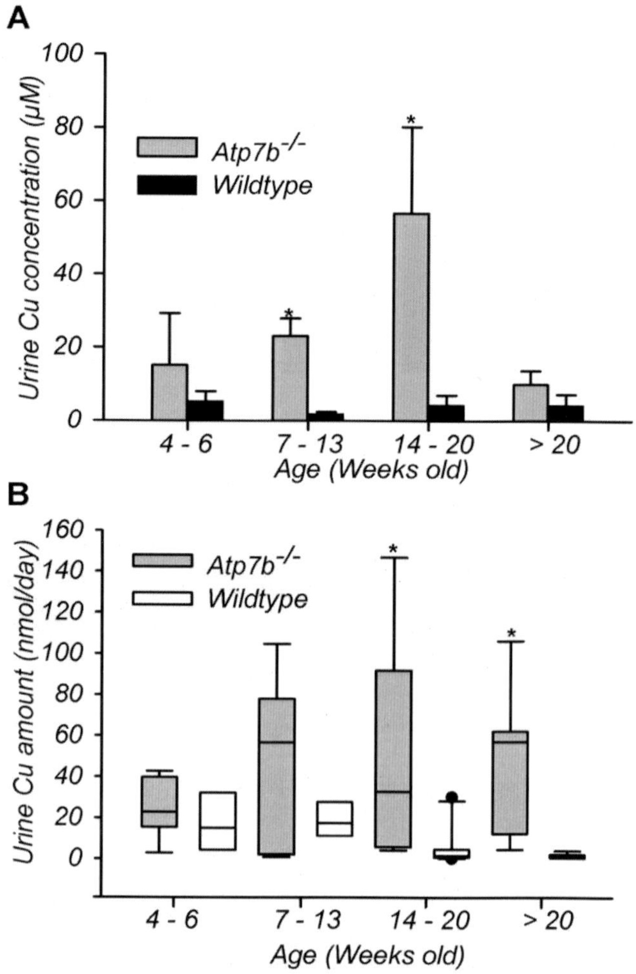

Figure 1. *Atp7b* inactivation induces age-dependent changes in urine copper content. (A) Urinary copper concentration and (B) total amount from wild-type (WT) and *Atp7b*$^{-/-}$ (KO) mice at different ages. Urine collected over 24 hours and measured by atomic absorption. Data reported as mean concentration ± SD, n = 3 to 13, animals per age group. *$P<0.05$ versus age-matched wild type. Boxplot middle horizontal bar represents the median; the dotted horizontal line signifies the mean. The while upper and lower box values signify the 75th and 25th percentiles, whiskers represent the 10th and 90th percentiles. The black dots represent outliers (three SD from the mean).

explaining the decrease in urinary copper concentration at this age. Markedly increased urine volume suggested that renal function was altered in *Atp7b*$^{-/-}$ animals older than 20 weeks. This conclusion was confirmed by measuring protein amounts in the urine, which revealed proteinuria in *Atp7b*$^{-/-}$ mice older than 20 weeks, but not before this age (Figure S1, additional details in Information S1).

Longitudinal PET-CT using $^{64}CuCl_2$ demonstrates age-dependent changes in copper accumulation by Atp7b$^{-/-}$ liver

The age-dependent increase of urinary copper suggested that copper uptake and/or excretion by organs were altered in *Atp7b*$^{-/-}$ animals in an age-dependent manner. To test this hypothesis we conducted a longitudinal PET imaging of copper distribution in live *Atp7b*$^{-/-}$ mice, who received orally administered $^{64}CuCl_2$ at 7–8, 13, and 20 weeks of age. We first compared

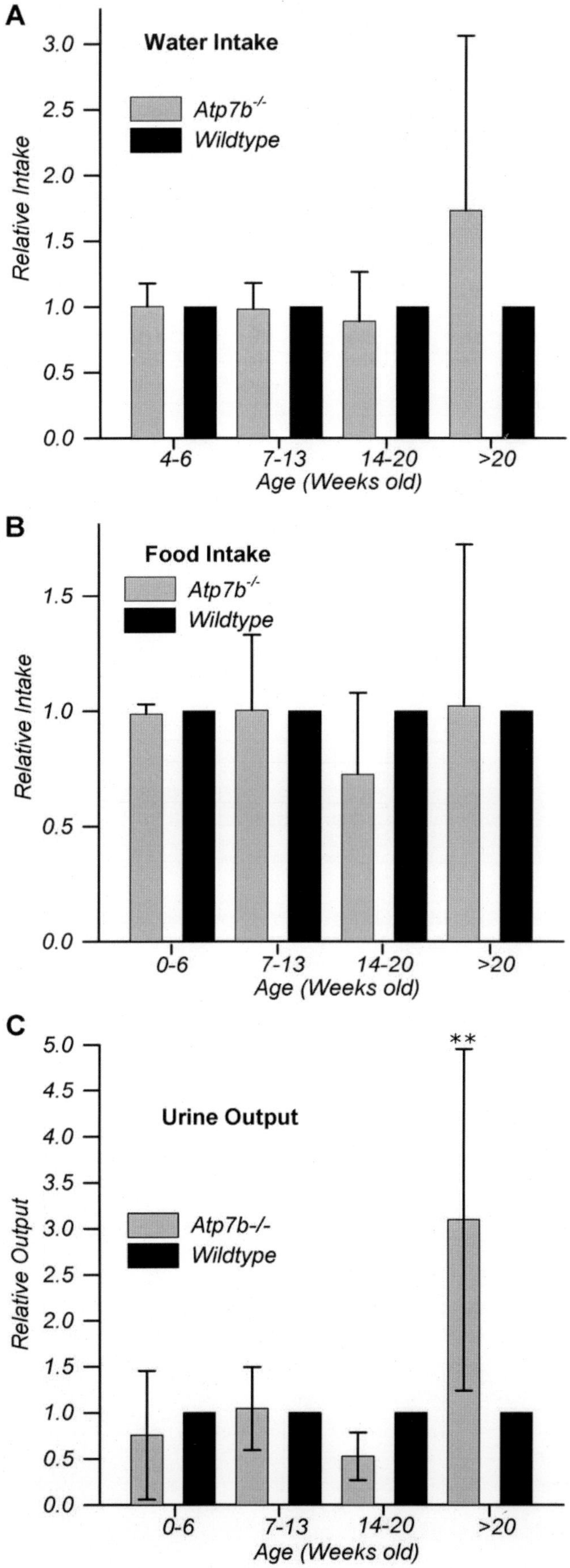

Figure 2. Renal function is altered in *Atp7b*$^{-/-}$ mice older than 20 weeks. Water intake (A), Food intake (B) and urine volume output (C) relative to age-matched wild-type mice were measured over a 24 hr period. Double asterisks denote $p \leq 0.003$. N = 3 to 7 age-matched pairs; data presented as mean ± SD; additional supporting data and details in Figure S1 and information S1.

copper accumulation in the liver at early (2 hours post administration) and late (24 hours post administration) phases (Figure S2 and Figure 3, respectively). At 2 hours, there was no measurable difference between ^{64}Cu radioactivity in the wild-type and *Atp7b*$^{-/-}$ livers (Figure S2 A, B). However, at 24 hours post oral administration of $^{64}CuCl_2$, hepatic ^{64}Cu radioactivity was noticeably higher in the *Atp7b*$^{-/-}$ mice compared to wild-type at all three ages (Figure 3A and B). Further quantitative analysis of PET data revealed a significantly higher accumulation/retention of copper by the *Atp7b*$^{-/-}$ liver in younger animals (7–8 weeks) compared to older animals (Figure 3C), $p<0.001$. No significant differences in hepatic copper accumulation were seen in wild-type animals of different ages ($p>0.5$).

Age-dependent changes in copper levels in Atp7b$^{-/-}$ kidneys are inverse to those in the liver and less pronounced

The apparent decrease in liver's ability to accumulate copper at 13–20 weeks and a concomitant increase of urinary copper pointed to the increasing involvement of kidneys in the export of copper from the body. To better understand the role of kidneys in copper processing, we performed quantitative PET analysis for both the kidneys and the bladder. We were able to measure large mean differences even though animal to animal-to-animal variation precluded significance. At 2 hours post ^{64}Cu administration, an average ^{64}Cu radioactivity in the *Atp7b*$^{-/-}$ kidneys was consistently lower compared to wild-type at all time-points (Figure S2). At 24 hours, radioactive copper in *Atp7b*$^{-/-}$ kidneys at 7–8 weeks was comparable to that of wild-types, but at 13 and 20 weeks copper levels showed a time-dependent increase and trended toward higher values than in the age matched wild-types (Figure 3D). Background ^{64}Cu radioactivity in the intestines made it difficult to compare actual values; nevertheless, the overall trend of increasing ^{64}Cu in the bladder of *Atp7b*$^{-/-}$ mice with age was evident and consistent with the atomic absorption (AA) measurements (Figure 3E). No such increase was observed in the bladder of wild-type mice, again supporting the AA data. It should be noted that although with increasing age, less ^{64}Cu is found in the *Atp7b*$^{-/-}$ liver and more ^{64}Cu radioactivity is detected in the *Atp7b*$^{-/-}$ kidneys, renal copper levels remain considerably lower compared to the liver pointing to tissue-specific differences in the mechanisms of maintaining copper balance (see discussion).

Selective and non-selective phases in urinary copper elevation

Our studies revealed two phases in elevation of urinary copper excretion: an initial phase prior to 20 weeks, when urine volume (and presumably kidney function) were normal, and a later phase (after 20 weeks) when urine volume was markedly increased. To understand the mechanism behind initial copper elevation, we focused on 13–20 weeks animals. We reasoned that elevated urinary copper along with diminished hepatic retention could be due to nonspecific leakage of copper from necrotic *Atp7b*$^{-/-}$ hepatocytes since necrosis is observed in the *Atp7b*$^{-/-}$ liver [11]. Alternatively, a lower retention of copper in the liver and increase in the urine could be due to specific transport processes such as

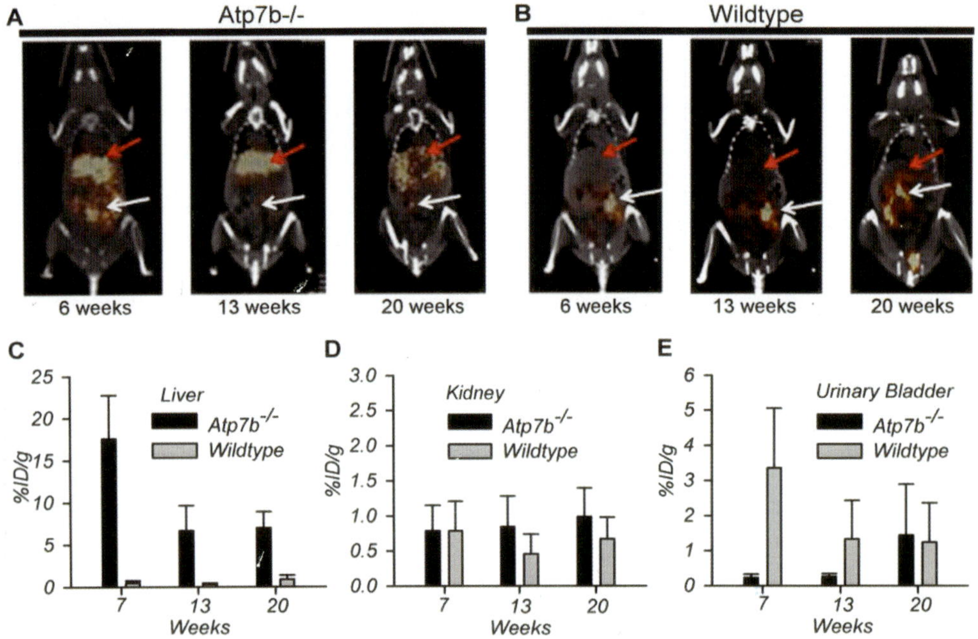

Figure 3. PET-CT analysis of ^{64}Cu distribution in live mice at 24 hrs after oral administration of $^{64}CuCl_2$. Representative PET-CT images of (A) *Atp7b*$^{-/-}$ and (B) wild-type mice at 24 hours post oral administration (PO) of $^{64}CuCl_2$. Orange-brown color denotes ^{64}Cu radioactivity. Red arrows and white arrows identify liver and gastrointestinal tract ^{64}Cu radioactivity, respectively. (C) Hepatic ^{64}Cu radioactivity in *Atp7b*$^{-/-}$ and wild-type mice at 24 hrs PO ($p<0.001$). Age-dependent ^{64}Cu radioactivity in the (D) kidneys ($p = 0.38$ for group effect) and (E) urinary bladder of wild-type and *Atp7b*$^{-/-}$ mice at 24 hr PO. %ID/g, percentage of administration dose per gram. Data presented as mean $\pm$ SD. N = 5, number of mice with same age and genotype. Additional data and details in Figure S2 and Information S1.

reduced copper uptake or facilitated export from the liver into circulation. To discriminate between these scenarios, we measured content of several metals in the urine (Figure 4). Specific excretion was expected to produce a selective increase in copper concentration, whereas a mechanism in which hepatic cell death is the primary pathway would likely change levels of several metals [12,13]. ICP-MS analysis confirmed that Cu levels were high in *Atp7b*$^{-/-}$ urine, compared with wild-type and increased with age (Figure 4A). In contrast, the concentration of all other elements did not change significantly between 6 and 20 weeks (Figure 4B). Fluctuations in the total output for all elements but copper showed strong correlation with the changes in urine volume (Table S1, additional details in Information S1), whereas copper was elevated independently of urine volume. Thus, the primary cause of high copper in the urine prior to 20 weeks is a specific change in the inter-organ copper fluxes, consistent with the PET data. In contrast, at 65 weeks of age, all metals showed high levels, especially iron and zinc (Figure 4C). This non-selective change in the urinary elemental content was followed by a marked increase in urine volume and was not explored further.

Copper in the urine is bound to a Small Copper Carrier (SCC)

The increase in copper but no other metals raised the question about the molecular form in which copper is exported into the urine. To address this issue, we fractionated urinary copper. Filtering urine through a 3 kDa cut-off filter demonstrated that more than 74% of copper in wild-type and 83% of copper in the urine of *Atp7b*$^{-/-}$ mice was associated with a low molecular weight fraction. (i.e. found in the flow-through, Figure 5B). High-resolution size-exclusion chromatography of the 3 kDa cut-off ultra-filtrate identified urinary copper in a fraction containing molecules with an apparent molecular weight of 2 kDa (Figure 5A). Subsequent analysis by fractionating $CuCl_2$ (to find elution time for free copper), tryptophan (to determine elution time for free amino-acid), and glycyl-L-histidyl-L-lysine copper-binding peptide, GHK (to find elution time for very short peptides) demonstrated that Cu is neither free ion nor bound to free amino-acids, since it elutes earlier, i.e. as a larger molecule (Figure 5C). We hypothesize that the majority of urinary copper binds to a specific Small Copper Carrier(s), which we named SCC.

CTR1 protein levels show specific age-dependent decrease in the Atp7b$^{-/-}$ liver, whereas ATP7A is unchanged

The predominant appearance of copper in one peak indicated that copper was bound to a single molecule or a limited number of molecules of a similar size, and implied the involvement of a specific transporter in this process. ATP7A is a copper transporter that can be up-regulated in the liver [14] and thus facilitate copper efflux. Consequently we examined *Atp7a* expression in the *Atp7b*$^{-/-}$ liver by real-time PCR and western blotting (Figure 6A,B) when urinary copper levels were near their peak. We found neither significant change in relative mRNA expression nor detectable ATP7A protein in the *Atp7b*$^{-/-}$ livers. (Figure 6A,B)

We have previously found that the mRNA levels for the copper transporter *Ctr1* are decreased in *Atp7b*$^{-/-}$ livers [15]. CTR1 is primarily responsible for the high-affinity copper uptake by various tissues, including liver [16]. If the decreased amount of *Ctr1* mRNA is associated with lower protein levels, this would result in a lower copper uptake, explaining (at least in part) the PET data. Consequently, we evaluated the CTR1 protein levels in the wild-type and *Atp7b*$^{-/-}$ livers at 6, 13, and 20 weeks by Western blot (Figure 6C). When compared to the age-matched

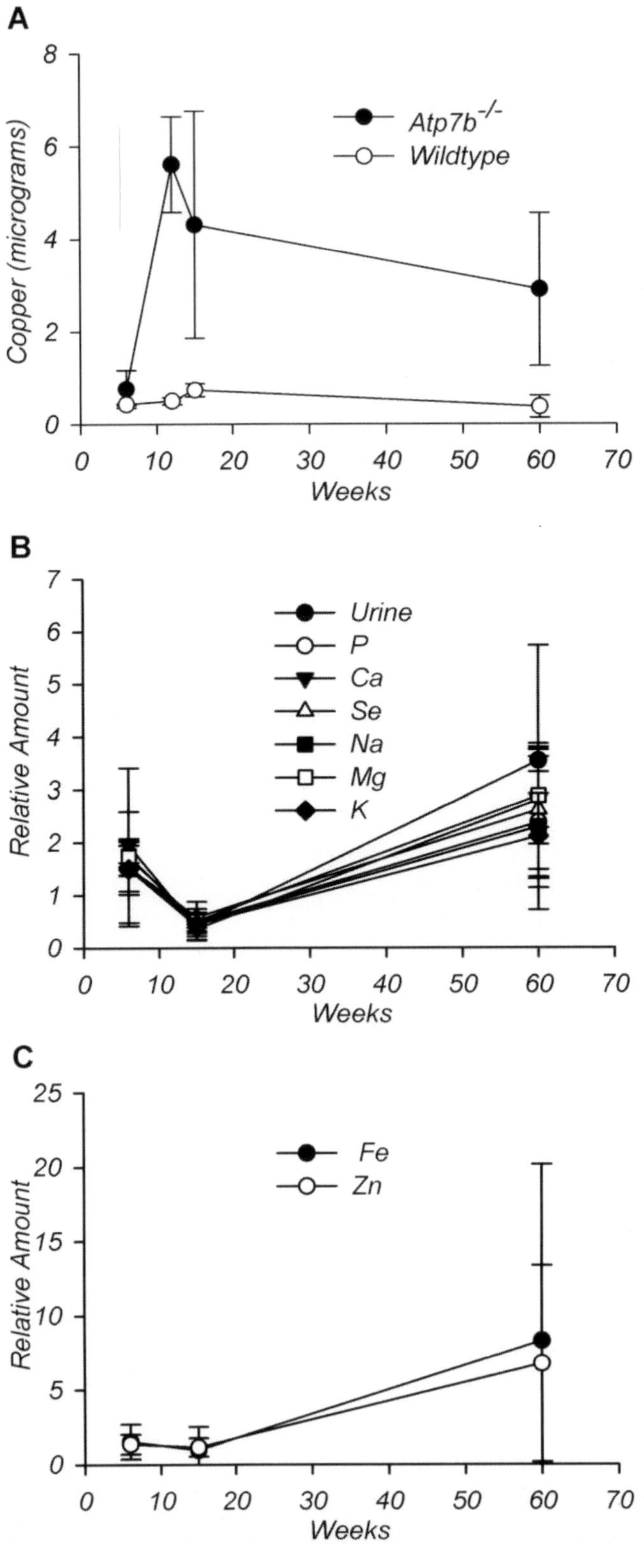

Figure 4. Elemental content of wild-type and *Atp7b*$^{-/-}$ urine during disease progression. ICP-MS analysis of urine collected over 24 hours from age-matched wild-type and *Atp7b*$^{-/-}$ mice. (A) Comparison of WT and KO copper amounts at different ages. (B) Urine amounts of Na, Mg, P, K, Ca, Se, and urine volume (relative to wild-type) at different ages. (C) Amounts of Fe and Zn at different ages (relative to wild type). N = 2 to 4 age-match WT/KO pairs for each time point. Data presented as mean ± SD, $^{**}P \leq 0.003$. The data points (from left to right) in Panel A represent 6 weeks, 12 weeks, 15 to 20 weeks, and 60 to 65 weeks. Panels B and C data points (from left to right) represent 6 to 12 weeks, 15 to 20 weeks, and 60 to 65 weeks. Correlation coefficients found in Table S1.

wild-types, the *Atp7b*$^{-/-}$ livers showed age-dependent decrease in CTR1 protein expression. These changes were specific for the liver, since similar analysis of kidney samples showed no significant changes in CTR1 protein compared to those of the wild-type controls (Figure 6D).

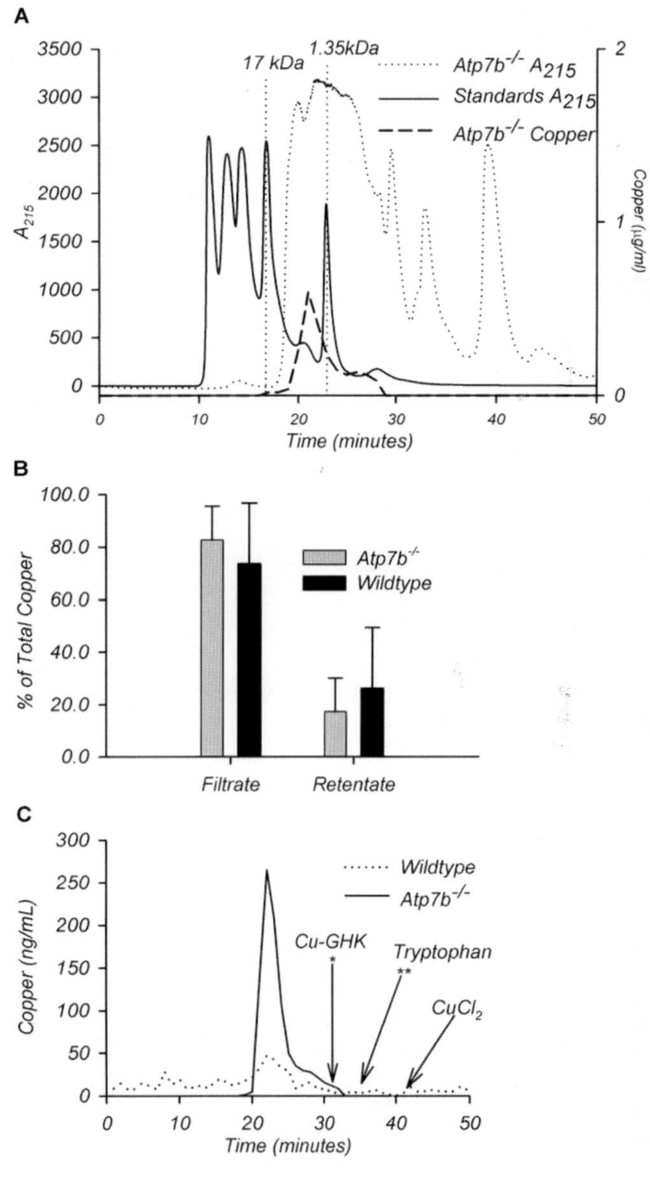

Figure 5. Characterization of urine copper component(s). (A) Representative graph of gel filtration analysis on 20 µl of *Atp7b*$^{-/-}$ urine along with copper levels in resulting fractions. (B) % of total copper found in the filtrate or retentate of wild-type and *Atp7b*$^{-/-}$ urine after application of whole urine to a filter with 3 kDa cutoff. Ages varied from 6 to 65 weeks. Data presented as % of total copper ± SD, n = 21 age-matched wild-type/*Atp7b*$^{-/-}$ pairs. (C) Representative graph of copper profile from gel filtration of 3 kDa filtrate from wild-type and *Atp7b*$^{-/-}$ urine. Arrows point to the elution time of indicated compounds.

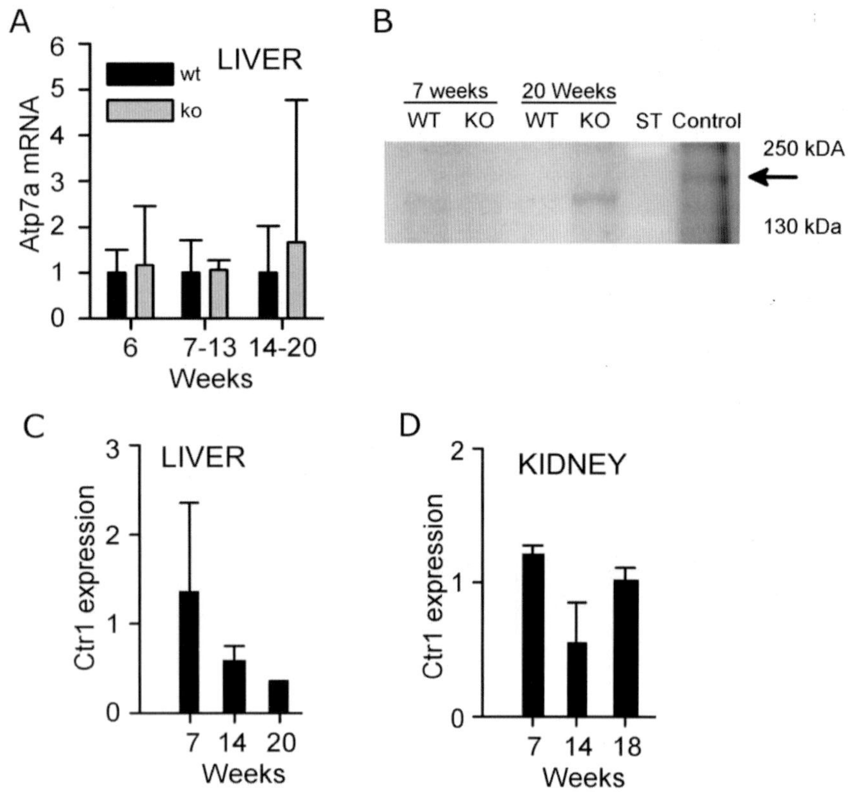

Figure 6. Ctr1 and Atp7A levels in the liver and kidney of Atp7b$^{-/-}$ and wild-type mice. (A) Real-time PCR analysis of Atp7A mRNA levels in the liver of wild-type and Atp7b$^{-/-}$ mice at different ages. Data presented as mean ± SD, n = 3 to 4 different samples of each genotype and age. (B) Representative Western blot illustrating ATP7A protein expression in the livers of wild-type and *Atp7b*$^{-/-}$ mice at 7 and 20 weeks. Twenty weeks old *Atp7b*$^{-/-}$ kidneys were used as a positive control for ATP7A protein expression. "ST" denotes molecular weight standards. Black arrow points to ATP7A band. Weak bands in the liver samples are due to non-specific staining (C, D) Quantitation of CTR1 protein levels by Western blot analysis and densitometry (relative to wild type) in liver and kidneys of wild-type and *Atp7b*$^{-/-}$ mice at different ages. Band intensity in each sample was normalized to a β-actin loading control. Data presented as mean ± SD. n = 2 for each genotype per age group.

Liver-specific down-regulation of CTR1 is associated with the elevation of copper-bound SCC in the urine

The apparent correlation between CTR1 down-regulation in the liver and elevation of SCC in the urine suggested that these events might be linked. Specifically, we hypothesized that SCC could be a normal source of exchangeable copper in the serum and that Cu-SCC became elevated in the urine because less CTR1 is available to accept copper from SCC and transport into hepatocytes. To test this hypothesis, we examined the urinary copper components of mice that have normal *Atp7b*, but lack *Ctr1* specifically in the liver. These animals do not have liver disease yet have elevated urinary copper [16]. Gel filtration analysis of urine from the liver –specific *Ctr1* knock-out mice showed a single peak of elevated copper that has the same elution time as SCC from *Atp7b*$^{-/-}$ mice (Figure 7A).

SCC competes with radioactive ^{64}Cu for uptake via CTR1

To further test our hypothesis that SCC represents a source of exchangeable copper in the serum, we measured total and exchangeable copper in wild-type and *Atp7b*$^{-/-}$ serum at 20 weeks and attempted to detect SCC in the serum. We observed an increase in a fraction of exchangeable copper in Atp7b$^{-/-}$ serum compared to wild-type (Figure S3, additional details Information S1), however we were unable to directly link it to SCC, presumably due to the association of serum copper with a fraction of high-molecular weight proteins (we found that in the mouse sera, copper-bound small molecular weight complexes, such as copper-bound chelators, do not elute with their apparent molecular weight in gel filtration chromatography but rather associate with higher-molecular weight proteins, data not shown).

Consequently, to examine whether SCC can transfer copper to CTR1 we measured competition between Cu-SCC and free Cu using ^{64}Cu uptake assays in HEK293 cells stably over-expressing CTR1. Identical volume from the corresponding elution fraction of the wild-type urine served as a control. ^{64}Cu uptake was gradually reduced in the presence of increasing amounts of SCC from KO urine. No such competition was seen using the wild-type fractions (Figure 7B).

Discussion

Genetic mutations in the copper transporter ATP7B disrupt biliary copper excretion resulting in a massive hepatic copper accumulation and Wilson's disease (WD). Using *Atp7b*$^{-/-}$ mice, an animal model for WD, we demonstrate that *Atp7b* inactivation also up-regulates an available but underutilized secondary pathway for copper removal from the body, which produces a clinically well-known phenomenon of high urinary copper in WD patients. *Atp7b*$^{-/-}$ mice show an age-dependent increase of urinary copper that does not directly follow known changes in liver pathology. This increase is selective for copper in animals under 20 weeks of age, which strongly suggests that urinary copper excretion is a specific mechanism to protect against hepatic copper

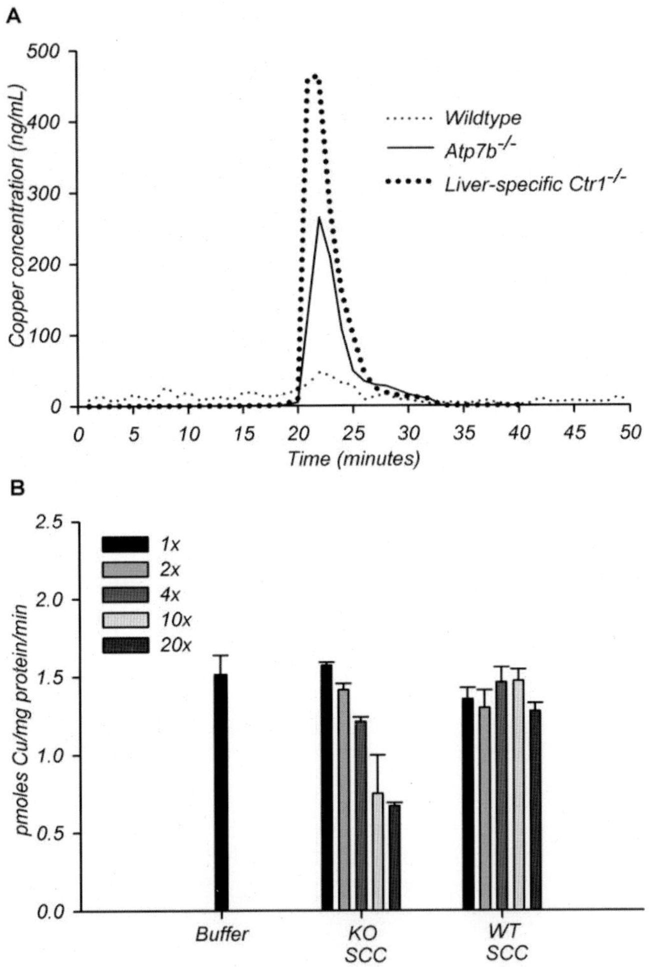

Figure 7. Functional interaction of SCC and CTR1. (A) Copper concentrations in fractions obtained from gel filtration of wild-type, *Atp7b*$^{-/-}$, and liver-specific *Ctr1*$^{-/-}$ urine. (B) 64Cu uptake assay by HEK293 cells stably overexpressing hCtr1 in the presence of increasing concentrations of gel filtration purified SCC from urine of *Atp7b*$^{-/-}$ and wild-type mice. Radioactive copper-64 was kept constant at 0.25 μM. Sodium phosphate buffer pH 7.4 was used as the buffer control. 1× is equal to a copper concentration of 0.25 μM for *Atp7b*$^{-/-}$ SCC and 2× to 20× are multiples of the original 1× concentration. The volumes used for the assays were set to achieve the desired 1× to 20× concentrations specifically for *Atp7b*$^{-/-}$ SCC. The wild-type SCC 1× to 20× assays are done with the same volumes of SCC utilized for corresponding *Atp7b*$^{-/-}$ SCC assays, thus wild-type concentrations used are low due to inherent lower copper levels in WT SCC. Data presented as mean ± SD, performed in triplicates. See Figure S3.

overload. A similar increase in urinary copper has been documented in WD patients as they transition from asymptomatic to symptomatic stage of the disease [5].

Older *Atp7b*$^{-/-}$ mice show changes of several metal ions and a markedly increased urine volume. This latter change is associated with an increased water intake and proteinuria, suggestive of glomerular damage. The time-dependent kidney damage could be either due to increased amounts of copper being filtered through kidney or, more likely, due to inactivation of renal *Atp7b* and copper misbalance in kidney cells. *Atp7b* is normally expressed in kidneys at relatively high levels [17–19] and inactivation of *Atp7b* is likely to alter normal copper homeostasis. It is interesting that despite loss of ATP7B function and gradual accumulation of copper in the kidney, renal copper overload is modest compared to the liver. This is likely due to the presence in kidneys of another copper-transporter, ATP7A, which is likely to facilitate copper release partially compensating for the loss of ATP7B function [20].

We have found that copper in the urine is bound to a previously unknown small carrier, SCC, with an apparent molecular weight of 2 kDa; SCC is larger than free amino-acids or the tripeptide GHK, but smaller than metallothionein. Sensitivity of copper-bound SCC to pH and organic solvents has complicated purification using standard protocols, and we are developing new approaches for SCC identification. Importantly, a similar small copper carrier complex is present at lower levels in wild-type urine, which suggest a role for SCC in normal copper metabolism. One such role could be copper sequestration and excretion via renal filtration when hepatic copper uptake is saturated. However, the SCC's ability to compete with ^{64}Cu for uptake via CTR1 strongly suggests that its normal physiological function could also be to deliver copper to cells. The highly similar copper profiles of urine from the *Atp7b*$^{-/-}$ and liver-specific *Ctr1*$^{-/-}$ mice further illustrates a functional interaction between SCC and CTR1.

Hepatic copper homeostasis is normally achieved by regulation of copper uptake (CTR1), sequestration (MT), and export (ATP7B). In the absence of ATP7B, MT levels are significantly elevated in WD patients and Atp7b$^{-/-}$ mice [10] yet elevation of MT alone cannot explain why copper is shuttled away from the liver as disease progresses. It was suggested in the literature that WD hepatocytes may release the MT-Cu complex [21], however our data are inconsistent with this hypothesis. ATP7A, which is not ordinarily seen in the adult mouse liver, under certain conditions can be upregulated in the liver [14] and pump copper across the basolateral surface back into the blood. Increased ATP7A levels could readily explain the age-dependent increase in serum copper levels observed in *Atp7b*$^{-/-}$ mice [11]. In the Atp7b$^{-/-}$ mice, we previously documented elevation of ATP7A in the kidney and brain, where ATP7A is assumed to replace some of the biosynthetic functions of ATP7B [20,22]. Additionally, specific genetic ablation of *Ctr1* in the heart, results in the elevation of ATP7A in the adult mouse liver [14]. However, in the liver of *Atp7b*$^{-/-}$ mice we did not find any changes in ATP7A protein or mRNA expression. These results agree with the PET data, showing higher copper retention in *Atp7b*$^{-/-}$ liver at all time-points despite time-dependent decrease of copper uptake transporter, *Ctr1*.

Walshe has insightfully suggested that in WD patients copper retention by the liver decreases as disease progresses [14]. Longitudinal PET-CT imaging of live *Atp7b*−/− animals allowed direct measurements of copper accumulation in their liver at different ages and tested this hypothesis. It is apparent that radioactive copper found in the liver 24 hours post injection decreases with age. The major copper entry pathway into the liver is through CTR1. CTR1 is known to be regulated by copper at the level of protein stability [23], trafficking [24–26], and transcription [27,28]. We found in the *Atp7b*$^{-/-}$ mouse liver, CTR1 protein and mRNA levels decrease in an age-dependent manner. The ablation of Ctr1 specifically in the liver of mice does not induce visible pathology in the liver, but is associated with elevation of urinary copper and no other metals [16]. Since no other metal increases in the urine prior to 20 weeks of age, we have concluded that down-regulation of CTR1 and increased filtration of SCC (rather than hepatocytes death) are primarily responsible for the initial phase of urinary copper elevation.

In is important to emphasize that our results do not exclude some contribution of copper from necrotic cells and may reflect a situation when the disease is relatively mild. In humans, the course of WD varies greatly from mild inflammation to a sudden liver failure. Whether the origin and/or molecular identity of urinary copper are the same in these conditions is unclear. The LPP rats, another model of WD, die invariably from liver failure that was linked to mitochondria destruction [29]. Mitochondria matrix contains a small copper ligand CuL [30], which upon mitochondria rupture and cell necrosis would presumably be released. In *Atp7b*$^{-/-}$ mice, the course of disease does not include liver failure and the selective mechanism discussed in present work better accommodates our results. Further characterization of copper-carrying small molecules will greatly contribute to our understanding of hepatic copper homeostasis and may help WD diagnosis and monitoring.

In conclusion, elevated urinary copper in *Atp7b*$^{-/-}$ mice is the result of a redundant and copper-selective mechanism based upon homeostatic control of CTR1 that is turned on to maintain systemic copper balance when liver copper homeostasis is compromised. The redirection of copper flow from the liver to kidneys in WD is mediated by a small copper carrier SCC, which is distinct from free amino acids, tripeptide GHK, or a full-length metallothionein. Functional interactions between SCC and CTR1 may control copper distribution between tissues.

Materials and Methods

Materials

Doubly deionized water (ddH_2O) was used in preparation of buffers and reagents. All buffers were treated with metal-ion chelating agent, Chelex 100 (Bio-Rad) prior to use then subsequently vacuumed degassed and filtered on a 0.45 μM FHLC filter (Millipore). Gel filtration standards were from Bio-Rad Laboratories.

Animal husbandry and urine collection

Urine was collected from *Atp7b* knockout (*Atp7b*$^{-/-}$), *Ctr1* knockout and wild-type (WT) littermate control mice. The generation of these mice was previously described [16,31]. The animals were housed at the Johns Hopkins University School of Medicine Animal Care Facility according to National Institute of Health guidelines. For urine collection, age matched *Atp7b*$^{-/-}$ and WT mice of both genders were placed for 48 hours in individual metabolic cages (Tecniplast). Animals were allowed to acclimate to their new environment for the first 24 hours, and then urine was collected for the subsequent 24 hour period. During collection, the mice had free access to food and water. Urine volume as well as water and food intake were measured. The urine was centrifuged at 4,000×g for 5 minutes at 4°C to remove debris. Urine was either used immediately or stored at −80°C. The above experimental protocols were approved by the Institutional Animal Care and Use Committee (IACUC) of JHU. Urine collection from the liver specific Ctr1−/− mice was performed as previously described [16] using protocols approved by the IACUC of University of Nebraska-Lincoln. Subsequent analysis of urine from both animal strains was performed under identical conditions, as described below.

Tissue preparation and analysis

Tissues were dissected after whole animal perfusion with phosphate-buffered saline (pH 7.4; PBS), frozen in liquid nitrogen, and stored at −80°C until use. Protein extracts were prepared on ice by homogenizing liver and kidney in the lysis buffer (50 mM Hepes (pH 7.4), 0.1% Igepal,150 mM NaCl, 1 mM AEBSF, 250 mM sucrose) containing EDTA-free protease inhibitor cocktail (Roche). The tissue homogenates were centrifuged at 700× g for 15 minutes to remove debris and the supernatant was spun at 22,000× g for 35 minutes to obtain a membrane pellet. The pellet was then dissolved in the Laemmli gel sample buffer. For SDS-PAGE, 1 μg and 25 μg of membrane protein were separated on 7.5% and 4–20% polyacrylamide gels to analyze Atp7A and Ctr1, respectively. Proteins were transferred onto polyvinyldifluoride (PVDF) membrane and probed with rabbit anti-CTR1 (1:1000) and rabbit anti-ATP7A (1:500) antibody. Staining was detected by goat anti-rabbit HRP secondary antibody (Santa Cruz Biotechnology, 1:20,000) and HRP-conjugated anti-mouse β-actin (Sigma,1:10,000) using West Pico Chemiluminescence (Pierce) according to the manufacturer's instructions. Staining with anti-β-actin antibody was used as a loading control. Band intensity was measured with Image J and quantified after normalization to β-actin.

Longitudinal PET-CT

The PET imaging experiments were conducted under the protocol approved by the Institutional Animal Care and Use Committee, UT Southwestern Medical Center at Dallas. The mice were administered with $^{64}CuCl_2$ [74 kBq (2 μCi)/g body weight] in a volume of 25 μl by oral feeding. The dose of $^{64}CuCl_2$ supplied in 0.1 N HCl was diluted in 25 μl of normal saline containing 0.9% sodium chloride. PET of the mice was performed with a Siemens Inveon microPET/CT system, using a protocol published recently [32]. Briefly, the mice were anesthetized using 3% isoflurane at room temperature and placed in spread-supine position on the imaging bed under 2% isoflurane anesthesia for the duration of the imaging. Static whole body imaging was performed at 2 and 24 hours post oral administration of the tracer, respectively, which consisted of two overlapping frames of 15 min duration for each frame. As part of the PET imaging protocol, CT data was acquired (80 kV, 500 μA) for attenuation correction and anatomical localization. PET images were subsequently reconstructed using the 3D OSEM algorithm and scatter as well as attenuation correction. All images were analyzed using the Inveon Research Workplace (IRW) software (Siemens). Following re-slicing of fused PET/CT images into arbitrary views, regions of interest (ROIs) for liver, kidneys, and urinary bladder were drawn to obtain quantitative measurements of the ^{64}Cu tracer activity expressed as percentage of administration dose per gram (%ID/g).

Size-Exclusion Chromatography of urine filtrates

Urine was ultrafiltered on a Microcon YM-3 (MWCO 3000, Bedford MA) at 14,000×g for 200 min at 4°C. One hundred microliters of urine filtrate was loaded onto a size-exclusion column (Phenomenex Bio-Sep S-2000, 7.5×200, 10 μM), equilibrated with 50 mM sodium phosphate buffer, pH 7.5. Samples were fractionated isocratically with the same buffer at a flow rate of 0.5 ml per min, and 0.5 ml fractions were collected over 50 minutes. Absorbance was monitored at 215 and 280 nm. Calibration of size exclusion column was done using molecular weight standards (Bio-Rad, Thyroglobulin 670 KDa; γ-globulin 158 KDa; Ovalbumin 44 KDa; Myoglobin 17 KDa; Vitamin B12 1,350 Da), reduced L-glutathione (307 Da), tryptophan (~204 Da), Copper Chloride (~64 Da). All standards were prepared in 50 mM sodium phosphate buffer pH 7.5.

Atomic Absorption Spectrophotometry

The copper concentration of the urine, filtrate, and in the chromatography fractions was determined using a Shimadzu 6650 graphite furnace atomic absorption spectrophotometer (AA) equipped with an ASC-6100 autosampler. Briefly, samples were diluted with ddH_2O (1:10 or 1:500 for fractionated and unfractionated urine, respectively) to be in the linear absorption range of the calibration curve [1–10 parts per billion (ppb)]. Each sample was measured 2 to 3 times, and the concentration of copper was derived by comparing absorption with a calibration curve. All values are reported as means.

Inductively coupled plasma mass spectrometry (ICP MS)

Analysis was performed using an Agilent 7700× equipped with an ASX 250 autosampler. The system is operated at a radio frequency power of 1550 W, an argon plasma gas flow rate of 15 L/min, Ar carrier gas flow rate of 1.04 L/min. All elements were measured in kinetic energy discrimination (KED) mode using He gas (4.3 ml/min). Urine samples were diluted into 1% HNO_3, (trace metal grade, Fisher Scientific). Data were quantified using a 10-point calibration curve (0–5000 ppb (ng/L)) with external standards for Na, Mg, P, K, Ca, Fe, Cu, Zn, in 1% HNO3, (to match the sample matrix). For each sample, data were acquired in triplicates and averaged. An internal standard was used to correct for plasma instabilities and differences in total ion concentrations, triplicate measurements of a 10 ppb Cu solution as well as a blank (containing diluent only) was used as quality control. To ensure maximum recovery of elements from the sample certified NIST standard reference materials (serum (SRM 1598a), and water (SRM 1643e)) were prepared and analyzed by the same method as the samples. Time-points presented in Figure 4 represent different ages of mice plotted as one time point; the "6 week" time-point represents the average of data for 6–12 week old urine, the "15 week" timepoint is the average of 15–20 week samples, and the 60 week timepoint is the average of 60–65 week old urine. Four age-matched wild-type/*Atp7b*$^{-/-}$ pairs were used to generate data for each of the 6 and 15 timepoints; two age-matched wild-type/*Atp7b*$^{-/-}$ pairs were used for the 60 week time-point.

Real-Time PCR

Total RNA was isolated from 100 mg of mouse liver using Trizol Reagent (Invitrogen). RNA quality was assessed by Agilent 2100 Bioanalyzer with all samples having RIN values greater than 8.6. For real-time PCR, cDNA was synthesized with QuantiTect Reverse Transcription Kit (Qiagen) from 1 µg of RNA. The target and control genes were amplified in 20 µL reactions using Applied Biosystems (ABI) Taq-Man Universal PCR Master Mix and Taq-Man gene expression primers on an ABI 7500 Real-time PCR system. RT-PCR data was analyzed using the ΔΔCT method. GAPDH was used for normalization.

Copper uptake. HEK293 cells containing tetracycline-regulated N-Terminal FLAG-tagged hCTR1 was previously described [33]. The cells were grown at 37°C and 5% CO_2 in DMEM (Mediatech) containing 10% FBS (Atlanta Biologicals), 25 mM Hepes and 1% PSF (Invitrogen) with the following selective antibiotics: 10 µg/ml blasticidin and 400 µg/ml hygromycin B. hCTR1 protein expression was induced by the addition of 1 µg/ml of tetracycline to the medium for 48 hours.

One day prior to Cu uptake assay HEK/hCTR1-FLAG tagged cells were seeded onto 12-well tissue culture plates at a density of 0.6×10^6 cells/well. Prior to the uptake assay the media was removed from the cells and replaced with transport media, DMEM+10%FBS, to which either gel filtration fraction of Atp7b$^{-/-}$ urine was added at 0.25–5 µM Cu or the same volume of the fractionated wild-type urine was added in a final volume of 0.5 ml. Control cells were those to which no urine sample was added. Copper uptake was performed by the addition of at 0.25 µM $CuCl_2$ containing ^{64}Cu (Washington University, St. Louis, MO) to the cells for 45 minutes at 37°C. Cu uptake was halted by the addition of ice-cold stop buffer (150 mM NaCl, 5 mM KCl, 2.5 mM $MgCl_2$ 10 mM EDTA, 25 mM Hepes, pH 7.4) to the cells; they were subsequently washed twice with stop buffer. The cells were then lysed in lysis buffer (0.4% Triton X-100, 5 mM DTT, 20 mM Tris pH 8 and 2 mM EDTA) and an aliquot of the cell lysate was added to EcoLume Scintillation fluid and counted using a Beckman LS 6500 scintillation counter. The protein concentration of the cell lysate was calculated after radioactive decay and the copper uptake per well was calculated as pmoles Cu/mg protein/min and the average of triplicate measurements per treatment were expressed as pmoles Cu/mg protein/min.

Statistical analysis

Values are expressed as mean ± SD. Statistical significance was evaluated using unpaired t-test and among more than two groups by analysis of one-way ANOVA. Differences were considered significant at $p<0.05$. PET quantitative values are expressed as mean of %ID/g ± SD. In order to assess significant differences in ^{64}Cu tracer activity among liver, kidneys, and urinary bladder between *Atp7b*$^{-/-}$ and C57BL wild-type mice, a 2× (3) mixed-design analysis was conducted, where the between-subjects factor represents the group (*Atp7b*$^{-/-}$, C57BL mice) and the within-subjects factor represents the three time-points (7–8, 13, 20 weeks). Analyses were performed separately for the 3 regions of interest (liver, kidneys, urinary bladder). The overall test was subsequently followed-up by post-hoc unpaired t-tests between the two groups for individual time-points. A p value<0.05 was considered to represent statistical significance. Box plot outliers were determined by multiplying the interquartile range by 1.5 and subtracting the obtained value from either the first quartile or third quartile, to determine the lower and upper limits; all measurements beyond these limits are considered outliers.

Supporting Information

Figure S1 Related to Figure 2: Proteinuria is apparent in *Atp7b*$^{-/-}$ mice older than 20 weeks. Comparison of protein amounts from urine of Atp7b$^{-/-}$ and wildtype mice at different ages. The solid horizontal bar within in the box represents the median, while upper and lower bars signify the 75th and 25th percentiles, respectively. The dotted horizontal line signifies the mean. The whiskers represent the 10th and 90th percentiles. The black dots represent outliers. #P value = 0.088. See supporting information for experimental details (Information S1).

Figure S2 Related to Figure 3. Representative PET-CT imaging and quantitative analysis of wildtype and Atp7b$^{-/-}$ mice at 2 hours post oral administration of ^{64}Cu. Pet-CT images of (A) wildtype and (B) Atp7b−/− mice at indicated ages. Quantitative analysis of radioactivity of (C) liver and (D) kidneys of wildtype and Atp7b$^{-/-}$ mice at indicated ages ($p = 0.27$ for group effect). Data presented as mean ± SD. n = 5, per genotype. Red arrows indicate the position of the liver and white arrows indicate ^{64}Cu radioactivity in the gastrointestinal tract.

Figure S3 Related to Figure 7: Exchangeable copper in the serum of wild-type and Atp7b$^{-/-}$ mice. Data presented as mean ± SD. n = 2 per genotype. See supporting information for experimental details (Information S1).

Table S1 Related to Figure 4: Correlation between changes in urine volume and amounts of urinary elements with disease progression. *Spearman ranked coefficients with significance $p<0.05$. $n=6$. See supporting information for description of statistical analysis (Information S1).

Information S1 Supplementary experimental procedures.

Acknowledgments

We thank Dr. Martina Ralle (OHSU) for ICP-MS measurements and Dr. Stephen Kaler (NIH) for the anti-ATP7A antibody.

Author Contributions

Conceived and designed the experiments: LWG FP SAM JHK SL. Performed the experiments: LWG FP SAM VSP AM OM JL. Analyzed the data: LWG FP SAM VSP AM OM JHK SL. Wrote the paper: LWG FP SL.

References

1. Tumer Z, Moller LB (2010) Menkes disease. Eur J Hum Genet 18: 511–518.
2. Pfeiffer RF (2011) Wilson's disease. Handb Clin Neurol 100: 681–709.
3. Kaplan JH, Lutsenko S (2009) Copper transport in mammalian cells: special care for a metal with special needs. J Biol Chem 284: 25461–25465.
4. Huster D (2010) Wilson disease. Best Pract Res Clin Gastroenterol 24: 531–539.
5. Walshe JM (2011) The pattern of urinary copper excretion and its response to treatment in patients with Wilson's disease. QJM 104: 775–778.
6. Frommer DJ (1981) Urinary copper excretion and hepatic copper concentrations in liver disease. Digestion 21: 169–178.
7. Melichar B, Jandik P, Malir F, Tichy M, Bures J, et al. (1994) Increased urinary zinc and copper excretion in colorectal cancer. J Trace Elem Electrolytes Health Dis 8: 209–212.
8. Wilken H (1961) [Urinary copper excretion in pregnancy]. Klin Wochenschr 39: 147–149.
9. Burkhead JL, Gray LW, Lutsenko S (2011) Systems biology approach to Wilson's disease. Biometals 24: 455–466.
10. Huster D, Purnat TD, Burkhead JL, Ralle M, Fiehn O, et al. (2007) High copper selectively alters lipid metabolism and cell cycle machinery in the mouse model of Wilson disease. J Biol Chem 282: 8343–8355.
11. Huster D, Finegold MJ, Morgan CT, Burkhead JL, Nixon R, et al. (2006) Consequences of copper accumulation in the livers of the Atp7b−/− (Wilson disease gene) knockout mice. Am J Pathol 168: 423–434.
12. Afridi HI, Kazi TG, Kazi NG, Jamali MK, Sarfaraz RA, et al. (2009) Determination of copper and iron in biological samples of viral hepatitis (A–E) female patients. Biol Trace Elem Res 129: 78–87.
13. Afridi HI, Kazi TG, Shah F, Sheikh HU, Kolachi NF (2011) Evaluation of arsenic, cadmium, lead, and nickel in biological samples (scalp hair, serum, blood, and urine) of Pakistani viral hepatitis (A–E) patients and controls. Clin Lab 57: 847–857.
14. Kim BE, Turski ML, Nose Y, Casad M, Rockman HA, et al. (2010) Cardiac copper deficiency activates a systemic signaling mechanism that communicates with the copper acquisition and storage organs. Cell Metab 11: 353–363.
15. Ralle M, Huster D, Vogt S, Schirrmeister W, Burkhead JL, et al. (2010) Wilson disease at a single cell level: intracellular copper trafficking activates compartment-specific responses in hepatocytes. J Biol Chem 285: 30875–30883.
16. Kim H, Son HY, Bailey SM, Lee J (2009) Deletion of hepatic Ctr1 reveals its function in copper acquisition and compensatory mechanisms for copper homeostasis. Am J Physiol Gastrointest Liver Physiol 296: G356–364.
17. Tanzi RE, Petrukhin K, Chernov I, Pellequer JL, Wasco W, et al. (1993) The Wilson disease gene is a copper transporting ATPase with homology to the Menkes disease gene. Nat Genet 5: 344–350.
18. Petrukhin K, Fischer SG, Pirastu M, Tanzi RE, Chernov I, et al. (1993) Mapping, cloning and genetic characterization of the region containing the Wilson disease gene. Nat Genet 5: 338–343.
19. Bull PC, Thomas GR, Rommens JM, Forbes JR, Cox DW (1993) The Wilson disease gene is a putative copper transporting P-type ATPase similar to the Menkes gene. Nat Genet 5: 327–337.
20. Linz R, Barnes NL, Zimnicka AM, Kaplan JH, Eipper B, et al. (2008) Intracellular targeting of copper-transporting ATPase ATP7A in a normal and Atp7b−/− kidney. Am J Physiol Renal Physiol 294: F53–61.
21. Elmes ME, Clarkson JP, Mahy NJ, Jasani B (1989) Metallothionein and copper in liver disease with copper retention–a histopathological study. J Pathol 158: 131–137.
22. Barnes N, Tsivkovskii R, Tsivkovskaia N, Lutsenko S (2005) The copper-transporting ATPases, menkes and wilson disease proteins, have distinct roles in adult and developing cerebellum. J Biol Chem 280: 9640–9645.
23. Nose Y, Wood LK, Kim BE, Prohaska JR, Fry RS, et al. (2010) Ctr1 is an apical copper transporter in mammalian intestinal epithelial cells in vivo that is controlled at the level of protein stability. J Biol Chem 285: 32385–32392.
24. Molloy SA, Kaplan JH (2009) Copper-dependent recycling of hCTR1, the human high affinity copper transporter. J Biol Chem 284: 29704–29713.
25. Petris MJ, Smith K, Lee J, Thiele DJ (2003) Copper-stimulated endocytosis and degradation of the human copper transporter, hCtr1. J Biol Chem 278: 9639–9646.
26. Ooi CE, Rabinovich E, Dancis A, Bonifacino JS, Klausner RD (1996) Copper-dependent degradation of the Saccharomyces cerevisiae plasma membrane copper transporter Ctr1p in the apparent absence of endocytosis. EMBO J 15: 3515–3523.
27. Liang ZD, Tsai WB, Lee MY, Savaraj N, Kuo MT (2012) Specificity protein 1 (sp1) oscillation is involved in copper homeostasis maintenance by regulating human high-affinity copper transporter 1 expression. Mol Pharmacol 81: 455–464.
28. Song IS, Chen HH, Aiba I, Hossain A, Liang ZD, et al. (2008) Transcription factor Sp1 plays an important role in the regulation of copper homeostasis in mammalian cells. Mol Pharmacol 74: 705–713.
29. Zischka H, Lichtmannegger J, Schmitt S, Jagemann N, Schulz S, et al. (2011) Liver mitochondrial membrane crosslinking and destruction in a rat model of Wilson disease. J Clin Invest 121: 1508–1518.
30. Cobine PA, Pierrel F, Bestwick ML, Winge DR (2006) Mitochondrial matrix copper complex used in metallation of cytochrome oxidase and superoxide dismutase. J Biol Chem 281: 36552–36559.
31. Buiakova OI, Xu J, Lutsenko S, Zeitlin S, Das K, et al. (1999) Null mutation of the murine ATP7B (Wilson disease) gene results in intracellular copper accumulation and late-onset hepatic nodular transformation. Hum Mol Genet 8: 1665–1671.
32. Peng F, Lutsenko S, Sun X, Muzik O (2011) Imaging Copper Metabolism Imbalance in Atp7b (−/−) Knockout Mouse Model of Wilson's Disease with PET-CT and Orally Administered (64)CuCl (2). Mol Imaging Biol.
33. Maryon EB, Molloy SA, Kaplan JH (2007) O-linked glycosylation at threonine 27 protects the copper transporter hCTR1 from proteolytic cleavage in mammalian cells. J Biol Chem 282: 20376–20387.

8

The Role of Fibrocytes in Sickle Cell Lung Disease

Joshua J. Field[2], Marie D. Burdick[1], Michael R. DeBaun[3], Brett A. Strieter[1], Ling Liu[1], Borna Mehrad[1], C. Edward Rose, Jr.[1], Joel Linden[4], Robert M. Strieter[1]*

1 Department of Medicine, Division of Pulmonary and Critical Care Medicine, The University of Virginia School of Medicine, Charlottesville, Virginia, United States of America, **2** Blood Center of Wisconsin, Blood Research Institute, Milwaukee, Wisconsin, United States of America, **3** Departments of Pediatrics and Medicine, Division of Hematology and Oncology, Vanderbilt University School of Medicine, Nashville, Tennessee, United States of America, **4** La Jolla Institute for Allergy & Immunology, La Jolla, California, United States of America

Abstract

Background: Interstitial lung disease is a frequent complication in sickle cell disease and is characterized by vascular remodeling and interstitial fibrosis. Bone marrow-derived fibrocytes have been shown to contribute to the pathogenesis of other interstitial lung diseases. The goal of this study was to define the contribution of fibrocytes to the pathogenesis of sickle cell lung disease.

Methodology/Principal Findings: Fibrocytes were quantified and characterized in subjects with sickle cell disease or healthy controls, and in a model of sickle cell disease, the NY1DD mouse. The role of the chemokine ligand CXCL12 in trafficking of fibrocytes and phenotype of lung disease was examined in the animal model. We found elevated concentration of activated fibrocytes in the peripheral blood of subjects with sickle cell disease, which increased further during vaso-occlusive crises. There was a similar elevations in the numbers and activation phenotype of fibrocytes in the bone marrow, blood, and lungs of the NY1DD mouse, both at baseline and under conditions of hypoxia/re-oxygenation. In both subjects with sickle cell disease and the mouse model, fibrocytes expressed a hierarchy of chemokine receptors, with CXCR4 expressed on most fibrocytes, and CCR2 and CCR7 expressed on a smaller subset of cells. Depletion of the CXCR4 ligand, CXCL12, in the mouse model resulted in a marked reduction of fibrocyte trafficking into the lungs, reduced lung collagen content and improved lung compliance and histology.

Conclusions: These data support the notion that activated fibrocytes play a significant role in the pathogenesis of sickle cell lung disease.

Editor: Neeraj Vij, Johns Hopkins School of Medicine, United States of America

Funding: This work was supported by the National Heart, Lung, and Blood Institute HL08710 (JJF), HL079937 (MRD), HL073848 (BM), HL098329 (BM, RMS), HL066027 and HL098526 (RMS). The funders had no role in study design, data collection and analysis, decision to publish, or preparation of the manuscript.

Competing Interests: The authors have declared that no competing interests exist.

* E-mail: mdb5b@virginia.edu

Introduction

Sickle cell disease (SCD) is the most common monogenic inherited disorder in African-Americans [1]. The two most common complications of SCD, vaso-occlusive pain crises (VOC) and acute chest syndrome (ACS), are the major risk factors for the development of interstitial lung disease (ILD) [2], a risk for morbidity and mortality in patients with SCD [2,3]. ILD is characterized by parenchymal and vascular remodeling among patients with SCD and has been associated with the development of pulmonary hypertension and, potentially through this mechanism, with increased mortality [2,4]. Although most studies of SCLD have focused on vascular remodeling and pulmonary hypertension [5], patients with SCD have long been recognized to develop a progressive restrictive ventilatory defect and interstitial markings on chest radiographs [2,6,7]. While many adults with SCD do not exhibit all features of SCLD, a restrictive pattern on pulmonary function tests is the most consistent clinical feature; for example, 74% of adults in a large prospective cohort study SCD had restrictive lung disease [6]. These studies underscore the need to better understand the pathogenesis of ILD in patients with SCD.

Fibrotic lung diseases are associated with dysregulated repair in response to persistent or recurrent injury, leading to loss of alveolar-capillary basement membrane integrity and remodelling of the lung airpace, interstitial and vascular compartments [8,9,10,11,12]. The fibroblasts involved in this process are known to be derived, in part, from proliferation of resident lung fibroblasts. More recent evidence has implicated a bone marrow-derived circulating mesenchymal progenitor cell, the fibrocyte, in lung fibrosis and has changed the perspective of lung repair [13,14,15]. Fibrocytes express the hematopoietic stem cell antigen CD34, the common leukocyte marker CD45, the myeloid markers CD11b and CD13, and fibroblast markers vimentin, collagen I, collagen III and fibronectin, as well as several chemokine receptors [16,17,18]. Only a subset of circulating fibrocytes expresses CD34, and the expression of both CD34 and CD45 on fibrocytes decreases when the cells are cultured or after they enter tissue. Since there is no single marker unique for the identification of fibrocytes, the co-expression of collagen production and CD34 or CD45 has been commonly used to identify these cells [16,17,18]. Fibrocytes are important in mediating pulmonary fibrosis in murine models of lung injury [7,13,19,20,21,22] and are elevated in the blood and lungs of patients with idiopathic pulmonary fibrosis (IPF) [23,24,25]. Moreover, the number of circulating fibrocytes is a predictor of prognosis in patients with IPF [25]. Given the role of fibrocytes in the pathogenesis of lung remodelling in other diseases, we postulated that these cells are important in the development of ILD in patients with SCD.

Methods

Peripheral blood samples from adult patients with SCD or race-matched controls and bone marrow, blood and lungs of NY1DD mice or congenic C57BL/6 mice were processed for quantification and characterization of fibrocytes, as previously described [19,23] (See the online supplement for additional details of methods used). In some experiments, animals were exposed to hypoxia-reoxygenation (3 h at 8% oxygen/92% nitrogen followed by 4 h at 21% oxygen/79% nitrogen) before tissue harvest. CXCL12 was neutralized in vivo as previously described [13,26]. Lung mechanics of animals were assessed by FlexiVent using Quasi-static pressure-volume (PV) curve to calculate total lung compliance and elastance, and forced oscillatory measurements to measure frequency dependence of parenchymal tissue impedance and parenchymal tissue elastance according to manufacturer's instructions. Plasma samples were analyzed for cytokines by Luminex multiplex protein analysis as previously described [13]. Lung collagen content was quantified using the Sircol assays (Biocolor Ltd., Belfast, United Kingdom) according to the manufacturer's instructions [27] and using morphometric analysis of histological samples after picrosirius red staining [28]. To quantify picrosirius red stains, lungs were inflated, fixed and sectioned; photomicrographs were then obtained from 10 randomly selected medium power fields from the lung periphery in each slide. By obtaining images from the lung periphery only, we excluded fields that included large blood vessels or airways. In human subjects, fibrocyte concentrations were not distributed normally and were compared using the Mann-Whitney U test;. Subject demographics and SCD characteristics were analyzed with Chi-Square tests for categorical variables and either Student's t or Mann-Whitney U tests for continuous variables that were normally or non-normally distributed, respectively. Mouse fibrocyte data were normally distributed and were compared using Student's t test. Paired measurements were compared using Wilcoxon matched-pairs signed-ranks test. Probability values were considered statistically significant if they were less than 0.05. Data analysis was performed in SAS version 9.1 (SAS Institute, Cary, NC).

The Institutional Review Board (IRB) at Washington University and the University of Virginia approved all human protocols and written informed consent was obtained in accordance with the Declaration of Helsinki. IRB approval numbers are PRO00014330 and 15598. The animal studies were carried out in accordance with the recommendations in the Guide for the Care and Use of Laboratory Animals of the National Institutes of Health and were approved by the Committee on the Ethics of Animal Experiments of the University of Virginia (Permit Number: 3549).

Refer to Supplemental Information S1 for detailed methods.

Results

Fibrocytes are markedly elevated and activated in the circulation of patients with SCD at baseline

Since previous studies had demonstrated that elevated fibrocytes can be found in the circulation of patients with ILD [23,25], we wanted to determine whether fibrocytes were present in patients with SCD under similar conditions (i.e., routine clinic visit with no clinical evidence of VOC). From a cohort of patients with SCD at

Table 1. Baseline demographics, SCD characteristics and fibrocyte levels in SCD subjects with severe SCD phenotypes (HbSS/Sβ-thalassemia^0) compared to milder SCD phenotypes (HbSC/Sβ-thalassemia$^+$).

	SCD cohort n = 114	HbSS/Sβthal^0 n = 82	HbSC/Sβthal$^+$ n = 32	*P* value
Demographics				
Age, median (IQR)	30.9 (17)	28.5 (14)	39.3 (21)	**0.03**
Gender, % male	46	47	44	0.28
SCD characteristics				
Hemogloblin (g/dL), mean (SD)	9.1 (1.8)	8.5 (1.4)	10.5 (1.8)	**<0.001**
WBC (cells/µL), mean (SD)	11.2 (3.3)	11.7 (3.2)	9.8 (3.1)	**0.004**
LDH (IU/L), median (IQR)	311 (194)	360 (231)	244 (102)	**<0.001**
Hydroxyurea, %	33	44	6	**<0.001**
Supplemental oxygen, %	19	26	3	**0.006**
Fibrocytes/ml × 10^5, median (IQR)				
CD45+Col1+	3.47 (6.78)	3.58 (6.90)	2.63 (6.28)	0.49
CD45+Col1+CXCR4+	2.25 (6.15)	2.30 (6.54)	2.05 (6.18)	0.71
CD45+Col1+CCR2+	0.68 (1.54)	0.66 (1.67)	0.74 (1.58)	0.98
CD45+Col1+CCR7+	0.45 (1.46)	0.45 (1.55)	0.43 (1.14)	0.68
CD45+Col1+αSMA+	0.58 (1.81)	0.66 (1.90)	0.56 (1.58)	0.93
CD45+Col1+pSMAD2/3+	1.05 (3.56)	1.05 (3.75)	1.02 (3.51)	0.62

IQR, inter-quartile range; LDH, lactate dehydrogenase; SCD, sickle cell disease; SD, standard deviation; WBC, white blood cell.

Washington University in St. Louis, samples from 114 unique SCD patients along with 19 African American controls were collected and shipped overnight to the laboratory at UVA (RMS). Mean age was 34±12 years for the SCD cases and 41±4 years for the controls. Fifty-four percent of the SCD subjects were female, whereas 88% of the control participants were female. Among the SCD cases, 73% percent had HbSS or HbSbeta-thalassemia^0; the remainder had HbSC and HbSbeta-thalassemia$^+$. Nineteen percent of SCD subjects required home oxygen either continuously or at night. When subjects with more and less severe SCD phenotypes were compared (HbSS/HbSβ-thalassemia^0 vs. HbSC/HbSβ-thalassemia$^+$), there were no differences in circulating fibrocyte levels (Table 1).

We assessed de novo the circulating levels of fibrocytes (CD45+Col1+ cells) in these patients using quantitative FACS analysis as previously described [23,25]. We chose to first gate on CD45+ rather than CD34+ cells, because we have historically found that the number of CD34+Col1+ fibrocytes in the circulation is an order of magnitude lower than CD45+Col1+ fibrocytes (data not shown). Fibrocyte levels were significantly higher in SCD cases compared to controls (median: 3.47×10^5 cells/ml vs. 1.49×10^5 cells/ml; $p=0.001$) (Figure 1A). Further analysis of SCD cases demonstrated a hierarchy of chemokine receptor expression (CXCR4≫CCR2>CCR7) (Figure 1B, 1C, and 1D). While tissue myofibroblasts can arise from cells other than fibroytes, prior literature indicated that in both in vitro studies and animal models, fibrocytes represent a progenitor cell that can differentiate into αSMA-expressing myofibroblast-like cells [13,29,30] and human lungs contain fibrocytes expressing the myofibrobast marker αSMA [24]. We therefore also determined whether the elevation in circulating fibrocytes in the SCD patients was associated with increased numbers of αSMA+ fibrocytes in circulation by quantitative FACS analysis as previously described [23,25,30]. SCD patients had a higher number of αSMA+ fibrocytes compared to controls (Figure 1E). We previously determined that TGF-b stimulation of fibrocytes via activation of receptor Smads (Smad2/3) is critical to initiate signal transduction and induction of αSMA in these cells [29]. On this

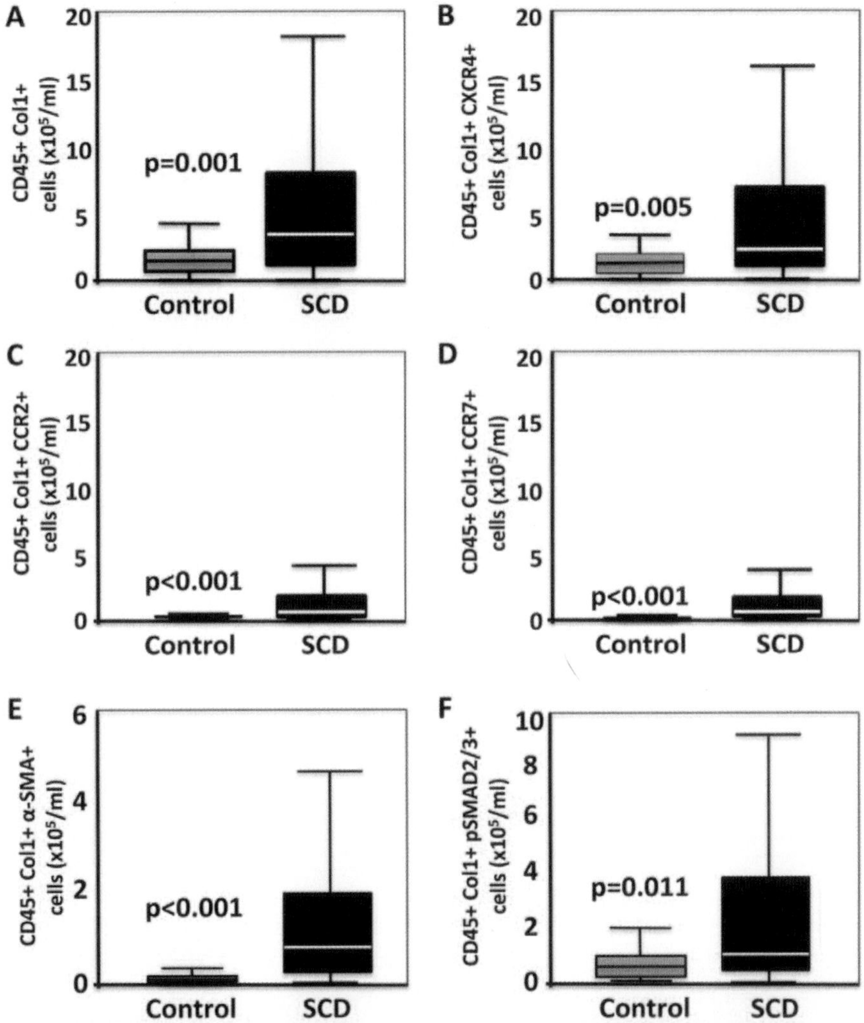

Figure 1. Fibrocytes are markedly elevated and activated in the circulation of patients with SCD at baseline compared to healthy African American controls. A) fibrocytes defined as CD45+Col1+ cells were elevated in number in the circulation of patients with SCD, as compared to control subjects. B–D) demonstrates that fibrocytes in the circulation of patients with SCD, as compared to control subjects express a chemokine receptor hierarchy (i.e., CXCR4+>CCR2+>CCR7+). E–F) demonstrates that fibrocytes in the circulation of patients with SCD, as compared to control subjects represent an activated phenotype of αSMA+ and pSmad2/3+ cells, respectively, compatible with fibrocytes pre-systemically activated by TGF-b.

basis, we developed a strategy in our laboratory to detect activated receptor Smads (pSmad2/3) by quantitative FACS analysis, which we confirmed by using Western Blot analysis of cells stimulated with TGF-b. Fibrocytes in circulation of SCD patients were subsequently analyzed for activated receptor Smads (pSmad2/3) and were found to be significantly higher than controls (Figure 1F).

Fibrocytes increase significantly over baseline level in patients with SCD under conditions of VOC

Blood from 9 SCD patients were analyzed at baseline and at time of admission to the hospital for VOC. Average age in this subset of patients was 35±9 years. Six subjects were female and 7 had HbSS/Sβ-thalassemia^0. Notably, there were no significant differences in age, gender, SCD genotype or baseline fibrocyte levels between those SCD subjects with and without paired measurements (data not shown). During a vaso-occlusive episode compared to baseline, there were significant increases the number of circulating fibrocytes ($p = 0.021$), αSMA+ fibrocytes ($p = 0.008$), and pSmad2/3+ fibrocytes (0.015) (Figure 2A–C).

NY1DD SCD mice demonstrated increased deposition of extracellular matrix in their lungs under baseline conditions

To more fully elucidate the role of fibrocytes in the development of ILD among patients with SCD, we next focused our studies on a murine model of SCD [31]. Prior studies have shown that significant injury from microvascular occlusion occurs during baseline conditions in the NY1DD mouse, including lung injury [31]. Since the NY1DD mice displayed evidence for marked lung injury under baseline conditions, we sought evidence of pulmonary fibroproliferation. Using the Sircol assay as previously described [13,32] to measure total soluble collagen in the lungs of NY1DD mice at 6 to 8 weeks; we determined that these mice have increased levels of soluble collagen in their lungs, as compared to controls (Figure 3A). These findings were confirmed by morphometric analysis of the lungs by the collagen-specific dye picrosirius red (Figure 3B). To put into context the levels of soluble collagen in the lungs of these SCD mice with other mouse models of pulmonary fibrosis, we compared these lung soluble

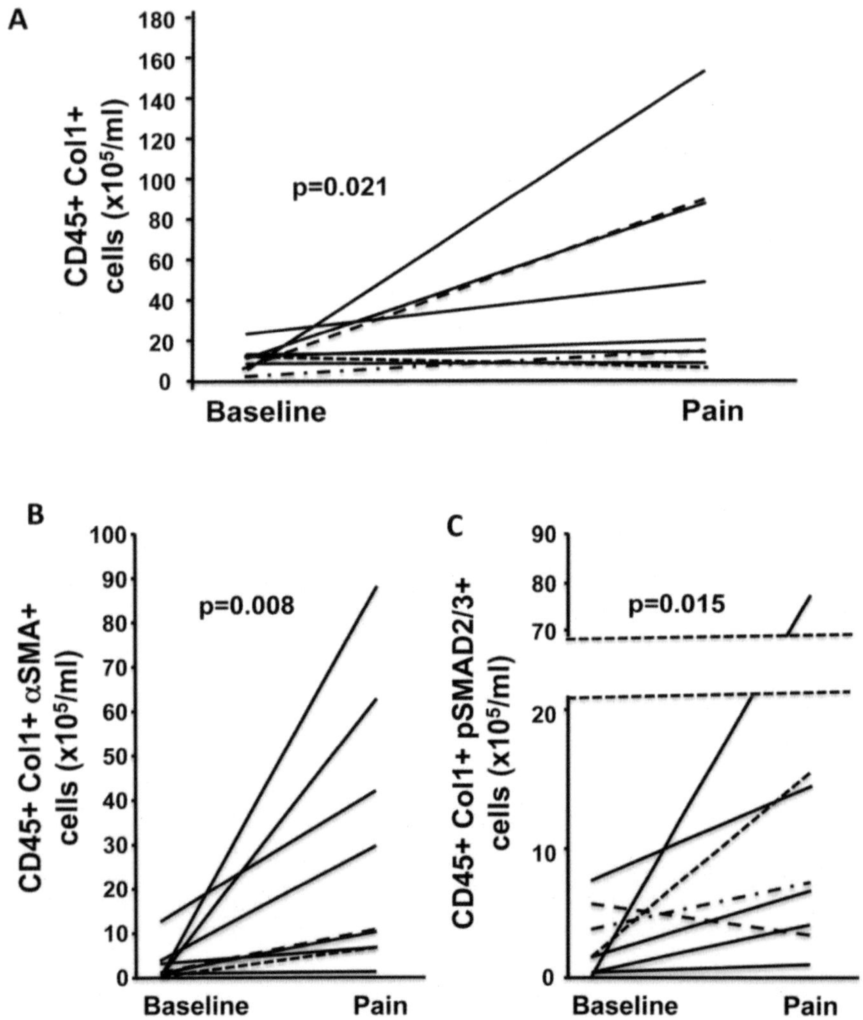

Figure 2. Fibrocytes increase significantly over baseline level in patients with SCD under conditions of VOC. A) Fibrocytes defined as CD45+Col1+ cells in nine SCD patients were markedly increased from baseline during an episode of VOC. B–C) demonstrates that the fibrocytes in the circulation of SCD patients undergoing a VOC represent an activated phenotype of αSMA+ and pSmad2/3+ cells, respectively, compatible with fibrocytes systemically pre-activated by TGF-b.

collagen levels to C57BL/6 mice that had been exposed to bleomycin for 16 days to produce pulmonary fibrosis [32,33]. Levels of soluble collagen in bleomycin-exposed mice were similar to the baseline levels of soluble collagen in the lungs of NY1DD mice (Figure 3A).

NY1DD SCD mice displayed increased numbers of fibrocytes in their bone marrow, circulation, and lungs under baseline conditions

To determine whether the pathogenesis of increased fibroproliferation in the lungs of the NY1DD mice was due to the presence of fibrocytes, we next assessed the quantitative levels of fibrocytes in the bone marrow, circulation (i.e., buffy coat cells), and lungs of these animals, as compared to controls. Fibrocytes were markedly expanded in the bone marrow, increased in the circulation, and increased in the lungs of NY1DD mice (Figure 4A, 4B, and 4C, respectively). The same chemokine receptor hierarchy was found on fibrocytes from the bone marrow, circulation, and lungs, CXCR4≫CCR2>CCR7 (Figure 4A, 4B, and 4C, respectively). To further confirm that these were fibrocytes and not

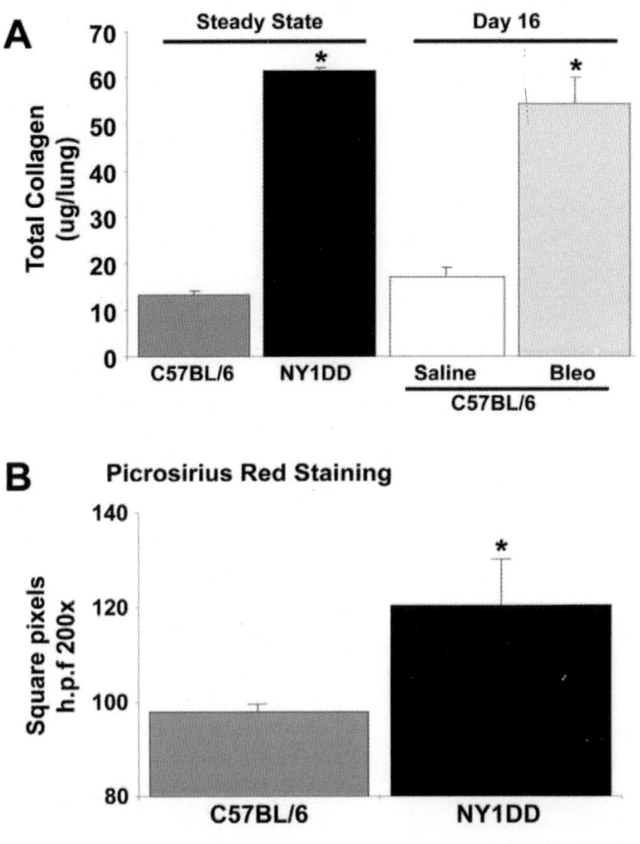

Figure 3. NY1DD SCD mice demonstrated increased deposition of extracellular matrix in their lungs under baseline conditions. A) NY1DD SCD mice, as compared to appropriate strain (C57Bl/6) and age-matched mice, demonstrate elevated levels of total collagen in their lungs under baseline (normoxia) conditions. The levels of total collagen in the lungs of NY1DD mice at baseline are equivalent to C57Bl/6 mice exposed to the pulmonary fibrotic agent, bleomycin, at day 16. B) NY1DD mice, as compared to appropriate strain and age-matched mice demonstrate elevated levels of collagen, as assessed by morphometric analysis of picrosirius red staining of lung tissue. N = six mice in each group. * $p<0.05$.

macrophages that had phagocytized collagen, FACS analysis was performed on these same cells to detect intracellular pro-collagen type I and III by using specific antibodies that detect the C-terminus and N-terminus of type I pro-collagen and the C-terminus of pro-collagen III. CD45+ pro-collagen type I and III positive cells were expanded in the bone marrow, increased in the circulation and lungs of NY1DD mice (Figure 4D, 4E, and 4F, respectively). In addition, we found increased numbers of fibrocytes that appeared to be undergoing differentiation to αSMA+ cells in the bone marrow, circulation, and lungs of NY1DD SCD mice (Figure 4G, 4H, and 4I, respectively).

NY1DD SCD mice displayed increased numbers of fibrocytes in their bone marrow, circulation, and lungs under conditions simulating VOC (hypoxia followed by reoxygenation)

To determine whether NY1DD SCD mice experience worsening of their chronic ILD with hypoxia followed by reoxygenation (normoxia) similar to patients with SCD that experience VOC, we placed NY1DD SCD mice and wild type (C57BL/6) mice in hypoxia (8% oxygen) for 3 hrs followed by return to normoxia for 4 hrs using a modification as previously described [31]. Hypoxia followed by reoxygenation in NY1DD SCD mice resulted in marked worsening histopathology of the lungs of NY1DD SCD (Figure 5A and 5B), as compared to normoxic-exposed mice, consisting of areas of fibrosis and inflammation. These findings recapitulated what we had found in our previous studies using this mouse model of SCD [31]. To determine whether the marked change in pathology under conditions of hypoxia/reoxygenation was associated with a change in the number of fibrocytes, we measured fibrocytes under the above conditions in the bone marrow, circulation, and lungs of these mice. We found a marked increase in numbers of fibrocytes in the bone marrow, circulation, and lungs under conditions of hypoxia followed by normoxia, as compared to NY1DD SCD mice exposed only to normoxia or to control mice (Figure 5C, 5D, and 5E, respectively). The chemokine receptor hierarchy that was found expressed on fibrocytes under these conditions in the bone marrow, circulation, and lungs demonstrated the persistent expression pattern of CXCR4≫CCR2>CCR7 (Figure 5C, 5D, and 5E, respectively).

NY1DD SCD mice have increased lung levels of CXCL12 and other cytokines that are relevant to fibrocyte biology

On the basis of the presence of increased fibrocytes expressing CXCR4 as the predominant chemokine receptor in the lungs of NY1DD mice under either baseline or hypoxia/normoxic conditions, we next determined whether CXCL12, the putative ligand to CXCR4, was elevated in the lungs of NY1DD mice under baseline conditions. We found that CXCL12 in lung homogenates of NY1DD mice is markedly elevated and similar to the levels of CXCL12 that we had found in bleomycin exposed lungs on days 8 to 20, which also correlated with maximal extracellular matrix deposition in this model (Figure 6A) [13]. Immunohistochemistry for CXCL12 in the lungs of NY1DD mice demonstrated that CXCL12 was localized to a variety of cells in the lung parenchyma that included type II pneumocytes. Moreover, when we measured other cytokines thought to be relevant to fibrocyte biology [34,35], we found elevated levels of PDGF and M-CSF in the lungs of these animals (Figure 6B).

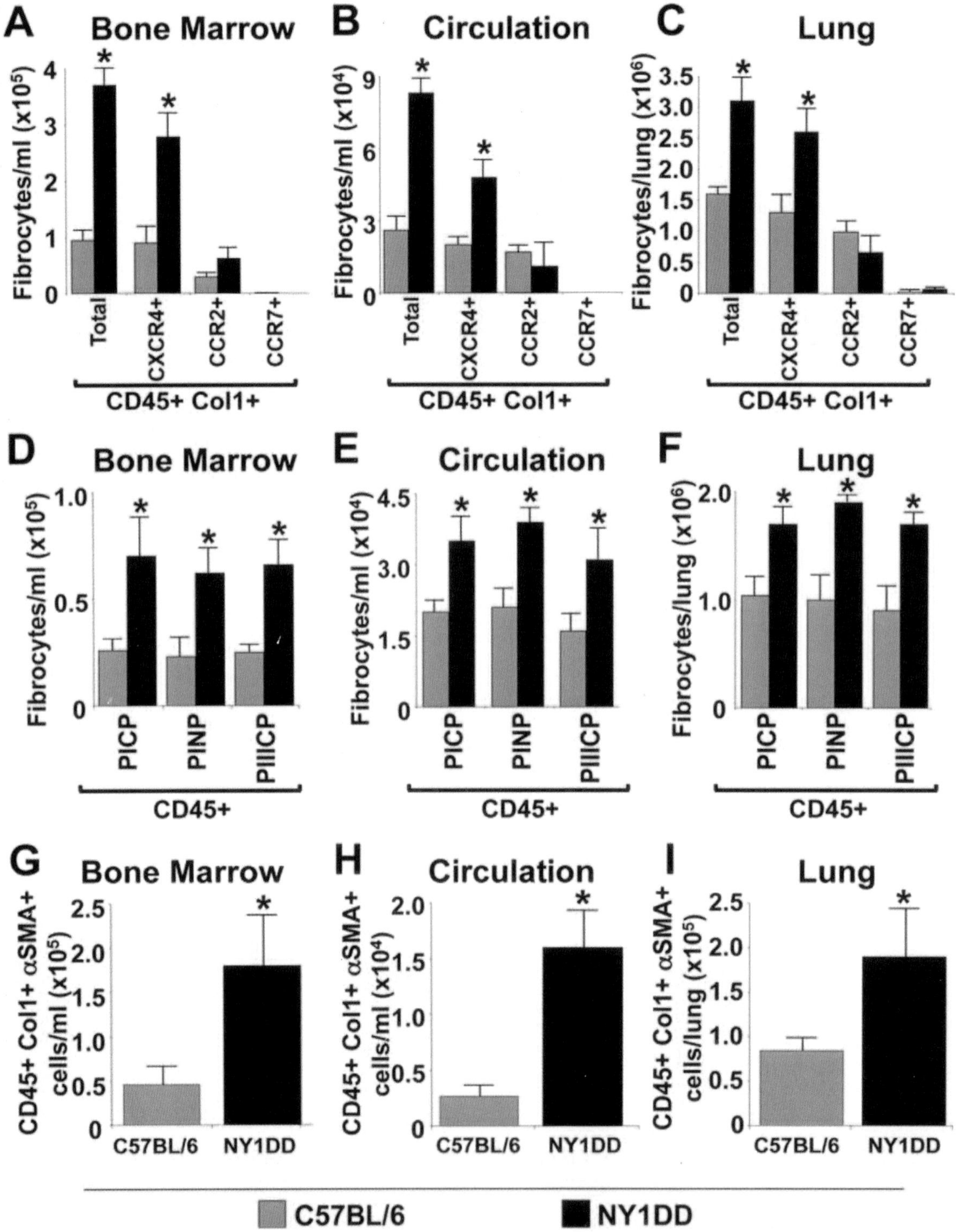

Figure 4. NY1DD SCD mice displayed increased numbers of fibrocytes in their bone marrow, circulation, and lungs under baseline conditions. A–C) demonstrates that fibrocytes are elevated in the bone marrow, circulation, and lungs of NY1DD SCD mice, as compared to strain and age-matched control mice. In addition, A–C) demonstrates that fibrocytes in the bone marrow, circulation, and lungs of NY1DD mice, as compared to strain and age-matched mice express a chemokine receptor hierarchy (i.e., CXCR4+≫CCR2+>CCR7+). D–F) demonstrates that elevated fibrocytes in the bone marrow, circulation, and lungs of NY1DD mice, as compared to appropriate strain and age-match mice express pro-collagens I and III (pro-collagen type I N and C-terminus = PINP and PICP, respectively; pro-collagen type III C-terminus = PIIICP). G–I) NY1DD SCD mice displayed increased numbers of fibrocytes (CD45+Col1+ cells) in their bone marrow, circulation, and lungs under baseline conditions that represent an activated phenotype (αSMA+ cells) compared to appropriate strain and age-match mice. N = six mice in each group. * $p<0.05$.

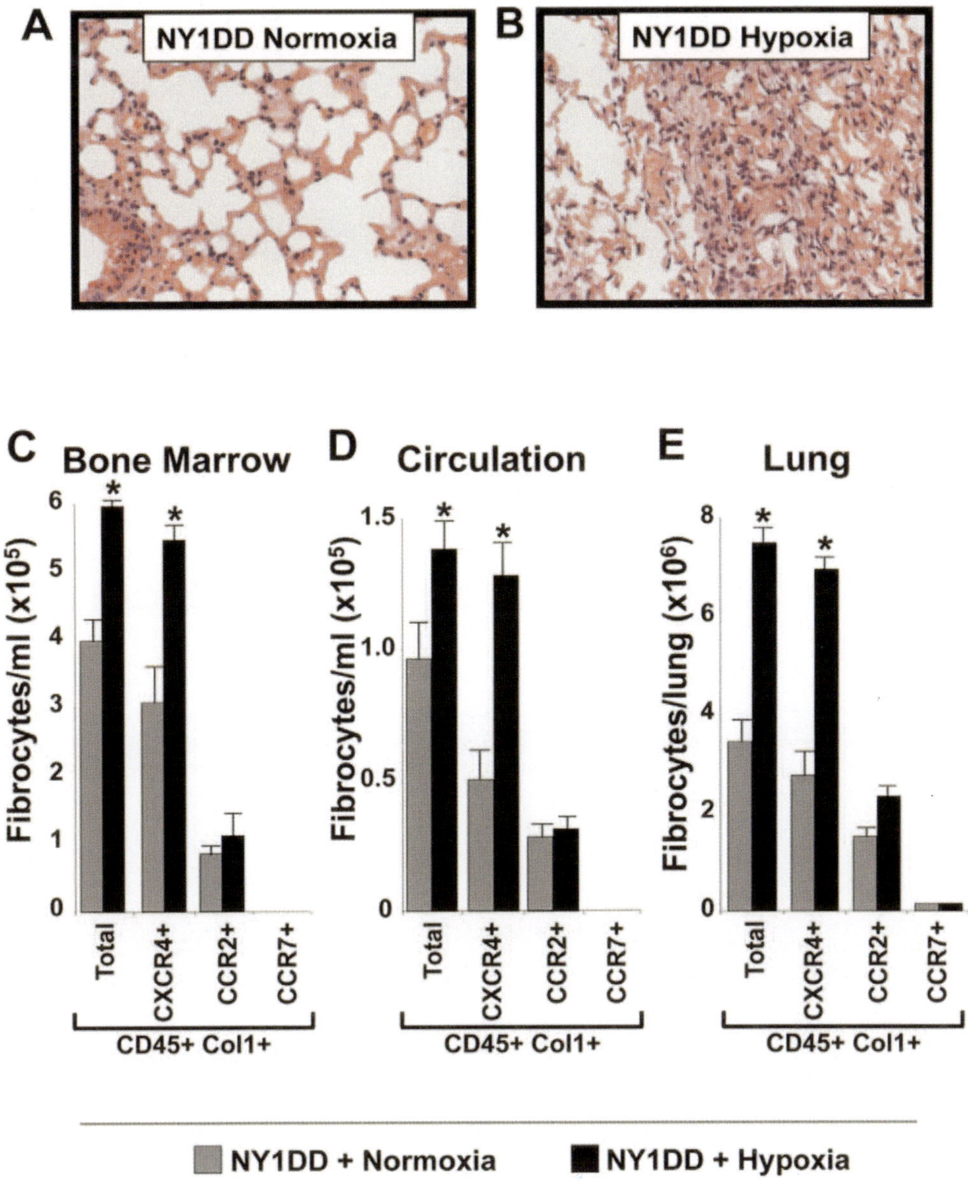

Figure 5. NY1DD SCD mice displayed marked lung fibrosis and inflammation under conditions simulating VOC (hypoxia followed by reoxygenation) (B), as compared to NY1DD mice exposed to normoxic conditions alone (A). Photomicrographs are representative H&E of lungs from six mice in each group, under 400×. NY1DD SCD mice displayed increased numbers of fibrocytes in their bone marrow, circulation, and lungs under conditions simulating VOC (hypoxia followed by reoxygenation). C–E) demonstrates that fibrocytes are elevated in the bone marrow, circulation, and lungs of NY1DD SCD mice under conditions simulating VOC (hypoxia followed by reoxygenation), as compared to NY1DD mice exposed to normoxic conditions alone. In addition, C–E) demonstrates that fibrocytes in the bone marrow, circulation, and lungs of NY1DD SCD mice under conditions simulating VOC (hypoxia followed by reoxygenation), as compared to NY1DD mice exposed to normoxic conditions alone express a chemokine receptor hierarchy (i.e., CXCR4+ ≫ CCR2+ > CCR7+). N = six mice in each group. * $p = < 0.05$.

Depletion of CXCL12 under baseline conditions in NY1DD SCD mice reduces the number of fibrocytes, and this is correlated with a reduction in collagen deposition and improvement in lung compliance and histopathology

On the basis of the presence of CXCL12 in the lungs of NY1DD mice under homeostatic conditions that directly correlated with the presence of increased numbers of CXCR4+ fibrocytes, we next examined whether depletion of CXCL12 would impact on extravasation of fibrocytes into the lungs of NY1DD mice, and whether this would have a direct effect on the magnitude of collagen deposition. NY1DD mice under baseline conditions were treated with neutralizing anti-CXCL12 or control antibodies (i.p. Q48 hrs) for a period of 7 days at which point they were sacrificed and their lungs assessed for levels of fibrocytes by quantitative FACS and soluble collagen by the Sircol assay as previously described [13,30]. We found a marked attenuation of CD45+Col1+CXCR4+ fibrocytes in the lungs of the NY1DD mice that had been depleted of CXCL12 (Figure 7A), which directly correlated with a reduction in soluble collagen (Figure 7B). Moreover, when we assessed the impact of this therapeutic strategy on other populations of leukocytes in the lungs of these mice, we found no significant impact on CD4, CD8, NK cells,

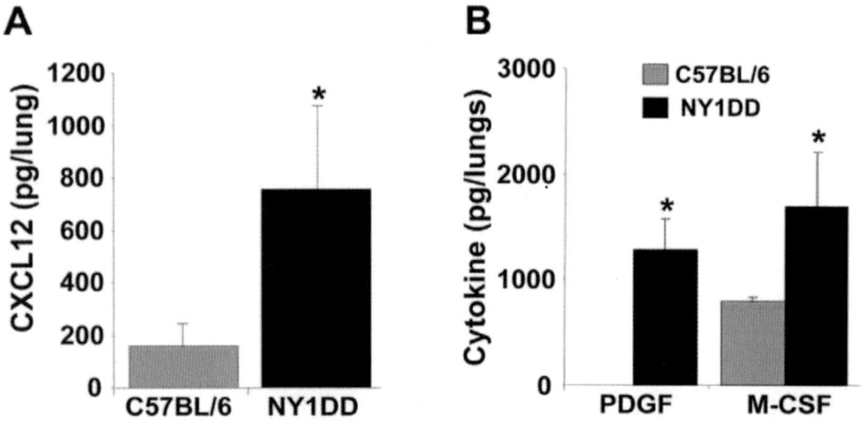

Figure 6. NY1DD SCD mice have increased lung levels of CXCL12 and other cytokines that are relevant to fibrocyte biology. A) demonstrates that the ligand to CXCR4, CXCL12, is markedly elevated in the lungs of NY1DD mice under baseline conditions compared to appropriate strain and age-match mice. B) demonstrates that the growth factor (PDGF) and colony stimulating factor (M-CSF) are significantly elevated in the lungs of NY1DD mice under baseline conditions compared to appropriate strain and age-match mice. N = six mice lungs in each group. * p = <0.05.

neutrophils, or macrophages (Table 2). These findings suggest that the lungs of NY1DD mice are undergoing collagen deposition under baseline conditions that appears to be related to extravasation of CXCR4+ fibrocytes into their lungs. In conjunction with these studies we measured lung compliance (i.e., using FlexiVent) under both conditions of closed chest and open diaphragm and found that blocking CXCL12 resulted in improved lung compliance (Figure 7C and 7D) that was associated with markedly less ILD histopathology (Figure 7E and 7F).

Discussion

This study provides the first evidence that circulating CD45+Col I+CXCR4+ fibrocytes, recruited through the CXCL12/CXCR4 axis, contribute to the expansion of the fibroblast/myofibroblast-like cell population in people and mice with SCD. At baseline, NY1DD mice have increased fibrocytes in the bone marrow, circulation and lungs compared to controls and, similar to studies of subjects with IPF, the fibrocytes express the hierarchy of chemokine expression CXCR4≫CCR2>CCR7. The CXCR4 ligand, CXCL12, is critical to CXCR4+ fibrocyte trafficking and neutralizing CXCL12 prevents fibrocyte extravasation into the lungs. These findings in NY1DD mice complement our initial findings in adult patients with SCD providing preliminary evidence for a role for fibrocytes in the development of human ILD.

The pathogenesis of ILD in patients with SCD is poorly understood. Previously, ILD in this patient population was thought to be solely the result of repetitive infarcts occurring during ACS episodes [2]. Recently, a new paradigm has emerged for the understanding of vascular occlusion and end-organ damage in SCD, suggesting that SCD should be viewed as a disease characterized by subclinical, ongoing microvascular occlusion and punctuated by clinically apparent exacerbations [31,36,37]. In this model of SCD pathogenesis, end organ damage in SCD results from the total injury that occurs from clinical exacerbations plus ongoing, subclinical events. The findings of this study demonstrating organ damage and elevated levels of circulating fibrocytes at baseline in NY1DD mice support this notion of chronic microvascular occlusion, systemic inflammation and ongoing injury and repetitive repair, and provide a novel mechanism for the understanding of lung fibroproliferation in chronic ILD in patients with SCD.

Since the initial observations of ILD in patients with SCD were published [2], newer data describing the role of nitric oxide depletion, hemolysis and pulmonary hypertension in pathogenesis of SCD has emerged [4,5]. In a prior study, Powars et al describe chronic sickle cell lung disease as a disorder characterized by pulmonary fibrosis, pulmonary hypertension and a mean survival of 5 years [2]. More recently, several large studies have demonstrated an increased risk of death associated with pulmonary hypertension in adults with SCD [5,38,39]. Potentially, the mortality risk associated with chronic sickle cell lung disease in the prior study was due to pulmonary hypertension and not pulmonary fibrosis. However, examining the etiology of ILD in patients with SCD is important, because ILD has been shown to contribute to the development of pulmonary hypertension in SCD [40]. Although the findings in current study implicate fibrocytes in the pathogenesis of ILD, future studies should focus on the potential role of fibrocytes in the vascular remodeling of pulmonary hypertension in SCD.

Circulating fibrocytes contribute to the fibroproliferation in the lung seen in NY1DD mice. At baseline, there is increased collagen deposition in the lung of NY1DD mice compared to control mice demonstrating the active fibroproliferation in the lungs of NY1DD mice. In the bone marrow, circulation and lungs of NY1DD mice, fibrocytes are increased compared to controls and there is a subpopulation of αSMA+ cells, consistent with a fibroblast/myofibroblast-like cell. Although we cannot define the lineage of αSMA+ cells based on our data, the presence of elevated αSMA+ fibrocytes in the bone marrow of NY1DD mice suggests that these cells are beginning to undergo differentiation to a fibroblast/myofibroblast-like cells in the bone marrow. Consistent with our findings of CXCR4 predominance on circulating fibrocytes in other mouse models of pulmonary fibrosis [23,24], the majority of fibrocytes in NY1DD mice express CXCR4. The only known ligand for CXCR4, CXCL12, was markedly elevated in the lungs of NY1DD mice compared to controls, and neutralizing CXCL12 attenuated extravasation of fibrocytes into the lungs of NY1DD mice and reduced lung collagen deposition. Taken together, these findings support the notion that, at baseline, fibrocytes are expanded in the bone marrow, mobilized to the circulation, home

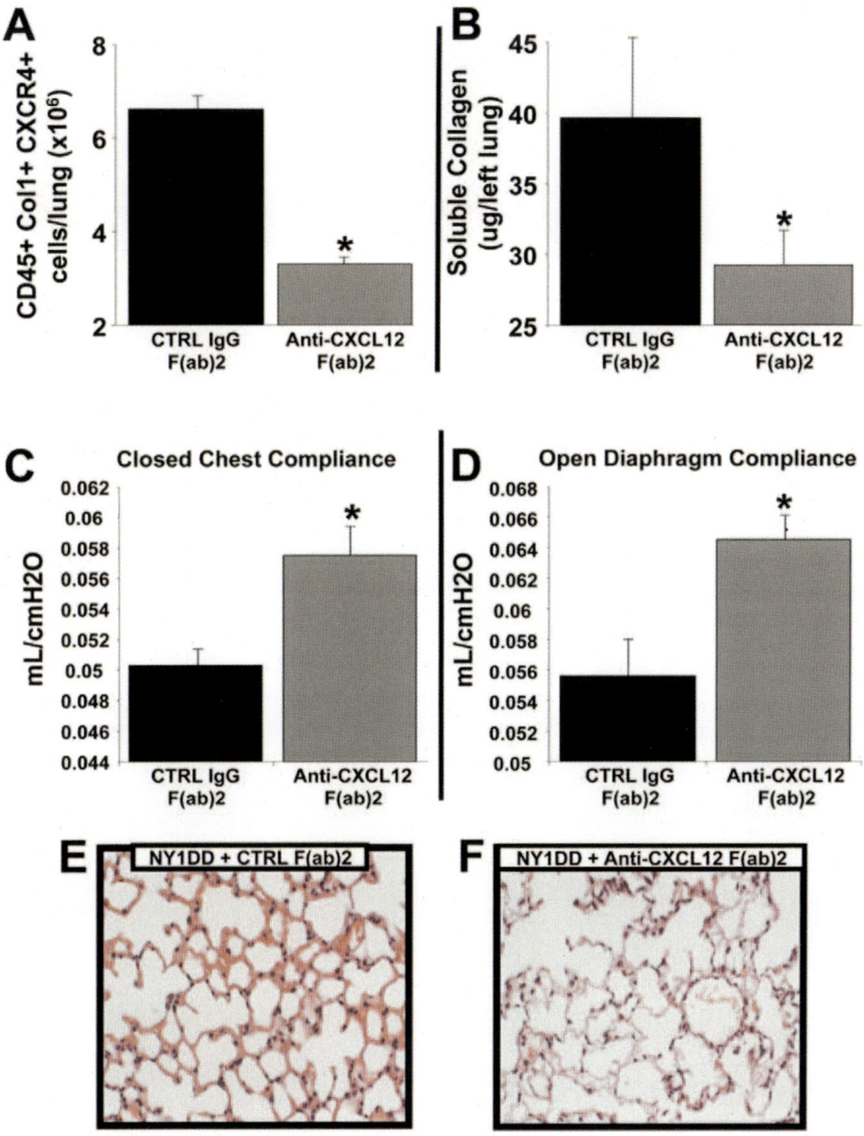

Figure 7. Depletion of CXCL12 under baseline conditions in NY1DD SCD mice reduces the number of fibrocytes within their lungs, and this is correlated with a reduction in collagen deposition and improvement in lung compliance and histopathology. A) demonstrates that passive immunization of NY1DD mice with anti-CXCL12, as compared to appropriate control F(ab)2 antibodies markedly attenuates the presence of fibrocytes in the lungs of NY1DD mice under baseline conditions. B) demonstrates that passive immunization of NY1DD mice with anti-CXCL12, as compared to appropriate control F(ab)2 antibodies reduces the amount of soluble collagen in the lungs of NY1DD mice under baseline conditions. C–D) demonstrates that passive immunization of NY1DD mice with anti-CXCL12, as compared to appropriate control F(ab)2 antibodies improves the compliance of the lungs of NY1DD mice under baseline conditions. E–F) demonstrates that passive immunization of NY1DD mice with anti-CXCL12 (F), as compared to appropriate control F(ab)2 antibodies (E) improves the histopathology of the lungs as demonstrated by the H&E photomicrographs. N = six mice in each group for A–D, lung photomicrographs (E–F) are representative of six lungs from each group. * p = <0.05.

and extravasate in the lung of SCD mice dependent upon the CXCR4/CXCL12 chemokine axis.

In NY1DD mice, fibrocytes increase during hypoxia/reoxygenation compared to levels during normoxic conditions. Although no animal model fully recapitulates human disease, inducing hypoxia in NY1DD mice is thought to be analogous to a VOC in patients with SCD [31,36]. Given that the natural history of SCD is characterized by disease exacerbations or VOC [41], hypoxia/reoxygenation in the mouse model approximates human disease. The current data suggest that VOC causes increased fibrocyte mobilization into circulation in both human SCD and the mouse model, and potentially promotes increased lung fibrosis.

Similar to findings in the NY1DD mouse, fibrocytes are elevated at baseline in patients with SCD compared to healthy control subjects. The chemokine hierarchy of CXCR4≫CCR2>CCR7 was also present in patients with SCD, suggesting that the CXCR4/CXCL12 chemokine axis is used for fibrocyte trafficking. Although circulating CXCL12 was higher in patients with SCD compared to controls, this did not reach statistical significance. CXCL12 was only measured in a subset of our patients and this may have limited our ability to

Table 2. Passive immunization of NY1DD mice with anti-CXCL12, as compared to appropriate control F(ab)2 antibodies does not alter the extravasation of populations of other leukocytes into the lungs of these mice under baseline conditions.

		Positive cells/Right Lung ($\times 10^5$)	
		Anti-CXCL12 F(ab)2	Control IgG F(ab)2
CD3 T-cells	CD3+	17.2+/−2.3	19.8+/−0.62
CD4 T-cells	CD3+ CD4+	6.6+/−0.61	8.2+/−0.99
CD8 T-cells	CD3+ CD8+	7.1+/−1.1	8.6+/−0.59
NK cells	CD3+ NK1.1+	6.1+/−0.31	9.5+/−1.4
Neutrophils	CD11b+ Ly6g+	21.4+/−1.5	28.3+/−2.1
Macrophages	MAC3+CD11b-CD11c+	23.3+/−2.5	26.6+/−4.2

detect a difference between cases and controls. Moreover, the lung should be the site for elevated levels of CXCL12 in order to promote a "chemotactic gradient" for CXCR4+ fibrocytes; and we found elevated levels of CXCL12 in the lungs of NY1DD mice. However, since plasma levels of CXCL12 were not significantly different between SCD subjects and controls, we can only postulate that in human SCD the CXCR4/CXCL12 chemokine axis and the gradient of CXCL12 in the lung is responsible for fibrocyte homing. During a VOC, fibrocyte levels within SCD subjects increased significantly over baseline and demonstrated an activated phenotype. Repeat measurements within an individual using a longitudinal study design provides assurance that the findings are not due to inter-individual variation. Our study was not designed to determine cause and effect between VOC and fibrocyte levels in patients with SCD. We can only report an association. Regardless of whether vaso-occlusion causes increased fibrocyte levels or vice versa, higher levels of fibrocytes in association with VOC may promote fibroproliferation and end organ damage. These data are consistent with NY1DD mice and support the notion that disease exacerbations (i.e., VOC) significantly contribute to the development of end organ disease. Furthermore, these data provide preliminary evidence that the pathophysiology and pathology we found in the NY1DD mouse can be translated to patients with SCD.

Taken together, our data in NY1DD mice and supported by evidence in patients with SCD suggests a novel model of ILD pathogenesis in SCD. This new paradigm for understanding the mechanism of pulmonary fibrosis in SCD implicating bone-marrow-derived fibrocytes is consistent with findings in IPF. Based on the data from this study, we postulate that inflammatory "signals" (i.e., CXCL12) generated in the lung communicate with the bone marrow leading to expansion of fibrocytes. The condition of vaso-occlusion (i.e., either subclinical or VOC) in the bone marrow creates an environment that is hypoxic in nature, which favors the induction of CXCR4 expression on fibrocytes that ultimately enhances their homing and extravasation at the target organ site (i.e., lung) in response to CXCL12. These circulating fibrocytes, largely CXCR4+, will only home and extravasate into an end-organ (i.e., lung) if there is the appropriate "address" signal, such as lung-specific expression of a chemokine ligand (i.e., CXCL12) to CXCR4. Once fibrocytes home and extravasate into the lung dependent on the CXCL12/CXCR4 biological axis, the data from our NY1DD mice suggests that they play a major role in functioning as mesenchymal progenitor cells for the production of extra-cellular matrix and contribution to fibrosis in the lungs of patients with SCD.

In summary, our results provide a new basis for understanding the pathogenesis of ILD in patients with SCD, a common and serious complication in this patient population [2,3,6]. The findings of our study offer the opportunity to therapeutically target fibrocytes by attenuating their recruitment into the lung in order to prevent pulmonary fibrosis.. Future studies are needed to examine strategies to attenuate fibrocytes and determine the impact on the longitudinal development of ILD in patients with SCD.

Author Contributions

Conceived and designed the experiments: RMS. Performed the experiments: MDB BAS LL. Analyzed the data: MDB JJF. Contributed reagents/materials/analysis tools: JJF. Wrote the paper: JJF RMS. Contributed to conception, experimental design, interpretation of results and manuscript editing: MRD BM CER JL.

References

1. Ashley-Koch A, Yang Q, Olney RS (2000) Sickle hemoglobin (HbS) allele and sickle cell disease: a HuGE review. American Journal of Epidemiology 151: 839–845.
2. Powars D, Weidman JA, Odom-Maryon T, Niland JC, Johnson C (1988) Sickle cell chronic lung disease: prior morbidity and the risk of pulmonary failure. Medicine (Baltimore) 67: 66–76.
3. Powars DR, Chan LS, Hiti A, Ramicone E, Johnson C (2005) Outcome of sickle cell anemia: a 4-decade observational study of 1056 patients. Medicine (Baltimore) 84: 363–376.
4. Gladwin MT, Vichinsky E (2008) Pulmonary complications of sickle cell disease. N Engl J Med 359: 2254–2265.
5. Gladwin MT, Sachdev V, Jison ML, Shizukuda Y, Plehn JF, et al. (2004) Pulmonary hypertension as a risk factor for death in patients with sickle cell disease. N Engl J Med 350: 886–895.
6. Klings ES, Wyszynski DF, Nolan VG, Steinberg MH (2006) Abnormal pulmonary function in adults with sickle cell anemia. Am J Respir Crit Care Med 173: 1264–1269.
7. McMillan TR, Moore BB, Weinberg JB, Vannella KM, Fields WB, et al. (2008) Exacerbation of established pulmonary fibrosis in a murine model by gammaherpesvirus. Am J Respir Crit Care Med 177: 771–780.
8. Strieter RM (2001) Mechanisms of pulmonary fibrosis: conference summary. Chest 120: 77S–85S.
9. Strieter RM (2008) What differentiates normal lung repair and fibrosis? Inflammation, resolution of repair, and fibrosis. Proc Am Thorac Soc 5: 305–310.
10. Strieter RM, Gomperts BN, Keane MP (2007) The role of CXC chemokines in pulmonary fibrosis. J Clin Invest 117: 549–556.
11. Fukuda Y, Ishizaki M, Masuda Y, Kimura G, Kawanami O, et al. (1987) The role of intraalveolar fibrosis in the process of pulmonary structural remodeling in patients with diffuse alveolar damage. Am J Pathol 126: 171–182.
12. Marshall R, Bellingan G, Laurent G (1998) The acute respiratory distress syndrome: fibrosis in the fast lane. Thorax 53: 815–817.
13. Phillips RJ, Burdick MD, Hong K, Lutz MA, Murray LA, et al. (2004) Circulating fibrocytes traffic to the lungs in response to CXCL12 and mediate fibrosis. J Clin Invest 114: 438–446.
14. Metz CN (2003) Fibrocytes: a unique cell population implicated in wound healing. Cell Mol Life Sci 60: 1342–1350.
15. Bucala R, Spiegel LA, Chesney J, Hogan M, Cerami A (1994) Circulating fibrocytes define a new leukocyte subpopulation that mediates tissue repair. Mol Med 1: 71–81.
16. Keeley EC, Mehrad B, Strieter RM (2011) The role of fibrocytes in fibrotic diseases of the lungs and heart. Fibrogenesis Tissue Repair 4: 2.
17. Strieter RM, Keeley EC, Hughes MA, Burdick MD, Mehrad B (2009) The role of circulating mesenchymal progenitor cells (fibrocytes) in the pathogenesis of pulmonary fibrosis. J Leukoc Biol.

18. Keeley EC, Mehrad B, Strieter RM (2009) Fibrocytes: bringing new insights into mechanisms of inflammation and fibrosis. Int J Biochem Cell Biol 42: 535–542.
19. Gomperts BN, Strieter RM (2007) Fibrocytes in lung disease. J Leukoc Biol 82: 449–456.
20. Moore BB, Kolodsick JE, Thannickal VJ, Cooke K, Moore TA, et al. (2005) CCR2-mediated recruitment of fibrocytes to the alveolar space after fibrotic injury. Am J Pathol 166: 675–684.
21. van Deventer HW, Wu QP, Bergstralh DT, Davis BK, O'Connor BP, et al. (2008) C-C chemokine receptor 5 on pulmonary fibrocytes facilitates migration and promotes metastasis via matrix metalloproteinase 9. Am J Pathol 173: 253–264.
22. Pilling D, Roife D, Wang M, Ronkainen SD, Crawford JR, et al. (2007) Reduction of bleomycin-induced pulmonary fibrosis by serum amyloid P. J Immunol 179: 4035–4044.
23. Mehrad B, Burdick MD, Zisman DA, Keane MP, Belperio JA, et al. (2007) Circulating peripheral blood fibrocytes in human fibrotic interstitial lung disease. Biochem Biophys Res Commun 353: 104–108.
24. Andersson-Sjoland A, de Alba CG, Nihlberg K, Becerril C, Ramirez R, et al. (2008) Fibrocytes are a potential source of lung fibroblasts in idiopathic pulmonary fibrosis. Int J Biochem Cell Biol 40: 2129–2140.
25. Moeller A, Gilpin SE, Ask K, Cox G, Cook D, et al. (2009) Circulating fibrocytes are an indicator of poor prognosis in idiopathic pulmonary fibrosis. Am J Respir Crit Care Med 179: 588–594.
26. Phillips RJ, Burdick MD, Lutz M, Belperio JA, Keane MP, et al. (2003) The stromal derived factor-1/CXCL12-CXC chemokine receptor 4 biological axis in non-small cell lung cancer metastases. Am J Respir Crit Care Med 167: 1676–1686.
27. Blease K, Schuh JM, Jakubzick C, Lukacs NW, Kunkel SL, et al. (2002) Stat6-deficient mice develop airway hyperresponsiveness and peribronchial fibrosis during chronic fungal asthma. Am J Pathol 160: 481–490.
28. Keane MP, Belperio JA, Arenberg DA, Burdick MD, Xu ZJ, et al. (1999) IFN-gamma-inducible protein-10 attenuates bleomycin-induced pulmonary fibrosis via inhibition of angiogenesis. J Immunol 163: 5686–5692.
29. Hong KM, Belperio JA, Keane MP, Burdick MD, Strieter RM (2007) Differentiation of human circulating fibrocytes as mediated by transforming growth factor-beta and peroxisome proliferator-activated receptor gamma. J Biol Chem 282: 22910–22920.
30. Mehrad B, Burdick MD, Strieter RM (2009) Fibrocyte CXCR4 regulation as a therapeutic target in pulmonary fibrosis. Int J Biochem Cell Biol 41: 1708–1718.
31. Wallace KL, Marshall MA, Ramos SI, Lannigan JA, Field JJ, et al. (2009) NKT cells mediate pulmonary inflammation and dysfunction in murine sickle cell disease through production of IFN-gamma and CXCR3 chemokines. Blood 114: 667–676.
32. Phillips RJ, Mestas J, Gharaee-Kermani M, Burdick MD, Sica A, et al. (2005) Epidermal growth factor and hypoxia-induced expression of CXC chemokine receptor 4 on non-small cell lung cancer cells is regulated by the phosphatidylinositol 3-kinase/PTEN/AKT/mammalian target of rapamycin signaling pathway and activation of hypoxia inducible factor-1alpha. J Biol Chem 280: 22473–22481.
33. Burdick MD, Murray LA, Keane MP, Xue YY, Zisman DA, et al. (2005) CXCL11 attenuates bleomycin-induced pulmonary fibrosis via inhibition of vascular remodeling. Am J Respir Crit Care Med 171: 261–268.
34. Maeda A, Hiyama K, Yamakido H, Ishioka S, Yamakido M (1996) Increased expression of platelet-derived growth factor A and insulin-like growth factor-I in BAL cells during the development of bleomycin-induced pulmonary fibrosis in mice. Chest 109: 780–786.
35. Baran CP, Opalek JM, McMaken S, Newland CA, O'Brien JM, Jr., et al. (2007) Important roles for macrophage colony-stimulating factor, CC chemokine ligand 2, and mononuclear phagocytes in the pathogenesis of pulmonary fibrosis. Am J Respir Crit Care Med 176: 78–89.
36. Kaul DK, Hebbel RP (2000) Hypoxia/reoxygenation causes inflammatory response in transgenic sickle mice but not in normal mice. J Clin Invest 106: 411–420.
37. Osarogiagbon UR, Choong S, Belcher JD, Vercellotti GM, Paller MS, et al. (2000) Reperfusion injury pathophysiology in sickle transgenic mice. Blood 96: 314–320.
38. De Castro LM, Jonassaint JC, Graham FL, Ashley-Koch A, Telen MJ (2008) Pulmonary hypertension associated with sickle cell disease: clinical and laboratory endpoints and disease outcomes. Am J Hematol 83: 19–25.
39. Ataga KI, Moore CG, Jones S, Olajide O, Strayhorn D, et al. (2006) Pulmonary hypertension in patients with sickle cell disease: a longitudinal study. Br J Haematol 134: 109–115.
40. Anthi A, Machado RF, Jison ML, Taveira-Dasilva AM, Rubin LJ, et al. (2007) Hemodynamic and functional assessment of patients with sickle cell disease and pulmonary hypertension. Am J Respir Crit Care Med 175: 1272–1279.
41. Platt OS, Thorington BD, Brambilla DJ, Milner PF, Rosse WF, et al. (1991) Pain in sickle cell disease. Rates and risk factors. N Engl J Med 325: 11–16.

9

Applying Microsatellite Multiplex PCR Analysis (MMPA) for Determining Allele Copy-Number Status and Percentage of Normal Cells within Tumors

Carles Garcia-Linares[1], Jaume Mercadé[1], Bernat Gel[1], Josep Biayna[1], Ernest Terribas[1], Conxi Lázaro[2], Eduard Serra[1]*

1 Institute of Predictive and Personalized Medicine of Cancer (IMPPC), Badalona, Barcelona, Spain, **2** Programa de Diagnòstic Molecular de Càncer Hereditari, Laboratori de Recerca Translacional, Institut Català d'Oncologia (ICO) – IDIBELL, L'Hospitalet de Llobregat, Barcelona, Spain

Abstract

The study of somatic genetic alterations in tumors contributes to the understanding and management of cancer. Genetic alterations, such us copy number or copy neutral changes, generate allelic imbalances (AIs) that can be determined using polymorphic markers. Here we report the development of a simple set of calculations for analyzing microsatellite multiplex PCR data from control-tumor pairs that allows us to obtain accurate information not only regarding the AI status of tumors, but also the percentage of tumor-infiltrating normal cells, the locus copy-number status and the mechanism involved in AI. We validated this new approach by re-analyzing a set of Neurofibromatosis type 1-associated dermal neurofibromas and comparing newly generated data with results obtained for the same tumors in a previous study using MLPA, Paralog Ratio Analysis and SNP-array techniques. Microsatellite multiplex PCR analysis (MMPA) should be particularly useful for analyzing specific regions of the genome containing tumor suppressor genes and also for determining the percentage of infiltrating normal cells within tumors allowing them to be sorted before they are analyzed by more expensive techniques.

Editor: Jörg D. Hoheisel, Deutsches Krebsforschungszentrum, Germany

Funding: This work was supported by grants from the Spanish Health Research Foundation: Instituto de Salud Carlos III (PI051155, PI081871, PI10/01422 and ISCIII-RTICC RD06/0020/1050; RD06/0020/1051); the Government of Catalonia (2009SGR290); the Asociación Española Contra el Cáncer (AECC) that recognizes and supports our group as a Grupo Estable de Investigación Oncológica 2010. The authors would like to especially acknowledge the Asociación Española de Afectados de Neurofibromatosis for their constant support to our research. The funders had no role in study design, data collection and analysis, decision to publish, or preparation of the manuscript.

Competing Interests: The authors have declared that no competing interests exist.

* E-mail: eserra@imppc.org

Introduction

Cancer development and progression is partly driven by the acquisition of somatic genetic alterations [1]. Both DNA copy-number changes and copy-neutral events have traditionally been identified by detecting the presence of allelic imbalances (AIs). These are significant deviations from the 1:1 allelic ratio of any heterozygous marker in a diploid cell, which are often reported as a loss of heterozygosity (LOH) when analyzing tumor-control tissue DNA pairs. Different techniques have been used to specifically detect copy-number changes in tumor DNA, such as semi-quantitative [2] or quantitative [3] PCR reactions, Multiplex Ligation-dependent Probe Amplification (MLPA) [4], Multiplex Amplicon Quantification (MAQ) [5] or array-CGH [6]. However, these techniques are not able to detect copy-neutral events, such as homologous recombination, which often reduce mutated tumor suppressor genes to homozygosity [7]. Fluorescent multiplex microsatellite PCR has been developed, semi-automatized and used in tumor AI analysis for a long time [8], and is still used now [9]. Determining the quotient between tumor-control tissue allelic ratios for a given heterozygous marker identifies AI. Guidelines on how to score and interpret AI analysis using microsatellite multiplex have been developed (see for instance [10]) as well as methodological modifications and statistical refinement (see for instance [11]). However, in order to differentiate whether an AI in a given locus is caused by a loss of DNA material or by a copy-neutral event, the use of an additional technique is required to determine the copy-number status of the locus. In addition, one of the problems of genetic analysis of tumors is the presence of high percentages of normal cells infiltrating the tumors. Since the development of microsatellite PCR for tumor AI analysis the presence of normal (non-AI) cells has been identified by the remaining signal of the lost allele, and grossly estimated by a simple allele ratio. This approximation is quite accurate in the case of an AI caused by a true loss of DNA material but it is not a good method in the case of copy-neutral events.

Today SNP-array analysis is the only single technique that can provide high resolution genome scale information on allele-specific copy-number, map and evaluate copy-neutral LOH, and accurately model the fractions of normal and tumor cells in tumor samples [12]. However, SNP-array analysis is not the preferred technique when analyzing just a few loci (e.g. to evaluate the status of specific tumor suppressor gene locus) or when performing a screening of many samples to make a tumor triage for further analysis, because of the high cost.

In this study we describe how, by applying simple calculations to an analysis of a microsatellite multiplex PCR (here referred to as MMPA), it is possible to obtain accurate information regarding not

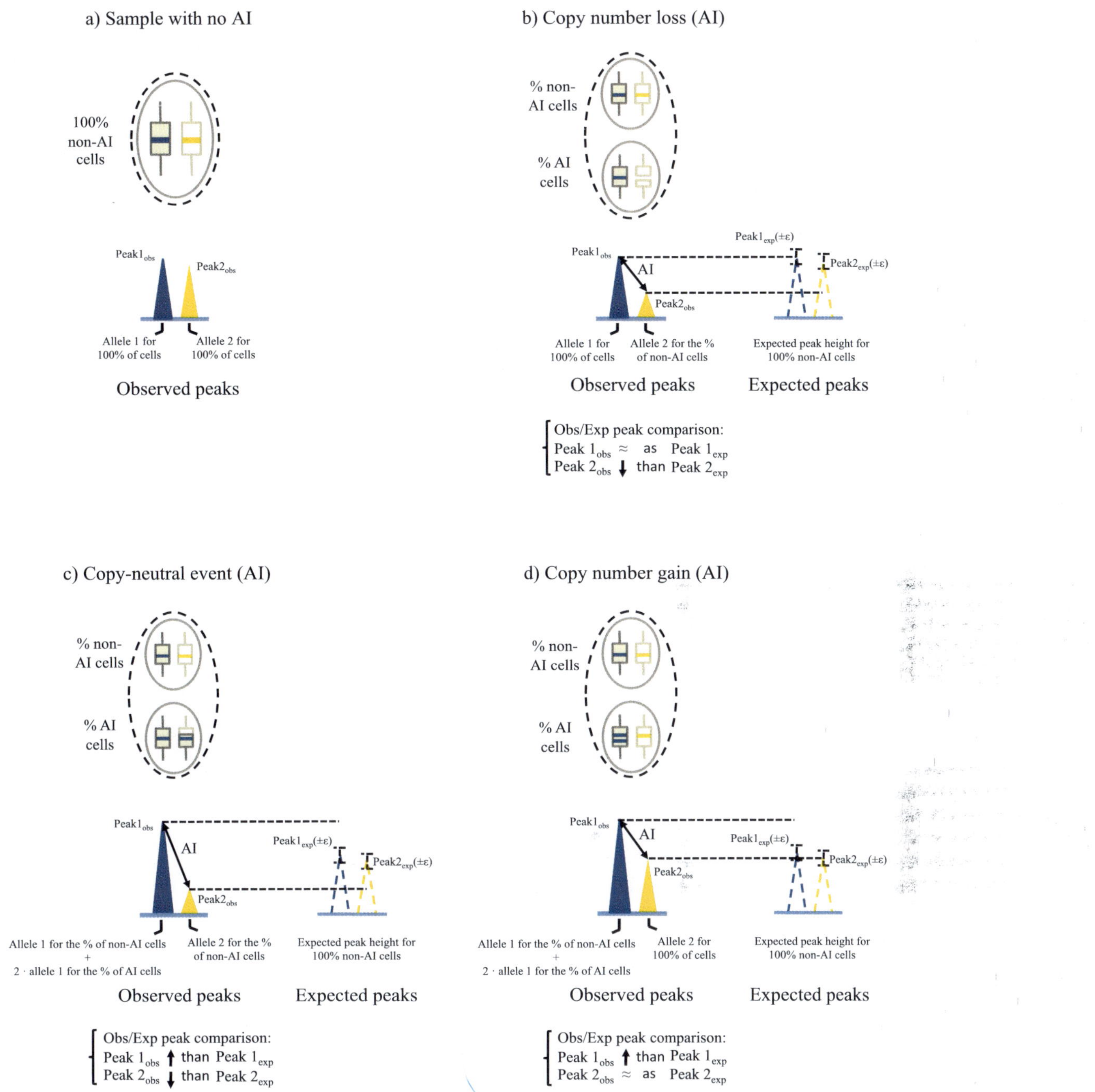

Figure 2. $Peak_{obs}$ vs. $peak_{exp}$ comparison for 1 heterozygous microsatellite in the analysis of AIs generated by different mutational mechanisms. Dashed line circles represent sample tissues (normal or tumor) and solid line circles represent types of genetically distinct cells within tissues. Blue and orange solid lines within chromosome-representing boxes indicate alleles of a heterozygous microsatellite marker. Solid color peaks represent allele peak heights obtained from microsatellite electropherograms after a theoretical MMPA. Dashed color peaks indicate expected peak heights in the case that 100% of the cells were non-AI, with the interval of peak height values indicated. Underneath allele peaks there is a short explanation of the source of peak height intensities regarding the number of amplified alleles according to the percentage of AI and non-AI cells. The Obs/Exp peak comparisons are also shown for the different mechanisms: a) Sample with no AI; b) Tumor sample with AI due to a copy-number loss; c) Tumor sample with AI due to a copy-neutral event; d) Tumor sample with AI due to a copy-number gain. Note that identical AI values for a given microsatellite in examples b and c will reflect distinct percentages of AI-cells within tumor samples.

Applying MMPA analysis to determine the *NF1* locus status in neurofibromas

Our group previously characterized a large set of neurofibromas for the presence/absence of AI in the *NF1* region by applying microsatellite analysis [13]. In the same study, the copy-number status of the same region was determined by either MLPA, PRA or SNP-array analysis [13]. After developing the MMPA calculations presented here, we re-analyzed a set of 29 dermal neurofibromas with the newly established microsatellite multiplex PCR conditions and obtained data regarding the percentage of non-AI cells within

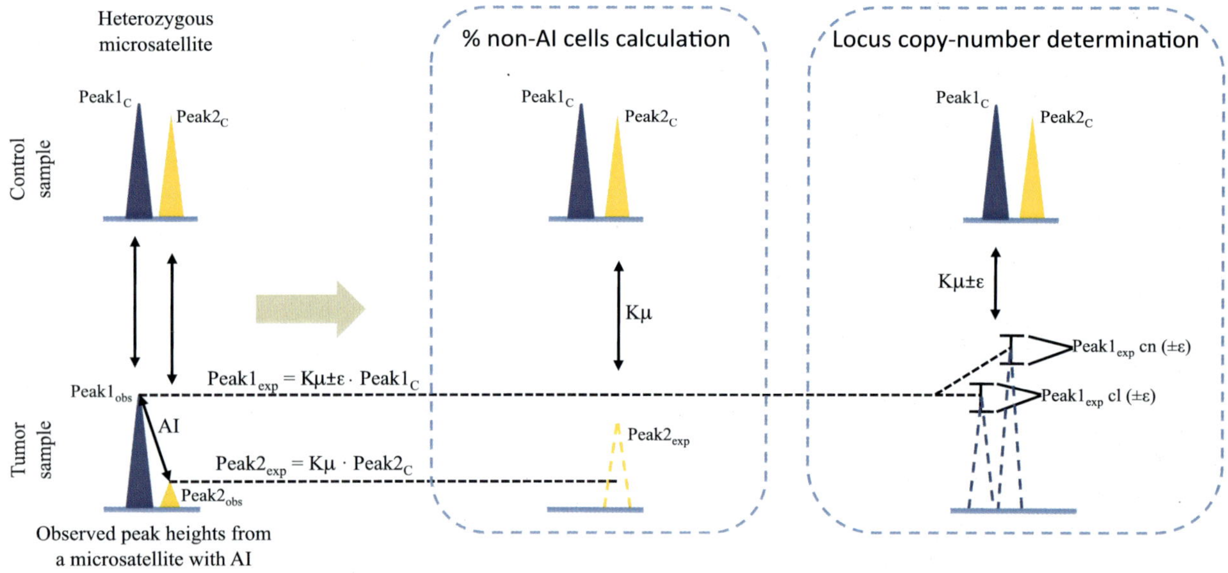

Figure 3. Calculating the percentage of non-AI cells and the locus copy-number of AI-cells from markers with allelic imbalance caused by copy-loss or copy-neutral events. Schematic view of the different use of both microsatellite alleles comparing observed vs. expected allele peak heights, concerning the calculation of the percentage of non-AI cells and the locus copy-number determination. Solid color peaks represent allele peak heights obtained from microsatellite electropherograms after a theoretical MMPA. Dashed color peaks indicate expected peak heights in the case 100% of the cells were non-AI. cl, copy-loss; cn, copy-neutral.

these tumors and the *NF1* locus copy-number. We compared the new MMPA generated data with that previously obtained in [13] for these 29 neurofibromas (Tables 1 and 2).

In 26 out of 29 neurofibromas MMPA calculations correctly determined locus copy-number and AI-mechanism, considering all informative microsatellites (Table 1). In addition, AI-mechanism was correctly determined in all neurofibromas, considering that they had at least 3 informative AI-microsatellites (27/29), and taking into account a correct result when at least 60% of all informative microsatellites were indicating the correct mechanism (Table 1). Overall 144 microsatellites showing AI were identified in these 29 neurofibromas: AI-mechanism was correctly determined after MMPA in 116 (80.5%); 25 (17.4%) were out of range (OOR) meaning that the $peak_{obs}$ value was not fitting within any of the expected intervals; and only 3 (2.1%) were incorrectly determined (Table 1). We included samples P009-1N and P102-4N (marked with an * in Table 1) in the analysis. These tumor samples contained high percentages of non-AI cells, making copy-number analysis impossible by MLPA, as shown in Garcia-Linares et al. (2011). However, they were considered to bear a deletion in the *NF1* locus, based in the similarity with other tumor samples bearing the same localized AI (only affecting the *NF1* gene and surrounding regions). MMPA calculations in these samples determined a deletion, supporting that this might be the actual mechanism generating AIs in these tumors. Copy-number ascertainment by MMPA calculations was possible due to the higher sensitivity of this technique when dealing with tumors containing high percentages of non-AI cells (Figure S5 and S8). Regarding the presence of normal cells within tumors, we calculated the percentage of AI/non-AI cells for 9 neurofibromas using previously generated SNP-array data [13] by applying the GPHMM algorithm [16]. We compared these data with the percentages obtained for the same tumors by applying MMPA calculations (Table 2). The results showed a good agreement between both techniques since, for all tumor samples but one, the calculated percentages of non-AI cells present in neurofibromas did not differ more than 8%.

In order to facilitate the calculations of the MMPA assay, we developed an automated analysis script that outputs the different parameters of an MMPA reaction together with the different calculations explained above (see Material and Methods; Script S1). This script is also freely downloadable at http://www.imppc.org/research-activities/genetic-variation-and-cancer/mmpa.html and can be easily customized to any MMPA design.

Discussion

In this study we present a set of simple calculations (MMPA) applied to a microsatellite multiplex PCR to gain information on the percentage of normal cells present in a tumor, the copy-number status of specific alleles of heterozygous loci showing AI and the mechanisms that generate these AIs. Previously, to obtain the same type of tumor genetic information, the use of microsatellite PCR had to be complemented with additional techniques. A global view of this new approach is summarized in Figure S7.

All information that can be obtained by applying an MMPA is based on the use of a constant of proportionality (Kμ) between a multiplex PCR reaction of a tumor DNA and its matching control pair. Thus, one of the key factors when using MMPA calculations is to design and set up a robust multiplex reaction controlling all aspects that affect Kμ to minimize variation in its value and in that way minimize the errors in the estimation of expected peak heights (see supplementary information). DNA quality is also an important aspect for the correct performance of MMPA, as it could affect DNA amplification and increase Kμ dispersion. Bad quality DNA can make MMPA calculations impossible. In addition, it is important to precisely quantify and always analyze the same amount of DNA for all samples. K values from microsatellites with no AI considerably different from 1 could indicate genetic alterations causing copy-number gains or losses without generating

Table 1. MMPA validation of the NF1 locus copy-number.

	MMPA calculations (present work)			Garcia-Linares et al. 2011		
Tumor samples	MMPA copy-number determination	Correct microsatellite determination/Total microsatellites with AI	Non determined microsatellites	(Copy-number assessment)		
				MLPA	PRA	SNP-array
P001-1N	Two copies	6/7	1 OOR	Two copies		
P009-1N	One copy	4/4		*		
P011-16N	Two copies	4/5	1 OOR	Two copies		Two copies
P022-19N	Two copies	3/5	2 OOR	Two copies		
P022-21N	Two copies	1/6	5 OOR	Two copies		
P023-14N	Two copies	6/8	2 OOR		Two copies	Two copies
P023-6N	One copy	3/4	1 RH	One copy	One copy	One copy
P023-97N	One copy	3/5	2 OOR	One copy	One copy	One copy
P030-2N	Two copies	4/5	1 OOR	Two copies		
P039-1N	One copy	4/4		One copy		One copy
P047-1N	Two copies	4/5	1 OOR	Two copies		
P054-1N	Two copies	6/6			Two copies	
P062-11N	One copy	2/2		One copy		
P079-1N	One copy	3/3		One copy		One copy
P081-1N	One copy	5/5		One copy		
P082-6N	One copy	5/5			One copy	One copy
P090-3N	One copy	3/3		One copy		One copy
P095-1N	One copy	2/3	1 OOR	One copy		One copy
P102-3N	One copy	4/5	1 OOR	One copy		
P102-4N	One copy	1/2	1 OOR	*		
P102-5N	Two copies	8/9	1 OOR	Two copies		
P102-18N	Two copies	9/9		Two copies	Two copies	Two copies
P103-5N	Two copies	5/5		Two copies	Two copies	Two copies
P103-21N	Two copies	4/6	2 OOR	Two copies		Two copies
P109-1N	Two copies	4/5	1 Del	Two copies		
P109-5N	Two copies	3/5	1 OOR, 1 Del	Two copies		
P109-6N	Two copies	4/4				Two copies
P109-7N	Two copies	3/4	1 OOR	Two copies		
P112-4N	Two copies	3/5	2 OOR	Two copies		

*see text for details.
Analysis of the copy number status of the *NF1* locus in 29 neurofibromas using newly developed MMPA calculations and comparison with previous data obtained for the same tumors using MLPA, PRA and SNP-array techniques (13).

allelic imbalances, as happens in cases where the two copies of a given locus were lost (e.g. nullosomy) or gained (e.g. tetrasomy).

Since $K\mu$ is calculated from control microsatellites, it is desirable to have at least three informative control microsatellites in the MMPA. Previous knowledge about the degree of genetic instability and the recurrence of altered and non-altered genomic regions would facilitate the inclusion of pre-established control markers in the MMPA design. This should not be a problem when analyzing specific genomic regions in tumors with a low or intermediate degree of recurrent copy-number alterations. However, in tumors with a highly altered genome, it will not be possible to determine upfront which markers could be used as control microsatellites, and only after doing MMPA calculations could those not exhibiting AI (and Ks close to 1) be used as control markers.

In addition, during the MMPA analysis, special care should be paid to heterozygous dinucleotide microsatellites when both alleles only differ in one repeat (2 bp). In these cases, the slippage of the DNA polymerase during PCR amplification can hamper the correct analysis of peak height values of smaller alleles, thus affecting the calculations of copy-number and percentage of AI-cells in markers showing AI. In the MMPA setup presented here, we decided not to use heterozygous microsatellite markers with a difference in length of only 2 bp for the MMPA calculations. However in the case that these microsatellites were required, a correction on the peak height values of the smaller alleles could be applied [10].

The interpretation of the information produced by an MMPA is based on a simple model in which tumors are composed of two cell populations: normal 2n cells and cells containing allelic imbalanc-

generated by multiple differential amplifications will show both observed allele peak heights higher than their expected peak heights. In both scenarios there is no observed peak height lower than expected. (**b**) Determination of allele locus copy-number for the two scenarios described. Only allele peak heights higher than expected will be used (Peak 1_{obs} in copy-gain and Peak 1_{obs} or Peak 2_{obs} for multiple amplification). In these cases, observed peak height values will fall inside the interval of expected peak height values [$Peak_{exp}$ cg ($\pm\varepsilon$)] obtained by using the actual number of copies of the locus, represented by the variable X. The percentage of AI/non-AI cells used for these calculations will need to be obtained from a different microsatellite marker showing AI generated by either copy-loss or copy-neutral events.

Figure S7 MMPA Workflow.

Figure S8 We performed an assay to determine the limit on the percentage of 2n cells present within tumor samples at which MMPA calculations are still reliable for the analysis of control/tumor pairs. The example illustrates the case of an AI caused by a copy-loss. To reproduce this situation two different DNA samples were mixed at different proportions. One DNA was from a normal individual and the other was from his son with Neurofibromatosis type 1 caused by a deletion of the *NF1* gene (maternal origin) and adjacent regions (already characterized and published elsewhere). For all microsatellites located within the deleted region the son was missing the maternal allele and only the remaining paternal allele was present. DNAs were mixed raging from proportions of 0% father's DNA-100% son's DNA, to exactly the opposite (100% father's DNA-0% son's DNA), in steps of 10% increasing proportions of father's DNA. Alleles from heterozygous markers, outside the deleted region and shared by both father and son, were used as controls since, independently of the DNA admixture, they were always present in a 100% proportion (Figure S8c). To reproduce the presence of normal cells within tumors, heterozygous paternal alleles not present in the son and mapping within the deleted region were quantified (see boxed alleles in Figure S8c). A control sample with 100% father's DNA was independently paired with each of the different DNA admixtures. Kμ and the different calculations were generated for each pair of samples. The real percentages of DNA admixtures were compared to the calculated percentages obtained by applying MMPA. Copy number analysis and the mechanism generating AI was also determined. a) Results (in triplicate) of the % of non-AI cells and the mechanism generating AI obtained by applying an MMPA to the different DNA admixtures. MMPA technique was able to calculate the percentage of non-AI cells present in the DNA admixtures up to 70–80% while still detecting the presence of a deletion (see also Figures S4 and S5). b) Regression analysis indicating a good correlation between the real percentages of non-AI cells present in the DNA admixtures and the percentages calculated by applying MMPA. Blue dots represent the percentage of non-AI cells calculated using MMPA of each replica vs. the real percentage of non-AI cells. c) Examples of the electropherograms obtained for control and AI microsatellites for the different DNA admixtures.

Table S1 Combination of primers used in the Microsatellite Multiplex PCR Assay exemplified in this work.

Script S1 Semi-automated analysis of MMPA results. In order to facilitate the calculations of the MMPA assay, we developed an automated analysis script that outputs the different parameters of an MMPA reaction together with the different calculations. Script S1 contains files required to perform the MMPA analysis and a short Script guide.

Acknowledgments

The authors would like to thank Miquel Àngel Peinado, Sergio Alonso, Anna Díez and other people from IMPPC for their comments and suggestions on the presented work, and Harvey Evans for corrections on the manuscript. We also thank the support of Elisabeth Castellanos, Imma Rosas, Juani Fernández, Gabriel Capellá and Ignacio Blanco and the continuous support and encouragement of the Spanish association of Patients with Neurofibromatosis (Asociación de Afectados de Neurofibromatosis) and the Asociación Española Contra el Cáncer (AECC).

Author Contributions

Conceived and designed the experiments: CGL ES. Performed the experiments: CGL JM BG JB ET. Analyzed the data: CGL JM BG ES. Contributed reagents/materials/analysis tools: CGL JM BG CL ES. Wrote the paper: CGL ES.

References

1. Beroukhim R, Mermel CH, Porter D, Wei G, Raychaudhuri S, et al. (2010) The landscape of somatic copy-number alteration across human cancers. Nature 463: 899–905.
2. Brandt B, Vogt U, Harms F, Bosse U, Zanker KS, et al. (1995) Double-differential PCR for gene dosage estimation of erbB oncogenes in benign and cancer tissues and comparison to cellular DNA content. Gene 159: 29–34.
3. Bieche I, Olivi M, Champeme MH, Vidaud D, Lidereau R, et al. (1998) Novel approach to quantitative polymerase chain reaction using real-time detection: application to the detection of gene amplification in breast cancer. Int J Cancer 78: 661–666.
4. Postma C, Hermsen MA, Coffa J, Baak JP, Mueller JD, et al. (2005) Chromosomal instability in flat adenomas and carcinomas of the colon. J Pathol 205: 514–521.
5. Kumps C, Van Roy N, Heyrman L, Goossens D, Del-Favero J, et al. (2010) Multiplex Amplicon Quantification (MAQ), a fast and efficient method for the simultaneous detection of copy number alterations in neuroblastoma. BMC Genomics 11: 298.
6. Pinkel D, Segraves R, Sudar D, Clark S, Poole I, et al. (1998) High resolution analysis of DNA copy number variation using comparative genomic hybridization to microarrays. Nat Genet 20: 207–211.
7. Serra E, Rosenbaum T, Nadal M, Winner U, Ars E, et al. (2001) Mitotic recombination effects homozygosity for NF1 germline mutations in neurofibromas. Nat Genet 28: 294–296.
8. Cawkwell L, Lewis FA, Quirke P (1994) Frequency of allele loss of DCC, p53, RBI, WT1, NF1, NM23 and APC/MCC in colorectal cancer assayed by fluorescent multiplex polymerase chain reaction. Br J Cancer 70: 813–818.
9. Dworkin AM, Ridd K, Bautista D, Allain DC, Iwenofu OH, et al. (2010) Germline variation controls the architecture of somatic alterations in tumors. PLoS Genet 6.
10. Skotheim RI, Diep CB, Kraggerud SM, Jakobsen KS, Lothe RA (2001) Evaluation of loss of heterozygosity/allelic imbalance scoring in tumor DNA. Cancer Genet Cytogenet 127: 64–70.
11. Slebos RJ, Umbach DM, Sommer CA, Horner GA, Choi JY, et al. (2004) Analytical and statistical methods to evaluate microsatellite allelic imbalance in small amounts of DNA. Lab Invest 84: 649–657.
12. Goransson H, Edlund K, Rydaker M, Rasmussen M, Winquist J, et al. (2009) Quantification of normal cell fraction and copy number neutral LOH in clinical lung cancer samples using SNP array data. PLoS One 4: e6057.
13. Garcia-Linares C, Fernandez-Rodriguez J, Terribas E, Mercade J, Pros E, et al. (2011) Dissecting loss of heterozygosity (LOH) in neurofibromatosis type 1-associated neurofibromas: Importance of copy neutral LOH. Hum Mutat 32: 78–90.
14. Hahn M, Matzen SE, Serth J, Pingoud A (1995) Semiautomated quantitative detection of loss of heterozygosity in the tumor suppressor gene p53. Biotechniques 18: 1040–1047.
15. Solomon E, Voss R, Hall V, Bodmer WF, Jass JR, et al. (1987) Chromosome 5 allele loss in human colorectal carcinomas. Nature 328: 616–619.

10

High-Content Chemical and RNAi Screens for Suppressors of Neurotoxicity in a Huntington's Disease Model

Joost Schulte[1]*, Katharine J. Sepp[1], Chaohong Wu[2], Pengyu Hong[2], J. Troy Littleton[1]

1 Department of Biology, Department of Brain and Cognitive Sciences, The Picower Institute for Learning and Memory, Massachusetts Institute of Technology, Cambridge, Massachusetts, United States of America, **2** Department of Computer Science, National Center for Behavioral Genomics, Brandeis University, Waltham, Massachusetts, United States of America

Abstract

To identify Huntington's Disease therapeutics, we conducted high-content small molecule and RNAi suppressor screens using a *Drosophila* primary neural culture Huntingtin model. *Drosophila* primary neurons offer a sensitive readout for neurotoxicty, as their neurites develop dysmorphic features in the presence of mutant polyglutamine-expanded Huntingtin compared to nonpathogenic Huntingtin. By tracking the subcellular distribution of mRFP-tagged pathogenic Huntingtin and assaying neurite branch morphology via live-imaging, we identified suppressors that could reduce Huntingtin aggregation and/or prevent the formation of dystrophic neurites. The custom algorithms we used to quantify neurite morphologies in complex cultures provide a useful tool for future high-content screening approaches focused on neurodegenerative disease models. Compounds previously found to be effective aggregation inhibitors in mammalian systems were also effective in *Drosophila* primary cultures, suggesting translational capacity between these models. However, we did not observe a direct correlation between the ability of a compound or gene knockdown to suppress aggregate formation and its ability to rescue dysmorphic neurites. Only a subset of aggregation inhibitors could revert dysmorphic cellular profiles. We identified *lkb1*, an upstream kinase in the mTOR/Insulin pathway, and four novel drugs, Camptothecin, OH-Camptothecin, 18β-Glycyrrhetinic acid, and Carbenoxolone, that were strong suppressors of mutant Huntingtin-induced neurotoxicity. Huntingtin neurotoxicity suppressors identified through our screen also restored viability in an *in vivo Drosophila* Huntington's Disease model, making them attractive candidates for further therapeutic evaluation.

Editor: Mark R. Cookson, National Institutes of Health, United States of America

Funding: This work was supported by NIH grants to JTL and R01 EB007042 to PH. The funders had no role in study design, data collection and analysis, decision to publish, or preparation of the manuscript.

Competing Interests: JS, KJS, and JTL are listed as authors on a provisional U.S. patent application (61419157) filed by the Massachusetts Institute of Technology on 02-DEC-2010. This does not alter the authors' adherence to all the PLoS ONE policies on sharing data and materials.

* E-mail: jschulte@mit.edu

Introduction

Huntington's Disease (HD) is a dominantly inherited fatal neurodegenerative disorder. It results from expansion of a polygluatamine (polyQ) tract in the Huntingtin (Htt) protein which alters its conformation and function [1]. Neuropathological hallmarks of the disease include Htt aggregation, early-onset striatal neurodegeneration, and late-stage cortical thinning [2,3]. Mammalian models of HD indicate that neuron-specific dysregulation of cellular physiology contributes to the underlying neuropathology, although subcortical white matter degeneration may also suggest a glial contribution [4–7]. Mutant Htt has been suggested to disrupt transcription, proteasome activity, axonal transport, synaptic function, signaling cascades (including the mTOR/Insulin pathway) and other physiological processes in a variety of neuronal subtypes [8].

PolyQ tract length accounts for approximately 70% of the variance in the age-of-onset of Huntington's disease [9], with the remaining variance attributed to disease-modifying agents such as environmental factors or genetic background. Linkage analysis using large affected families is the gold standard for identifying disease modifying loci [10]. However, these investigations require lengthy study periods and considerable resources. *In vitro* genetic or chemical suppressor screens offer another avenue to rapidly identify suppressors. The suitability of cell-based screening models encompasses several considerations. Htt is ubiquitously expressed, yet deleterious effects of mutant polyQ expansion are observed primarily in the central nervous system of HD patients. In conducting suppressor screens, it is therefore desirable to use neuronal systems. Stable neuronal cell lines can change their characteristics over continued passages, and thus may not retain HD phenotypes. In addition, stable cell lines continually divide, which may alter regulation of cell survival and death pathways that are relevant to the human disease state in quiescent neurons. Primary neuronal disease models have many advantages, since cellular growth and differentiation states are more similar to the *in vivo* situation, yet they are amenable to high-throughput chemical and genetic suppressor screens.

Huntingtin is conserved in *Drosophila*, and orthologs of many interacting proteins exist [11–13]. Suppressor screening with first generation exon 1 Htt fragments has generated important candidate disease modifying agents [14,15]. However, protein

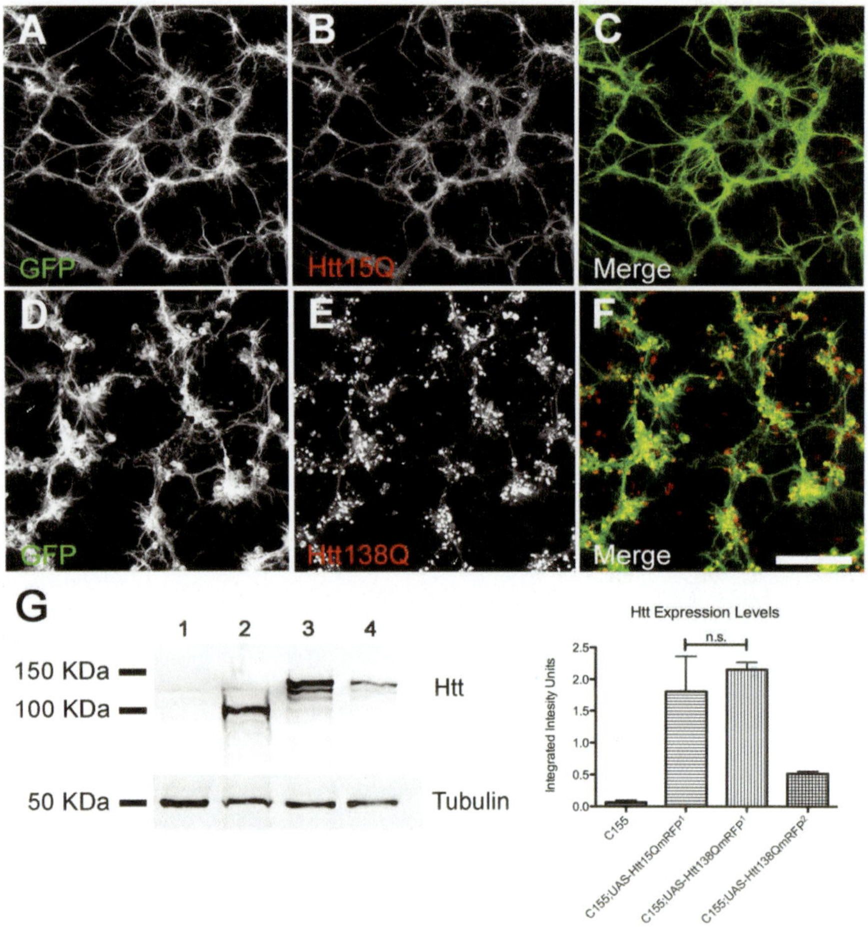

Figure 1. Confocal microscopy images of Htt15Q (A–C) and Htt138Q (D–F) expressing *Drosophila* primary neural cultures plated on glass coverslips. The subcellular distribution of Htt (red channel), morphology of Htt expressing primary cultures (green channel, UAS-CD8GFP), and merged images are shown. Htt15Q (**B**) has a diffuse cytoplasmic distribution and fills most processes of cultured neurons, while Htt138Q forms large insoluble aggregates that accumulate in neurites and within cell bodies of neuromere clusters (**E**). Htt15Q and Htt138Q expressing cultures also display different neuronal morphologies. Htt15Q cultures have long straight neurites (**A**), while Htt138Q cultures have shorter neurites that fail to extend from neuromere clusters leading to a club-like appearance (**B**). (**G**) Quantitative Western blot (n = 4) showing that the relative expression level of Htt15Q[1] and Htt138Q[1] is comparable in strains used for primary culture screening (compare lanes 2 and 3). A Htt138Q strain with weaker expression is also shown (lane 4, Htt138Q[2]). The strain genotypes that are listed on the bar graph (left to right) correspond to lanes 1–4 of the blot. Tubulin was used as a loading control. $p<0.05$. Scale bar: 100 µm.

context has been shown to be an important component of mutant Htt pathogenesis, and therefore there is a need to conduct additional screens using larger Htt constructs in more physiologically relevant systems [16]. To this end, we have developed a *Drosophila* primary neural culture system for HD, using a large human Htt fragment (exons 1–12, 588 amino acids in addition to the polyQ tract). The methodology is suited to high throughput small molecule and RNAi suppressor screening, and offers a desirable balance between physiological relevance and technical tractability.

We demonstrate that a 588 amino acid human Htt fragment containing an expanded polyQ tract (138Q) readily forms cytoplasmic aggregates in primary neurons, in addition to causing aberrant neuronal morphology when compared to non-expanded human Htt controls (15Q). From a screen of approximately 2600 small molecules and a whole genome kinase/phosphatase RNAi library, we identified four new compounds that could revert the mutant phenotype (Camptothecin, 10-Hydroxycamptothecin, 18β-Glycyrrhetinic acid, Carbenoxolone) and knockdown of the *lkb1* kinase, that can suppress polyQ Htt aggregation and revert morphological profiles towards control states. In addition, we identified several previously studied polyQ Htt aggregation inhibitors. This *Drosophila* HD model represents an attractive system for future large-scale suppressor screening. In addition, the current candidates provide new avenues to define pathogenic mechanisms in HD.

Results

Drosophila Primary Neural Culture Screening System for Huntington's Disease

We have previously described a *Drosophila* Huntington's Disease model which displays many characteristics of human HD, including neurodegeneration, disrupted axonal transport, and decreased longevity [17]. To extend our studies of HD pathology, we generated a new monomeric Red Fluorescent Protein (mRFP) N-terminal tag variant for *in vivo* imaging of Htt distribution (Htt-RFP). The Htt-RFP construct encompasses the caspase-6 cleavage fragment important for Htt toxicity [18] and includes either a non-pathogenic (15Q) or pathogenic (138Q) polyQ tract. This fragment corresponds to exons 1–12 of human Htt and is 588 amino acids in length (~80 kDa), excluding the polyQ domain and RFP tag. For our studies, we used the GAL4/UAS system [19] to drive expression of the constructs in the nervous system using the pan-neuronal GAL4 driver *Elav*^{c155} (*C155*). We selected *UAS-Htt15QmRFP* and *UAS-Htt138QmRFP* strains that had comparable expression levels (i.e. Htt15Q^1 and Htt138Q^1) when crossed to *C155* as demonstrated by quantitative Western blotting (Figure 1G). Prominent bands of ~109 kDa and ~125 kDa were observed for the Htt15Q^1 and Htt138Q^1 strains, respectively, in agreement with the predicted molecular weights of the RFP-fusion proteins. Pan-neuronal expression of *Htt138Q*^{1} using C155 causes pupal lethality, while *Htt15Q*^{1} controls are viable and have normal longevity (see detailed analysis below). For downstream behavioral analysis, we selected an additional UAS-Htt138QmRFP strain (Htt138Q^2) that has reduced Htt138Q protein expression (Figure 1G) and is adult viable. The decreased longevity observed in the *Htt138Q*^{1} strain is more severe than that observed in our earlier studies [17] and may be related to an increased polyQ length in the new construct (138Q vs. 128Q), a larger Htt N-terminal fragment (588 a.a. vs. 548 a.a.), or differences in Htt expression levels. The severity of the *Htt138Q*^{1} allele suggests that this model may correspond to juvenile-onset HD observed in humans [20]. In juvenille-onset HD, the CAG repeats often exceed 55 and phenotypes develop prior to adulthood.

To conduct a small molecule and RNAi screen to identify suppressors of Huntington toxicity we prepared primary neuronal cultures from control (*C155;Htt15QmRFP*^{1}, abbreviated as *Htt15Q*) and mutant (*C155;UAS-Htt138QmRFP*^{1}, abbreviated as *Htt138Q*) Huntingtin strains that simultaneously expressed membrane associated-GFP (*UAS-CD8GFP*) in all neurons. This dual labeling approach enabled us to track the subcellular distribution of mRFP-tagged Huntingtin, while simultaneously monitoring the general morphology of cultured neurons (Fig. 1 A–F). Visualization of Htt-RFP localization demonstrated that Htt138Q readily forms aggregates which accumulate in cell bodies and neurites, while Htt15Q is soluble and has a more uniform cytoplasmic distribution (Fig. 1, compare 1B, 1E). In addition, we found that Htt138Q-expressing neurons display morphological indicators of reduced neuronal health [21,22], including smaller neuromeres, increased branching, and reduced axonal connectivity, as monitored by membrane associated-GFP (Fig. 1, compare 1A, 1D). Neurite morphology and Htt aggregation were quantified in cultures plated in 384-well format using custom algorithms developed to process digital images collected via automated microscopy [23]. Population analysis of Htt15Q and Htt138Q replicate wells revealed that eight morphology features (small, medium, large, and average neuromere size, and short, medium, long, and average neurite length) provided robust data content to generate effective separation of Htt15Q control from Htt138Q mutant neuronal morphology. Differences in Htt aggregation were also readily detectable between mutant and control cultures using these algorithms. To screen for suppressors of HD toxicity we therefore monitored the presence of Htt aggregates, as well as morphology, to evaluate overall neuron health.

Small Molecule/RNAi Suppressor Screens Using HD Primary Cultures

We performed dual RNAi and small molecule screens to identify HD toxicity suppressors, and assayed for suppression of Htt138Q aggregate formation, in addition to reversion of mutant Htt138Q morphology towards Htt15Q controls. For RNAi screening, we wanted to identify novel targets for HD therapeutic development, and focused on a kinase/phosphatase RNAi library (468 genes) that would potentially contain targets of high value for chemical inhibition. For small-molecule screening, we tested libraries enriched for FDA-approved drugs, including the NINDS Custom Collection 2, BIOMOL ICCB Known Bioactives Collection and the Prestwick 1 Collection. This allowed screening of ≈2600 approved compounds, potentially facilitating the advancement of screen hits to clinical trials. For compound screening, we verified that addition of 0.2% DMSO to primary cultures does not significantly alter neuronal morphology or Htt138Q aggregation characteristics (Table 1). Known suppressors of Htt polyQ aggregation, including *C2-8*, *GW5074*, *Juglone*, *Radicicol*, and *Rapamycin*, were tested for efficacy in our assay [24–28]. Although all control compounds reduced Htt138Q aggregation, none reverted the morphology profiles of Htt138Q expressing neurons towards Htt15Q controls (Table 1). Instead, these compounds caused reduced axon outgrowth, neuromere size, and suppressed GFP expression over a wide concentration range, suggesting these compounds have neurotoxic properties.

To identify new potential therapeutic compounds that were not neurotoxic, but that were able to suppress mutant Htt toxicity in our model, we conducted RNAi/compound screens in duplicate. All wells were visually scored independently by two investigators to identify agents that either suppressed aggregation, or reverted mutant Htt138Q neural profiles towards Htt15Q controls. From the visual-based screens, three novel suppressors of Htt polyQ toxicity were identified: 1 RNAi hit (*lkb1*), and 2 compounds (Camptothecin and 10-Hydroxycamptothecin). Lkb1 is a known tumor suppressor and a negative regulator of the mTOR/Insulin pathway, which has important roles in autophagy and nutrient sensing [29,30], while the Camptothecins function as DNA Topoisomerase 1 (*Top1*) inhibitors [31]. In addition to visual inspection of the screen plates, automated microscopy was used to record images of the compound-treated plates for subsequent morphometric analysis using custom algorithms. For automated microscopy, three images per well were taken at different sites for each channel (GFP/RFP) to facilitate hit identification and increase statistical power. Htt138Q aggregation was first quantified, leading to the identification of 62 compounds that significantly suppressed Htt aggregate formation (Fig. 2, Table S1). Subsequently, wells where aggregate formation was inhibited were re-evaluated to determine if any treatments were able to revert the mutant Htt138Q morphology profiles towards that of Htt15Q controls. Of the 62 compounds that were found to inhibit Htt138Q aggregate formation, 8 compounds were identified that improved the Htt138Q induced morphological defects (Fig. 3A, Table 2). Unmasking of the identities of the 8 compounds revealed that 4 compounds were Camptothecins, in agreement with the visual scoring observations. In addition, two Na+/K+ ATPase inhibitors, and a Glutathione-S-Transferase inhibitor were also identified as being capable of suppressing aggregate formation and rescuing the mutant Htt138Q culture morphologies towards the control state (Table 2). We subsequently validated screen hits, focusing on the targets that overlapped in both the visual scoring and morphometric computational analysis. The Lkb-1 target was validated with three independent dsRNAs (amplicons DRSC16481, DRSC36925, DRSC36926). Each amplicon improved Htt138Q mutant morphology with statistical significance, but did not inhibit aggregate formation (Table 3). The Camptothecin and 10-Hydroxy-camptothecin small molecules are structural analogues, and were found to reduce aggregate formation in addition to partially reverting dystrophic morphology profiles over a range of concentrations (56 µM, 5.6 µM) (Fig. 4). These compounds alter Htt138Q localization within neurons, such that it more closely resembles the distribution of Htt15Q in control cultures (Fig. 4).

Table 1. Effect of positive control compounds on Htt138Q aggregate formation and neurite morphology (p-values listed) in *Drosophila* primary neural culture system.

Compound	CAS#	Well Conc. (mM)	Htt Culture	Mutant Htt 138Q aggregation*	Mutant Htt138Q morphology rescue**	n =
C2-8	300670-16-0	2	138Q	***0.0072745***	0	6
C2-8		0.4	138Q	0.216406	0	6
C2-8		0.08	138Q	0.0679971	0	6
C2-8		0.016	138Q	0.381982	0	6
C2-8		0.0032	138Q	0.436453	0	6
GW5074	220904-83-6	2	138Q	***0.000242646***	0	6
GW5074		0.4	138Q	0.414394	0	6
GW5074		0.08	138Q	0.859258	0	6
GW5074		0.016	138Q	0.193046	0	6
GW5074		0.0032	138Q	0.062019	2.54 E-14	6
Juglone	481-39-0	100	138Q	***0.00062262***	0.00000361	6
Juglone		20	138Q	0.999965	0	6
Juglone		4	138Q	0.999994	0	6
Juglone		0.8	138Q	0.908447	0	6
Juglone		0.16	138Q	0.640557	1.26 E-11	6
Radicicol	12772-57-5	100	138Q	***9.17E-66***	0	6
Radicicol		20	138Q	***0.0000587***	0	6
Radicicol		4	138Q	0.671473	0	6
Radicicol		0.8	138Q	***0.0313196***	0	6
Radicicol		0.16	138Q	***0.0116727***	0	6
Rapamycin	53123-88-9	4	138Q	***0.00161737***	0	6
Rapamycin		0.8	138Q	0.134587	0	6
Rapamycin		0.16	138Q	0.151829	0	6
Rapamycin		0.032	138Q	0.382367	0	6
Rapamycin		0.0064	138Q	0.290667	0	6
DMSO	67-68-5	0.2%	138Q	1	0	360
DMSO	67-68-5	0.2%	15Q	0	1	144

*p<0.05 indicates Htt138Q aggregate formation is inhibited (bold, italics).
**p>0.05 indicates Htt138Q drug-treated culture have morphology similar to Htt15Q control cultures.

Genetic and Pharmacological Validation of Screen Hits

To further examine the RNAi/small molecule screen hits, we assayed *in vivo* efficacy by testing their ability to rescue lethality in our *Drosophila* HD model. Htt138Q expression in the nervous system results in late stage pupal lethality when animals are reared on standard media. Animals undergo metamorphosis but fail to eclose. In liquid culture, the longevity of the Htt138Q expressing animals is reduced and larvae perish during the 2nd instar stage, likely due to drowning from decreased motility. Rapamycin, a well characterized mTOR inhibitor [25], suppresses neurodegeneration in various HD models, and we found it enhanced viability of Htt138Q expressing larvae reared in liquid culture in a dose-dependant fashion compared to DMSO-treated controls (Fig. 5A). Using this assay, we found that Camptothecin and 10-Hydroxycamptothecin also increased larval longevity *in vivo*, but to a lesser extent than Rapamycin (Fig. 5A). 10-Hydroxycamptothecin is more efficacious than Camptothecin, possibly due to solubility differences since Camptothecin readily precipitates when added to cultures. Specific inhibitors of Lkb1 were not available for *in vivo* testing. Given its role as an upstream regulatory kinase of the mTOR/Insulin pathway, we tested additional pharmacological agents that regulate this pathway, including Metformin (an mTOR pathway activator and oral anti-diabetic drug) [32,33] and 18β-Glycyrrhetinic acid (a putative mTOR inhibitor that acts through PI3K/AKT) [34,35]. Metformin could not revert Htt138Q-incuded lethality. However, 18β-Glycyrrhetinic acid was almost as efficacious as Rapamycin (Fig. 5A). We also tested an analogue of 18β-Glycyrrhetinic acid that has increased solubility: Carbenoxolone, and found it to have comparable activity. 18β-Glycyrrhetinic acid is non-toxic and has been used as a commercial sweetener, making it an attractive candidate for future studies for suppressive effects in mammalian HD models. Rapamycin, in contrast, has numerous toxic side-effects that can impact kidney and lung function, cause increased risk of infection, and lead to hyperlipidemia [36–40].

To further examine the role of the Lkb1/Insulin pathway in the suppression of HD toxicity, we conducted genetic interaction studies with *lkb1* loss-of-function mutations. While pan-neuronal expression of Htt138Q[1] causes pupal lethality, the introduction of a heterozygous *lkb1* null mutation into the Htt138Q background suppresses lethality. We observed no C155/+; UAS-Htt138Q/+ adult escapers at 25°C (n = 83 pupae), however, the introduction

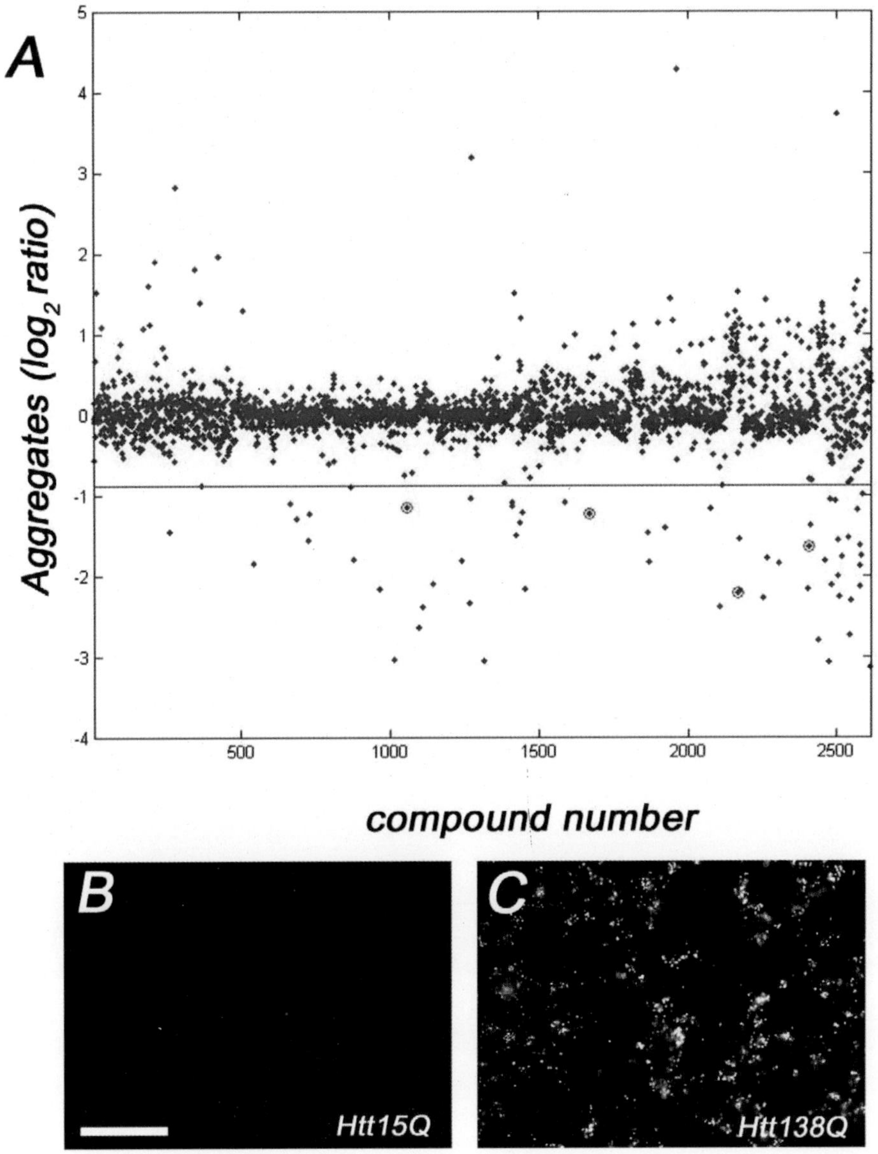

Figure 2. Htt138Q aggregation inhibition screening in primary neural cultures using custom algorithms. (**A**) Scatter plot indicating the extent of Htt138Q aggregation following treatment with ~2600 small molecules. Log_2 ratio of Htt138Q aggregates (small molecule treated well/DMSO treated well from the same screen plate) is plotted. The red line denotes two standard deviations from the mean Log_2 ratio observed in the screen data set. Circled wells correspond to compounds that suppress aggregate formation and were subsequently analyzed in downstream validation studies. (**B,C**) Representative data set images collected via automated microscopy and analyzed with algorithms. (**B**) Htt15Q control cultures have few aggregates, while mutant Htt138Q cultures (**C**) have numerous aggregates. The exposure time used for image collection was optimized for Htt aggregate detection, which has a higher signal intensity than soluble Htt. This avoided pixel saturation at the upper end of the aggregate dynamic range, ensuring accurate aggregate quantification, although soluble Htt is not readily detectable in automated microscopy images. Image analysis was performed as described in the materials and methods. Scale bar: 200 μm.

of an *Lkb1*$^{4B1-11}$/+ or *Lkb1*$^{4A4-2}$/+ allele into this background led to an adult escaper frequency of 1.8% (n = 110 pupae) and 3.7% (n = 81 pupae) respectively. Using quantitative Western blot analysis, we found that the introduction of *lkb1* trans-heterozygous alleles does not reduce Htt138Q protein levels (Fig. 5D), suggesting the suppressive effects are not tied to altering Htt expression. This is in contrast to another rescuing deficiency we identified in an independent screen, *Df(3L)vin7*, which significantly decreases Htt138Q expression and yields an escaper frequency of 25.9% (n = 85 pupae). The *Lkb1* heterozygous animals expressing Htt138Q are viable and have relatively normal walking ability, although they do not inflate their wings (Fig. 5C, Movie S1). To further investigate the relationship between *lkb1* and mutant Htt138Q toxicity, we introduced the *Lkb1*$^{4A4-2}$/+ allele into a weaker Htt138Q expressing strain (C155/+; UAS-Htt138QmRFP^2/+) which is adult viable so that we could evaluate climbing behavior as an indicator of motor performance. From negative geotaxis assays performed on 25-day old flies, we found that introduction of an *Lkb1*$^{4A4-2}$/+ mutant background enhanced performance only in the C155:Htt138Q background, but had no effect on either C155 or C155:Htt15Q control backgrounds (Fig. 5E). This suggests that the toxicity effects of

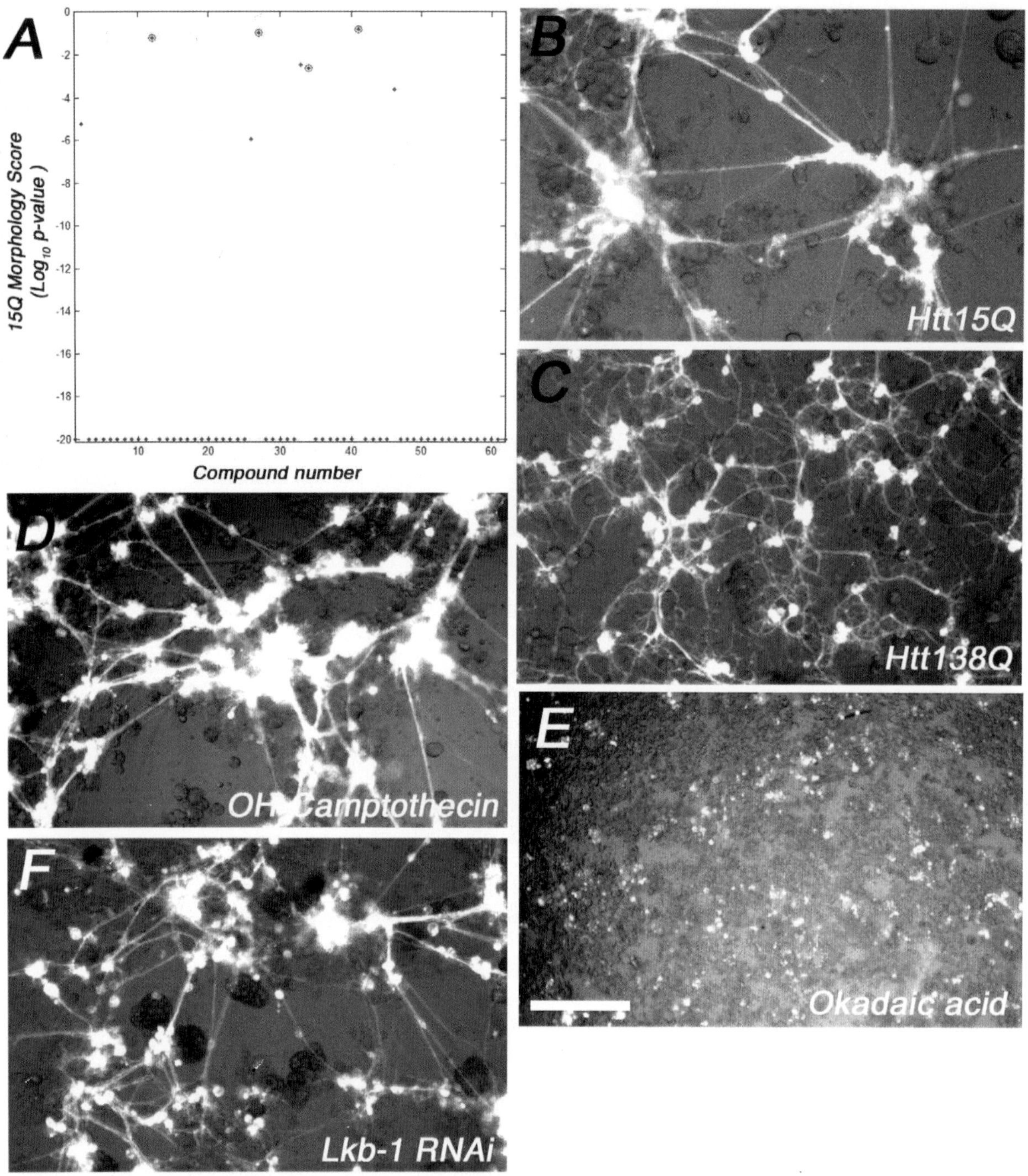

Figure 3. Morphological analysis of Htt138Q aggregation inhibitors. (**A**) P-value scatter plot illustrating the ability of a subset of Htt138Q aggregation inhibitors to revert neuronal morphology towards Htt15Q controls. Circled compounds are the Camptothecin aggregation inhibitors. For morphological analysis, neurite (short, medium, long and average neurite length) and neuromere features (small, medium, large, average neuromere area) were used to compute statistical significance. (**B–E**) Representative automated microscopy images showing the neuronal morphology profiles of *Drosophila* primary neural cultures plated on plastic, optical-bottom, 384-well plates. (**C**) Htt138Q primary neural cultures have dysmorphic neuronal profiles relative to Htt15Q controls (**B**). (**D, F**) Rescue of Htt138Q mutant morphology by treatment with 10-Hydroxy Camptothecin or Lkb-1 knockdown via RNAi. (**E**) An example of a small molecule (Okadaic acid) found to suppress Htt138Q aggregation, but which exacerbates the mutant Htt138Q mutant morphology. Scale bar: 200 μm.

Htt138Q in neurons, is associated with Lkb-1 signaling. Since RNAi knockdown, as performed in our primary culture screening assay, is representative of a hypomorphic situation, and the *in vivo* *lkb1* rescue studies we conducted were haplo-insufficient, partial knockdown screening can be advantageous to uncover therapeutic targets. Full knockdown of *lkb1* would not have revealed beneficial effects, as homozygous *lkb1* null mutants are lethal and have cell polarity defects [41].

To investigate the mechanism of action of Camptothecins in suppression of Htt138Q neurotoxicity, we performed genetic loss-

Table 2. Compounds found to inhibit mutant Htt138Q aggregation and revert primary culture morphology towards Htt15Q controls*.

I.D.	Compound	CAS#	Function	Htt Culture	Htt138Q Aggregate Log_2 ratio	Aggregate Suppression Significance** (p-value)	Morphology Statistical Significance*** (p-value)	Library	ICCB Plate I.D., Well #	Well Conc
1	**Camptothecin**	7689-03-4	topoisomerase I inhibitor, antineoplastic	138Q	−1.637238	0.00000365	0.151249	BIOMOL2	1791, N06	26 uM
2	**Camptothecin**	7689-03-4	topoisomerase I inhibitor, antineoplastic	138Q	−1.22608	0.00000927	0.109087	Prestwick	1568, H21	10 uM
3	**Camptothecin**	7689-03-4	topoisomerase I inhibitor, antineoplastic	138Q	−1.152003	0.00000000	0.06008	NINDS	1921, N08	20 uM
4	Etoposide	33419-42-0	topoisomerase II inhibitor, antineoplastic	138Q	−0.881592	0.00003212	0.003217	Prestwick	1569, O13	6.8 uM
5	**10-OH-Camptothecin**	64439-81-2	topoisomerase 1 inhibitor, antineoplastic	138Q	−2.21028	0.00000012	0.00242	BIOMOL2	1791, B06	26 uM
6	Ouabain	630-60-4	Na+/K+-ATPase inhibitor	138Q	−1.050767	0.00000268	0.000246	BIOMOL2	1792, B13	17 uM
7	Proscillaridin A	466-06-8	Na+/K+-ATPase inhibitor	138Q	−0.876806	0.00020794	0.000006	Prestwick	1571, E13	7.5 uM
8	Ethacrynic acid	58-54-8	GST inhibitor	138Q	−1.088665	0.00003454	0.000001	Prestwick	1568, D20	13.2 uM

*Compounds listed correspond to hits shown in Figure 3A. Bolded compounds are the circled hits.
**$P<0.05$ indicates that Htt138Q aggregate formation is inhibited.
***$P>0.05$ indicate mutant Htt138Q neurite morphology is reverted towards Htt15Q controls.

of-function studies with target effector proteins. Since Camptothecins function as *Top1* inhibitors, we reasoned that *Top1* RNAi knockdown in primary cultures should phenocopy Camptothecin treatment and suppress HD pathology. RNAi knockdown of *Top1* or other annotated *Drosophila Top* genes (*Top2, 3α or 3β*), either singularly or in combination, did not suppress Htt aggregation (Table 3). Knockdown of the Tops did, however, partially revert the mutant Htt138Q neurite morphology towards controls. To extend these studies *in vivo* we introduced a heterozygous *Top1* null allele into the HD model background, but this had no effect on Htt138Q-induced pupal lethality, as no adult escapers were observed. Given that Camptothecins have a robust effect on Htt138Q aggregation inhibition, while Top-knockdown does not, these results suggest that Camptothecins may act through a Top1-independent pathway to suppress Htt138Q aggregation.

The compounds that suppress Htt138Q aggregate formation, and/or rescue neurite morphology in our system, can be grouped into two classes based on their structures (Figure S1). The Camptothecins, GW5074, Radicicol, and Etoposide form one class that have partially overlapping backbone ring-

Table 3. RNAi validation. Effect of Lkb-1 or Top knockdown on Htt138Q aggregate formation and rescue of mutant culture morphology.

Gene Target	dsRNA amplicon	Off-targets	Htt Culture	Aggregate Suppression Significance (p-value)*	Morphology Statistical Significance (p-value)**	n=
LKB-1	DRSC16481	0	138Q	0.995894	0.152692	12
LKB-1	DRSC36925	0	138Q	0.730001	0.979141	12
LKB-1	DRSC36926	0	138Q	0.89236	0.702101	12
Top 1	DRSC36056	0	138Q	0.833703	0.428127	12
Top 1	DRSC20295	0	138Q	0.968551	0.015374	12
Top 2	DRSC36057	0	138Q	0.993983	0.208051	12
Top 2	DRSC03459	0	138Q	0.960684	0.35244	12
Top 3α	DRSC03460	0	138Q	0.980167	0.102255	12
Top 3α	DRSC37672	0	138Q	1	0	12
Top 3β	DRSC18724	0	138Q	0.288516	0.331471	12
Mock	N/A	N/A	138Q	1	0	12
Mock	N/A	N/A	15Q	0	1	72

*Htt Aggregates. $P<0.05$ Indicates suppression of Htt138Q aggregate formation.
**$P>0.05$ indicates mutant Htt138Q neurite morphology is reverted towards Htt15Q controls.

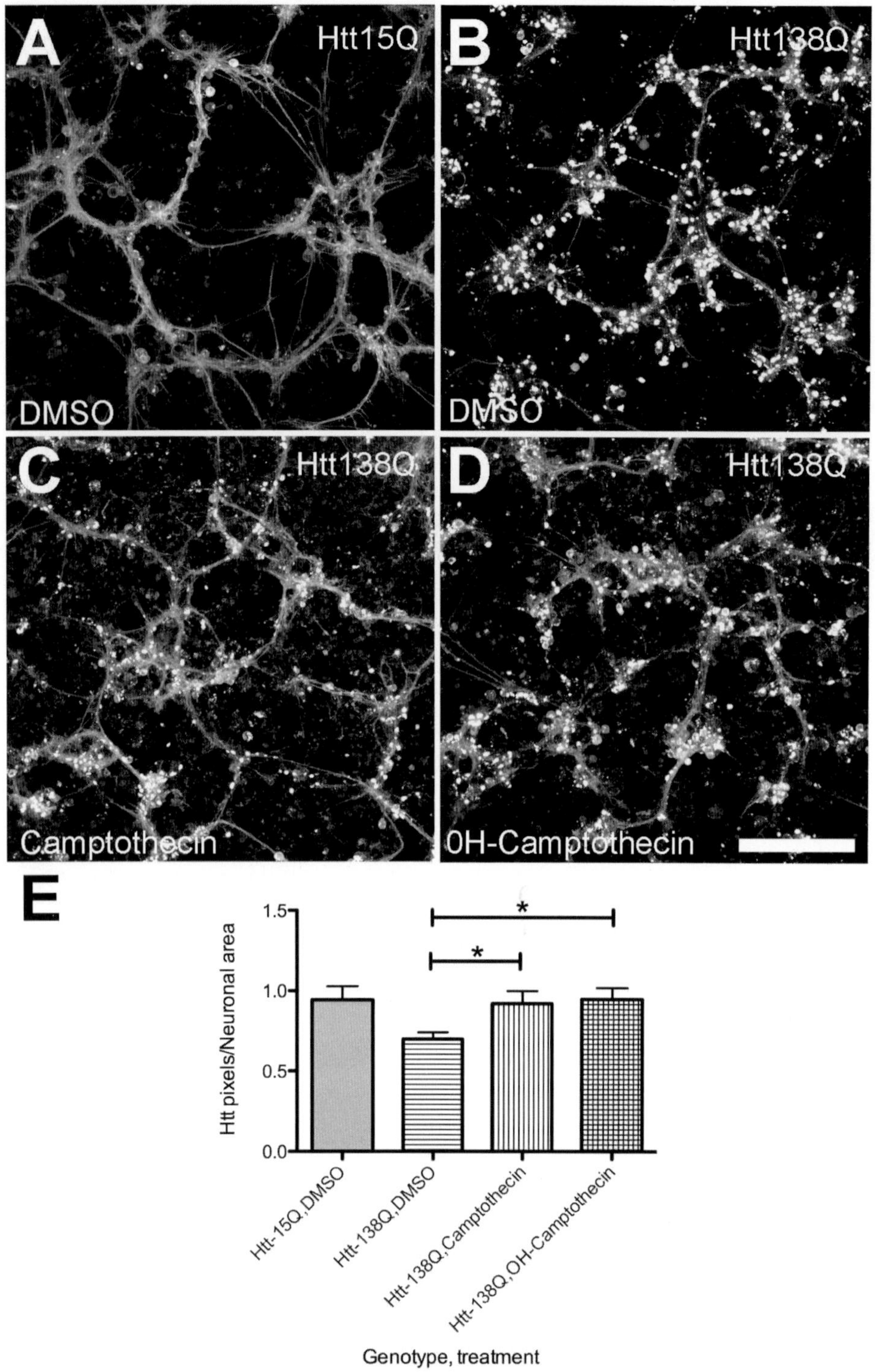

Figure 4. *In vitro* validation of small molecule screen hits. Confocal microscopy images of primary cultures plated on glass coverslips and treated with either DMSO (**A,B**) or test compounds (**C,D**). Primary neural cultures expressing Htt138Q have numerous aggregates in neurite processes and surrounding the cell bodies (**B**), while control Htt15Q expressing cultures do not (**A**). Htt15Q is soluble and fills most neurite processes. Treatment of Htt138Q expressing cultures with Camptothecin (**C**) or 10-OH-Camptothecin (**D**) at 56 μM reduces aggregate formation and increases the proportion of soluble Htt138Q which fills neurite processes. (**E**) Quantification of altered Htt138Q distribution following Camptothecin treatment. An increase in the number of Htt138Q pixels/neuronal area (Htt-RFP pixels/neuromere and neurite GFP pixels) is observed in mutant cultures, suggesting an increase in Htt138Q solubility after drug treatment. * $p<0.05$, $n=4$, Scale bar: 100 μm.

structures, while 18β-Glycyrrhetinic acid, Ouabain and Proscillaridin-A form a second class that share a similar steroid-like backbone. It will be interesting to conduct further structure-function analysis to determine a minimal architecture that is required for these compounds to rescue Htt138Q-induced pathology.

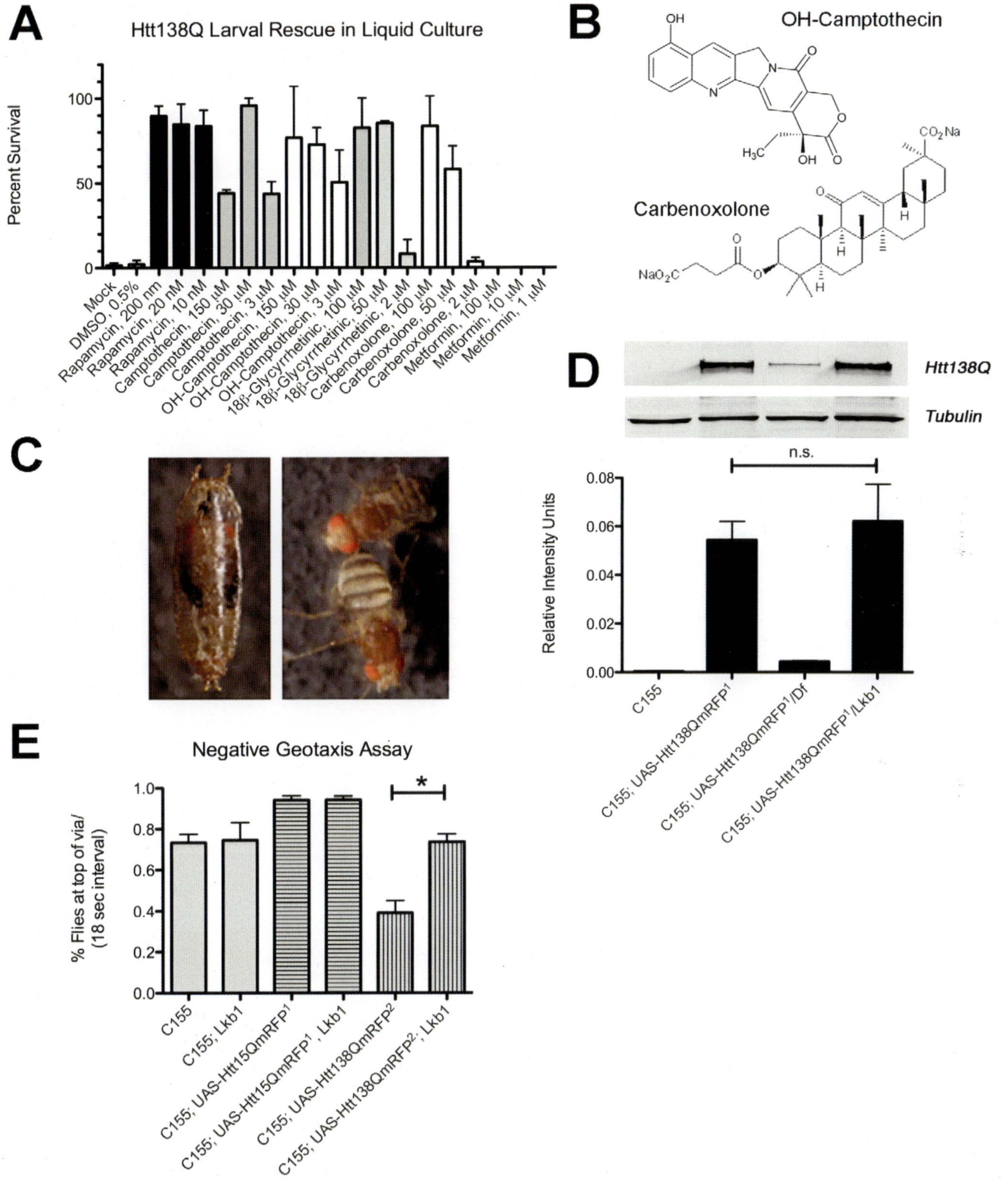

Figure 5. *In vivo* validation of screen hits. (**A**) Survival frequency scores for HD larvae (*Elav*^{c155}*-GAL4; UAS-Htt138Q*^{2}*/+*) after 5-day drug dosing in liquid culture. (**B**) Chemical structures of the Camptothecin and 18β-Glycyrrhetinic acid class of small molecules found to rescue Htt138Q toxicity *in vivo*. (**C–E**) Genetic interaction studies to assess the effect of *lkb1* kinase reduction on Htt138Q toxicity. (**C**) Pan-neuronal expression of Htt138Q^{1} causes pupal lethality (left) which can be rescued with the introduction of an *lkb1* heterozygous background. (**D**) Quantitative Western blot analysis demonstrating *lkb1*-rescued HD adults have normal Htt138Q expression levels. A control deficiency, *Df(3L)vin*, which reduces Htt138Q expression is shown for comparison. (**E**) *Lkb1* mutation rescues the climbing behavior of HD flies. 25 day-old Htt138Q flies (*C155;UAS-Htt138QmRFP*^{2}) have impaired climbing behavior as compared to controls. Introduction of an *Lkb1*$^{4A4\text{-}2}$ trans-heterozygous mutation into the *Htt138Q*^{2} background improves climbing ability. * $p<0.05$.

Discussion

We have used *Drosophila* primary neural cultures isolated from an HD model to screen for RNAi and small molecule suppressors of expanded polyQ Htt-induced toxicity. Cultures expressing a 588 amino acid fragment of human Htt containing an expanded polyQ domain (138Q) display robust cytoplasmic Htt aggregates, and have dystrophic neurites compared to Htt15Q control cultures. To identify supressors of expanded polyQ Htt toxicity, we screened for compounds and RNAi targets that reduce aggregate formation and revert morphological defects towards the control state. Our screening resulted in the identification of *lkb1*, an upstream kinase regulator of the mTOR/Insulin pathway, as a suppressor of mutant Htt toxicity. We also identified multiple compounds that have promising HD therapeutic efficacy: 18β-Glycyrrhetinic acid, Carbenoxolone, and the Camptothecins. Due to the efficiency of conducting screens in cell culture, and the increased physiological relevance of primary neurons, this methodology represents a powerful approach to identify modifiers for other neurodegenerative disorders.

LKB-1 knockdown was found to suppress mutant Htt toxicity in our system, as it rescued the dysmorphic primary neural culture morphology *in vitro* and restored viability *in vivo*. LKB-1 has been extensively studied, and mutations in the locus result in the Peutz Jeghers Syndrome (PJS) [42,43]. In *Drosophila*, loss of LKB-1 in the embryonic nervous system blocks apoptosis and results in hyperplasia [44]. How a partial LKB-1 knockdown elicits its beneficial effect in our system is still uncertain, although decreased levels of LKB-1 may reduce apoptosis caused by mutant Htt. LKB-1 lies upstream of many pathways that have previously been implicated in HD, including the mTOR/autophagy pathway [25,45,46] and the Insulin/AMPK signaling network [47,48]. Recently our findings were corroborated in vertebrates as activation of AMPK, the main kinase target of LKB-1, was found to potentiate striatal neurodegeneration in HD [49].

Several compounds that suppressed mutant Htt toxicity in our primary culture system have previously been shown to have neuroprotective effects in mammalian systems, indicating that the assay with *Drosophila* primary cultured neurons has translational capacity. Compound GW5074 inhibited mutant Htt aggregate formation in our system, and also reduced striatal degeneration in the NP-3 mouse HD model [28]. Similarly, 18β-Glycyrrhetinic acid, which rescued HD toxicity *in vivo* in our *Drosophila* assays, has been shown to suppresses neurotoxicity in a PC12 cellular stress model [34].

By analyzing the molecular structures and mechanisms of action of the small molecules identified as mutant Htt suppressors, new avenues to investigate the biology of HD pathogenesis have been uncovered. 18β-Glycyrrhetinic acid, and Carbenoxolone, which were used to pharmacologically manipulate LKB-1 dependent pathways and rescue HD toxicity *in vivo*, have also been reported to block gap junction activity [50]. Although this mechanism was not further investigated, it is an intriguing approach for future characterization in HD pathology. Recently there have been several reports that mutant Htt expressed in glia can trigger neuronal defects [7,51–53]. In addition, postmortem analysis of HD patient brain samples revealed increased activated astrocytes and reactive microglia in the striatum and cortex compared to similar aged non-diseased brains [54]. Gap junctions allow astrocytes to communicate via elaborate networks, and there is evidence that cell death signals can be propagated through gap junction networks [55]. Therefore, modulating gap junction activity with non-toxic compounds such as 18β-Glycyrrhetinic acid or Carbenoxolone might have neuroprotective benefits. 18β-Glycyrrhetinic acid derivatives are particularly interesting because they have already been evaluated in two clinical trials for other indications (ClinicalTrials.gov Identifier: NCT00384384 and NCT00759525), and are widely used as commercial sweeteners. Recently, an 18β-Glycyrrhetinic acid derivative was found to be efficacious in the treatment of two mouse models of Amyotrophic Lateral Scleosis (ALS) and an Alzheimer's Disease model, further supporting the potential therapeutic value of this class of compounds for neurodegenerative diseases [56].

Camptothecins were very effective at suppressing the dystrophic neuronal profiles and mutant Htt aggregation in our assay. Camptothecins are potent anti-cancer drugs that block cell division through several mechanisms including the introduction of DNA replication-dependant double-stranded breaks which trigger apoptosis, and down regulation of Top-1 by activation of proteasome pathways. In quiescent neurons, Camptothecins most likely cause transcriptional repression as a result of collisions between RNA polymerase and immobilized Top-1/Camptothecin complexes linked to the DNA. In our system, the benefit of Camptothecin treatment could theoretically be related to decreased Htt transgene expression, although we did not observe any decrease in Htt-mRFP fluorescence, even after one week of continuous exposure to the drug. Since targeted knockdown of mutant Htt via siRNA has been found to be effective at reversing disease progression in mouse models, small molecule transcriptional repressors may offer another therapeutic avenue to control HD [57]. Although toxicity issues have been reported in neural cultures following Camptothecin treatment, we did not observe morphological defects in our *Drosophila* HD model [58]. Camptothecins have been reported to regulate a number of different pathways, including activation of the ubiquitin/proteasome system and upregulation of mitochondrial biogenesis. These secondary Camptothecin effects could alleviate toxic Htt cellular stress by removing toxic Htt species or restoring energy homeostatis [59–62].

There has been debate in field about the contribution of Htt aggregates to disease pathology for many years. Several studies have shown that Htt aggregates accumulate in fine neuronal processes such as axons and dendrites, and block axon-transport to negatively impact cell heath [17,63–65]. Real-time imaging experiments have suggested that soluble Htt, and not aggregates, correlate better with cellular toxicity [66]. Given this controversy, we chose not to use aggregate suppression as the sole metric to identify small molecules and RNAi knockdown probes that have therapeutic value and included an additional parameter: neurite morphology. We found that neurite processes are sensitive to mutant polyQ-expanded Htt and offer a means of identifying drugs and RNAi knock-downs that have non-specific toxicity effects. Using this assay we were able to identify compounds and RNAi knockdowns that have potential therapeutic value. Although our studies cannot conclusively demonstrate a physiological link between aggregate inhibition and improved neuronal health, we did discover compounds that improved neurite morphology in addition to reducing mutant Htt aggregation, providing anecdotal evidence that in some cases aggregates may have toxic properties.

Drosophila models of neurodegenerative disease have been a powerful tool for understanding mechanisms of neurodegeneration for more than a decade, and have more recently been applied directly to drug discovery as well [67–74]. Aside from genetic tools in *Drosophila* and the host of neurodegenerative disease models available, it is an attractive model for conducting suppressor screens given the lack of gene redundancy often observed in mammals. While single gene knock-down studies often fail to produce robust phenotypes in mammals, this is not the case in

Drosophila [75,76]. We have found that the complex neural morphologies of *Drosophila* primary cultures can also provide sensitive information about the general cell physiological status of a disease model. The algorithms that we have used in this study can help quantify complex morphologies can also facilitate the identification of disease modifying genes [23]. Live imaging, as presented here, has the advantage over traditional cell staining experiments in that the fine neurite morphology of cultures is preserved. Detergents and washes needed for immunofluorescence-based assays can disrupt fine cellular processes and introduce artifacts, which reduce assay sensitivity and introduce noise. Live-cell imaging also makes it possible to collect different time points in a single experiment, which not only reduces labor but also enables one to track the effect of a compound or gene knockdown over time. Because of the ease and speed of conducting RNAi and compound screens in *Drosophila* primary culture systems, this methodology offers an attractive approach to identify disease-modifying agents for neurodegenerative diseases.

Methods

Primary Cell Culture

Elav^{c155}-GAL4 virgins were collected en masse and crossed to either *UAS-Htt138QmRFP^{1},UAS-mCD8-GFP* or *UAS-Htt15Qm RFP^{1},UAS-mCD8GFP* males to generate embryos for primary culture preparation. Neuroblasts were isolated as previously described [22].

Western Blotting

Embryonic lysates (n = 4/genotype) were prepared from control and Htt expressing strains (50 mM Tris, pH 8.0, 150 mM NaCl, 0.1% SDS, 1.0% NP-40 (IgePal), 0.1% sodium deoxycholate plus protease inhibitors (cOmplete-mini, Roche)), and protein content was quantified using a BCA kit (Pierce). Protein samples (10 µg/lane) were analyzed using standard SDS-PAGE/Western blotting techniques, and quantified using an Odyssey Infrared Imaging System (Li-Cor). For immunoblotting, antibodies were used at the following concentrations: mouse anti-Tubulin (6-11B-1, Sigma-Aldrich T7451) at 1/60,000, mouse anti-human Htt (MAb 2166, Chemicon) at 1/1,000, and goat-anti-mouse IR800 secondary (LI-COR 926-32210) at 1/3,000.

Compound screening

Primary cultures were re-suspended directly in Shields and Sang M3 media (Sigma) supplemented with 10 U/mL penicillin, 10 µg/mL streptomycin, 200 ng/mL insulin, and 5% fetal bovine serum. 100 nL of compounds from arrayed small-molecule libraries (NINDS Custom Collection 2, Prestwick1 Collection, BIOMOL2 ICCB-Longwood Known Bioactives High Concentration, various concentration from 1–15 mM in DMSO) were applied to 50 µL of cultures 24 hours after plating on optical bottom 384-well plates (Corning 3712). The neuroblast density was 18,500 cells/well. The primary screen was carried out in duplicate and hits were validated with 12 additional replicate wells.

RNAi Screening

dsRNAs (250 ng/well) were aliquoted onto microscopy plates and then 10 µL of neuroblasts were applied to a density of 18,500 cells/well. Cultures were incubated for 3 days with dsRNAs to achieve gene knockdown. Shields and Sang M3 media (Sigma) supplemented with 10 U/mL penicillin, 10 µg/mL streptomycin, 200 ng/mL insulin, and 5% fetal bovine serum was then added to cultures to bring assay volume to 50 µL. The *Drosophila* RNAi Screening Center (DRSC) whole genome kinase/phosphatase library (468 genes, 3 amplicons/gene) was screened in duplicate, and hits were validated using additional dsRNA amplicons containing no off-targets. For RNAi validation studies, dsRNAs were synthesized from T7-tailed DNA templates using the MEGAshortscript T7 transcription kit (Ambion). Synthesized dsRNAs were purified with RNeasy kits (Qiagen) before use in cell culture experiments. The T7-tailed oligonucleotides used to generate DNA templates from w^{1118} genomic DNA are as follows: Lkb-1: DRSC16481 (GCCGTCAAGATCCTGACTA/CTCCG-CTGGACCAGATG), DRSC36925 (GCAACTCCACGGTGA-TACCT/ATGCAGGACGTCAGCTTCTT), DRSC36926 (AT-TGCGGCGAACTTACTTTG/TAATCCTCACCAGGCACA-CA); Top-1: DRSC36056 (GAGAATGTGCAGGGACAGGT/GTCGATGAAGTAAAGGGCCA), DRSC20295 (GGAGGAG-GAGAAGCGTG/GCGCCGCTTGATCATG); Top2: DRSC 36057 (CACAGCGACAGAAGCATCAT/TTCTTGTATTCC-CTCGTGGC), DRSC3459 (TTTGCCAGAGCGATATCTC/CCATAGTGGCTCGATCTTTT); Top3α: DRSC3460 (TTAA-ACGTGGCTGAGAAGAA/GCCCACGCCCTTTTTCA), DR SC37672(GTGGTCCTGACCGAACAGAT/AGGTTTTGTA-CCAACCGCTG); Top3β: DRSC18724(GCGGACTTCGGT-GAGGA/CGCTGGCAGATGTTGTTG).

Microscopy

For high-content screening, mature 7-day old cultures were imaged with an ImageXpress^{MICRO} robotic microscope (Molecular Devices, Sunnyvale, CA) using a 10× objective and FITC/Cy3 filter sets. Images were 1392×1040 pixels, or 897×670 micrometers. Laser-based autofocusing was used to locate plate bottoms, and then image-based focusing was used to resolve fluorescently labeled neurons over a 48 µm range. The GFP and mRFP channels were imaged in the same focal plane, with exposure times of 850 and 400 ms respectively. Three sites were imaged per well for each treatment group, and the screen was done in duplicate. For confocal microscopy of primary cultures, neuroblsts were plated on poly-L-lysine coated chambered cover slips (LabTekII, 0.8 cm^2/well) at 18,300 cells/well in 50 µL volume. Small molecules were added to cultures 24 hours after plating, incubated for 7 days, and then imaged with a Leica TCS-SP2 confocal LSM microscope.

Digital Image Analysis of High Content Screening Data Sets

Neuronal morphological analysis and Htt aggregate quantification for automated microscopy images was performed as previously described [23,77]. In brief, Htt138Q aggregates were quantified as the total number of pixels/image with intensity higher than an empirically set threshold. To quantify neuronal morphologies, cell body clusters (neuromeres) and neurites were extracted from images using our custom algorithms [21]. The log_2 transformed areas of cell body clusters were found to fit a Gaussian mixture model (GMM) and therefore were separated into three bins (small, medium, and large). Absolute counts of neuromeres/bin were tabulated for all images. Neurite segment lengths were similarly clustered into three groups (short, medium, and long) using the *K*-means method and then quantified. Cell cluster and neurite counts were converted into percentages to control for any variation in cell number between wells arising from pipetting error. Mean neuromere area and neurite length for each image were also calculated to give a total of eight morphological metrics for image morphology quantification. For statistical analysis, *p*-values for each morphological feature were calculated using a two sample *t*-test (e.g. small neuromere feature of Htt138Q drug-treated cultures *versus* small neuromere feature of Htt15Q DMSO cultures). The resultant morphological *p*-values for individual features were then integrated into a single *p*-value using the Fisher method [78] defined by the equation $\chi^2 = -2\Sigma_{i=1}^{k}\log_e(p_i)$, where k represents independent tests, p_i is the *p*-value of the *i*-th feature. The combined statistic has a χ^2 distribution with $2k$ degrees of freedom under the joint null hypothesis. This method works well in cases where the evidence against the null-hypothesis is spread across different features. Excluded from analysis were compound-treated wells with <6 images, out-of-focus images, or images that lacked cell profiles altogether.

In vivo Rescue studies

For small molecule *in vivo* rescue studies, *Elav^{c155}; UAS-Htt138QmRFP^{1},UAS-mCD8-GFP/+* 1st instar larvae were collected en-masse and dispensed into liquid media (10 larvae/well) containing different concentrations of test compounds (n = 8 replicas/concentration). The cultures were reared at 21°C for 5 days, and the mean number or living Htt138Q larvae (i.e. GFP^{+}, Htt138QmRFP^{+}, and mobile) was tabulated, and expressed as a percentage of total larvae/well. For genetic rescue studies with *lkb1*, two Htt138Q strains were utilized: a strong expressing line, *UAS-Htt138QmRFP^{1}* which is pharate lethal when crossed to *Elav^{c155}*, and a weaker expressing line, *UAS-Htt138QmRFP^{2}* which survives to adulthood and is viable for a number of weeks. Using the strong line, pharate lethality at 25°C was calculated after *lkb1* (*lkb1^{4B1-11}* and *lkb1^{4A4-2}* alleles) was introduced into an Elav^{c155},UAS-Htt/+ background. *Lkb1^{4B1-11}* is a premature truncation allele (Q98>Stop), and *lkb1^{4A4-2}* is an EMS null allele (589 b.p. deletion removing 150 b.p. of the 5′ UTR, the start codon and the beginning of the open reading frame). For Top1 *in vivo* analysis, Elav^{c155},*Top^{112}* recombinants were generated and crossed to *UAS-Htt138QmRFP^{1}*.

Negative Geotaxis Assay

Lkb1^{4A4-2} was crossed into the Elav^{c155}, *UAS-Htt138QmRFP^{2}* which is adult viable and has weaker Htt138Q expression. Virgin female *Drosophila* were collected and flipped onto fresh media two times per week until the start of the assay. 25 day-old flies (10–15 flies/vial, 4 vials/genotype) were gently tapped to the base of vials, and climbing behavior was video-recorded for 18 seconds (trial). The percentage of flies to reached the top of a vial was tabulated and averaged after 4 trails. Vials were back-lit with a light box to enhance the resolution of the fly climbing trajectories. Statistical analysis was performed using a t-test.

Supporting Information

Figure S1 Selective compounds tested for their ability to suppress *Htt138Q* neuronal toxicity.

Table S1 Compounds found to inhibit Htt138Q aggregate formation in *Drosophila* primary neural culture screen.

Movie S1 *Elav^{c155}-GAL4;UAS-Htt138QmRFP^{1}/lkb1^{4A4-2}* rescued adult *Drosophila.* While *Elav^{c155}-GAL4;UAS-Htt138QmRFP^{1}/+* adults are pharate lethal, introduction of a heterozygous *lkb1^{4A4-2}* allele suppresses Htt138Q toxicity and results in the emergence of viable escapers. Escapers have normal walking ability, but are unable to unfurl and inflate their wings.

Acknowledgments

The authors thank C. Shamu, M. Booker, S. Mohr at the Institute of Chemistry and Cell Biology-Longwood (ICCB-L) and the *Drosophila* RNAi Screening Center (DRSC) at Harvard Medical School for their advice and use of screening facilities and compound/RNAi libraries. The *lkb1^{4A4-2}* and lkb1^{4B1-11} alleles were obtained from the St. Johnston lab, and other stocks were obtained from the Bloomington Stock Center.

Author Contributions

Conceived and designed the experiments: JS KJS. Performed the experiments: JS KJS. Analyzed the data: JS KJS CW PH. Contributed reagents/materials/analysis tools: JTL. Wrote the paper: JS KJS. Designed the software used in the analysis: CW PH.

References

1. Kim MW, Chelliah Y, Kim SW, Otwinowski Z, Bezprozvanny I (2009) Secondary structure of Huntingtin amino-terminal region. Structure 17: 1205–1212.
2. Halliday GM, McRitchie DA, Macdonald V, Double KL, Trent RJ, et al. (1998) Regional specificity of brain atrophy in Huntington's disease. Exp Neurol 154: 663–672.
3. Nopoulos PC, Aylward EH, Ross CA, Johnson HJ, Magnotta VA, et al. (2010) Cerebral cortex structure in prodromal Huntington disease. Neurobiol 40: 544–554. Epub 2010 Aug 2012.
4. Gu X, Li C, Wei W, Lo V, Gong S, et al. (2005) Pathological cell-cell interactions elicited by a neuropathogenic form of mutant Huntingtin contribute to cortical pathogenesis in HD mice. Neuron 46: 433–444.
5. Paulsen JS, Nopoulos PC, Aylward E, Ross CA, Johnson H, et al. (2010) Striatal and white matter predictors of estimated diagnosis for Huntington disease. Brain 82: 201–207. Epub 2010 Apr 2010.
6. Gu X, Andre VM, Cepeda C, Li SH, Li XJ, et al. (2007) Pathological cell-cell interactions are necessary for striatal pathogenesis in a conditional mouse model of Huntington's disease. Mol Neurodegener 2: 8.
7. Shin JY, Fang ZH, Yu ZX, Wang CE, Li SH, et al. (2005) Expression of mutant huntingtin in glial cells contributes to neuronal excitotoxicity. J Cell Biol 171: 1001–1012.
8. Roze E, Saudou F, Caboche J (2008) Pathophysiology of Huntington's disease: from huntingtin functions to potential treatments. Curr Opin Neurol 21: 497–503.
9. Wexler NS, Lorimer J, Porter J, Gomez F, Moskowitz C, et al. (2004) Venezuelan kindreds reveal that genetic and environmental factors modulate Huntington's disease age of onset. Proc Natl Acad Sci U S A 101: 3498–3503. Epub 2004 Mar 3491.
10. Gayan J, Brocklebank D, Andresen JM, Alkorta-Aranburu G, Zameel Cader M, et al. (2008) Genomewide linkage scan reveals novel loci modifying age of onset of Huntington's disease in the Venezuelan HD kindreds. Genet Epidemiol 32: 445–453.
11. Zhang S, Feany MB, Saraswati S, Littleton JT, Perrimon N (2009) Inactivation of Drosophila Huntingtin affects long-term adult functioning and the pathogenesis of a Huntington's disease model. Dis Model Mech 2: 247–266. Epub 2009 Apr 2006.
12. Li SH, Li XJ (2004) Huntingtin-protein interactions and the pathogenesis of Huntington's disease. Trends Genet 20: 146–154.
13. Li Z, Karlovich CA, Fish MP, Scott MP, Myers RM (1999) A putative Drosophila homolog of the Huntington's disease gene. Hum Mol Genet 8: 1807–1815.
14. Doumanis J, Wada K, Kino Y, Moore AW, Nukina N (2009) RNAi screening in Drosophila cells identifies new modifiers of mutant huntingtin aggregation. PLoS One 4: e7275.
15. Zhang S, Binari R, Zhou R, Perrimon N (2010) A genomewide RNA interference screen for modifiers of aggregates formation by mutant Huntingtin in Drosophila. Genetics 184: 1165–1179. Epub 2010 Jan 1125.
16. Robertson AL, Bottomley SP (2010) Towards the treatment of polyglutamine diseases: the modulatory role of protein context. Curr 17: 3058–3068.
17. Lee W-CM, Yoshihara M, Littleton JT (2004) Cytoplasmic aggregates trap polyglutamine-containing proteins and block axonal transport in a Drosophila model of Huntington's disease. Proc Natl Acad Sci USA. pp 3224–3229.
18. Graham R, Deng Y, Slow E, Haigh B, Bissada N, et al. (2006) Cleavage at the caspase-6 site is required for neuronal dysfunction and degeneration due to mutant huntingtin. Cell. pp 1179–1191.
19. Brand AH, Perrimon N (1993) Targeted gene expression as a means of altering cell fates and generating dominant phenotypes. Development 118: 401–415.
20. Roos RA (2010) Huntington's disease: a clinical review. Orphanet J Rare Dis 5: 40.
21. DiFiglia M, Sapp E, Chase K, Davies S, Bates G, et al. (1997) Aggregation of huntingtin in neuronal intranuclear inclusions and dystrophic neurites in brain. Science. 1990 p.
22. Sepp KJ, Hong P, Lizarraga SB, Liu JS, Mejia LA, et al. (2008) Identification of neural outgrowth genes using genome-wide RNAi. PLoS Genet 4: e1000111.

23. Wu C, Schulte J, Sepp KJ, Littleton JT, Hong P (2010) Automatic robust neurite detection and morphological analysis of neuronal cell cultures in high-content screening. Neuroinformatics 8: 83–100.
24. Wang J, Gines S, MacDonald ME, Gusella JF (2005) Reversal of a full-length mutant huntingtin neuronal cell phenotype by chemical inhibitors of polyglutamine-mediated aggregation. BMC Neurosci 6: 1.
25. Ravikumar B, Vacher C, Berger Z, Davies J, Luo S, et al. (2004) Inhibition of mTOR induces autophagy and reduces toxicity of polyglutamine expansions in fly and mouse models of Huntington disease. Nat Genet. pp 585–595.
26. Hay DG, Sathasivam K, Tobaben S, Stahl B, Marber M, et al. (2004) Progressive decrease in chaperone protein levels in a mouse model of Huntington's disease and induction of stress proteins as a therapeutic approach. Hum Mol Genet 13: 1389–1405. Epub 2004 Apr 1328.
27. Zhang X, Smith DL, Meriin AB, Engemann S, Russel DE, et al. (2005) A potent small molecule inhibits polyglutamine aggregation in Huntington's disease neurons and suppresses neurodegeneration in vivo. Proc Natl Acad Sci U S A 102: 892–897. Epub 2005 Jan 2010.
28. Chin PC, Liu L, Morrison BE, Siddiq A, Ratan RR, et al. (2004) The c-Raf inhibitor GW5074 provides neuroprotection in vitro and in an animal model of neurodegeneration through a MEK-ERK and Akt-independent mechanism. J Neurochem 90: 595–608.
29. Inoki K, Corradetti MN, Guan KL (2005) Dysregulation of the TSC-mTOR pathway in human disease. Nat Genet 37: 19–24.
30. Shaw RJ, Bardeesy N, Manning BD, Lopez L, Kosmatka M, et al. (2004) The LKB1 tumor suppressor negatively regulates mTOR signaling. Cancer Cell 6: 91–99.
31. Hertzberg R, Busby R, Caranfa M, Holden K, Johnson R, et al. (1990) Irreversible trapping of the DNA-topoisomerase I covalent complex. Affinity labeling of the camptothecin binding site. Journal of Biological Chemistry. 19287 p.
32. Shaw R, Lamia K, Vasquez D, Koo S, Bardeesy N, et al. (2005) The kinase LKB1 mediates glucose homeostasis in liver and therapeutic effects of metformin. Science. 1642 p.
33. Hardie D (2006) Neither LKB1 nor AMPK are the direct targets of metformin. Gastroenterology. pp 973–973.
34. Kao TC, Shyu MH, Yen GC (2009) Neuroprotective effects of glycyrrhizic acid and 18beta-glycyrrhetinic acid in PC12 cells via modulation of the PI3K/Akt pathway. J Agric Food Chem 57: 754–761.
35. Zoncu R, Efeyan A, Sabatini DM (2010) mTOR: from growth signal integration to cancer, diabetes and ageing. Nat 12: 21–35. Epub 2010 Dec 2015.
36. Morrisett JD, Abdel-Fattah G, Hoogeveen R, Mitchell E, Ballantyne CM, et al. (2002) Effects of sirolimus on plasma lipids, lipoprotein levels, and fatty acid metabolism in renal transplant patients. J Lipid Res 43: 1170–1180.
37. Letavernier E, Bruneval P, Mandet C, Duong Van Huyen JP, Peraldi MN, et al. (2007) High sirolimus levels may induce focal segmental glomerulosclerosis de novo. Clin J Am Soc Nephrol 2: 326–333.
38. Kuypers DR (2005) Benefit-risk assessment of sirolimus in renal transplantation. Drug Saf 28: 153–181.
39. Pham PT, Pham PC, Danovitch GM, Ross DJ, Gritsch HA, et al. (2004) Sirolimus-associated pulmonary toxicity. Transplantation 77: 1215–1220.
40. Maroto JP, Hudes G, Dutcher JP, Logan TF, White CS, et al. (2011) Drug-related pneumonitis in patients with advanced renal cell carcinoma treated with temsirolimus. J Clin Oncol 29: 1750–1756.
41. Martin S, St Johnston D (2003) A role for Drosophila LKB1 in anterior-posterior axis formation and epithelial polarity. Nature. pp 379–384.
42. Jenne DE, Reimann H, Nezu J, Friedel W, Loff S, et al. (1998) Peutz-Jeghers syndrome is caused by mutations in a novel serine threonine kinase. Nat Genet 18: 38–43.
43. van Veelen W, Korsse SE, van de Laar L, Peppelenbosch MP (2011) The long and winding road to rational treatment of cancer associated with LKB1/AMPK/TSC/mTORC1 signaling.
44. Lee JH, Koh H, Kim M, Park J, Lee SY, et al. (2006) JNK pathway mediates apoptotic cell death induced by tumor suppressor LKB1 in Drosophila. Cell Death Differ 13: 1110–1122.
45. Sarkar S, Perlstein EO, Imarisio S, Pineau S, Cordenier A, et al. (2007) Small molecules enhance autophagy and reduce toxicity in Huntington's disease models. Nat Chem Biol 3: 331–338. Epub 2007 May 2007.
46. Fleming A, Noda T, Yoshimori T, Rubinsztein DC (2011) Chemical modulators of autophagy as biological probes and potential therapeutics. Nat 7: 9–17.
47. Yamamoto A, Cremona M, Rothman J (2006) Autophagy-mediated clearance of huntingtin aggregates triggered by the insulin-signaling pathway. Journal of Cell Biology. 719 p.
48. David DC, Ollikainen N, Trinidad JC, Cary MP, Burlingame AL, et al. (2010) Widespread protein aggregation as an inherent part of aging in C. elegans. PLoS 8: e1000450.
49. Ju TC, Chen HM, Lin JT, Chang CP, Chang WC, et al. (2011) Nuclear translocation of AMPK-{alpha}1 potentiates striatal neurodegeneration in Huntington's disease. J Cell Biol 194: 209–227.
50. Juszczak GR, Swiergiel AH (2009) Properties of gap junction blockers and their behavioural, cognitive and electrophysiological effects: animal and human studies. Prog Neuropsychopharmacol Biol Psychiatry 33: 181–198. Epub 2009 Jan 2001.
51. Tamura T, Sone M, Yamashita M, Wanker EE, Okazawa H (2009) Glial cell lineage expression of mutant ataxin-1 and huntingtin induces developmental and late-onset neuronal pathologies in Drosophila models. PLoS One 4: e4262. Epub 2009 Jan 4223.
52. Bradford J, Shin JY, Roberts M, Wang CE, Sheng G, et al. (2010) Mutant huntingtin in glial cells exacerbates neurological symptoms of Huntington disease mice. J 285: 10653–10661. Epub 12010 Feb 10659.
53. Kretzschmar D, Tschape J, Bettencourt Da Cruz A, Asan E, Poeck B, et al. (2005) Glial and neuronal expression of polyglutamine proteins induce behavioral changes and aggregate formation in Drosophila. Glia 49: 59–72.
54. Sapp E, Kegel KB, Aronin N, Hashikawa T, Uchiyama Y, et al. (2001) Early and progressive accumulation of reactive microglia in the Huntington disease brain. J Neuropathol Exp Neurol 60: 161–172.
55. Lin JH, Weigel H, Cotrina ML, Liu S, Bueno E, et al. (1998) Gap-junction-mediated propagation and amplification of cell injury. Nat Neurosci 1: 494–500.
56. Takeuchi H, Mizoguchi H, Doi Y, Jin S, Noda M, et al. (2011) Blockade of gap junction hemichannel suppresses disease progression in mouse models of amyotrophic lateral sclerosis and Alzheimer's disease. PLoS One 6: e21108.
57. DiFiglia M, Sena-Esteves M, Chase K, Sapp E, Pfister E, et al. (2007) Therapeutic silencing of mutant huntingtin with siRNA attenuates striatal and cortical neuropathology and behavioral deficits. Proc Natl Acad Sci U S A 104: 17204–17209. Epub 12007 Oct 17216.
58. Lang-Rollin IC, Rideout HJ, Noticewala M, Stefanis L (2003) Mechanisms of caspase-independent neuronal death: energy depletion and free radical generation. J Neurosci 23: 11015–11025.
59. Kluza J, Marchetti P, Gallego MA, Lancel S, Fournier C, et al. (2004) Mitochondrial proliferation during apoptosis induced by anticancer agents: effects of doxorubicin and mitoxantrone on cancer and cardiac cells. Oncogene 23: 7018–7030.
60. Reipert S, Berry J, Hughes MF, Hickman JA, Allen TD (1995) Changes of mitochondrial mass in the hemopoietic stem cell line FDCP-mix after treatment with etoposide: a correlative study by multiparameter flow cytometry and confocal and electron microscopy. Exp Cell Res 221: 281–288.
61. Fu X, Wan S, Lyu YL, Liu LF, Qi H (2008) Etoposide induces ATM-dependent mitochondrial biogenesis through AMPK activation. PLoS One 3: e2009.
62. Thomas CJ, Rahier NJ, Hecht SM (2004) Camptothecin: current perspectives. Bioorg Med Chem 12: 1585–1604.
63. Sapp E, Penney J, Young A, Aronin N, Vonsattel JP, et al. (1999) Axonal transport of N-terminal huntingtin suggests early pathology of corticostriatal projections in Huntington disease. J Neuropathol Exp Neurol 58: 165–173.
64. Gunawardena S, Her LS, Brusch RG, Laymon RA, Niesman IR, et al. (2003) Disruption of axonal transport by loss of huntingtin or expression of pathogenic polyQ proteins in Drosophila. Neuron 40: 25–40.
65. Trushina E, Dyer RB, Badger JD, 2nd, Ure D, Eide L, et al. (2004) Mutant huntingtin impairs axonal trafficking in mammalian neurons in vivo and in vitro. Mol Cell Biol 24: 8195–8209.
66. Arrasate M, Mitra S, Schweitzer ES, Segal MR, Finkbeiner S (2004) Inclusion body formation reduces levels of mutant huntingtin and the risk of neuronal death. Nature 431: 805–810.
67. Ambegaokar SS, Roy B, Jackson GR (2010) Neurodegenerative models in Drosophila: polyglutamine disorders, Parkinson disease, and amyotrophic lateral sclerosis. Neurobiol 40: 29–39. Epub 2010 May 2031.
68. Lim KL (2010) Non-mammalian animal models of Parkinson's disease for drug discovery. Expert Opin Drug Discov 5: 165–176.
69. O'Kane CJ (2011) Drosophila as a Model Organism for the Study of Neuropsychiatric Disorders.
70. Bilen J, Bonini NM (2005) Drosophila as a model for human neurodegenerative disease. Annu Rev Genet 39: 153–171.
71. Agrawal N, Pallos J, Slepko N, Apostol BL, Bodai L, et al. (2005) Identification of combinatorial drug regimens for treatment of Huntington's disease using Drosophila. Proc Natl Acad Sci U S A 102: 3777–3781.
72. Steffan JS, Bodai L, Pallos J, Poelman M, McCampbell A, et al. (2001) Histone deacetylase inhibitors arrest polyglutamine-dependent neurodegeneration in Drosophila. Nature 413: 739–743.
73. Auluck PK, Bonini NM (2002) Pharmacological prevention of Parkinson disease in Drosophila. Nat Med. pp 1185–1186.
74. Min KT, Benzer S (1999) Preventing neurodegeneration in the Drosophila mutant bubblegum. Science 284: 1985–1988.
75. Banovic D, Khorramshahi O, Owald D, Wichmann C, Riedt T, et al. (2010) Drosophila neuroligin 1 promotes growth and postsynaptic differentiation at glutamatergic neuromuscular junctions. Neuron 66: 724–738.
76. Williams R (2006) Development: Neuroligin knockouts: form but no function. Nature Reviews Neuroscience 7: 831.
77. Schulte J, Sepp KJ, Jorquera RA, Wu C, Song Y, et al. (2010) DMob4/Phocein regulates synapse formation, axonal transport, and microtubule organization. J Neurosci 30: 5189–5203.
78. Fisher RA (1932) Statistical Methods for Research Workers; Oliver, Boyd, eds. Edinburgh.

11

Losses of Both Products of the *Cdkn2a/Arf* Locus Contribute to Asbestos-Induced Mesothelioma Development and Cooperate to Accelerate Tumorigenesis

Deborah A. Altomare[1,¶,¤], Craig W. Menges[1,¶], Jinfei Xu[1], Jianming Pei[1], Lili Zhang[1], Ara Tadevosyan[1], Erin Neumann-Domer[1], Zemin Liu[1], Michele Carbone[2], Ilse Chudoba[3], Andres J. Klein-Szanto[1], Joseph R. Testa[1]*

1 Cancer Biology Program, Fox Chase Cancer Center, Philadelphia, Pennsylvania, United States of America, **2** Thoracic Oncology Program, Cancer Research Center of Hawaii, University of Hawaii, Honolulu, Hawaii, United States of America, **3** MetaSystems, Altlussheim, Germany

Abstract

The *CDKN2A/ARF* locus encompasses overlapping tumor suppressor genes *p16(INK4A)* and *p14(ARF)*, which are frequently co-deleted in human malignant mesothelioma (MM). The importance of *p16(INK4A)* loss in human cancer is well established, but the relative significance of *p14(ARF)* loss has been debated. The tumor predisposition of mice singly deficient for either *Ink4a* or *Arf*, due to targeting of exons 1α or 1β, respectively, supports the idea that both play significant and nonredundant roles in suppressing spontaneous tumors. To further test this notion, we exposed *Ink4a*(+/−) and *Arf*(+/−) mice to asbestos, the major cause of MM. Asbestos-treated *Ink4a*(+/−) and *Arf*(+/−) mice showed increased incidence and shorter latency of MM relative to wild-type littermates. MMs from *Ink4a*(+/−) mice exhibited biallelic inactivation of *Ink4a*, loss of Arf or p53 expression and frequent loss of p15(Ink4b). In contrast, MMs from *Arf*(+/−) mice exhibited loss of Arf expression, but did not require loss of Ink4a or Ink4b. Mice doubly deficient for *Ink4a* and *Arf*, due to deletion of *Cdkn2a/Arf* exon 2, showed accelerated asbestos-induced MM formation relative to mice deficient for *Ink4a* or *Arf* alone, and MMs exhibited biallelic loss of both tumor suppressor genes. The tumor suppressor function of Arf in MM was p53-independent, since MMs with loss of Arf retained functional p53. Collectively, these *in vivo* data indicate that both *CDKN2A/ARF* gene products suppress asbestos carcinogenicity. Furthermore, while inactivation of Arf appears to be crucial for MM pathogenesis, the inactivation of both *p16(Ink4a)* and *p19(Arf)* cooperate to accelerate asbestos-induced tumorigenesis.

Editor: Ralf Krahe, University of Texas M. D. Anderson Cancer Center, United States of America

Funding: This research was supported by grants from the National Cancer Institute (P01CA114047 to J.R.T., M.C., CA06927 to J.R.T., A.J.K.-S.), and CA009035 (C.W.M.), by the Commonwealth of Pennsylvania (Fox Chase Cancer Center), and by the Local No. 14 Mesothelioma Fund of the International Association of Heat and Frost Insulators & Allied Workers (J.R.T.). The funders had no role in study design, data collection and analysis, decision to publish, or preparation of the manuscript.

Competing Interests: One of the authors (I.C.) is employed by a commercial company (MetaSystems, Altlussheim, Germany). This fact does not alter the authors' adherence to all the PLoS ONE policies on sharing data and materials. The remaining authors declare that no competing interests exist.

* E-mail: joseph.testa@fccc.edu

¶ These authors contributed equally to this work.

¤ Current address: Burnett School of Biomedical Sciences, University of Central Florida, Orlando, Florida, United States of America

Introduction

CDKN2A/ARF is among the most commonly mutated loci in human cancer, encoding two different tumor suppressors translated from alternatively spliced mRNAs. *p16(INK4A)* is composed of exons 1α, 2 and 3, and is designated here as *INK4A* (inhibitor of cyclin dependent kinase 4). Human *p14(ARF)* is encoded by exon 1β and alternate reading frames of *CDKN2A/ARF* exons 2 and 3, herein referred to as *ARF* (alternate reading frame). Knockout mice with targeted deletion of specific *Cdkn2A/Arf* exons have disrupted *p16Ink4a*, *p19Arf* or both genes [1,2,3,4] and develop a different spectrum of spontaneous tumors, although not malignant mesotheliomas (MMs). A differential impact of heterozygous loss of *Ink4a* or *Arf* to the induction of MM by asbestos has not been previously addressed. The studies presented here provide genetic evidence for the significance of *Ink4a* and *Arf* alterations in MM by directly comparing susceptibility to tumor induction by asbestos in *Ink4a*-deficient, *Arf*-deficient and doubly heterozygous *Ink4a;Arf* mice in a common genetic background. The enhanced tumor susceptibility of mice singly deficient for either *p16(Ink4a)* or *p19(Arf)* supports the view that both play significant and nonredundant roles in suppressing malignant transformation. The fact that mice deficient for both tumor suppressors have accelerated tumor development indicates that inactivation of both *p16(Ink4a)* and *p19(Arf)* cooperate to promote asbestos carcinogenicity.

Results

Using a genetic approach, we assessed the relative contribution of Ink4a and Arf deficiency to induction of asbestos-induced tumor formation. MM incidence was increased and latency decreased in *Ink4a*(+/−) and *Arf*(+/−) mice relative to wild-type littermates (Fig. 1, Supporting File S1). Mice doubly deficient for *Ink4a;Arf* had accelerated asbestos-induced MMs relative to mice deficient for *Ink4a* or *Arf* alone. As in prior studies [5,6,7], MM did not develop in TiO_2-treated mice (Supporting File S1). Median latency for MM detection after initial asbestos exposure was 29.6 weeks for *Ink4a;Arf*(+/−), 34.6 weeks for *Ink4a*(+/−), 38.0 weeks for *Arf*(+/−), and 49.4 weeks for wild-type mice. *Ink4a-*, *Arf- and Ink4a;Arf*-deficient mice had decreased survival compared to wild-type mice (Fig. 1). Tumor latency for *Ink4a-* and *Arf*-deficient mice was not significantly different, whereas latency was decreased in *Ink4a;Arf*-deficient mice ($p<0.0001$).

Sarcomatoid MMs were prevalent in all asbestos-treated mice (Fig. 2), although biphasic and epithelial morphology were occasionally observed. MMs frequently presented with ascites, occasional spheroids, and diffuse peritoneal seeding of the serosal lining. Most tumors in wild-type mice were early-stage MMs, whereas tumors in *Ink4a*(+/−), *Arf*(+/−), and *Ink4a;Arf*(+/−) mice generally were more advanced. Extensive disease was most evident in doubly heterozygous mice. In a few cases, diagnosis was difficult because MMs may arise anywhere in the abdominal cavity and may not be obvious in the sampled tissues. Thus, where possible, tumor cells from ascites or peritoneal lavage were tested with markers to verify MM (Supporting File S1).

Using early passage (≤6) MM cells, we found biallelic inactivation of the predisposing tumor suppressor gene in all MMs tested (Fig. 3A). In most (4 of 5 tested) MMs from *Ink4a*(+/−) mice, there also was loss of *Arf* and *p15(Ink4b)*, the latter located near the *Cdkn2a/Arf* locus. Tumor #200, from an *Ink4a*(+/−) mouse, retained expression of Arf but did not express p53 protein. Interestingly, in MM cells with loss of Arf, the p53 pathway appeared to remain functional intact based on their response to DNA damage with etoposide (100 μM) or UV irradiation (80 J/m^2) (Fig. 3C).

MMs from *Arf*(+/−) mice consistently exhibited loss of Arf protein. In 4 of 5 samples tested, the mutant *Arf* allele was retained, as determined by RT-PCR (Supplemental Fig. S2); insertion of the *neo*-selectable marker used in the *Arf* targeting strategy results in a stop codon and no Arf protein expression (Fig. 3). *Arf*(+/−) mice showed loss of Ink4a expression in 3 of 6 MM cultures, whereas p15(Ink4b) was retained in 5 of 6 cultures (Fig. 3). Similarly, inactivation of Ink4a and p15(Ink4b) were not required for MM formation in a C57Bl/6 *Arf*(+/−) model [6].

MMs from *Ink4a;Arf* doubly heterozygous mice exhibited biallelic inactivation of *Ink4a* and *Arf*, whereas *Ink4b* was retained in 6 of 7 MM samples tested. Expression of Nf2 and p53 was retained in nearly all MM cultures from *Ink4a*(+/−), *Arf*(+/−), and *Ink4a;Arf*(+/−) mice (Fig. 3).

Cytogenetic analyses were performed on two randomly-selected MM cultures from each mouse model. As in the human disease counterpart, MMs from *Ink4a-*, *Arf-*, and *Ink4a;Arf*-deficient mice typically showed numerous chromosome alterations. No consistent alteration was seen, although 3 of 6 tumors had extra copies of chromosome 19, including a MM from an *Ink4a*(+/−) mouse (#264), in which gain of chromosome 19 was the only abnormality observed. MM cultures from *Arf-* and *Ink4a;Arf*-deficient mice typically had numerous clonal structural rearrangements (Fig. 4A). Furthermore, aCGH analysis revealed a homozygous deletion encompassing the *Cdkn2a/Arf* locus (Fig. 4B).

Discussion

Previous studies have shown that *Arf*(−/−) and *Ink4a*(−/−) mice are more prone to spontaneous tumors than wild-type animals, but each less so than *Ink4a;Arf*(−/−) mice [8]. The *in vivo* carcinogenesis studies reported here evaluated the contribution of heterozygous mutations of *Arf* and *Ink4a*, as well as a both tumor suppressor genes, to the induction of MM by asbestos, a well-established cause of this malignancy. *In vivo* genetic models were used to investigate the relative impact of *Arf* versus *Ink4a* deficiency in a common genetic background. By analogy, our findings suggest that *p14(ARF)*, like *p16(INK4A)*, is an important target of 9p21 deletions in human MM. Moreover, the data indicate that co-deletion of *Arf* and *Ink4a* can cooperate to accelerate tumorigenesis.

In previous studies of heterozygous *Arf* mice, spontaneous tumors exhibited loss of the residual wild-type *Arf* allele [2], consistent with a classical two-hit tumor suppressor gene. We found asbestos-induced MMs from heterozygous *Ink4a*, *Arf* and *Ink4a;Arf* mice required biallelic inactivation of the predisposing tumor suppressor genes, and MMs were detected faster in the

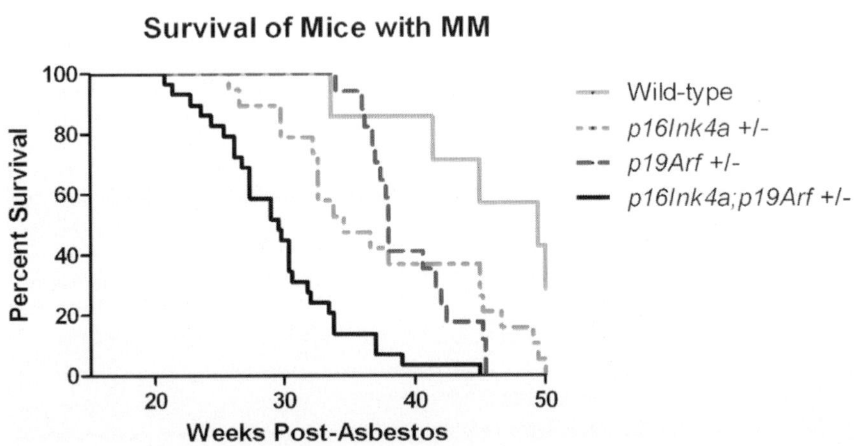

Figure 1. Accelerated asbestos-induced MM in mice deficient for *Ink4a, Arf,* or *Ink4a;Arf.* Kaplan-Meier survival curves (GraphPad Prism 5). Mice with no tumors or with incidental tumors were censored. A log-rank test verified significant differences between wild-type and *Ink4a-*, *Arf-* and *Ink4a;Arf*-deficient groups (p-value = 0.0342, 0.0312, and <0.0001, respectively).

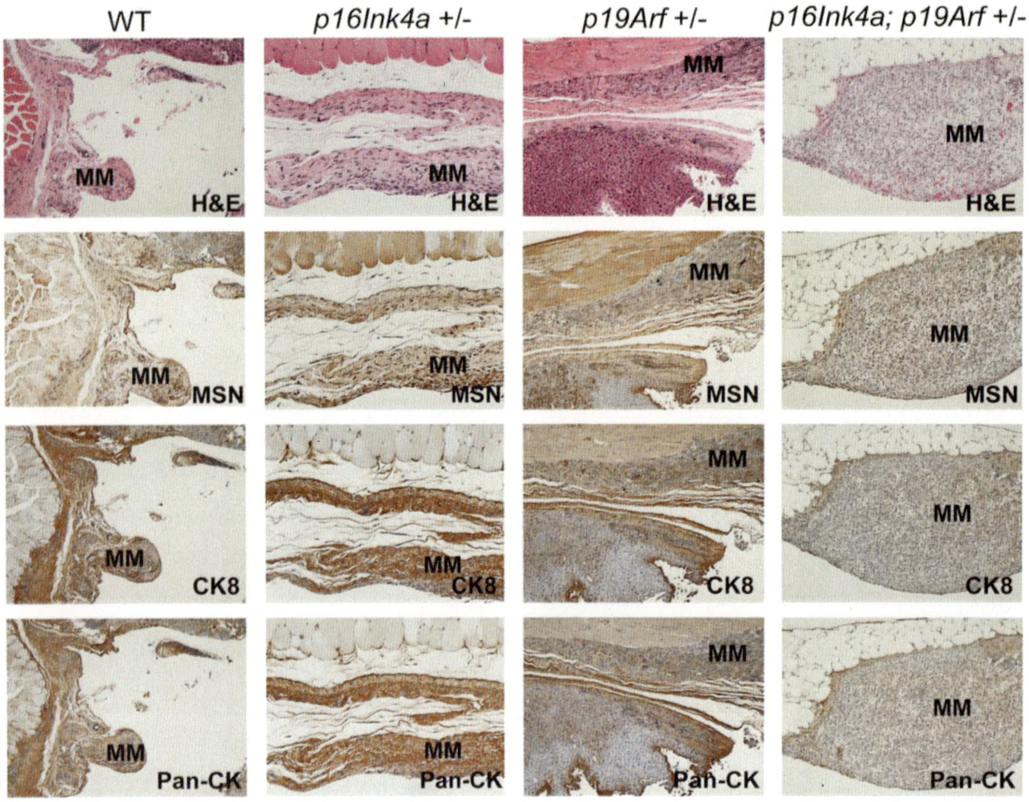

Figure 2. Representative histopathology of asbestos-induced MMs. Sections were stained with hematoxylin and eosin (H&E) or with antibodies against mesothelin (MSN), cytokeratin (CK8), and pan-cytokeratin (Pan-CK).

doubly deficient model. The importance of these tumor suppressors is in accordance with an investigation using conditional knockout mice [9], in which adeno-Cre-mediated homozygous excision of *Ink4a;Arf* was sufficient to induce MM in the absence of asbestos exposure.

Notably, while tumor cells from *Ink4a*(+/−)-deficient mice acquired loss of Arf or p53 expression, loss of p16(Ink4a) was observed in only 3 of 6 MMs from *Arf*(+/−) mice. Similarly, in our earlier studies of *Arf*-deficient mice in a different (C57Bl/6) genetic background, all 11 MMs analyzed showed loss of Arf, although loss of p16(Ink4a) was identified in only two tumors. Collectively, these data imply that inactivation of Arf or p53 may be crucial for MM pathogenesis, whereas inactivation of p16(Ink4a) is not.

Since MMs analyzed here retained expression of p15Ink4b, loss of this gene is not critical for induction of MM by asbestos. In addition, our deletion mapping studies of human MMs revealed that deletions of *p15INK4B* occur less frequently than losses of *CDKN2A/ARF* and never occurred in the absence of a homozygous loss in the *CDKN2A/ARF* locus [5].

Also similar to our earlier study of *Arf*-deficient mice in a different (C57Bl/6) background, we rarely observed loss of Nf2 in MMs arising in *Ink4a*-, *Arf*- or *Ink4a;Arf*-deficient mice. Inactivation of the *NF2* tumor suppressor gene is postulated to facilitate cell cycle progression and tissue invasion/metastasis [10], and *Nf2*-deficient mice are predisposed to asbestos-induced MM and contribute to its invasiveness and spreading [5,11]. However, NF2/merlin loss does not appear to be required for development of MM in mice having this genotype and/or background.

Lastly, we found retention of functional p53 expression in MM cells that exhibit loss of Arf expression. Only one of the 20 asbestos-induced MMs showed loss of p53 expression (Fig. 3B), and that single sample retained expression of Arf, consistent with our previous work showing a reciprocal pattern of inactivation of Tp53 in asbestos-induced MMs from *Nf2*(+/−) mice that had retained expression of Arf [5,6]. Interestingly, in MM cells with loss of Arf, the p53 pathway appeared to remain functional based on response to DNA damage (Fig. 3C). These results from genetic model systems suggest that Arf loss can contribute to MM pathogenesis via p53-independent pathway(s), as previously noted in human MM cells [12], and that an intact p53 pathway remains a potential target for the treatment of this highly aggressive, chemo-resistant malignancy.

In summary, this is the first report directly assessing the relative importance of *Ink4a* and *Arf* in the susceptibility to asbestos-induced MM. Collectively, these *in vivo* data indicate that both *Cdkn2A/Arf* gene products suppress asbestos carcinogenicity. Furthermore, while Arf inactivation appears to be critical for MM pathogenesis and genomic instability (Fig. 4), the inactivation of both *p16(Ink4a)* and *p19(Arf)* cooperate to accelerate asbestos-induced tumorigenesis. Thus, future therapeutic approaches for MM should consider targeting pathways cooperatively regulated by both tumor suppressor genes.

Materials and Methods

Animals and treatments

Ink4a (01XE4, FVB.129-$Cdkn2a^{tm2.1Rdp}$) [3] and *Ink4a;Arf* (01XB2, FVB/N.129-$Cdkn2a^{tm1Rdp}$) [4] mice were from the Mouse

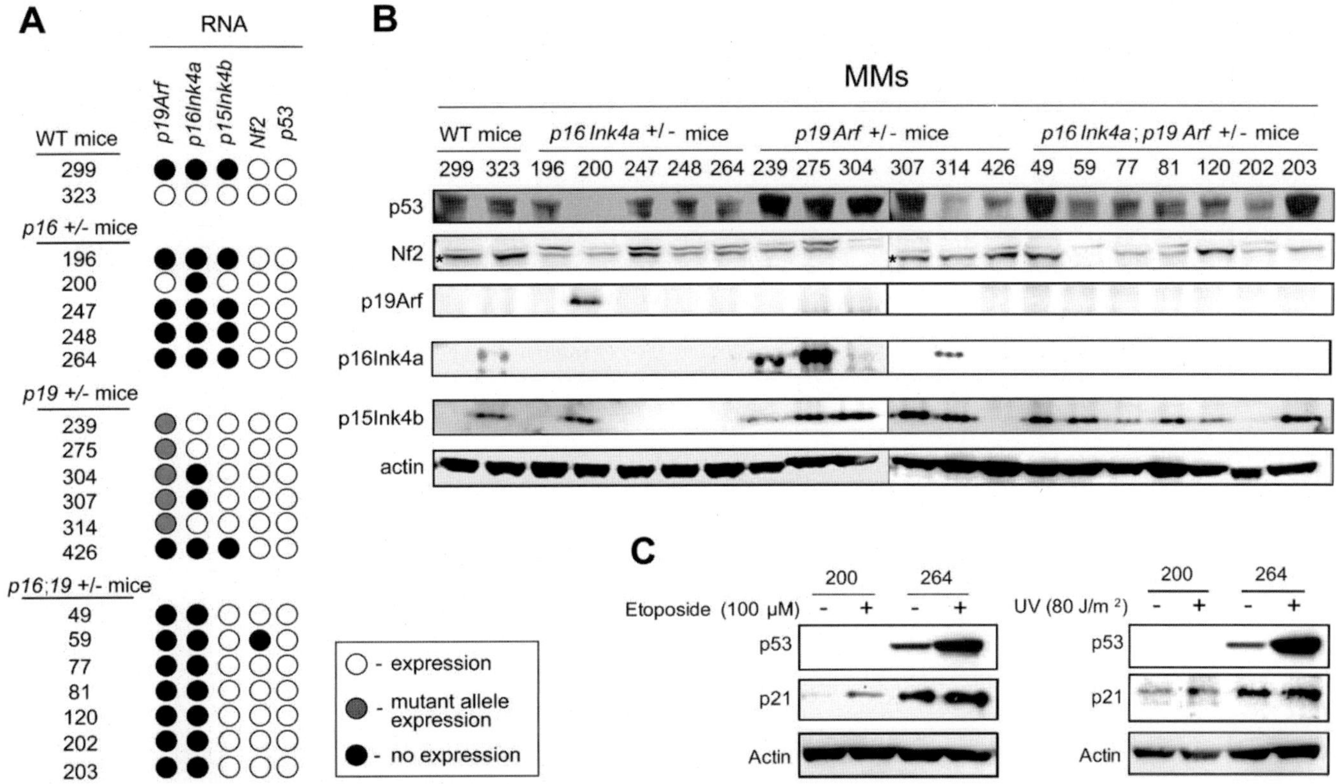

Figure 3. Biallelic inactivation of predisposing *Ink4a* and *Arf* tumor suppressor genes in MM. *A*, Composite depicting RT-PCR for *Arf* exon 1β, *Ink4a* exon 1α, *Ink4b*, *Nf2* and *Tp53* from primary MM cells (passage ≤5). *B*, Immunoblotting of MM cells. Note that Arf was lost in nearly all tumors, with p53 expression being absent in the only tumor (#200) retaining Arf expression. Two bands were observed in the Nf2 immunoblot (panel 3). An asterisk beside the lower band depicts Nf2, with a non-specific band accounting for the upper signal. Actin was a loading control. *C*, Immunoblot of MM cells treated with Etoposide (100 μM) or UV irradiation (80 J/m^2) 24 hours post-treatment.

Models of Human Cancers Consortium. Mice lacking *Arf* (a gift of N. Sharpless) were generated with Cre-mediated excision of the neomycin selection cassette, similar to *Ink4a* mice [3]. All mice were in a comparable genetic background [8]. Mice were backcrossed at least two additional generations with FVB/N mice for uniformity and genotyped as described (MMHCC and [8]). Procedures were compliant with the NIH *Guide for the Care and Use of Laboratory Animals*.

6–8 week-old mice were injected intraperitoneally every 3 weeks with 400 μg crocidolite (UICC, SPI Supplies) (total, 3.2 mg/mouse), or with equivalent control TiO_2 particles (Aldrich) [5,6]. Mice were scored as having MM based on histological evidence and/or if tumor cells exhibited a combination of three or more MM markers, including mesothelin, as assessed by reverse transcriptase-PCR (RT-PCR) and/or immunohistochemistry (Supplemental tables in File S1, Supplemental Fig. S1). This study was carried out in strict accordance with the recommendations in the Guide for the Care and Use of Laboratory Animals of the National Institutes of Health. The protocol was approved by the Committee on the Ethics of Animal Experiments of the Fox Chase Cancer Center (protocol number: 00-26). All surgery was performed under sodium pentobarbital anesthesia, and all efforts were made to minimize suffering.

Immunohistochemistry

Slides of formalin-fixed, paraffin-embedded samples were incubated with antibodies against pan-cytokeratin and cytokeratin 8 (Sigma) and mesothelin (Santa Cruz Biotechnology), which were detected with biotinylated secondary antibodies. Sections were stained with DAB and counterstained with hematoxylin.

Primary cell cultures. Primary MM cells were isolated from ascitic fluid and/or peritoneal lavage, as described [5]. All primary cell cultures used for the molecular analyses were from passages ≤6. PCR analysis was conducted on all cultures that expressed mesothelial markers, and immunoblot analysis was performed on a random set of cultures to validate the PCR results. To test for p53, sub-confluent mouse MM cells (>passage 6) were treated with Etoposide (100 μM) or UV irradiation (80 J/m^2) and harvested 24 hours post-treatment for immunoblotting.

PCR

RT-PCR was used to evaluate tumor cells for expression of E-cadherin, N-cadherin, cytokeratin 18 and cytokeratin 19 [5]. Control *Gapdh* was used to assess template integrity [6]. RT-PCR for mesothelin used primers 5′-ATCAAGACATTCCTGGGTGGG-3′ and 5′-CGGTTAAAGCTGGGAGCAGAG-3′. Oligonucleotides for genomic and RT-PCR of *Ink4a*, *Ink4b*, *Nf2* and *p53* were as described [5,6]. Primers for *p19(Arf)* exon 1β were based on National Center of Biotechnology Information (NCBI) sequences.

Immunoblotting

Immunoblots were prepared with 15–30 μg of protein/sample, as described [5,6]. Antibodies included anti-Arf (Abcam), anti-p53 (NCL-p53-505, Novocastra), and anti-Ink4a (M-156), -Nf2 (H-260), and -β-actin (I-19) (Santa Cruz).

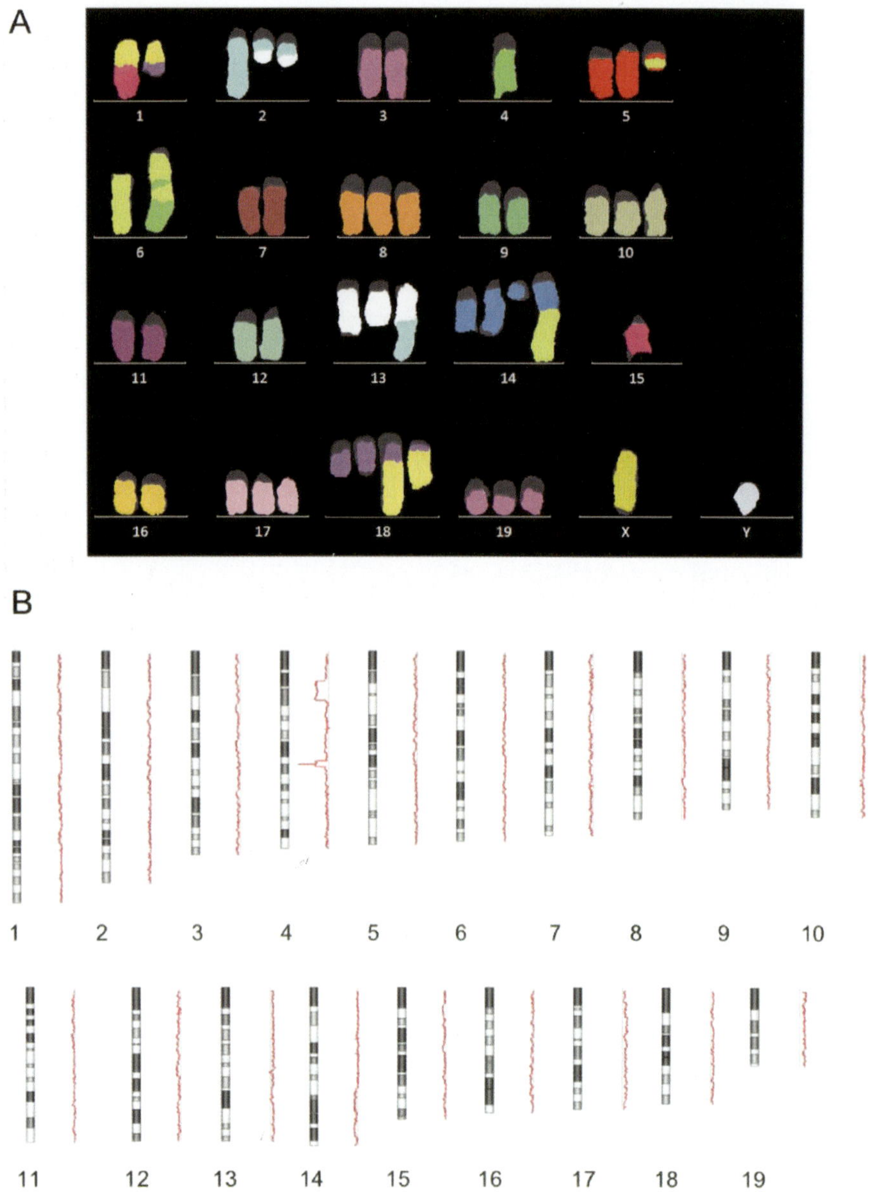

Figure 4. Chromosomal analyses of MM cells from an *Arf*-deficient mouse. *A*, mFISH revealed one or more copies of 1;15, 1;18, 2;13, 5;6, and 6;14 rearrangements; der(6) composed of (from centromere to telomere) segments of chromosomes 6, 4, 6, and 4; deletion of chromosome 14; and trisomies of chromosomes 8, 10, 17 and 19. *B*, aCGH analysis showed gains of chromosomes 8, 10, 13, 17, 18, and 19; and deletions of two regions of chromosome 4, one of which (*lower*) represents a homozygous deletion encompassing the *Cdkn2a/Arf* locus embedded within a hemizygous deletion.

Karyotypic and M-FISH Analysis

Preparation of metaphases and G-banding were performed as reported [13]. Guidelines for karyotypic designations of mouse metaphase chromosomes are found at http://www.pathology.washington.edu/research/cytopages/idiograms/mouse/. Metaphase preparations were hybridized using a 21Xmouse mFISH kit (MetaSystems). Image capturing/processing utilized a Zeiss AxioImager Z2 fluorescence microscope, with single band pass filters (Chroma Technology) appropriate for each fluorochrome and an Isis/mFISH image analysis system (MetaSystems).

Array-CGH

Genomic DNA was isolated from primary MM cell cultures at passages ≤6. Agilent 244K Genomic DNA Arrays and scanner were used for DNA copy number analysis. Data were extracted using Feature Extraction Software, and output was imported into CGH Analytics for DNA Copy Number Analysis (Agilent).

Supporting Information

Figure S1 Immunohistochemical staining of a MM tumor with anti-mesothelin (MSN) or anti-MSN plus blocking peptide to show specificity of staining.
(TIF)

Figure S2 Retention of mutant *Arf* allele in MMs from *Arf* (+/−) mice. *A*, Abnormally large RT-PCR product amplified with *Arf*-specific primers for exon 1β. Samples are from MM cells of five *Arf*

(+/−) mice (lanes 1–5); lane 6 is from wild-type mouse embryonic fibroblasts. *B*, Sequencing of PCR products revealed an 84-bp insertion (grey italicized letters) in the mutated *Arf* allele (Mu.) replacing an AG (underlined) in the wild-type allele (Wt.). The insertion generates a predicted stop codon (marked in black), which would result in unsuccessful translation of the p19(Arf) protein.
(TIF)

File S1 MM Markers for primary cell cultures derived from asbestos-treated mice.
(DOC)

Acknowledgments

The following Fox Chase Cancer Center shared facilities were used: Laboratory Animal, Biostatistics, Biotechnology, Cell Culture, and Genomics.

Author Contributions

Conceived and designed the experiments: DAA CWM JRT. Performed the experiments: DAA CWM JX JP LZ AT EN-D ZL IC. Analyzed the data: DAA CWM JP IC MC AJK-S JRT. Wrote the paper: DAA CWM JRT.

References

1. Kamijo T, Zindy F, Roussel MF, Quelle DE, Downing JR, et al. (1997) Tumor suppression at the mouse INK4a locus mediated by the alternative reading frame product p19[ARF]. Cell 91: 649–659.
2. Kamijo T, Bodner S, van de Kamp E, Randle DH, Sherr CJ (1999) Tumor spectrum in *ARF*-deficient mice. Cancer Res 59: 2217–2222.
3. Sharpless NE, Bardeesy N, Lee KH, Carrasco D, Castrillon DH, et al. (2001) Loss of p16Ink4a with retention of p19Arf predisposes mice to tumorigenesis. Nature 413: 86–91.
4. Serrano M, Lee H-W, Chin L, Cordon-Cardo C, Beach D, et al. (1996) Role of the *INK4a* locus in tumor suppression and cell mortality. Cell 85: 27–37.
5. Altomare DA, Vaslet CA, Skele KL, De Rienzo A, Devarajan K, et al. (2005) A mouse model recapitulating molecular features of human mesothelioma. Cancer Res 65: 8090–8095.
6. Altomare DA, Menges CW, Pei J, Zhang L, Skele-Stump KL, et al. (2009) Activated TNF-alpha/NF-kappaB signaling via down-regulation of Fas-associated factor 1 in asbestos-induced mesotheliomas from Arf knockout mice. Proc Natl Acad Sci U S A 106: 3430–3435.
7. Heintz NH, Janssen-Heininger YM, Mossman BT (2010) Asbestos, lung cancers, and mesotheliomas: from molecular approaches to targeting tumor survival pathways. Am J Respir Cell Mol Biol 42: 133–139.
8. Sharpless NE, Ramsey MR, Balasubramanian P, Castrillon DH, DePinho RA (2004) The differential impact of p16(INK4a) or p19(ARF) deficiency on cell growth and tumorigenesis. Oncogene 23: 379–385.
9. Jongsma J, van Montfort E, Vooijs M, Zevenhoven J, Krimpenfort P, et al. (2008) A conditional mouse model for malignant mesothelioma. Cancer Cell 12: 261–271.
10. Poulikakos PI, Xiao GH, Gallagher R, Jablonski S, Jhanwar SC, et al. (2006) Re-expression of the tumor suppressor NF2/merlin inhibits invasiveness in mesothelioma cells and negatively regulates FAK. Oncogene 25.
11. Fleury-Feith J, Lecomte C, Renier A, Matrat M, Kheuang L, et al. (2003) Hemizygosity of Nf2 is associated with increased susceptibility to asbestos-induced peritoneal tumours. Oncogene 22: 3799–3805.
12. Hopkins-Donaldson S, Belyanskaya LL, Simões-Wüst AP, Sigrist B, Kurtz S, et al. (2006) p53-induced apoptosis occurs in the absence of p14(ARF) in malignant pleural mesothelioma. Neoplasia 8: 551–559.
13. Testa JRGL, Salazar H, Liu Z, Handel LM, Godwin AK, Hamilton TC (1994) Spontaneous transformation of rat ovarian surface epithelial cells results in well to poorly differentiated tumors with a parallel range of cytogenetic complexity. Cancer Res 54: 2778–2784.

12

A High Degree of LINE-1 Hypomethylation Is a Unique Feature of Early-Onset Colorectal Cancer

Marina Antelo[1], Francesc Balaguer[2,3]*, Jinru Shia[4], Yan Shen[2], Keun Hur[2], Leticia Moreira[3], Miriam Cuatrecasas[3], Luis Bujanda[5], Maria Dolores Giraldez[3], Masanobu Takahashi[2], Ana Cabanne[1], Mario Edmundo Barugel[1], Mildred Arnold[2], Enrique Luis Roca[1], Montserrat Andreu[6], Sergi Castellvi-Bel[3], Xavier Llor[7], Rodrigo Jover[8], Antoni Castells[3], C. Richard Boland[2], Ajay Goel[2]*

1 Oncology and Pathology Sections, Hospital of Gastroenterology "Dr. C. B. Udaondo", Buenos Aires, Argentina, **2** Department of Internal Medicine, Division of Gastroenterology, Charles A. Sammons Cancer Center and Baylor Research Institute, Baylor University Medical Center, Dallas, Texas, United States of America, **3** Department of Gastroenterology, Hospital Clínic, Centro de Investigación Biomédica en Red de Enfermedades Hepáticas y Digestivas (CIBERehd), Institut d'Investigacions Biomediques August Pi i Sunyer (IDIBAPS), University of Barcelona, Barcelona, Catalonia, Spain, **4** Department of Pathology, Memorial Sloan Kettering Cancer Center, New York, New York, United States of America, **5** Department of Gastroenterology, CIBERehd, University of Country Basque, Donostia Hospital, San Sebastián, Spain, **6** Deparment of Gastroenterology, Hospital del Mar, Barcelona, Spain, **7** Department of Medicine and Cancer Center, University of Illinois at Chicago, Chicago, Illinois, United States of America, **8** Gastroenterology Unit, Hospital General Universitario, Alicante, Spain

Abstract

Objective: Early-onset colorectal cancer (CRC) represents a clinically distinct form of CRC that is often associated with a poor prognosis. Methylation levels of genomic repeats such as LINE-1 elements have been recognized as independent factors for increased cancer-related mortality. The methylation status of LINE-1 elements in early-onset CRC has not been analyzed previously.

Design: We analyzed 343 CRC tissues and 32 normal colonic mucosa samples, including 2 independent cohorts of CRC diagnosed ≤50 years old (n = 188), a group of sporadic CRC >50 years (MSS n = 89; MSI n = 46), and a group of Lynch syndrome CRCs (n = 20). Tumor mismatch repair protein expression, microsatellite instability status, LINE-1 and *MLH1* methylation, somatic *BRAF* V600E mutation, and germline *MUTYH* mutations were evaluated.

Results: Mean LINE-1 methylation levels (±SD) in the five study groups were early-onset CRC, 56.6% (8.6); sporadic MSI, 67.1% (5.5); sporadic MSS, 65.1% (6.3); Lynch syndrome, 66.3% (4.5) and normal mucosa, 76.5% (1.5). Early-onset CRC had significantly lower LINE-1 methylation than any other group ($p<0.0001$). Compared to patients with <65% LINE-1 methylation in tumors, those with ≥65% LINE-1 methylation had significantly better overall survival ($p = 0.026$, log rank test).

Conclusions: LINE-1 hypomethylation constitutes a potentially important feature of early-onset CRC, and suggests a distinct molecular subtype. Further studies are needed to assess the potential of LINE-1 methylation status as a prognostic biomarker for young people with CRC.

Editor: Anthony W.I. Lo, The Chinese University of Hong Kong, Hong Kong

Funding: The present work was supported by grants R01 CA72851 and CA129286 from the National Cancer Institute, National Institutes of Health; and funds from the Baylor Research Institute to CRB and AG. FB was supported by a grant from Fundación Alfonso Martín Escudero and from Instituto de Salud Carlos III (PI10/00384). MA was supported by a "Type I Postgraduate Scholarship" given by the CONICET (National Council of Scientific and Technical Investigations) dependent on the Argentine Ministry of Science and Technology. The funders had no role in study design, data collection and analysis, decision to publish, or preparation of the manuscript.

Competing Interests: The authors have declared that no competing interests exist.

* E-mail: ajay.goel@baylorhealth.edu (AG); fprunes@clinic.ub.es (FB)

Introduction

Colorectal cancer (CRC) is an important public health problem and represents the second most frequent cancer and the second greatest cause cancer-related mortality in most of the developed world. Each year, one million people develop CRC, and 40–50% of them will die within 5 years of diagnosis [1]. CRCs are highly heterogeneous both histopathologically, and at the molecular and genetic level. It appears that the biology and response to therapies is equally diverse. Understanding the molecular mechanisms of colorectal carcinogenesis is essential for the development of new strategies for prevention, diagnosis, treatment and prognosis. Although CRC has been a major focus of attention for basic and clinical research during the last 25 years, we still lack robust biomarkers that can be used for diagnosis and treatment of CRC.

The peak incidence of CRC is between 60–70 years old; however up to 10% of all cases occur before age 50. Moreover, recent epidemiological studies suggest that the incidence of early-onset CRC is increasing, representing an important clinical challenge [2]. Early-onset CRC often presents with advanced stage tumors, which contributes to a higher rate of mortality [3]. Since young people are not included in CRC screening programs, there is an urgent need to understand the biology of early-onset tumors, which could facilitate earlier detection and treatment of these cancers.

Although early-onset CRC raises the possibility of a hereditary risk factor, the known non-polyposis hereditary CRC syndromes (Lynch Syndrome and *MUTYH*-associated CRC) represents no more than 15–20% of cases in this group [4,5,6]. Lynch Syndrome accounts for about 3% of all CRC cases, and is caused by germline mutations of the DNA mismatch repair (MMR) genes (*MLH1, MSH2, MSH6* and *PMS2*) [7]. It is characterized by early-onset cancers arising in the colorectum and other organs, and there are currently several strategies and algorithms to predict the presence of a germline mutation in one of the MMR genes [8,9,10,11]. Biallelic mutations in the *MUTYH* gene (a member of the base excision repair system) accounts for<1% of all CRC, and usually causes an attenuated form of polyposis, although 30% of these patients can manifest as a non-polyposis CRC [12].Identifying individuals with germline mutations that predispose to CRC has significant implications for the clinical management of affected individuals and for their relatives.

The remaining 75–80% of early-onset CRC represents another group in which the genetic etiology has not yet been discovered. In contrast to CRC on older individuals, early-onset CRC is often characterized by more advanced stage, distal location (especially in rectum), mucinous and poorly differentiated tumors with signet ring cells, and a poorer prognosis [4,13,14]. The majority of these cancers do not show microsatellite instability (MSI), but rather are microsatellite stable (MSS). The molecular basis for the biological and behavioral differences in early-onset CRC is unclear.

Genome-wide DNA hypomethylation is a frequent epigenetic alteration that is an early event in CRC and has been associated with the activation of certain proto-oncogenes (i.e. MET) [15] and the presence of chromosomal instability [16,17]. Global DNA hypomethylation can be measured indirectly by assessing the methylation status of long interspersed nucleotide element-1 (LINE-1) repeat sequences [18]. The pyrosequencing assay for LINE-1 methylation has been found to be quantitative, robust and reproducible [19]. The degree of LINE-1 hypomethylation has been recognized as an independent factor for increased cancer-related mortality and overall mortality in CRC patients [20]. Although it has been suggested that LINE-1 hypomethylation is associated with CRC in younger patients [21], the specific association between methylation status of LINE-1 elements and early-onset CRC has not been further analyzed.

The aim of this study was to characterize the clinical, histological, and molecular features of a large cohort of early-onset CRCs in the context of the methylation status of LINE-1 elements. Our results indicate that LINE-1 hypomethylation in these tumors constitutes a unique and specific feature, which is suggestive of a distinct molecular subtype in these colorectal neoplasms. Our findings suggest that LINE-1 methylation status could be used as a prognostic biomarker for young people with CRC.

Patients and Methods

Ethics Statement

The study was approved by the Institutional Review Boards (IRB) of each participating center, including Hospital of Gastroenterology "Dr. C. B. Udaondo", Buenos Aires, Argentina, Baylor University Medical Center, Dallas, TX and the Epicolon consortium. A written informed consent was obtained from all patients.

Patients

We analyzed 343 CRCs from different clinic-pathological groups, and 32 normal colonic mucosa samples. We included a cohort of 118 retrospectively recruited CRC patients ≤50 years old seen at the Oncology Section of the Argentine Public Hospital of Gastroenterology between 1993 and 2009. Patients with colorectal polyposis or inflammatory bowel disease were excluded. Demographic and clinic-pathological features were collected from each patient's medical history, and family history of cancer in first and second degree relatives was obtained by personal interview. The median follow-up time was 39 months (range, 1.5–195 months). For the LINE-1 methylation analyses, as a validation group, we included a previously described cohort of 70 patients with CRC diagnosed ≤50 years old treated at two Spanish centers (Hospital Clinic of Barcelona and Hospital of Donostia) between 1995–2007 [4]. We also included a population-based cohort of sporadic CRCs>50 years recruited in Spain (Epicolon I study) [9] categorized by the presence of MSI ("sporadic MSI" due to somatic *MLH1* promoter hypermethylation [n = 46], and "sporadic MSS" [n = 89]); and a group of Lynch syndrome CRCs recruited at Baylor University Medical Center at Dallas (n = 20). We histologically analyzed normal colonic mucosa from 32 individuals undergoing colonic surgery for reasons other than cancer (i.e. diverticulosis) recruited in the Hospital Clinic of Barcelona, Spain.

DNA Isolation

Genomic DNA from each patient were extracted from formalin-fixed paraffin-embedded (FFPE) microdissected tumor tissues using the QiaAmp Tissue Kit (Qiagen, Courtaboeuf, France) according to the manufacturers' instructions. Peripheral blood DNA was extracted using the QiaAmpDNA blood Mini Kit (Qiagen, Courtaboeuf, France). For rectal tumors in which chemo-radiotherapy was administered, pre-treatment tissue samples were analyzed.

Tumor Mismatch Repair Protein Expression

One block of FFPE tumor tissue was selected per case and immunostaining was performed using standard protocols. The following mouse monoclonal antibodies were used: anti-MLH1 (clone G168-728, diluted 1:250, PharMingen, San Diego, CA), anti-MSH2 (clone FE11, diluted 1:50, Oncogene ResearchProducts, Cambridge, MA), anti-MSH6(clone GRBP.P1/2.D4, diluted 1:200; Serotec Inc, Raleigh, NC) and anti-PMS2 (clone A16-4, diluted 1:200, BD PharMingen, San Diego, CA). A tumor was deemed negative for protein expression only if the neoplastic epithelium lacked nuclear staining, while non-neoplastic epithelial or stromal cells retained normal expression of that protein.

Tumor Microsatellite Instability Analysis

MSI analysis was carried out using five mononucleotide repeat microsatellite targets (BAT-25, BAT-26, NR-21, NR-24 and NR-27) in a pentaplex PCR system. Primer sequences have been described previously [22]. Tumors with instability at ≥3 these markers were classified as microsatellite unstable (MSI) and those showing instability at ≤2 markers as microsatellite stable (MSS). The researchers scoring immunostaining were blinded to the MSI results, and vice versa.

Methylation Analyses

DNA was modified with sodium-bisulfite using the EZ Methylation Gold Kit (Zymo Research, Orange, CA). Methylation of LINE-1 sequences and the promoter of *MLH1* was analyzed by quantitative bisulfite pyrosequencing as described previously [23]. Primers are detailed in **Table S1**.

Germline MUTYH Gene Mutation Analysis

All patients were screened for the two most prevalent *MUTYH* mutations in Caucasian populations (p.G393D and p.Y176C) by pyrosequencing. Primers are detailed in **Table S1**. In heterozygotes for any of these mutations, the coding region and exon-intron boundaries of the *MUTYH* gene were screened by SSCP with sequencing of abnormal band shifts, as described previously [12].

Somatic BRAF V600Emutation Analysis

The *BRAF* V600E mutational analysis was performed by pyrosequencing. The PCR and sequencing primers are detailed in **Table S1**.

Statistical Analysis

Quantitative variables were compared using Student's test. Qualitative variables were compared using either the Chi Square or the Fisher's test when appropriate. For associations with MMR deficiency and LINE-1 methylation (treated as a binary variable) a multivariate analysis using a stepwise backward logistic regression procedure was performed to assess the independent associations. The Mann Whitney test was used to compare LINE-1 values. Overall survival associated with clinic-pathological and molecular variables (tumor stage, MMR deficiency, tumor location, family history of CRC, tumor differentiation, mucinous component, tumor infiltrating lymphocytes and LINE-1 methylation) were calculated by the Kaplan–Meier method (log rank test). A two sided p-value of <0.05 was regarded as significant. SPSS v17 software was used for statistical analysis.

Results

Patient's Characteristics

We recruited 118 patients with early-onset CRC. Clinico-pathological features are shown in **Table 1**. The mean age at diagnosis was 37 years (standard deviation (SD), 8.25), and 61 (51.7%) patients were female. In 34 (28.8%) the tumor was proximal to the splenic flexure, 35 (29.6%) were in the distal colon, and 49 (41.6%) were in the rectum. At presentation, 22 (18.6%) patients had 1–10 synchronous adenomas; 18 presented with 1–5 adenomas and 4 patients had 6–10 adenomas. Three cases (2.5%) had a synchronous tumor (2 CRC and 1 neuroendocrine tumor in the appendix), and 5 (4.2%) developed a metachronous tumor during follow-up (4 CRC and 1 urothelial carcinoma). The majority of cases (77; 65.3%) were diagnosed at advanced stages (III-IV). Poorly differentiated tumors were seen in 15 (13.1%) patients, 41 (34.7%) had mucinous features and 65 (55%) had pathological features suggestive of the MSI phenotype, with one or more of the following: signet ring cells, Crohn's-like lymphocytic reaction, tumor infiltrating lymphocytes, medullary growth pattern, or anaplastic features. More than 85% (n = 100) of the patients had experienced abdominal pain prior to diagnosis, 83 (70%) presented with an alteration in bowel habits, 71 (60%) had rectal bleeding and weight loss, 34 (29%) had iron deficiency anemia, 18 (15.5%) presented with bowel obstruction, and 6 (5%) with perforation. The average delay between initial symptoms and CRC diagnosis was 6.5±5 months. Fifteen patients (12.7%) had a family history of CRC or another Lynch syndrome-associated neoplasm in first or second-degree relatives. Three patients met Amsterdam I criteria, 3 patients met Amsterdam II criteria, 4 patients had one first degree relative with CRC, 3 patients had two or more second degree relatives with CRC, and 2 patients had one second degree relative with CRC.

Germline MUTYH Gene Mutation Analysis

Biallelic MUTYH mutations were found in 1/91 MMR-proficient cases (1.1%)(**Table S2**). This single case was a 29-year-old patient with a stage III rectal cancer and 2 synchronous adenomas. Two siblings of this patient had a history of attenuated polyposis and CRC (one presented with 30 adenomas and the other with 8 adenomas and an *in situ* carcinoma in the cecum); in both siblings total colectomies had been performed. Finally, we identified two p.G393D heterozygous patients that had no specific clinico-pathological features (**Table S2**).

Mismatch Repair Deficiency Analysis

MMR deficiency was evaluated by MSI analysis and immunohistochemistry, and was defined by the presence of MSI in a tumor, and/or loss of expression in any of the MMR proteins. Twenty seven (22.9%) tumors were classified as MMR deficient, and 25 of these showed loss of protein expression (8 for MLH1/PMS2, 1 for isolated MLH1, 4 for isolated PMS2, 11 for MSH2/MSH6, and 1 for isolated MSH6). Clinico-pathological features of patients with MMR deficiency are summarized in **Table 2**.

Nearly all cases of MSI had loss of protein expression; two cases with MSI retained normal expression of all four proteins. Likewise, 1 case with loss of MSH6 expression and one case with loss of PMS2 were MSS. The last patient was a 24 year-old woman who had CRC at age 15, a urothelial carcinoma at age 23, a metachronous CRC at age 24, and finally, a mediastinal B-cell lymphoma. Her CRC specimen showed loss of expression of PMS2 in tumor cells and in normal colonic surrounding tissue, leading to a presumptive diagnosis of constitutional MMR-deficiency syndrome due to bi-allelic PMS2 mutations.

As shown in **Table 1**, compared to MMR-proficient tumors, MMR-deficient tumors were more likely to be located in the proximal colon (59.3% *vs.* 19.8%, p = 0.0001), to be mucinous (63% *vs.* 26.4%, p = 0.0001), to have tumor infiltrating lymphocytes (59.3% *vs.* 11.5%, p = 0.0001), and to have MSI-suggestive pathology (81.5% *vs.* 47.2%, p = 0.002). MMR deficient tumors were also more likely to be diagnosed at a lower stage (stages I–II: 51.9% *vs.* 29.7%, p = 0.03), and to have less tumor recurrence or progression (22.2% *vs.* 44%, p = 0.042). Multivariate analysis showed that independent variables associated with MMR deficiency were: proximal location (OR = 3.86 [95%CI: 1.32–11.32]; p = 0.013), mucinous features (OR = 3.38 [95%CI: 1.16–9.84]; p = 0.025) and presence of tumor infiltrating lymphocytes (OR = 8.8 [95%CI: 2.93–26.31]; p = 0.0001). Although there was no difference in the age of CRC diagnosis between the 2 groups, the chance of having a MMR-deficient tumor was greater among younger patients (12–30 years: 8/27, 29.6%; 31–40 years: 9/45, 20%, 41–50 years: 10/46, 21.7%).

Somatic *BRAF* mutation was present in one MMR-deficient tumor (**Table 2**). This case was a 49-year-old male with an MSI tumor in the cecum that showed loss of MLH1 and PMS2 protein expression. This case showed high degree of *MLH1* promoter methylation (88%) and was therefore likely associated with CpG island methylator phenotype (CIMP) [24]. In the rest of the*MLH1*-deficient tumors, presumably carriers of *MLH1* germline mutations, 4 showed very low levels of methylation (range, 1–2%), and the other 4 showed intermediate levels (range, 25–51%).

Table 1. Clinical, pathological and molecular features of patients with mismatch repair deficiency.

Clinical, pathological or molecular feature	Cohort N = 118	MMR deficient[1] N = 27 (22.9%)	MMR proficient[2] N = 91 (77.1%)	p-value
Age at diagnosis, mean (standard deviation)	37 (8.25)	35 (10.06)	38 (7.55)	0.23
Age range	(29–45)	(25–45)	(30–45)	
Sex, n (%)				
Female	61 (51.7)	13 (48.1)	48 (52.7)	0.67
Male	57 (48.3)	14 (51.9)	43 (47.3)	
Tumor location, n (%)				
Rectum	49 (41.5)	6 (22.2)	43 (47.3)	0.0001
Distal to splenic flexure	35 (29.7)	5 (18.5)	30 (33)	
Proximal to splenic flexure	34 (28.8)	16 (59.3)	18 (19.8)	
Synchronous or metachronous CRC, n (%)				
Yes	6 (5.1)	3 (11.1)	3 (3.3)	0.132
No	112 (94.9)	24 (88.9)	96.7)	
Synchronous adenomas, n (%)				
0	81 (68.6)	18 (66.7)	63 (69.2)	0.589
1–5	18 (15.2)	6 (22.2)	12 (13.2)	
6–10	4 (3.4)	1 (3.7)	3 (3.3)	
Incomplete colonoscopy	15 (12.8)	2 (7.4)	13 (14.3)	
Synchronous hyperplastic polyps, n (%)				
0	95 (80.5)	24 (86.2)	71 (78.0)	0.644
1–5	7 (6)	1 (6.9)	6 (6.6)	
6–10	1 (0.70)	0 (0)	1 (1.1)	
Incomplete colonoscopy	15 (12.8)	2 (6.9)	13 (14.3)	
Family history of CRC or other Lynch syndrome associated neoplasia[3], n (%)				
Yes	15 (12.7)	5 (18.5)	10 (11.0)	0.30
No	103 (87.3)	22 (81.5)	81 (89.0)	
TNM tumor stage, n (%)				
I–II	41 (34.7)	14 (51.9)	27 (29.7)	0.03
III–IV	77 (65.3)	13 (48.1)	64 (70.3)	
Tumor differentiation, n (%)				
Well or moderate	100 (86.9)	24 (88.9)	76 (86.3)	1
Poor	15 (13.1)	3 (11.1)	12 (13.7)	
Mucinous component, n (%)				
>50%	41 (34.7)	17 (63)	24 (26.4)	0.0001
<50%	77 (65.3)	10 (37)	67 (73.6)	
Tumor infiltrating lymphocytes, n (%)				
Yes	26 (22.8)	16 (59.3)	10 (11.5)	0.0001
No	88 (77.2)	11 (40.7)	77 (88.5)	
Medullary growth pattern, n (%)				
Yes	11 (9.4)	3 (11.1)	8 (8.9)	0.714
No	106 (90.6)	24 (88.9)	82 (91.1)	
Tumors withCrohns reaction, n (%)				
Yes	12 (10.6)	5 (18.5)	7 (8.1)	0.154
No	101 (89.4)	22 (81.5)	79 (91.9)	
Pathology suggestive of MSI[4], n (%)				
Yes	65 (55)	22 (81.5)	43 (47.2)	0.002
No	53 (45)	5 (18.5)	48 (52.8)	
Somatic *BRAF* mutations, n (%)				
Wild-type	108 (96.4)	25 (96.2)	83 (96.5)	1
Mutated	4 (3.6)	1 (3.8)	3 (3.5)	

Table 1. Cont.

Clinical, pathological or molecular feature	Cohort N = 118	MMR deficient[1] N = 27 (22.9%)	MMR proficient[2] N = 91 (77.1%)	p-value
LINE-1 methylation, mean (standard deviation)	59.97 (6.57)	61.26 (6.13)	59.7 (6.68)	0.244
Progression/recurrence				
Yes	46 (39)	6 (22.2)	40 (44)	0.042
No	72 (61)	21 (77.8)	51 (56)	
Three-year overall survival	84.7%%	96.3%	83.5%	0.115

[1]MSI-H and/or loss of expression of MMR proteins by immunohistochemistry.
[2]MSS and normal expression of MMR proteins by immunohistochemistry.
[3]Including first and second degree relatives; Lynch syndrome-associated neoplasia includes: endometrium, stomach, ovaries, urinary tract, small intestine, pancreas, bile ducts, brain or sebaceous glands.
[4]Signet ring cells and/or Crohn's-like lymphocytic reaction and/or tumor infiltrating lymphocytes and/or medullary growth pattern and/or anaplastic tumor.

LINE-1 Methylation Analysis

We used the quantitative bisulfite pyrosequencing method to determine the methylation status of LINE-1 repetitive sequences in the CRCs. The average methylation in the CRCs was 59.97% (standard deviation, 6.57), which followed a normal distribution (**Figure S1**). Clinico-pathological features associated with LINE-1 methylation are shown in **Table 3**. A significant difference in LINE-1 methylation status was found according to tumor location, with lower levels of methylation in distal compared with proximal tumors (59.02% *vs.* 62.3%, p = 0.015). In addition, a trend towards lower levels of methylation was found in females (58.87% *vs.* 60.93, p = 0.092) and in non-mucinous tumors (59.24% *vs.* 61.41%, p = 0.096). No differences in LINE-1 methylation status were found for any of the other clinic-pathological features.

We then compared the LINE-1 methylation levels in this series with another independent cohort of patients with CRC diagnosed at <50 years of age recruited in Spain [4], 2 groups of patients with sporadic CRC diagnosed >50 year-old categorized by the presence or absence of MSI (MSI, n = 46; mean age: 70.2+13.9 years old; and MSS, n = 89; mean age: 70.6±11.4 years old), a group of Lynch Syndrome CRCs (n = 20), and normal colonic mucosa from individuals without tumors (n = 32) (**Figure 1** and **Table 4**). Clinico-pathological features of both cohorts of early-onset CRCs are depicted in **Table S3**. Both cohorts were similar in terms of tumor location and tumor pathological features. As expected, the average LINE-1 methylation levels in normal colonic mucosa were higher than in tumor tissues for all groups. LINE-1 methylation levels in early-onset CRCs was 59.9% (SD, 6.5) and 51.1% (SD, 9.2) for the Argentinian and the Spanish cohorts, respectively. The mean methylation level in the combined cohort of early-onset CRCs (n = 185) was 56.6% (SD, 8.6). Interestingly, tumor LINE-1 methylation levels in the two independent cohorts of early-onset CRC were significantly lower than that observed in older-onset CRCs and Lynch syndrome tumors (**Table 4**), suggesting that this represents a unique feature of this subgroup of tumors (p<0.0001 for all comparisons). LINE-1 hypomethylation levels were similar in older-onset sporadic MSI tumors (67.1%, SD 5.5), Lynch syndrome CRCs (66.3%, SD 4.5), and sporadic MSS tumors (65.1%, SD 6.3).

Survival Analyses

Follow-up was available on all 118 patients, ranging from 1.5 to 195 months, with a mean of 39 months. The 3-year survival rate for all 118 patient in this series was 84.7%; 46 patients (39%) relapsed or had progression of disease, 22 (18.6%) died, and 3 patients were lost to follow-up. Advanced tumor stage was significantly associated with a worse 3-year overall survival (stages I-II: 92.9% vs. stages III-IV: 82.9%;p = 0.046, log rank test) and a trend was observed for better survival in patients with mucinous tumors (95.1% vs. 82.9%; p = 0.077, log rank test) or with tumor infiltrating lymphocytes (96.2% vs. 85.2%; p = 0.16, respectively; log rank test). Patients with MMR-deficient tumors showed a trend towards a better 3-year overall survival (96.3% *vs.* 83.5%; p = 0.1, log rank).

Next, we evaluated the effect of LINE-1 hypomethylation on the overall survival of CRC patients. With the aim of identifying a cut-off value of LINE-1 that could distinguish a group of patients with worse prognosis, several cut-offs starting from the lowest level of LINE-1 methylation were evaluated. We found that in comparison to patients with <65% LINE-1 methylation, those with ≥65% LINE-1 methylation had significantly better overall survival (83.5% vs. 100%; p = 0.026, log rank test; p = 0.039, Fisher's exact test; **Figure 2**). Comparison of clinico-patological and molecular features of patients according to the level of LINE-1 methylation is shown in **Table 5**. Interestingly, tumors with LINE-1 methylation ≥65% were more frequently mucinous (60.9% vs 24.5%, p = 0.003) and those patients had higher frequency of synchronous or metachronous tumors (13% vs 2.2%, p = 0.054). Multivariate analysis showed mucinous tumors as the only variable associated with tumor with LINE-1≥65% (OR = 4.32 (95%CI: 1.65–11.34); p = 0.003), independently of the MMR deficiency status.

Discussion

Several studies have suggested that early-onset CRC constitutes a biologically distinct disease that is frequently associated with advanced stage, distal tumors, and poor prognosis. We and others have shown that the known hereditary cancer syndromes only explain a minority of early-onset CRC cases [2,4,5,13]; consequently, the pathogenic mechanism in the majority of cases remains unknown. In this study we aimed to gain further insight into the pathogenesis of early-onset CRC by assessing the clinic-pathological and molecular features of 118 patients with early-onset CRC. The most interesting and novel result we observed is that LINE-1 hypomethylation constitutes a unique feature of early-onset CRC patients. LINE-1 hypomethylation is a surrogate marker for genome-wide hypomethylation and is associated with increased chromosomal instability [16,17]; therefore, this finding may help explain some of the biological mechanisms underlying early-onset CRC. In addition, we found that the frequency of

Table 2. Clinicopathological and molecular features of patients with MMR deficiency.

Case	Age/Sex	Location	Stage	MSI	Immunohistochemistry*				Other tumors	Family history[2]	*BRAF status*	*MLH1* methylation	LINE-1 methylation (%)
					MLH1	PMS2	MSH2	MSH6				*(%)*	
2ARG	46 F	Ascending	II	MSI	P	P	L	L	Colon (46)	No	wt		53
63ARG	12 M	Rectum	IV	MSI	P	P	L	L	No	No	wt		53
90ARG	19 M	Caecum	IV	MSI	P	P	L	L	No	No	wt		59
24ARG	34 M	Hepatic flexure	I	MSI	P	P	L	L	No	No	wt		69
23ARG	30 F	Sigmoid	III	MSI	P	P	L	L	No	No	ND		71
71ARG	38 F	Rectum	II	MSI	P	P	L	L	No	Pancreas (mother, 52); Colon (uncle, 55); Colon (cousin, 44)	wt		60
16ARG	52 F	Caecum	III	MSI	P	P	L	L	No	No	wt		63
97ARG	54 F	Ascending	II	MSI	P	P	L	L	No	No	wt		59
84ARG	56 M	Rectum	I	MSI	P	P	L	L	Colon (40)	Colon (sister, 37 and 49); Colon (father, 37)	wt		66
62ARG	57 F	Rectum	III	MSI	P	P	L	L	No	No	wt		49
76ARG	53 M	Caecum	II	MSI	P	P	L	L	No	No	wt		51
77ARG	59 F	Ascending	III	MSS	P	P	P	L	No	Colon (grandmother, 65)	wt		62
19ARG	37 F	Caecum	II	MSI	L	L	P	P	No	No	wt	2	66
101ARG	43 F	Descending	II	MSI	L	L	P	P	No	No	wt	27	64
46ARG	42 M	Caecum	II	MSI	L	L	P	P	No	No	wt	25	59
93ARG	33 M	Splenic flexure	II	MSI	L	L	P	P	No	No	wt	1	61
49ARG	43 M	Caecum	II	MSI	L	L	P	P	No	No	wt	26	63
37ARG	49 F	Caecum	III	MSI	L	L	P	P	No	No	mutated	88	64
38ARG	50 M	Descending	III	MSI	L	L	P	P	No	No	wt	2	66
115ARG	55 F	Rectum	II	MSI	L	L	P	P	No	No	wt	51	64
21ARG	15 F	Caecum	III	MSS	P	L	P	P	No	No	wt		71
113ARG	36 M	Descending	III	MSI	P	L	P	P	No	No	wt		47
18ARG	58 M	Hepatic flexure	II	MSI	P	L	P	P	No	No	wt		62
79ARG	51 M	Transverse	III	MSI	P	L	P	P	No	Colon (aunt, 76)	wt		61
108ARG	41 M	Ascending	II	MSI	L	P	P	P	No	No	wt	1	65
112ARG	28 F	Rectum	III	MSI	P	P	P	P	No	No	wt		63
82ARG	26 M	Caecum	III	MSI	P	P	P	P	No	Colon (mother, 52); Colon (aunt, 46)	wt		63

MMR: mismatch repair; MSI: microsatellite instability; MSS: microsatellite stability; ND: not determined; wt: wild-type; P: present; L: loss of expression.
[1]Solid cells indicate loss of protein expression,
[2]Affected relative and age at diagnosis are indicated between parentheses.

Table 3. LINE-1 methylation level in early-onset colorectal cancer.

Clinical, pathological or molecular features	Total (n)*	Mean	Standard deviation	p-value
Sex				
Male	61	60.93	6.598	0.092
Female	54	58.87	6.422	
Age				
>30 years	91	60.26	6.757	0.345
<30 years	24	58.83	5.791	
Body Mass Index (kg/m2)				
<30	100	59.71	6.029	0.728
>30	10	60.4	5.337	
Family history of CRC[1]				
Yes	16	59.68	6.005	0.246
No	99	61.75	9.40	
Tumor location				
Rectum	47	58.3	6.54	0.026
Distal to splenic flexure	35	60	5.46	
Proximal to splenic flexure	33	62.3	7.12	
Synchronous or metachronous CRC				
Yes	5	64.2	6.76	0.141
No	110	59.77	6.52	
TNM tumor stage				
I–II	40	59.63	6.054	0.687
III–IV	75	60.15	6.861	
Tumor differentiation				
Well or moderate	97	60.03	6.555	0.926
Poor	15	60.2	6.527	
Mucinous component				
>50%	39	61.41	5.959	0.096
<50%	75	59.24	6.824	
Medullary growth pattern				
Yes	11	61.36	4.905	0.453
No	103	59.79	6.748	
Crohns reaction				
Yes	12	62.75	3.545	0.128
No	98	59.63	6.908	
Tumor infiltrating lymphocytes				
Yes	26	60.88	5.443	0.447
No	85	59.74	7.004	
Microsatellite instability				
MSI	25	59.72	6.717	0.454
MSS	90	60.84	6.053	
Mismatch repair deficiency[2]				
Yes	27	61.26	6.137	0.244
No	88	59.7	6.680	

P value was calculated by t-test.
*Referred to patients with available information.
[1]Including first and second degree relatives.
[2]MSI-H and/or loss of expression of MMR proteins by immunohistochemistry.

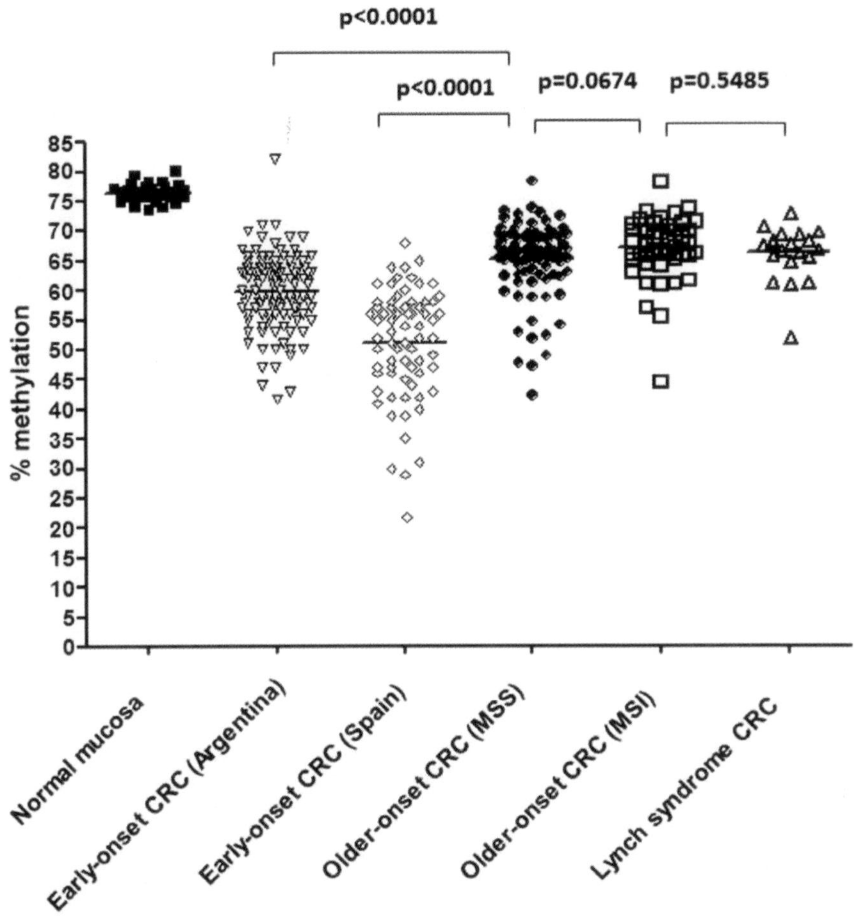

Figure 1. LINE-1 methylation analysis by bisulfite pyrosequencing in different CRC subsets. Bisulfite pyrosequencing of LINE-1 in colorectal tissues; Normal mucosa (n = 32), early-onset CRC from Argentina (n = 116), early-onset CRC from Spain (n = 70), older onset CRC with microsatellite stability (MSS; n = 89), older onset CRC with microsatellite instability (MSI) associated with *MLH1* promoter hypermethylation (n = 46) and Lynch syndrome CRCs (n = 20).The black horizontal bar indicates the mean methylation level.

MMR deficiency in this cohort is ~20%, which is consistent with previous reports that characterized such populations [4,5,6]. Finally, we found that *MUTYH* deficiency accounts for ~1% of MMR-proficient CRCs. This work and the previous work help exclude a number of possible explanations for early-onset CRC.

Cancer is a complex disease, which arises as a result of both genetic and epigenetic alterations. Human CRCs often display changes in DNA methylation, and it has been known for decades that genome-wide hypomethylation is a consistent biochemical characteristic of human colorectal tumors [16,17,25]. In mice, DNA hypomethylation is sufficient to induce T cell lymphomas [26]. Genome-wide hypomethylation plays a causative role in cancer through different mechanisms: genomic instability, transcriptional activation of proto-oncogenes, activation of endogenous retroviruses and transposable elements, and the induction of inflammatory mediators. All these mechanisms have been

Table 4. LINE-1 methylation results in different clinical subgroups.

	Mean % LINE-1 methylation (SD)	Range	p-value[1]	p-value[2]
Normal colonic mucosa (n = 32)	76.5 (1.5)	73.5–80.2		
Earlyonset CRC (n = 185)	56.6 (8.6)	22–82	<0.0001	
Lynch syndrome CRC (n = 20)	66.3 (4.5)	52.1–73.1	<0.0001	<0.0001
Older onset sporadic MSI (n = 46)	67.1 (5.5)	44.7–78.3	<0.0001	<0.0001
Older onset sporadic MSS (n = 89)	65.1 (6.3)	42.5–78.4	<0.0001	<0.0001

CRC, colorectal cancer; SD, standard deviation.
Mann Whitney test was used to compare the LINE-1 values.
[1]Values for comparison between normal colonic mucosa and other groups of CRC.
[2]Values for comparison between early onset CRC (n = 185) and other groups of CRC.

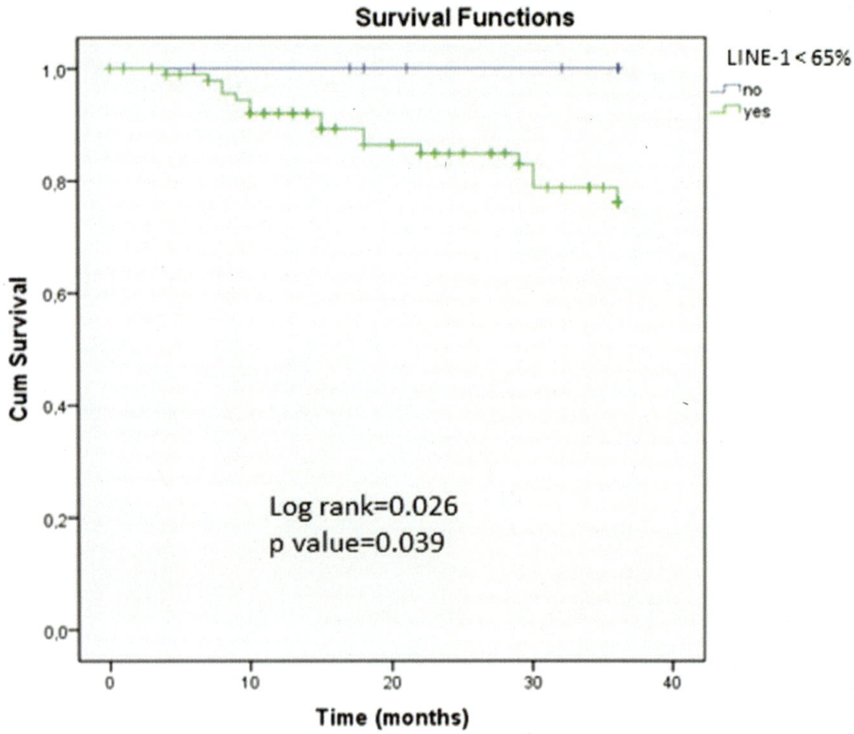

Figure 2. Kaplan–Meier survival curves depicting the effect of LINE-1 methylation on 3-year overall survival in early-onset CRC patients. *Vertical tick marks* indicate censored events. The green line represents survival in CRCs with LINE-1 hypomethylation <65% (n = 92) and the blue line represents LINE-1 methylation ≥65% (n = 23). p value for log rank and Fisher's exact test are shown.

associated with DNA hypomethylation, poor prognosis and tumor aggressiveness [26,27,28,29,30,31]. Repetitive nucleotide elements, including long interspersed nucleotide elements-1 (i.e., LINE-1) contain numerous CpG sites, and prior studies have established that the level of LINE-1 methylation is an accurate indicator of cellular 5-methylcytosine content [18], which reflects global DNA methylation. In recent years, it has been suggested that LINE-1 methylation may identify different molecular subtypes of CRC. CIMP and MSI are inversely associated with DNA hypomethylation, suggesting that genomic hypomethylation represents an alternative pathway for CRC progression, and may reflect a fundamentally different disease process [32,33]. Moreover, LINE-1 hypomethylation has been associated with poorer survival among patients with CRC, and represents an independent factor for increased cancer-related mortality and overall mortality [20]. Therefore, evaluation of tumoral LINE-1 methylation and its correlation with clinical and pathological features is important to determine the potential clinical value of this biomarker.

We used a quantitative pyrosequencing assay for LINE-1 methylation, which is a robust, accurate and reproducible method to precisely quantitate this in individual tumors [18]. Compared to older-onset colorectal tumors, we found significantly lower levels of LINE-1 methylation in early-onset CRCs. This observation was validated in an independent set of early-onset CRC patients, reinforcing the strength of our conclusions. In addition, we found that LINE-1 hypomethylation was associated with distal tumors and worse prognosis. Although there are no previous studies that have specifically examined LINE-1 methylation in early-onset CRC patients, a recent study suggested a relationship between greater LINE-1 hypomethylation in CRC and earlier onset of the cancer (<60 years) [21]. Overall these findings suggest the presence of a distinct subtype of CRC with a unique pathogenic mechanism [4,13]. Since the degree of LINE-1 hypomethylation is a prognostic marker in CRC and our data show that LINE-1 hypomethylation is a characteristic feature of early-onset CRC, this study provides a novel and previously unrecognized explanation for some of the biological differences (tumor location, prognosis and pathological features) involved in early-onset CRCs. These results provide an opportunity to improve our understanding of the mechanism behind early-onset CRC. In this regard, we are currently investigating whether LINE-1 hypomethylation causes direct transcriptional reactivation of certain proto-oncogenes in this setting, a unique feature that might help explain the aggressive clinical behavior of early-onset CRC. In addition, our results give rise to the hypothesis that the LINE-1 hypomethylation in peripheral blood could also be evaluated as a prognosis marker in early-onset CRCs.

Lynch syndrome is the most frequent hereditary cause of CRC, and accounts for approximately 1–3% of all CRCs [7]. It is an autosomal dominant condition caused by germline mutations in the DNA MMR genes (*MLH1, MSH2, MSH6, PMS2*), and *MSH2* and *MLH1* account for ~90% of identifiable families. This syndrome has a gene-dependent variable penetrance for CRC and endometrial carcinoma, and an increased risk for various other extracolonic tumors. The diagnosis of Lynch syndrome has been traditionally based on tumor MMR deficiency analysis when this disease is suspected [10,11], but the definitive diagnosis is established by finding a deleterious germline mutation in a DNA MMR gene. However, detecting Lynch syndrome is a particular challenge in the absence of a reliable family history. For this reason, universal screening with tumor MMR-deficiency analysis has been suggested [34,35]. We have previously shown that MMR deficiency accounts for up to 20% of early-onset CRC cases [4,5]. We also found that the pattern of MMR deficiency in early-onset

Table 5. Clinical, pathological and molecular features of patients according to the LINE-1 methylation levels.

Clinical, pathological or molecular features	LINE-1≥65% (n = 23)	LINE-1<65% (n = 92)	p-value
Sex, n (%)			
Male	9 (39.1)	45 (48.9)	0.4
Female	14 (60.9)	47 (51.1)	
Mean age (standard deviation)*	37.65 (8.3)	37.36 (8.3)	0.8
Family history of CRC[1], n (%)			
Yes	4 (17.4)	12 (13)	0.736
No	19 (82.6)	80 (87)	
Tumor location, n (%)			
Rectum	7 (30.4)	40 (43.5)	0.209
Distal to splenic flexure	6 (26.1)	29 (31.5)	
Proximal to splenic flexure	10 (43.5)	23 (25)	
Synchronous or metachronous CRC, n (%)			
Yes	3 (13)	2 (2.2)	0.054
No	20 (87)	90 (97.)8	
TNM tumor stage, n (%)			
I–II	9 (39.5)	31 (33.7)	0.625
III–IV	14 (60.9)	61 (66.3)	
Tumor differentiation, n (%)			
Well or moderate	18 (81.8)	79 (87.8	0.489
Poor	4 (18.2)	11 (12.2)	
Mucinous component, n (%)			
>50%	14 (60.9)	25 (27.5)	0.003
<50%	9 (39.1)	66 (72.5)	
Medullary growth pattern, n (%)			
Yes	2 (8.7)	9 (9.9)	1
No	21 (91.3)	82 (90.1)	
Crohns reaction, n (%)			
Yes	5 (21.7)	7 (8)	0.124
No	18 (78.3)	80 (92)	
Tumor infiltrating lymphocytes, n (%)			
Yes	5 (21.7)	21 (23.9)	0.83
No	18 (78.3)	67 (76.1)	
Microsatellite instability, n (%)			
MSI	6 (26.1)	19 (20.7)	0.572
MSS	17 (73.9)	73 (79.3)	
Mismatch repair deficiency[2], n (%)			
Yes	7 (30.4)	20 (21.7)	0.379
No	16 (69.6)	72 (78.3)	

*P value was calculated by t-test.
[1]Including first and second degree relatives.
[2]MSI-H and/or loss of expression of MMR proteins by immunohistochemistry.

CRC patients is not identical to that for all Lynch syndrome cases, and is characterized by in increased frequency of MSH6 and PMS2 deficiency. Another diagnostic challenge are MSH6-deficient CRC, as these might be missed if the screening algorithm relies entirely on MSI testing and does not include MMR immunohistochemistry [22]. In the present study, we evaluated the MMR status in an Argentinian population of early-onset CRC by analyzing both MSI and immunohistochemistry of the four MMR proteins. Twenty seven (22.9%) tumors were classified as MMR deficient. MSH2 and MLH1 deficiency accounted for the majority of cases, however, up to 20% were due to either MSH6 or PMS2 deficiency. One out of 9 MLH1-deficient cases had a *BRAF* mutation, which is typically associated with *MLH1* promoter hypermethylation. In the rest of the MLH1-deficient cases, 4 had different degrees of *MLH1* methylation, suggesting that promoter methylation might be the second hit in putative Lynch syndrome MLH1-type patients [36,37]. It is noteworthy that 2 patients had MSI tumors with normal DNA MMR protein expression, highlighting possible limitations when using either method, since these patients would not have otherwise been identified if immunohistochemistry had been used as the only screening technique. Our results also revealed that most patients with MMR-deficient tumors did not display any significant family history of CRC or other Lynch syndrome associated tumors. These facts underscore the importance of considering the diagnosis of Lynch syndrome in all early-onset CRC even in the absence of family history, given the important clinical implications for the management of affected individuals and their relatives [38].

We found only 1 case with biallelic germline mutations in the *MUTYH* gene (p.Y176C;p.W472S) in a 29-year-old female with no family history and a MSS rectal cancer. The p.W472S variant has not been previously described and is predicted to be probably damaging based on PolyPhen 2 software analysis [39]. Therefore, novel and previously unrecognized *MUTYH* mutations should also be considered when evaluating early-onset CRC.

In spite of all the strengths, there are potential limitations of this study. First of all, comparison between groups from different geographical areas can potentially induce a selection bias. However, we were able to find a unique molecular feature in two clinical and pathologically similar cohorts of early-onset CRC from different countries, and far from a limitation, we think that this actually constitutes one of the strengths of our investigation. The differences between LINE-1 methylation in the two cohorts of early-onset CRC patients remains unexplained in this article and actually gives rise to interesting hypothesis regarding tumor biology or environmental factors influencing LINE-1 methylation. Secondly, multivariate overall survival analysis was not performed because of the limited number of patients. Larger studies are needed in the future to further confirm the association between CRC DNA hypomethylation and poorer outcomes, specifically in the early-onset patients. Also, information about chemotherapy was not available and accordingly we could not analyze the predictive value of LINE-1. On the other hand, germline MMR genetic testing was not done in patients with MMR deficiency to confirm Lynch syndrome; for MLH1-deficient cases, we ruled out CIMP-associated tumors by analyzing the V600E *BRAF* mutation and *MLH1* methylation status. Since somatic inactivation of *MSH2*, *MSH6*, and *PMS2* are rare events, we hypothesized that most patients with MMR deficiency in this study are putative Lynch syndrome cases. Finally, we only studied the 2 most prevalent MUTYH mutations in Caucasian population, which account for >85% of cases. Despite the fact that in Argentina >75% of the population are European descendants, our results may be underestimated due to the presence of mutations other than G393D or Y176C.

In summary, we have studied a large cohort of early-onset CRC cases and found that LINE-1 hypomethylation in these tumors constitutes a unique and specific feature compared with older-onset CRC, which is suggestive of a distinct molecular subtype of these colorectal neoplasms. Our results suggest that the LINE-1 methylation status could be used as prognostic biomarker for young people with CRC. Future studies are needed to confirm this association and to understand the mechanisms by which DNA hypomethylation affects CRC prognosis, as well as to examine whether this feature could have therapeutic implications.

Supporting Information

Figure S1

Table S1 Pyrosequencing primer description.

Table S2 Clinicopathological and molecular features of *MUTYH* mutation carriers.

Table S3 Clinical, pathological and molecular features of early-onset CRC recruited in Spain and Argentina.

Author Contributions

Conceived and designed the experiments: M. Antelo FB AG. Performed the experiments: M. Antelo A. Cabanne MEB LB M. Arnold ELR M. Andreu XL. Analyzed the data: M. Antelo FB JS YS KH LM MDG MT MC. Contributed reagents/materials/analysis tools: A. Castells RJ XL M. Andreu SC-B. Wrote the paper: M. Antelo FB AG A. Castells CRB.

References

1. Jemal A, Siegel R, Ward E, Hao Y, Xu J, et al. (2009) Cancer statistics, 2009. CA Cancer J Clin 59: 225–249.
2. Siegel RL, Jemal A, Ward EM (2009) Increase in incidence of colorectal cancer among young men and women in the United States. Cancer Epidemiol Biomarkers Prev 18: 1695–1698.
3. Dozois EJ, Boardman LA, Suwanthanma W, Limburg PJ, Cima RR, et al. (2008) Young-onset colorectal cancer in patients with no known genetic predisposition: can we increase early recognition and improve outcome? Medicine (Baltimore) 87: 259–263.
4. Giraldez MD, Balaguer F, Bujanda L, Cuatrecasas M, Munoz J, et al. (2010) MSH6 and MUTYH deficiency is a frequent event in early-onset colorectal cancer. Clin Cancer Res 16: 5402–5413.
5. Goel A, Nagasaka T, Spiegel J, Meyer R, Lichliter WE, et al. (2010) Low frequency of Lynch syndrome among young patients with non-familial colorectal cancer. Clin Gastroenterol Hepatol 8: 966–971.
6. Gryfe R, Kim H, Hsieh ET, Aronson MD, Holowaty EJ, et al. (2000) Tumor microsatellite instability and clinical outcome in young patients with colorectal cancer. N Engl J Med 342: 69–77.
7. Lynch HT, de la Chapelle A (2003) Hereditary colorectal cancer. N Engl J Med 348: 919–932.
8. Kastrinos F, Steyerberg EW, Mercado R, Balmana J, Holter S, et al. (2011) The PREMM(1,2,6) model predicts risk of MLH1, MSH2, and MSH6 germline mutations based on cancer history. Gastroenterology 140: 73–81.
9. Pinol V, Castells A, Andreu M, Castellvi-Bel S, Alenda C, et al. (2005) Accuracy of revised Bethesda guidelines, microsatellite instability, and immunohistochemistry for the identification of patients with hereditary nonpolyposis colorectal cancer. Jama 293: 1986–1994.
10. Umar A, Boland CR, Terdiman JP, Syngal S, de la Chapelle A, et al. (2004) Revised Bethesda Guidelines for hereditary nonpolyposis colorectal cancer (Lynch syndrome) and microsatellite instability. J Natl Cancer Inst 96: 261–268.
11. Vasen HF, Watson P, Mecklin JP, Lynch HT (1999) New clinical criteria for hereditary nonpolyposis colorectal cancer (HNPCC, Lynch syndrome) proposed by the International Collaborative group on HNPCC. Gastroenterology 116: 1453–1456.
12. Balaguer F, Castellvi-Bel S, Castells A, Andreu M, Munoz J, et al. (2007) Identification of MYH mutation carriers in colorectal cancer: a multicenter, case-control, population-based study. Clin Gastroenterol Hepatol 5: 379–387.
13. Boardman LA, Johnson RA, Petersen GM, Oberg AL, Kabat BF, et al. (2007) Higher frequency of diploidy in young-onset microsatellite-stable colorectal cancer. Clin Cancer Res 13: 2323–2328.
14. Chan TL, Curtis LC, Leung SY, Farrington SM, Ho JW, et al. (2001) Early-onset colorectal cancer with stable microsatellite DNA and near-diploid chromosomes. Oncogene 20: 4871–4876.
15. Wolff EM, Byun HM, Han HF, Sharma S, Nichols PW, et al. Hypomethylation of a LINE-1 promoter activates an alternate transcript of the MET oncogene in bladders with cancer. PLoS Genet 6: e1000917.
16. Goelz SE, Vogelstein B, Hamilton SR, Feinberg AP (1985) Hypomethylation of DNA from benign and malignant human colon neoplasms. Science 228: 187–190.
17. Jones PA, Baylin SB (2007) The epigenomics of cancer. Cell 128: 683–692.
18. Yang AS, Estecio MR, Doshi K, Kondo Y, Tajara EH, et al. (2004) A simple method for estimating global DNA methylation using bisulfite PCR of repetitive DNA elements. Nucleic Acids Res 32: e38.

19. Irahara N, Nosho K, Baba Y, Shima K, Lindeman NI, et al. (2010) Precision of pyrosequencing assay to measure LINE-1 methylation in colon cancer, normal colonic mucosa, and peripheral blood cells. J Mol Diagn 12: 177–183.
20. Ogino S, Nosho K, Kirkner GJ, Kawasaki T, Chan AT, et al. (2008) A cohort study of tumoral LINE-1 hypomethylation and prognosis in colon cancer. J Natl Cancer Inst 100: 1734–1738.
21. Baba Y, Huttenhower C, Nosho K, Tanaka N, Shima K, et al. (2010) Epigenomic diversity of colorectal cancer indicated by LINE-1 methylation in a database of 869 tumors. Mol Cancer 9: 125.
22. Goel A, Nagasaka T, Hamelin R, Boland CR (2010) An optimized pentaplex PCR for detecting DNA mismatch repair-deficient colorectal cancers. PLoS One 5: e9393.
23. Goel A, Xicola RM, Nguyen TP, Doyle BJ, Sohn VR, et al. (2010) Aberrant DNA methylation in hereditary nonpolyposis colorectal cancer without mismatch repair deficiency. Gastroenterology 138: 1854–1862.
24. Weisenberger DJ, Siegmund KD, Campan M, Young J, Long TI, et al. (2006) CpG island methylator phenotype underlies sporadic microsatellite instability and is tightly associated with BRAF mutation in colorectal cancer. Nat Genet 38: 787–793.
25. Feinberg AP, Gehrke CW, Kuo KC, Ehrlich M (1988) Reduced genomic 5-methylcytosine content in human colonic neoplasia. Cancer Res 48: 1159–1161.
26. Gaudet F, Hodgson JG, Eden A, Jackson-Grusby L, Dausman J, et al. (2003) Induction of tumors in mice by genomic hypomethylation. Science 300: 489–492.
27. Yamada Y, Jackson-Grusby L, Linhart H, Meissner A, Eden A, et al. (2005) Opposing effects of DNA hypomethylation on intestinal and liver carcinogenesis. Proc Natl Acad Sci U S A 102: 13580–13585.
28. Karpf AR, Matsui S (2005) Genetic disruption of cytosine DNA methyltransferase enzymes induces chromosomal instability in human cancer cells. Cancer Res 65: 8635–8639.
29. Shahrzad S, Bertrand K, Minhas K, Coomber BL (2007) Induction of DNA hypomethylation by tumor hypoxia. Epigenetics 2: 119–125.
30. Rodriguez J, Frigola J, Vendrell E, Risques RA, Fraga MF, et al. (2006) Chromosomal instability correlates with genome-wide DNA demethylation in human primary colorectal cancers. Cancer Res 66: 8462–9468.
31. Esteller M (2008) Epigenetics in cancer. N Engl J Med 358: 1148–1159.
32. Estecio MR, Gharibyan V, Shen L, Ibrahim AE, Doshi K, et al. (2007) LINE-1 hypomethylation in cancer is highly variable and inversely correlated with microsatellite instability. PLoS One 2: e399.
33. Ogino S, Kawasaki T, Nosho K, Ohnishi M, Suemoto Y, et al. (2008) LINE-1 hypomethylation is inversely associated with microsatellite instability and CpG island methylator phenotype in colorectal cancer. Int J Cancer 122: 2767–2773.
34. Boland CR, Shike M (2010) Report from the Jerusalem workshop on Lynch syndrome-hereditary nonpolyposis colorectal cancer. Gastroenterology 138: 2197 e2191–2197.
35. Lindor NM, Petersen GM, Hadley DW, Kinney AY, Miesfeldt S, et al. (2006) Recommendations for the care of individuals with an inherited predisposition to Lynch syndrome: a systematic review. Jama 296: 1507–1517.
36. Ollikainen M, Hannelius U, Lindgren CM, Abdel-Rahman WM, Kere J, et al. (2007) Mechanisms of inactivation of MLH1 in hereditary nonpolyposis colorectal carcinoma: a novel approach. Oncogene 26: 4541–4549.
37. Rahner N, Friedrichs N, Steinke V, Aretz S, Friedl W, et al. (2008) Coexisting somatic promoter hypermethylation and pathogenic MLH1 germline mutation in Lynch syndrome. J Pathol 214: 10–16.
38. Jarvinen HJ, Renkonen-Sinisalo L, Aktan-Collan K, Peltomaki P, Aaltonen LA, et al. (2009) Ten years after mutation testing for Lynch syndrome: cancer incidence and outcome in mutation-positive and mutation-negative family members. J Clin Oncol 27: 4793–4797.
39. Adzhubei IA, Schmidt S, Peshkin L, Ramensky VE, Gerasimova A, et al. (2010) A method and server for predicting damaging missense mutations. Nat Methods 7: 248–249.

13

Bifunctional Anti-Huntingtin Proteasome-Directed Intrabodies Mediate Efficient Degradation of Mutant Huntingtin Exon 1 Protein Fragments

David C. Butler[1,2], Anne Messer[1,2]*

1 Wadsworth Center, New York State Department of Health, Albany, New York, United States of America, 2 Department of Biomedical Sciences, University at Albany, Albany, New York, United States of America

Abstract

Huntington's disease (HD) is a fatal autosomal dominant neurodegenerative disorder caused by a trinucleotide $(CAG)_n$ repeat expansion in the coding sequence of the huntingtin gene, and an expanded polyglutamine (>37Q) tract in the protein. This results in misfolding and accumulation of huntingtin protein (htt), formation of neuronal intranuclear and cytoplasmic inclusions, and neuronal dysfunction/degeneration. Single-chain Fv antibodies (scFvs), expressed as intrabodies that bind htt and prevent aggregation, show promise as immunotherapeutics for HD. Intrastriatal delivery of anti-N-terminal htt scFv-C4 using an adeno-associated virus vector (AAV2/1) significantly reduces the size and number of aggregates in HDR6/1 transgenic mice; however, this protective effect diminishes with age and time after injection. We therefore explored enhancing intrabody efficacy via fusions to heterologous functional domains. Proteins containing a PEST motif are often targeted for proteasomal degradation and generally have a short half life. In ST14A cells, fusion of the C-terminal PEST region of mouse ornithine decarboxylase (mODC) to scFv-C4 reduces htt exon 1 protein fragments with 72 glutamine repeats (httex1-72Q) by ~80–90% when compared to scFv-C4 alone. Proteasomal targeting was verified by either scrambling the mODC-PEST motif, or via proteasomal inhibition with epoxomicin. For these constructs, the proteasomal degradation of the scFv intrabody proteins themselves was reduced<25% by the addition of the mODC-PEST motif, with or without antigens. The remaining intrabody levels were amply sufficient to target N-terminal httex1-72Q protein fragment turnover. Critically, scFv-C4-PEST prevents aggregation and toxicity of httex1-72Q fragments at significantly lower doses than scFv-C4. Fusion of the mODC-PEST motif to intrabodies is a valuable general approach to specifically target toxic antigens to the proteasome for degradation.

Editor: Philipp J. Kahle, Hertie Institute for Clinical Brain Research and German Center for Neurodegenerative Diseases, Germany

Funding: National Institutes of Health/NINDS NS053912, NS 073415 and NS061257 Hereditary Disease Foundation (http://www.hdfoundation.org/home.php). The funders had no role in study design, data collection and analysis, decision to publish, or preparation of the manuscript.

Competing Interests: The authors have declared that no competing interests exist.

* E-mail: messer@wadsworth.org

Introduction

Huntington's disease (HD) is the most prevalent of nine known human neurodegenerative disorders linked to the expansion of polyglutamine (polyQ) tracts in specific disease-associated proteins [1]. The cellular localization of wild-type Huntingtin (htt) is predominantly cytosolic and diffuse; however, N-terminal fragments of mutant htt (mhtt) have been reported to form both intranuclear and cytoplasmic inclusions in HD [2,3,4]. N-terminal mhtt fragments can fold into several conformations resulting in different solubilities and pathological consequences [5,6]. Although the precise conformations of the toxic species are still a matter of debate, it is clear that various misfolded N-terminal cleavage products are a major early step in HD pathogenesis [7,8]. Because HD is a progressive genetic disorder with death occurring 10–20 years after diagnosis, early intervention therapies may significantly improve patient quality of life by slowing and/or reversing the course of the disease.

Intrabody-based therapies show significant potential for addressing the critical need to reduce the misfolded protein burden in HD [9]. These recombinant single-chain and single-domain variable fragments of full-length antibodies exhibit high specificity and affinity for targets, can be selected, engineered, and delivered as genes [10,11,12,13]. The N-terminal 17 amino acids of htt form a highly conserved amphipathic alpha helix immediately preceding the polyQ tract, and have been shown to be involved in membrane binding, subcellular localization, aggregation, and toxicity [14,15,16,17]. A naïve human spleen scFv phage-display library screened against the N-terminal 17 amino acids of htt generated the scFv-C4 intrabody, which successfully counteracts *in situ* length-dependent htt aggregation, in both cell culture [18,19,20,21] and *Drosophila* models of HD [22]. scFv-C4 preferentially binds to soluble mhtt N-terminal fragments. It is only weakly active against endogenous full-length mhtt and wild type htt, possibly due to epitope inaccessibility [20]. Intrastriatal delivery of scFv-C4, using the adeno-associated virus vector (AAV2/1), resulted in a significant reduction in the size and number of mhtt aggregates in B6.Cg-HDR6/1 transgenic mice. However, the neuroprotective effect weakened both with severity of disease at time of injection, and with age beyond 6 months, although it does not disappear entirely [23]. Additional optimization of scFv-C4 is required for this intrabody to be of future use in clinical applications.

In this study, we developed a bifunctional intrabody that prevented N-terminal htt exon 1 (httex1) protein fragments from aggregating while directing them to the proteasome for degradation. Proteins that contain enriched regions of amino acids Proline (P), Glutamic Acid (E) or Aspartic Acid (D), Serine (S), and Threonine (T), otherwise known as PEST regions, are targeted for proteasomal degradation and generally have a short half-life. Mouse Ornithine Decarboxylase (mODC), a cytosolic enzyme involved in the biosynthesis of polyamines, is rapidly degraded in mammalian cells [24]. Deletion of the C-terminal PEST motif from mODC stabilizes mODC independent of protein synthesis, with no detrimental effects on enzyme activity [24]. Transfer of the mODC-PEST motif (amino-acids 422–461) to the C-terminus of stable proteins such as green fluorescent protein [25] and Luciferase [26] significantly reduced their intracellular half-life. Although there is one report in the literature that a PEST-fused intrabody against β-galactosidase was unsuccessful in depleting its target, intrabodies and targets can vary greatly in their intracellular properties, and our system differs significantly from the one reported [27]. We have previously shown that fusion of a nuclear localization sequence (NLS) derived from SV40 Large T antigen to scFv-C4 was able to bind, transport, and sequester soluble httex1 protein fragments with 72 glutamine repeats fused to enhanced green florescent protein (httex1-72Q-GFP) into the nuclei [18,19]. Based on the ability of the scFv-C4-NLS fusion construct to redirect httex1-72Q-GFP protein to different subcellular compartments, we hypothesized that fusion of the proteolytic PEST signal sequence of mODC to scFv-C4 could affect the steady-state level of httex1-72Q-GFP by redirecting the antigen-antibody complex to the proteasome. Our current studies provide a strong proof of concept that PEST fusion can greatly enhance the functionality of our intrabody, with implications for multiple additional diseases.

Results

Anti-htt scFv-C4-PEST intrabody enhances degradation of httex1-72Q fragments

Our approach sought to harness the proteasomal machinery for the targeted degradation of httex1 protein fragments. To develop a bifunctional intrabody that redirected httex1 protein fragments to the proteasome for degradation, while preventing aggregation of mhtt, we fused the mODC-PEST motif (amino-acids 422–461) to the C-terminus of scFv-C4 intrabody to generate scFv-C4-PEST. Because the targeted epitope of scFv-C4 is the N-terminal 17 amino acids of htt, scFv-C4 and scFv-C4-PEST are likely to bind a variety of N-terminal mhtt fragments produced from the cleavage of full-length mhtt during HD pathology. We co-transfected intrabody constructs (empty vector, scFv-C4, and scFv-C4-PEST) with GFP-labeled huntingtin fragments of either non-pathological (httex1-25Q-GFP) or pathological (httex1-72Q-GFP) repeat lengths to determine if scFv-C4-PEST could redirect N-terminal htt fragments to the proteasome in ST14A striatal progenitor cells [28].

Live cell imaging of transfected cells (Fig. 1A) revealed that without intrabody, httex1-25Q-GFP remained diffuse throughout the cell compared to httex1-72Q-GFP, which formed punctate aggregates. In cells co-transfected with scFv-C4 and httex1-72Q-GFP, GFP-labeled mhtt was diffusely localized throughout the cell, as previously reported [20,21,29,30]. However, co-transfection of scFv-C4-PEST resulted in a dramatic reduction of observable httex1-25-QGFP and httex1-72Q-GFP fluorescence (Fig. 1A). Residual httex1-72Q-GFP seen after 4-fold overexposure of scFv-C4-PEST showed a phenotype consistent with native scFv-C4 (Data not shown). In agreement with live cell imaging, scFv-C4-PEST vs. scFv-C4 showed a 51% reduction of monomeric htt in httex1-25Q-GFP and a 78% reduction of httex1-72Q-GFP co-transfected cells by Western blot (Fig. 1B). To assess the effectiveness of our anti-htt intrabody based therapy on the biochemical formation of mhtt aggregates, we used agarose gel electrophoresis for resolving aggregates (AGERA). Unlike sodium dodecyl sulfate polyacrylamide gel electrophoresis (SDS-PAGE), where aggregated mhtt is trapped in the stacking gel, AGERA allows aggregated mhtt to be separated based on size, with larger aggregates remaining near the top of the gel [31]. In cells co-transfected with empty vector and httex1-72Q-GFP, there was a large smear of aggregated mhtt compared to cells co-transfected with scFv-C4; however, in cells co-transfected with scFv-C4-PEST aggregated htt was substantially reduced with respect to empty vector and scFv-C4 transfected cells (Fig. 1C, right panel). scFv-C4-PEST appeared to remove httex1-25Q-GFP as well, but presumably at the level of monomer (Fig. 1C, left panel).

scFv-C4-PEST inhibits polyQ-mediated toxicity of mutant httex1-72Q-GFP protein fragments

To further examine functionality, viability was assayed by flow cytometric analysis with propidium iodide (PI). As seen in previous studies, we observed an increase of PI-positive non-viable cells when empty vector was co-transfected with httex1-72Q-GFP compared to cells co-transfected with httex1-25Q-GFP (Fig. 2A) [18]. Both scFv-C4 and scFv-C4-PEST inhibited polyQ-mediated toxicity of mutant httex1-72Q-GFP protein fragments (Fig. 2A). In agreement with findings reported in Figure 1, scFv-C4-PEST significantly reduced the geometric mean fluorescence intensity (MFI) of GFP labeled httex1-25Q and httex1-72Q cells by 1.5 and 1.8-fold, respectively (Fig. 2B).

PEST scramble and specific inhibition of the proteasome eliminates the enhanced degradation of N-terminal httex1-72Q-GFP protein fragments

The solubility of human scFv intrabodies can be improved by an overall negative charge at cytoplasmic pH and increased hydrophilicity (as demonstrated by decreased grand average of hydropathicity, GRAVY score) [32]. Our previous data show that addition of a highly charged acidic 3×FLAG tag to aggregation-prone positively charged intrabodies resulted in increased intracellular solubility [32]. Because a PEST sequence is defined by hydrophilic stretches of amino acids greater than or equal to 12 residues in length [33], addition of a PEST motif to scFv intrabodies may enhance their intracellular solubility. Sequence analyses of scFv-C4 and estimation of net charge at pH 7.4 GRAVY hydrophilicity score predicted that fusion of hydrophilic PEST motif to scFv-C4 could increase solubility (Table 1). To determine if the enhanced clearance of httex1-72Q-GFP protein fragments was simply due to enhanced solubility of scFv-C4, we scrambled the PEST motif (scFv-C4-PEST-SCR), while maintaining the physico-chemical properties of scFv-C4. Because positively charged residues are not contained within PEST regions [33], we rearranged the PEST motif placing positively charged amino acids within the PEST motif. The subsequent PEST-FIND scores for scFv-C4-PEST and scFv-C4-PEST-Scramble were +5.16 and −2.41 respectively (Table 1).

To determine if the enhanced clearance of httex1-72Q-GFP protein fragments was due to enhanced scFv-C4-PEST intrabody protein solubility, we examined protein levels of the different intrabody constructs. There appears to be no qualitative difference in the solubility of HA tagged scFv-C4, scFv-C4-PEST, or scFv-

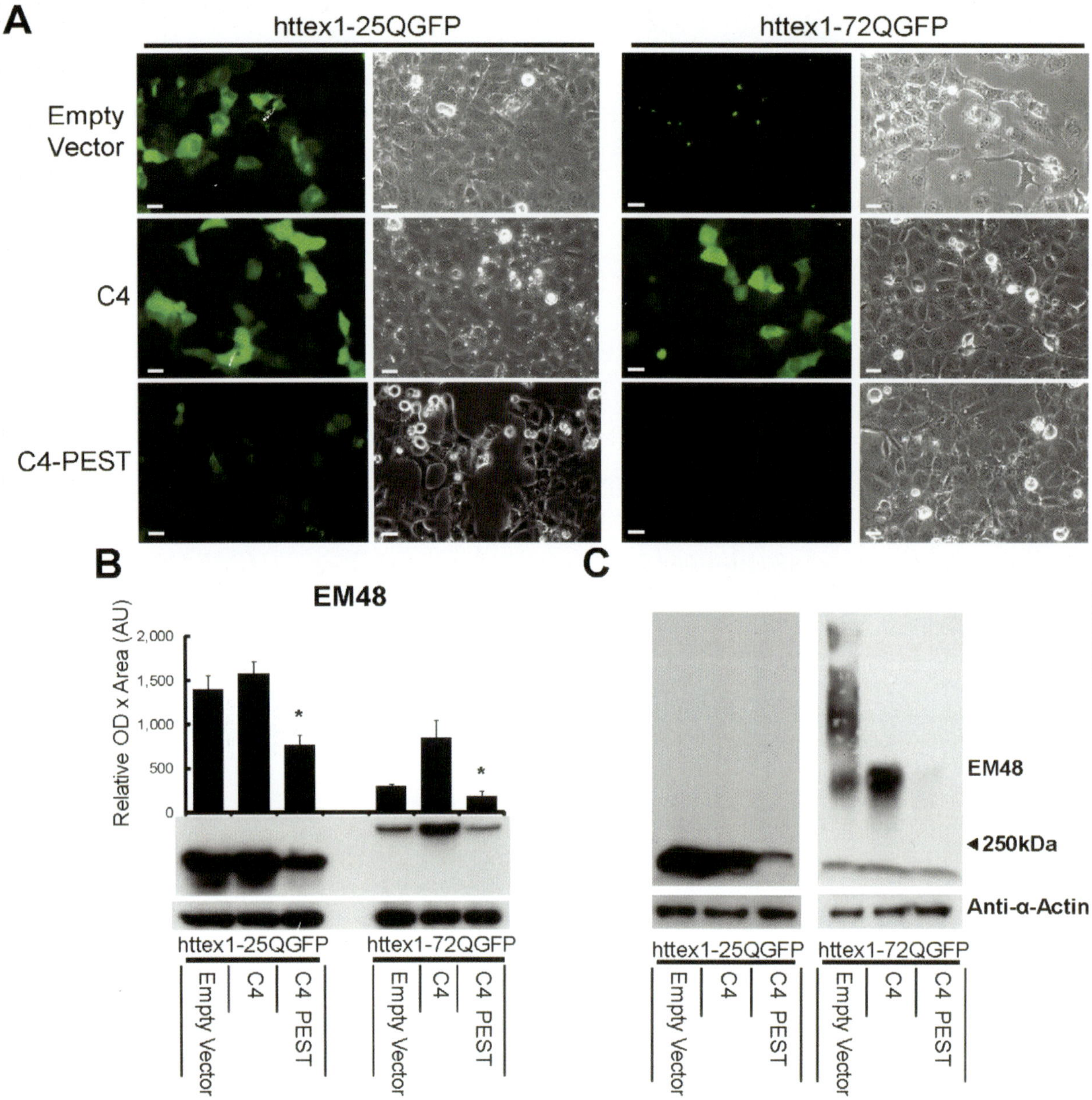

Figure 1. scFv-C4-PEST enhances degradation of GFP-tagged httex1 soluble and insoluble protein fragments. ST14A cells were co-transfected with GFP-tagged httex1-25Q (httex1-25Q-GFP) or (httex1-72Q-GFP), plus either empty vector, scFv-C4, or scFv-C4-PEST plasmids. **A**. Representative live cell imaging depicting reduction of httex1-72Q-GFP and httex1-25Q-GFP fluorescence in the scFv-C4-PEST co-transfected groups. Phase contrast confirms uniform cell integrity. 48 h; bar = 20 μm. **B**. SDS-PAGE Western blot and densitometry probed for htt (EM48), quantified vs. actin. Monomeric soluble mhttex1 protein fragments were quantitatively reduced in scFv-C4-PEST vs. scFv-C4 co-transfected cells. (Mean ± SEM; *$p<0.05$ comparing httex1-25Q-GFP co-transfections; *$p<0.05$ comparing httex1-72Q-GFP co-transfections) Note that **B** shows only soluble httex1-72Q fragment levels, which are low unless intrabody is present. **C**. Agarose Gel Electrophoresis for Resolving Aggregates (AGERA) shows the decrease of detergent-insoluble material in httex1-72Q-GFP to scFv-C4-PEST co-transfected cells compared to other groups.

C4-PEST-SCR intrabodies, based on biochemical fractionation into detergent-soluble and –insoluble cell lysates (Fig. 3B). These data suggest that enhanced solubility of scFv-C4-PEST is not a major factor in PEST-mediated enhanced target clearance.

Live cell imaging of scFv-C4-PEST-SCR produced similar results to scFv-C4 for inhibiting aggregation of httex1-72Q-GFP (Fig. 3A). In agreement with findings reported in Figure 1, monomeric mhtt was significantly reduced in empty vector control and scFv-C4-PEST detergent-soluble fractions (Fig. 3B). As expected, the levels of monomeric mhtt were similar between scFv-C4 and scFv-C4-PEST-SCR (Fig. 3B). The absence of monomeric mhtt from the insoluble fractions is due to aggregation of httex1-72Q-GFP, which is retained in the stacking gel. To address this issue, total cell lysates were analyzed by AGERA. Empty vector and httex1-72GFP co-transfected cells contain a substantial amount of detergent insoluble mhtt compared to all other groups (Fig. 3C, Left lane). As expected the levels of detergent insoluble mhtt are similar between scFv-C4-PEST-SCR and scFv-C4 compared to scFv-C4-PEST co-transfected cell lysates (Fig. 3C). Immunoblot quantification of this series showed

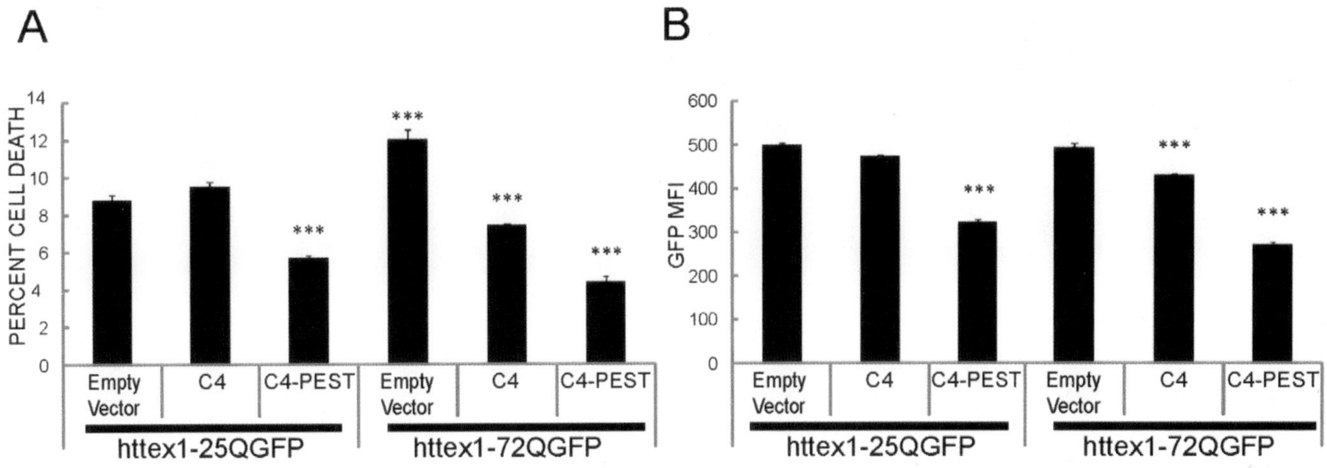

Figure 2. scFv-C4-PEST further enhances viability in ST14A co-transfection experiments compared to scFv-C4. Viability and GFP geometric mean fluorescent intensity (MFI) were assayed by flow cytometric analysis 48 h after transfection. For scFv-C4-PEST vs.scFv-C4: **A**. The percentage of propidium iodide (PI) positive nonviable cells is reduced. **B**. Total httex1-25Q-GFP and httex1-72Q-GFP reduction was confirmed. (means ± SEM; *** $p<0.001$ within groups.)

that there was a 90% reduction of soluble mhtt in scFv-C4-PEST cells compared to scFv-C4 and scFv-C4-PEST-SCR (Fig. 3D).

To further confirm that scFv-C4-PEST is acting in a proteasome-dependent manner, we treated cells with epoxomicin, a potent and selective proteasome inhibitor [34]. ST14A cells were co-transfected with httex1-72Q-GFP and scFv-C4-PEST. 36 h after transfection, cells were treated with 10 μM epoxomicin or vehicle control DMSO, and then harvested at 48 h. As expected, 12-h proteasome inhibition with epoxomicin resulted in reduced clearance of insoluble mhtt in scFv-C4-PEST and httex1-72Q co-transfected cells (Fig. 3E).

PEST fusion reduces steady-state scFv-C4 intrabody levels modestly, and independent of antigen

Sibler et al. reported that fusion of the mODC-PEST motif to the anti- β-galactosidase scFv-13R4 intrabody resulted in a destabilization of the intrabody-PEST construct in the absence of intracellular target [27]. The experiments above also allowed us to determine if fusion of the mODC-PEST motif to the C-terminus altered the steady state levels of anti-htt scFv-C4. In Fig. 4, we quantitatively compared the expression levels of scFv-C4 and scFv-C4-PEST with and without intracellular target httex1-72Q-GFP, using a hemagglutinin (HA) tag to identify the intrabodies. In contrast to scFv-13R4-PEST intrabody, our steady-state protein levels of scFv-C4-PEST were reduced by only 25% independent of antigen presence or absence. Likewise, the levels of a second intrabody, anti-fibrillar scFv-6E and scFv-6E-PEST are similar with and without intracellular target httex1-72Q-GFP (Fig. 5B). Interestingly, scFv-13R4, scFv-C4 and scFv-6E were derived from different intrabody libraries. These data suggest that not all classes of intrabodies are significantly destabilized by the addition of the mODC-PEST motif.

PEST mediated degragation of mhtt is specific to soluble monomeric, and not fibrillar, species

Insoluble polyQ protein aggregates are generally resistant to proteolytic degradation [35]. We fused the mODC-PEST motif to a fibril-specific scFv-6E intrabody [36], which does not bind to the soluble monomeric mhtt fragment [18], to investigate whether an aggregated/fibrillar htt-PEST complex is also resistant to proteolytic degradation. Previously, we reported that under slightly different conditions, scFv-6E modestly enhanced the aggregation propensity of httex1-72Q-GFP compared to httex1-25Q-GFP in ST14A cells [18]. As opposed to the soluble monomer binding scFv-C4 intrabody studies above, live cell imaging of httex1-72Q-GFP is qualitatively indistinguishable when PEST is fused to the anti-fibrillar scFv-6E intrabody (Fig. 5A). Western blotting confirmed that the levels of monomeric mhtt were comparable among empty vector, scFv-6E, and scFv-6E-PEST (Fig. 5B). Detergent-insoluble migration patterns of httex1-72Q-GFP resolved by AGERA were also similar between empty vector, scFv-6E, and 6E-PEST through the gel (Fig. 5C). These

Table 1. Physico-chemical properties of scFv-C4 intrabodies.

	Isoelectric point	Net Charge at pH 7.4	Gravy Score	PEST Find Score
scFv-C4	6.62	−0.5	−0.282	------
scFv-C4-PEST	5.24	−5.5	−0.328	5.16
scFv-C4-PEST-SCR	5.24	−5.5	−0.328	−2.41

Physico-chemical determinants of soluble intrabody expression. Solubility is improved by an overall negative charge at pH 7.4 and reduced GRAVY score. The GRAVY score is the average hydropathy score for all the amino acids in the protein, with a more negative score indicating increased hydrophilicity. The PEST-FIND program **http://emboss.bioinformatics.nl/cgi-bin/emboss/pestfind** objectively produces a score ranging from about −50 to +50. A score above +5 denotes a PEST region [33].

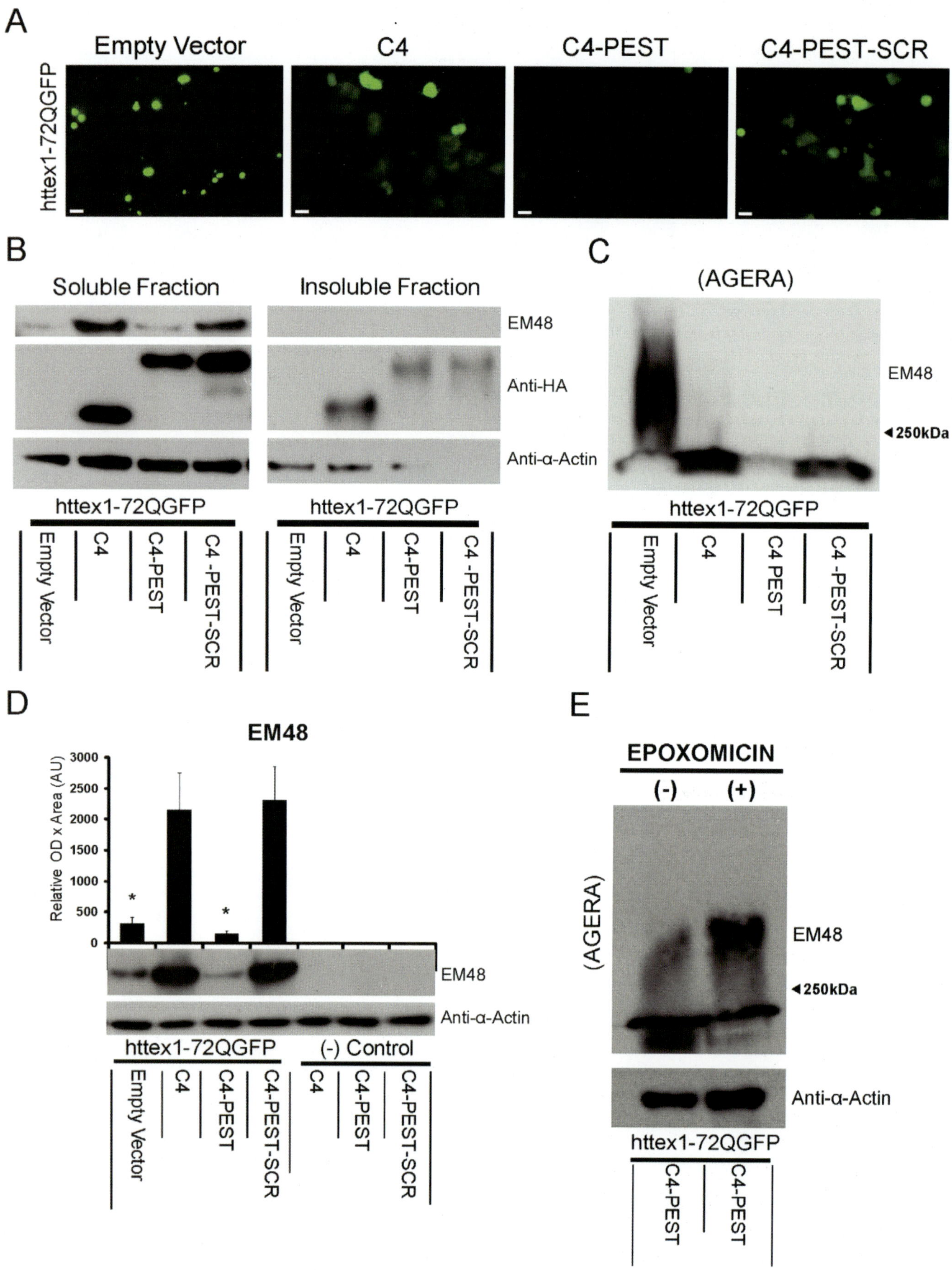
A
Empty Vector
C4
C4-PEST
C4-PEST-SCR
httex1-72QGFP
B
Soluble Fraction
Insoluble Fraction
EM48
Anti-HA
Anti-α-Actin
httex1-72QGFP
Empty Vector
C4
C4-PEST
C4 -PEST-SCR
C
(AGERA)
EM48
◄250kDa
httex1-72QGFP
Empty Vector
C4
C4-PEST
C4 -PEST-SCR
D
EM48
Relative OD x Area (AU)
3000
2500
2000
1500
1000
500
0
*
*
EM48
Anti-α-Actin
httex1-72QGFP
(-) Control
Empty Vector
C4
C4-PEST
C4-PEST-SCR
C4
C4-PEST
C4-PEST-SCR
E
EPOXOMICIN
(-)
(+)
(AGERA)
EM48
◄250kDa
Anti-α-Actin
httex1-72QGFP
C4-PEST
C4-PEST

Figure 3. Scrambling the PEST sequence and specific inhibition of the proteasome eliminates the enhanced degradation of httex1-72Q-GFP. A. Representative live cell images of dual transfections. Diffuse httex1-72Q-GFP fluorescence is similar between scFv-C4-PEST-SCR and scFv-C4 cells, and much higher than scFv-C4-PEST. **B**. Biochemical fractionation of HA-tagged fluorobodies from ST14A cells. Detergent-soluble and -insoluble cell lysates were prepared as described in Materials and Methods. Empty vector and scFv-C4-PEST transfected cells express minimal levels of monomeric htt, while scFv-C4-PEST-SCR and scFv-C4 transfected cells have similar levels of monmeric htt **C**. AGERA. There is an increase of detergent-insoluble material in scFv-C4-PEST-SCR transfected cells compared to scFv-C4-PEST. **D**. Western blotting of total protein. Monomeric mhtt levels do not differ between scFv-C4 and scFv-C4-PEST-SCR co-transfected cells. C4-PEST reduces soluble mhtt by ~90%, and empty vector control mhtt is insoluble **E**. Proteasome inhibition reduced clearance of insoluble httex1-72Q by scFv-C4-PEST. ST14A cells were co-transfected with httex1-72Q-GFP and scFv-C4-PEST. 36 h after transfection, cells were treated with 10 μM epoxomicin (+), a potent and selective proteasome inhibitor [34]; or DMSO vehicle control. Insoluble mhtt was assessed at 48 h using AGERA. Proteasome inhibition resulted in reduced clearance of htt exon1 protein fragments by scFv-C4-PEST.

data are consistent with previous studies that suggest aggregated htt is inefficiently degraded by the proteasome [37].

scFv-C4-PEST alters target at a lower dose than scFv-C4

A therapeutic range is especially advantageous for gene therapy. We therefore co-transfected ST14A cells with a 1:2 or a 1:5 ratio of intrabody to httex1-72Q-GFP. In contrast to previous experiments (see Fig. 1A), where intrabody and httex1-72Q-GFP were co-transfected at a 1:1 ratio, aggregation of httex1-72Q-GFP was present in scFv-C4 transfected cells at a 1:2 ratio and was noticeably elevated at a 1:5 ratio (Fig. 6A). However, scFv-C4-PEST transfected cells still enhanced the clearance of httex1-72Q-GFP at a 1:2 ratio of intrabody to httex1-72Q-GFP. At a 1:5 ratio of scFv-C4-PEST to httex1-72Q-GFP, scFv-C4-PEST maintained httex1-72Q-GFP in a mostly non-aggregated soluble state (Fig. 6A). Western blots of the dose response experiments confirmed the live cell observation that scFv-C4-PEST can counteract aggregation very effectively at 1:2, and still shows effects at 1:5 (Fig. 6B). Compared to scFv-C4, the levels of insoluble httex1-72Q-GFP were reduced at 1:2 and 1:5 ratio of scFv-C4-PEST to httex1-72Q-GFP (Fig. 6C).

Discussion

In HD, the initial pathogenic trigger is the misfolding of mhtt, which eventually leads to intracellular accumulation of a toxic N-terminal fragment of the mhtt protein with excess polyQ. Prevention of mhtt misfolding, or reducing its availability for abnormal intracellular interactions, should therefore offer significant protection. We and others have developed intrabodies that bind to the regions adjacent to the polyQ repeat [38,39,40], altered the protein context, and reduced the aggregation and toxicity of mhtt. One very promising candidate, the scFv intrabody scFv-C4, targets the N-terminal 17 amino acids of the htt protein, a domain of htt protein that is increasingly being recognized as pivotal in mediating physiological and pathological pathways in HD [41]. The human scFv-C4 is very effective at counteracting the misfolding and toxicity of mutant httex1 in transient transfection assays of multiple cell lines [10] and stressed organotypic brain slice cultures [21]. In an HD *Drosophila* model, the intrabody shows strong protective effects initially, and increases lifespan by 30%, although the mutant flies still die prematurely [42]. AAV2/1 delivery of this intrabody to the striatum of inbred B6.HDR6/1 mice also demonstrates phenotypic correction at the cellular level; however, scFv-C4 alone has been insufficient to produce amelioration of the full disease phenotype over a period of several months [23]. This could be due to targeting of a suboptimal epitope, gradual dilution of efficacy due to build-up of mhtt that escapes intrabody binding, and/or insufficient delivery of an otherwise effective reagent. Work here and elsewhere suggests that all three of these parameters impact long-term efficacy *in vivo*. Here, we addressed the first two factors by engineering fusions of scFv-C4 to heterologous proteolytic domains that can lead to rapid and irreversible turnover of the antigen-antibody complex. Inducing rapid turnover of the bound antigen reduces dependence on the precise functionality of the bound epitope, although the epitope must still be available. We show that fusion of scFv-C4 to a proteasomal PEST signal domain results in greatly enhanced degradation of soluble mutant httex1 protein fragments in a transiently-transfected striatal cell line. This in turn reduces both the aggregate burden and the toxicity of the mutant protein.

The goal of this study was to determine whether a bifunctional intrabody could manipulate the stability of its intracellular target. Because heterologous transfer of the mODC-PEST motif to the C-terminus of stable proteins significantly reduced their intracellular half-life [25,26], fusion of a PEST motif to scFv-C4 might destabilize the intrabody protein itself, thus reducing the amount of intrabody available to bind to its target. For this reason, we chose a specific mODC-PEST sequence that was known to induce

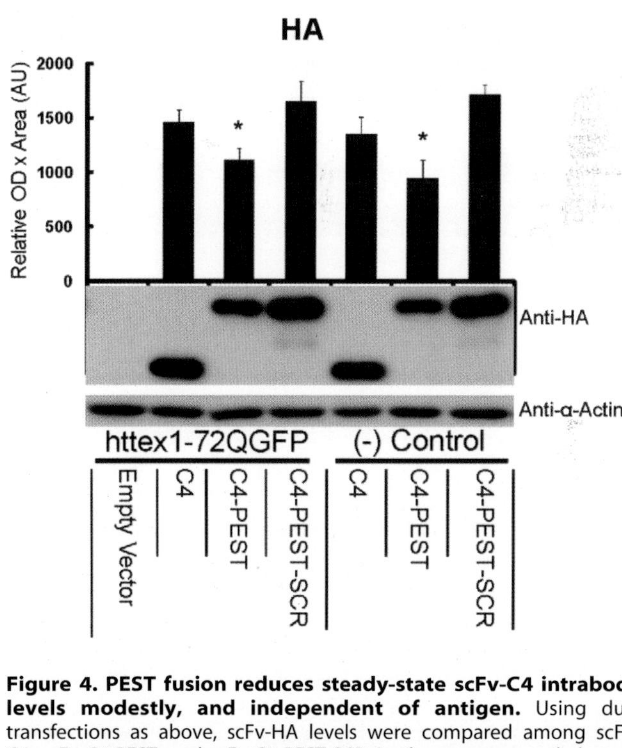

Figure 4. PEST fusion reduces steady-state scFv-C4 intrabody levels modestly, and independent of antigen. Using dual transfections as above, scFv-HA levels were compared among scFv-C4, scFv-C4-PEST, and scFv-C4-PEST-SCR, in the presence and absence of httex1-72Q-GFP. Levels of scFv-C4-PEST were reduced by ~25% when compared with scFv-C4 or the scrambled (inactive) PEST. The presence or absence of antigen had no significant effect on intrabody-PEST levels. (n = 4; mean ± SEM; *p<0.05. for C4 vs. C4-PEST/C4-PEST-SCR.)

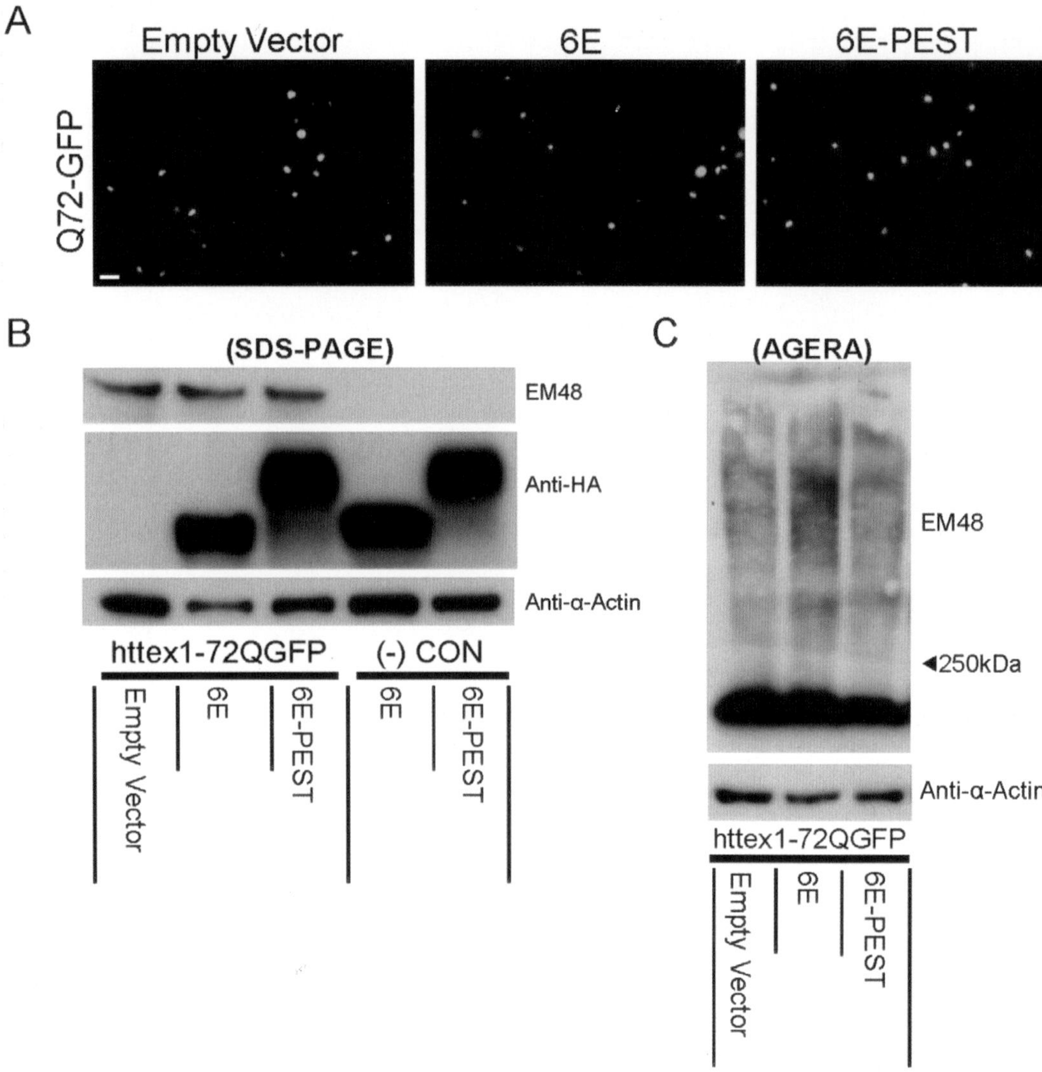

Figure 5. Fusion of PEST motif to anti htt fibril-specific scFv-6E intrabody does not degrade htt fragments in ST14A cells. ST14A cells co-transfected with httex1-72Q-GFP and either empty vector, scFv-6E, or scFv-6E-PEST plasmids. Cells imaged and processed at 48 h. **A**. Live cell imaging. scFv-6E-PEST does not appear to alter the aggregation of htt compared to empty vector or scFv-6E. **B**. Western blotting. Monomeric htt is similar between groups. HA-tagged intrabody levels are similar between groups. **C**. Detergent-insoluble material resolved by AGERA is similar between empty vector and 6E-PEST groups.

moderate, rather than very strong, turnover, based on destabilized GFP-PEST studies [25]. It was also important to consider the functional state of the proteasome in affected cells. The ubiquitin-proteasome system (UPS) has been implicated in the failure to degrade mhtt, leading to aggregate formation [43]. Proteasome impairment is thought to occur through sequestering of 20S proteasome subunits [37], failure of aggregated mhtt to enter the 20S proteasome core [44], or clogging of the proteasome with polyglutamine fragments [45]. Fortunately, *in vivo* studies have shown that 26S proteasome is not impaired in HDR6/2 mice [44], and it is the 26S proteasome that recognizes the PEST motif of mODC and processes it for degradation [46]. Therefore, our strategy was designed to take advantage of this conserved functionality.

The difference in the ratios of scFv-C4 to scFv-C4-PEST intrabody levels vs. httex1-72Q-GFP+scFv-C4 to httex1-72Q-GFP+scFv-C4-PEST was larger than expected. Our data suggest that this particular combination of intrabody and PEST does not lead to rapid degradation of the unliganded intrabody fused to PEST. With intrabody binding, the mhtt antigen appears to be delivered to the proteasome and degraded, while sufficient intrabody-PEST protein remains available for additional substrate. Qualitative comparisons of cellular protein levels of a second intrabody, scFv-6E, which binds only to aggregated fibrillar httex1, also show intrabody levels that appear even less reduced by fusion with this PEST motif. However, in this case the fibrillar antigen-antibody complex could not be degraded by the proteasome, which is in agreement with data suggesting that once htt has aggregated it is resistant to degradation by the UPS [35]. Published results suggest that these types of highly structured aggregates are degraded via autophagy [43,47].

For safety reasons, it would be valuable to use an intrabody that preferentially targets N-terminal mhtt fragments, because long-term reduction of full-length wild-type htt may exacerbate neurological degeneration, even in the presence of low levels of mhtt [48] We have previously shown that scFv-C4 preferentially

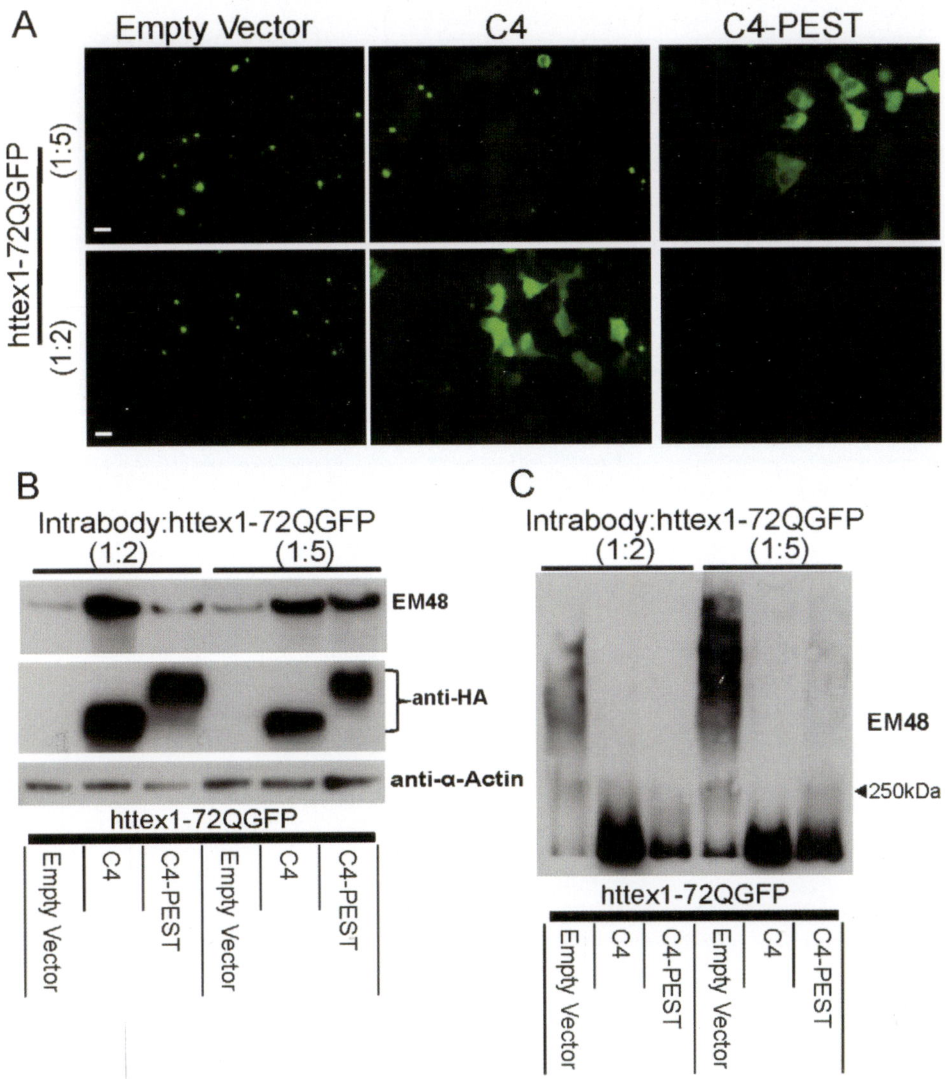

Figure 6. Targeted degradation of htt occurs in a dose-dependent manner. ST14A cells co-transfected with 1:2 or 1:5 transfection ratio of intrabody-PEST to httex1-72Q-GFP plasmids. **A.** Live cell imaging. Httex1-72Q is diffuse at 1:2, and being begins to form aggregates at a 1:5 transfection ratio of intrabody to httex1-72Q-GFP in scFv-C4 transfected cells. Fusion scFv-C4-PEST clears mhtt at 1:2, and keeps mhtt diffuse at 1:5. **B, C.** Western blots of EM48 immunoreactivity measuring the soluble (**B**; SDS-PAGE) and insoluble (**C**; AGERA) material to confirm live cell imaging.

binds to soluble mhtt N-terminal fragments, and is only weakly active against endogenous full-length mhtt and wild type htt, possibly due to epitope inaccessibility [20]. Pilot experiments using the scFv-C4-PEST construct in B6.Cg-R6/1 HD and wild-type mouse striatum have not shown excess transgene-induced toxicity up to 6 months after injection of AAV2/1-scFv-C4-PEST (data not shown). However, quantitation of the level of residual wild-type full-length htt will be necessary prior to extending these studies to clinical use.

An additional safety/efficacy issue for bifunctional intrabodies is subcellular localization. Soluble mhtt appears to be largely cytoplasmic, while aggregated mhtt is often found juxtaposed to the nucleus in ST14A cells [18]. In contrast to *in situ* studies of N-terminal mhttex1 fragment localization, aggregated mhtt is primarily localized in the nucleus of B6.Cg-R6/1 HD transgenic mice. Localization of htt is thought to be due primarily to a motif within the AA1–17 region that acts as a cytoplasmic retention signal [15,17,49,50,51]. Intrabodies that bind AA1–17 might influence this distribution by masking nuclear export or cytoplasmic retention signals, thereby increasing nuclear concentrations and toxicity. scFv-C4, which was selected against AA1–17, appears to bind to the far N-terminus, AAs 2–12 (Thumfort and Ingram, pers. Comm.). scFv-C4 does not lead to nuclear concentration of diffuse httex1-72Q-GFP, as shown here and in our previous studies. Another engineered intrabody, V_L12.3, was selected against a peptide that included AAs1–20 [29,30], and the epitope has recently been identified as including AAs 5–18 [52]. This binding therefore is likely to block the phosphorylation at serine 13 and serine 16, which fits well with *in situ* and *in vivo* observations that the V_L12.3-mhttex1 fragment complex is preferentially found in the nuclear compartment, and may not be protective *in vivo* reviewed in Butler et al 2011 [9]. It would be interesting to test whether a PEST fusion of this intrabody can utilize nuclear proteasomes for mhtt degradation.

We were able to confirm that N-terminal mutant httex1 fragment degradation is dependent upon proteasomal function, since epoxomicin, a potent and selective proteasome inhibitor [34], inhibited the turnover. The intrabody-PEST mediated turnover of intracellular target is dependent upon the specific order of key amino acids within mODC-PEST motif rather than enhanced solubility. The intracellular stability of scFv-intrabodies is notoriously poor due to macromolecular crowding and an unfavorable redox potential within the cellular cytoplasm [10,29,53]. We have previously reported that cis-acidification of a poorly soluble scFv-intrabody with a C-terminal 3X-Flag tag can enhance intrabody solubility and function [32], thus it is possible that the addition of this highly acidic domain would improve the scFv-C4 intrabody function via enhanced folding effects. However, a scrambled version of the PEST used here maintained the charge density without enhancing the intrabody-mediated turnover of its target. Since both scFv-C4 and scFv-6E are soluble in the cellular environment, it is unlikely that enhanced solubility contributed to the clearance of htt fragments.

Intrabody-mediated degradation with a PEST motif had been previously tested with a fusion intrabody scFv-13R4 against β-galactosidase [27]. In that case, PEST fusion rendered the intrabody-PEST protein itself unstable, and binding to its target stabilized the complex. The (β-gal) target protein is extremely large, which may account for the inability of cellular proteasomes to degrade the antigen-antibody complex. The scFv-13R4 intrabody itself also belongs to a different framework family than scFv-C4 [54]. The scFv-C4 intrabody was selected from a natural non-immune human library [55], while scFv-6E used a consensus framework [56,57]. The biophysical and intracellular properties of intrabodies are quite dependent upon both the frameworks and the complementary determining regions. This should carry over to the properties of the fusion intrabodies as well. We have previously reported that the anti-β-gal scFv-13R4 parent intrabody also differs from anti-htt scFv-C4 in solubility calculations [32]. In an attempt to circumvent the potential effect of a proteasomal targeting signal on steady-state intrabody levels, Mechionna and Cattaneo created inducible suicide intrabodies by fusion with IκBα, which must be activated by TNFα [58]. After activation, scFv-R4-IκBα reduced β-gal by 15–20%, while an anti-Tau scFv#2 reduced τ151–422 by 70–90%. However, as noted in their publication, the requirement to use a biologically active ligand is suboptimal, due to potential side-effects. It is clear from our work that there may be many classes of intrabodies that do not require exogenous activation in order to effectively degrade targets. Testing of constitutively active intrabody fusions is quite straightforward, allowing empirical determination of the most suitable fusions of intrabodies and PEST domains for specific targets. Once a sufficient number of studies have been performed on diverse constructs, it may also be possible to predict the behavior of fusions and engineer them to degrade targets without suicide. Fusion construct approaches should empower long-term intrabody-mediated correction, and may be more generally applicable to intrabody therapeutics of neurological diseases characterized by abnormal protein accumulation.

Materials and Methods

Expression plasmids

cDNA, previously described by Kvam et. al., [18] encoding scFv-C4 (GenBank accession number EU490426) was PCR amplified using complementary primers. The forward primer (5′-TGCTCTA-GACGCCATGGCCCAGGTG CAGC-3′) introduced an XbaI restriction site (underlined) prior to the existing 5′ Kozak sequence. The reverse primers (Standard: 5′-CCC**AAGCTT**TTACTACA-CATTG ATCCTAGCAGAAG CACAGGCTGCAGGGTGACG-GTCCATCCCGCTCTCCTGGGCACAAGACATGGGCAGC-GTGCCATCATCCTGCTCCTCCACCTCCGGCGGGAAGC-CATGGCTCGCGTAGTCTGGGACGTCG-3′; "Scramble": 5′-CCC**AAGCTT**TTACTACAGCCTGTGACGATGCACTGCA-GACATAGGGGCAGCAGAGTCCCCGCTCTGGATATTGG-CCTCACAAGCCATGGGCGTACAGAACTCATCCTCGCCA-TCCTCCACCGGCTGC GGGCTGCCCGCGTAGTCTGGGA-CGTCG-3′) introduced a standard or scrambled PEST motif corresponding to amino acids 422–461 from mouse ornithine decarboxylase (GenBank accession number NM_013614.2) and a HindIII (BOLD) restriction site immediately following the stop codon. The resulting PCR product was ligated into pAAV-MCS (Stratagene) at the corresponding XbaI and HindIII restriction sites using standard cloning techniques. scFv-6E (GenBank accession number FJ695518) was cloned into pAAV-MCS in a similar manner. To create fluorescently-labeled intrabodies, scFv-C4 -HA-PEST was PCR amplified using a complementary forward primer (5′-TGCTCTA-GACGCCATGGCCCAGG-3′) and a reverse primer that introduced a BamHI (underlined) restriction site (5′-CGGGATCCCACATT-GATCCT AGCAGAAGCAC-3′). The PCR removes the stop codon, allowing the scFv-C4 -HA-PEST construct to be ligated in-frame 5′ to a $(Gly_4Ser)_4$ flexible peptide repeat linked to a humanized enhanced green fluorescent protein (EGFP), all on a pcDNA3.1(-) plasmid backbone previously described by Kvam et al. [18]. The resulting expression plasmid cassette was the following: Kozak sequence-scFv-C4-HA-PEST-$(Gly_4Ser)_4$-EGFP-stop. Vectors for the expression of human httex1 with different polyglutamine repeat lengths labeled with either EGFP or RFP respectively, were described elsewhere (pcDNA3.1-Httex1-25Q-EGFP, pcDNA3.1-Httex1-72Q-EGFP [59], and pcDNA3.1-Httex1-25Q-RFP, pcDNA3.1-Httex1-72Q-RFP [60]. All expression plasmids were prepared using EndoFree Plasmid Maxi (Qiagen) and confirmed by DNA sequencing.

Cell culture and transfection

Undifferentiated ST14A cells were cultured according to standard protocols [28]. ST14A cells were transiently transfected with jetPEI DNA transfection reagent (Polyplus Transfection Inc.) as previously described [18]. For all transfections, intrabody plasmids were applied at equal (1:1) or lesser ratios (1:2 or 1:5) to httex1 plasmids, and cells were analyzed 48 hours post-transfection.

Cell fractionation, AGERA, and Western blot

Transiently transfected ST14A cells were collected from 6-well culture dishes by trypsinization and washed twice with PBS. Soluble and insoluble protein fractions were isolated as previously described [18]. Briefly, whole-cell lysates were extracted at 4°C in 50 uL/well of RIPA lysis buffer (50 mM Tris pH 7.5, 150 mM NaCl, 1% NP40, 0.25% sodium deoxycholate, 0.1% SDS) supplemented with complete protease inhibitor cocktail (Roche). Detergent-insoluble material was pelleted by microcentrifugation (13,000 rpm 610 min., 4°C). Soluble protein in the supernatant was quantified using Bio-Rad DC Protein Assay kit (Bio-Rad Laboratories). Lysates were adjusted to 1 mg/mL in 2X denaturing sample buffer (125 mM Tris, 4% SDS, 20% glycerol, 10% 2-mercaptoethanol, 0.02% bromophenol blue, pH 6.8) and boiled. Insoluble pellet fractions were washed with RIPA, resuspended in 50 μL/well of 2X denaturing sample buffer, and boiled for 15 min. Equal volumes of pellet and soluble fractions corresponding to, 20 μg of total protein (10 mL) were resolved by SDS-PAGE and transferred onto PVDF membranes (PerkinElmer).

Aggregated huntingtin was quantified by agarose gel electrophoresis for resolving aggregates (AGERA) method [31]. Briefly, samples were homogenized in 10 volumes (w/v) tris-saline (10 mM Tris-HCl, pH 8.0, 150 mM NaCl, 2% SDS) and complete protease inhibitor (Roche Diagnostics) and stored at −80°C. For 1.5% agarose gels, 1.5 g agarose (Invitrogen) was dissolved in 100 mL 375 mmol/L Tris-HCl, pH 8.8 and then boiled. After melting, SDS was added to a final concentration of 0.1% (w/v). Samples were diluted 1:1 into 2X non-denaturing sample buffer (150 mmol/L Tris-HCl pH 6.8, 33% glycerol, 1.2% SDS and bromophenol blue) and incubated for 5 min. at 95°C. Forty µg of protein was loaded per AGERA lane. After loading, gels were run in Laemmli running buffer (192 mmol/L glycine, 25 mmol/L Tris-base, 0.1% (w/v) SDS) at 100 V, 2 A until the bromophenol blue running front reached the bottom of the gel. A Transblot SD semi-dry electroblotter (BIORAD) was used to blot the gels on PDVF membranes (Millipore) at 200 mA for 1 hour. Membranes were then developed using mouse monoclonal EM48 (1:1000, Chemicon). HA-tagged intrabodies and endogenous actin were probed with monoclonal anti-HA (1:5,000, Covance) and anti-actin (1:1000, Sigma) Abs, respectively, labeled with HRP-conjugated goat-anti-mouse IgG (1:2000, Santa Cruz), and detected by ECL (PerkinElmer).

Live-cell imaging and aggregation counts

ST14A cells transfected with GFP- and/or mRFP-tagged reporters were imaged directly in 6-well culture dishes using an Olympus IX70 inverted microscope equipped with an Olympus IXFLA Inverted Reflected Light Fluorescence Observation attachment and RGB Mirror Cube filter wheel (Olympus). Cells were observed without fixation using a 406lens, and images were captured 48 hours post-transfection with a SPOT RT Color CCD camera using SPOT Advanced software (Diagnostic Instruments). Digital images were overlayed and cropped using Adobe Photoshop.

Flow cytometry

ST14A cells were seeded into 6-well culture dishes (2.50×10^5 cells/well) and transfected, 24 hours later, in triplicate wells, with plasmids encoding GFP (containing either normal or expanded polyglutamine repeat tracts) and either intrabody or empty vector. Approximately 48 hours post-transfection, cell medium was harvested and adherent cells were collected by trypsinization. Harvested cells and exhausted media were combined and passed through a 70 µm cell strainer (BD Biosciences). Cells were pelleted by centrifugation (800 rpm, 5 min.) and resuspended in 1 mL of FACS buffer (16 $Ca2^+$- and $Mg2^+$-free PBS, 10% FBS) containing 50 mM propidium iodide (PI; Sigma). Cells were stained for 20 min. in the dark and pelleted by centrifugation (4,000 rpm, 5 min.). Cell pellets were resuspended in 0.5 mL of FACS buffer/well and transferred to Falcon 5 mL round-bottom polystyrene FACS tubes. Labeled cells were sorted by fluorescence using a BD FACSCalibur Flow Cytometer (BD Biosciences) and a minimum of 30,000 events were recorded per sample using BD CellQuest Pro software. GFP was detected with an FL1 detector, and PI with FL3. Prior to each experiment, the flow cytometer was calibrated against three control groups: (1) unstained ST14A cells to gate autofluorescence, (2) unstained ST14A cells expressing httex1-25Q-eGFP alone to identify transfected cells, and (3) stained ST14A cells pre-treated with H_2O_2 for maximal PI uptake. Using BD CellQuest Pro software, data were displayed in two-color dotplot formats on a log-scale, and cell death was expressed as a percentage by dividing the number of cells that stained with PI by the total number of events. Because scFv-C4-PEST decreased the MFI of GFP, gating for GFP positive cells and PI-positive cells for viability was not possible.

Statistical analysis

All values represent the mean of at least three independent experiments, with multiple individual values per experiment. Statistical significance was determined by one-way ANOVA using Minitab or Statview statistical software. P values$<$0.05 were designated as statistically significant.

Acknowledgments

We thank Dr. Elena Cattaneo (Milano, Italy) for ST14A cells. We thank Kevin Manley, Abigail Snyder-Keller, and Shubhada Joshi for helpful discussions; and the Wadsworth Center Applied Genomic Technologies Core for sequencing, and Flow Cytometry Unit of Immunology Core for cell assays.

Author Contributions

Conceived and designed the experiments: DCB AM. Performed the experiments: DCB. Analyzed the data: DCB AM. Contributed reagents/materials/analysis tools: AM. Wrote the paper: DCB AM.

References

1. Gusella JF, MacDonald ME (2000) Molecular genetics: unmasking polyglutamine triggers in neurodegenerative disease. Nat Rev Neurosci 1: 109–115.
2. Sapp E, Schwarz C, Chase K, Bhide PG, Young AB, et al. (1997) Huntingtin localization in brains of normal and Huntington's disease patients. Ann Neurol 42: 604–612.
3. DiFiglia M, Sapp E, Chase KO, Davies SW, Bates GP, et al. (1997) Aggregation of huntingtin in neuronal intranuclear inclusions and dystrophic neurites in brain. Science 277: 1990–1993.
4. Becher MW, Kotzuk JA, Sharp AH, Davies SW, Bates GP, et al. (1998) Intranuclear neuronal inclusions in Huntington's disease and dentatorubral and pallidoluysian atrophy: correlation between the density of inclusions and IT15 CAG triplet repeat length. Neurobiol Dis 4: 387–397.
5. Davies SW, Turmaine M, Cozens BA, DiFiglia M, Sharp AH, et al. (1997) Formation of neuronal intranuclear inclusions underlies the neurological dysfunction in mice transgenic for the HD mutation. Cell 90: 537–548.
6. Slow EJ, Graham RK, Osmand AP, Devon RS, Lu G, et al. (2005) Absence of behavioral abnormalities and neurodegeneration in vivo despite widespread neuronal huntingtin inclusions. Proc Natl Acad Sci U S A 102: 11402–11407.
7. Ratovitski T, Gucek M, Jiang H, Chighladze E, Waldron E, et al. (2009) Mutant huntingtin N-terminal fragments of specific size mediate aggregation and toxicity in neuronal cells. J Biol Chem 284: 10855–10867.
8. Graham RK, Deng Y, Carroll J, Vaid K, Cowan C, et al. (2010) Cleavage at the 586 amino acid caspase-6 site in mutant huntingtin influences caspase-6 activation in vivo. J Neurosci 30: 15019–15029.
9. Butler DC, McLear JA, Messer A (2011) Engineered antibody therapies to counteract mutant huntingtin and related toxic intracellular proteins. Progress in Neurobiology: in Press.
10. Messer A, Lynch SM, Butler DC (2009) Developing intrabodies for the therapeutic suppression of neurodegenerative pathology. Expert Opin Biol Ther 9: 1189–1197.
11. Messer A, McLear J (2006) The therapeutic potential of intrabodies in neurologic disorders: focus on huntington and Parkinson diseases. Biodrugs 20: 327–333.
12. Cardinale A, Biocca S (2008) The potential of intracellular antibodies for therapeutic targeting of protein-misfolding diseases. Trends Mol Med 14: 373–380.
13. Perez-Martinez D, Tanaka T, Rabbitts TH (2010) Intracellular antibodies and cancer: new technologies offer therapeutic opportunities. Bioessays 32: 589–598.
14. Atwal RS, Xia J, Pinchev D, Taylor J, Epand RM, et al. (2007) Huntingtin has a membrane association signal that can modulate huntingtin aggregation, nuclear entry and toxicity. Hum Mol Genet 16: 2600–2615.
15. Cornett J, Cao F, Wang CE, Ross CA, Bates GP, et al. (2005) Polyglutamine expansion of huntingtin impairs its nuclear export. Nat Genet 37: 198–204.
16. Omi K, Hachiya NS, Tanaka M, Tokunaga K, Kaneko K (2008) 14-3-3zeta is indispensable for aggregate formation of polyglutamine-expanded huntingtin protein. Neurosci Lett 431: 45–50.
17. Rockabrand E, Slepko N, Pantalone A, Nukala VN, Kazantsev A, et al. (2007) The first 17 amino acids of Huntingtin modulate its sub-cellular localization, aggregation and effects on calcium homeostasis. Hum Mol Genet 16: 61–77.
18. Kvam E, Nannenga BL, Wang MS, Jia Z, Sierks MR, et al. (2009) Conformational targeting of fibrillar polyglutamine proteins in live cells escalates aggregation and cytotoxicity. PLoS One 4: e5727.
19. Lecerf J-M, Shirley TL, Zhu Q, Kazantsev A, Amersdorfer P, et al. (2001) Human single-chain Fv intrabodies counteract in situ huntingtin aggregation in cellular models of Huntington's disease. PNAS 98: 4764–4769.

20. Miller TW, Zhou C, Gines S, MacDonald ME, Mazarakis ND, et al. (2005) A human single-chain Fv intrabody preferentially targets amino-terminal huntingtin fragments in striatal models of Huntington's disease. Neurobiol Dis 19: 47–56.
21. Murphy RC, Messer A (2004) A single-chain Fv intrabody provides functional protection against the effects of mutant protein in an organotypic slice culture model of Huntington's disease. Brain Res Mol Brain Res 121: 141–145.
22. McLear JA, Lebrecht D, Messer A, Wolfgang WJ (2008) Combinational approach of intrabody with enhanced Hsp70 expression addresses multiple pathologies in a fly model of Huntington's disease. FASEB J 22: 2003–2011.
23. Snyder-Keller A, McLear JA, Hathorn T () Messer A Early or late-stage anti-N-terminal Huntingtin intrabody gene therapy reduces pathological features in B6.HDR6/1 mice. J Neuropathol Exp Neurol 69: 1078–1085.
24. Ghoda L, van Daalen Wetters T, Macrae M, Ascherman D, Coffino P (1989) Prevention of rapid intracellular degradation of ODC by a carboxyl-terminal truncation. Science 243: 1493–1495.
25. Li X, Zhao X, Fang Y, Jiang X, Duong T, et al. (1998) Generation of destabilized green fluorescent protein as a transcription reporter. J Biol Chem 273: 34970–34975.
26. Leclerc GM, Boockfor FR, Faught WJ, Frawley LS (2000) Development of a destabilized firefly luciferase enzyme for measurement of gene expression. Biotechniques 29: 590–591, 594–596, 598 passim.
27. Sibler AP, Courtete J, Muller CD, Zeder-Lutz G, Weiss E (2005) Extended half-life upon binding of destabilized intrabodies allows specific detection of antigen in mammalian cells. FEBS J 272: 2878–2891.
28. Ehrlich ME, Conti L, Toselli M, Taglietti L, Fiorillo E, et al. (2001) ST14A cells have properties of a medium-size spiny neuron. Exp Neurol 167: 215–226.
29. Colby DW, Chu Y, Cassady JP, Duennwald M, Zazulak H, et al. (2004) Potent inhibition of huntingtin aggregation and cytotoxicity by a disulfide bond-free single-domain intracellular antibody. Proc Natl Acad Sci U S A 101: 17616–17621.
30. Colby DW, Garg P, Holden T, Chao G, Webster JM, et al. (2004) Development of a human light chain variable domain (V(L)) intracellular antibody specific for the amino terminus of huntingtin via yeast surface display. J Mol Biol 342: 901–912.
31. Weiss A, Klein C, Woodman B, Sathasivam K, Bibel M, et al. (2008) Sensitive biochemical aggregate detection reveals aggregation onset before symptom development in cellular and murine models of Huntington's disease. J Neurochem 104: 846–858.
32. Kvam E, Sierks MR, Shoemaker CB, Messer A (2010) Physico-chemical determinants of soluble intrabody expression in mammalian cell cytoplasm. Protein Eng Des Sel 23: 489–498.
33. Rechsteiner M, Rogers SW (1996) PEST sequences and regulation by proteolysis. Trends Biochem Sci 21: 267–271.
34. Meng L, Mohan R, Kwok BH, Elofsson M, Sin N, et al. (1999) Epoxomicin, a potent and selective proteasome inhibitor, exhibits in vivo antiinflammatory activity. Proc Natl Acad Sci U S A 96: 10403–10408.
35. Verhoef LG, Lindsten K, Masucci MG, Dantuma NP (2002) Aggregate formation inhibits proteasomal degradation of polyglutamine proteins. Hum Mol Genet 11: 2689–2700.
36. Barkhordarian H, Emadi S, Schulz P, Sierks MR (2006) Isolating recombinant antibodies against specific protein morphologies using atomic force microscopy and phage display technologies. Protein Eng Des Sel 19: 497–502.
37. Jana NR, Zemskov EA, Wang G, Nukina N (2001) Altered proteasomal function due to the expression of polyglutamine-expanded truncated N-terminal huntingtin induces apoptosis by caspase activation through mitochondrial cytochrome c release. Hum Mol Genet 10: 1049–1059.
38. Southwell AL, Khoshnan A, Dunn DE, Bugg CW, Lo DC, et al. (2008) Intrabodies binding the proline-rich domains of mutant huntingtin increase its turnover and reduce neurotoxicity. J Neurosci 28: 9013–9020.
39. Southwell AL, Ko J, Patterson PH (2009) Intrabody gene therapy ameliorates motor, cognitive, and neuropathological symptoms in multiple mouse models of Huntington's disease. J Neurosci 29: 13589–13602.
40. Khoshnan A, Ko J, Patterson PH (2002) Effects of intracellular expression of anti-huntingtin antibodies of various specificities on mutant huntingtin aggregation and toxicity. Proc Natl Acad Sci U S A 99: 1002–1007.
41. Greiner ER, Yang XW () Huntington's disease: flipping a switch on huntingtin. Nat Chem Biol 7: 412–414.
42. Wolfgang WJ, Miller TW, Webster JM, Huston JS, Thompson LM, et al. (2005) Suppression of Huntington's disease pathology in Drosophila by human single-chain Fv antibodies. Proc Natl Acad Sci U S A 102: 11563–11568.
43. Zuccato C, Valenza M, Cattaneo E (2010) Molecular mechanisms and potential therapeutical targets in Huntington's disease. Physiol Rev 90: 905–981.
44. Bett JS, Goellner GM, Woodman B, Pratt G, Rechsteiner M, et al. (2006) Proteasome impairment does not contribute to pathogenesis in R6/2 Huntington's disease mice: exclusion of proteasome activator REGgamma as a therapeutic target. Hum Mol Genet 15: 33–44.
45. Bennett EJ, Shaler TA, Woodman B, Ryu KY, Zaitseva TS, et al. (2007) Global changes to the ubiquitin system in Huntington's disease. Nature 448: 704–708.
46. Murakami Y, Matsufuji S, Hayashi SI, Tanahashi N, Tanaka K (1999) ATP-Dependent inactivation and sequestration of ornithine decarboxylase by the 26S proteasome are prerequisites for degradation. Mol Cell Biol 19: 7216–7227.
47. Sarkar S, Rubinsztein DC (2008) Huntington's disease: degradation of mutant huntingtin by autophagy. FEBS J 275: 4263–4270.
48. Auerbach W, Hurlbert MS, Hilditch-Maguire P, Wadghiri YZ, Wheeler VC, et al. (2001) The HD mutation causes progressive lethal neurological disease in mice expressing reduced levels of huntingtin. Hum Mol Genet 10: 2515–2523.
49. Atwal RS, Xia J, Pinchev D, Taylor J, Epand RM, et al. (2007) Huntingtin has a membrane association signal that can modulate huntingtin aggregation, nuclear entry and toxicity. Hum Mol Genet 16: 2600–2615.
50. Benn CL, Landles C, Li H, Strand AD, Woodman B, et al. (2005) Contribution of nuclear and extranuclear polyQ to neurological phenotypes in mouse models of Huntington's disease. Hum Mol Genet 14: 3065–3078.
51. Landles C, Sathasivam K, Weiss A, Woodman B, Moffitt H, et al. (2010) Proteolysis of mutant huntingtin produces an exon 1 fragment that accumulates as an aggregated protein in neuronal nuclei in Huntington disease. J Biol Chem 285: 8808–8823.
52. Schiefner A, Chatwell L, Korner J, Neumaier I, Colby DW, et al. A Disulfide-Free Single-Domain V(L) Intrabody with Blocking Activity towards Huntingtin Reveals a Novel Mode of Epitope Recognition. J Mol Biol.
53. Miller TW, Messer A (2005) Intrabody applications in neurological disorders: progress and future prospects. Mol Ther 12: 394–401.
54. Martineau P, Jones P, Winter G (1998) Expression of an antibody fragment at high levels in the bacterial cytoplasm. J Mol Biol 280: 117–127.
55. Sheets MD, Amersdorfer P, Finnern R, Sargent P, Lindquist E, et al. (1998) Efficient construction of a large nonimmune phage antibody library: the production of high-affinity human single-chain antibodies to protein antigens. Proc Natl Acad Sci U S A 95: 6157–6162.
56. Tomlinson I, Holliger P (2000) Methods for generating multivalent and bispecific antibody fragments. Methods Enzymol 326: 461–479.
57. Holt LJ, Bussow K, Walter G, Tomlinson IM (2000) By-passing selection: direct screening for antibody-antigen interactions using protein arrays. Nucleic Acids Res 28: E72.
58. Melchionna T, Cattaneo A (2007) A protein silencing switch by ligand-induced proteasome-targeting intrabodies. J Mol Biol 374: 641–654.
59. Steffan JS, Kazantsev A, Spasic-Boskovic O, Greenwald M, Zhu YZ, et al. (2000) The Huntington's disease protein interacts with p53 and CREB-binding protein and represses transcription. Proc Natl Acad Sci U S A 97: 6763–6768.
60. Jach G, Pesch M, Richter K, Frings S, Uhrig JF (2006) An improved mRFP1 adds red to bimolecular fluorescence complementation. Nat Methods 3: 597–600.

Hdac6 Knock-Out Increases Tubulin Acetylation but Does Not Modify Disease Progression in the R6/2 Mouse Model of Huntington's Disease

Anna Bobrowska[1], Paolo Paganetti[2¤], Patrick Matthias[3], Gillian P. Bates[1]*

1 Department of Medical and Molecular Genetics, King's College London, London, United Kingdom, **2** Novartis Institutes for BioMedical Research, Neuroscience Discovery, Basel, Switzerland, **3** Friedrich Miescher Institute for Biomedical Research, Novartis Research Foundation, Basel, Switzerland

Abstract

Huntington's disease (HD) is a progressive neurodegenerative disorder for which there is no effective disease modifying treatment. Following-on from studies in HD animal models, histone deacetylase (HDAC) inhibition has emerged as an attractive therapeutic option. In parallel, several reports have demonstrated a role for histone deacetylase 6 (HDAC6) in the modulation of the toxicity caused by the accumulation of misfolded proteins, including that of expanded polyglutamine in an N-terminal huntingtin fragment. An important role for HDAC6 in kinesin-1 dependent transport of brain-derived neurotrophic factor (BDNF) from the cortex to the striatum has also been demonstrated. To elucidate the role that HDAC6 plays in HD progression, we evaluated the effects of the genetic depletion of HDAC6 in the R6/2 mouse model of HD. Loss of HDAC6 resulted in a marked increase in tubulin acetylation throughout the brain. Despite this, there was no effect on the onset and progression of a wide range of behavioural, physiological, molecular and pathological HD-related phenotypes. We observed no change in the aggregate load or in the levels of soluble mutant exon 1 transprotein. HDAC6 genetic depletion did not affect the efficiency of BDNF transport from the cortex to the striatum. Therefore, we conclude that HDAC6 inhibition does not modify disease progression in R6/2 mice and HDAC6 should not be prioritized as a therapeutic target for HD.

Editor: Koichi M. Iijima, Thomas Jefferson University, United States of America

Funding: This work was supported by a European Commission Marie Curie Initial Training Network (215618) Fellowship (AB) and the CHDI Foundation. The funders had no role in the study design, data collection and analysis, decision to publish or preparation of the manuscript. At the time that this study was performed, PP was an employee of Novartis Institutes for BioMedical Research and helped with experimental design, data analysis, and reading of the manuscript.

Competing Interests: At the time that this research was performed, PP was an employee of Novartis Institutes for BioMedical Research. There are no patents, products in development, or marketed products to declare. This does not alter the authors' adherence to all the PLoS ONE policies on sharing data and materials, as detailed online in the guide for authors.

* E-mail: gillian.bates@kcl.ac.uk

¤ Current address: AC Immune SA, Lausanne, Switzerland

Introduction

Huntington's disease (HD) is an autosomal dominant progressive neurodegenerative disorder with a mean age of onset of 40 years [1]. The most characteristic features of symptomatic HD patients are motor disorders, cognitive decline, psychiatric disturbances and weight loss. The disease progresses on average for 15–20 years and although the first symptomatic drug has recently been approved by the Federal Drug Administration, there is still no disease modifying treatment available [2]. The cause of HD is the expansion of a CAG trinucleotide repeat in the *HTT* gene, resulting in an expanded polyglutamine (polyQ) tract in the N-terminus of the huntingtin protein [3]. HD pathology is mostly observed in the brain with the striatum displaying pronounced atrophy, although other brain regions are also affected [4,5]. A prominent feature of HD is the presence of mutant huntingtin containing cytoplasmic aggregates and nuclear inclusions that are ubiquitin positive [6]. At the molecular level, many changes have been observed that may contribute to HD pathology including abnormal levels of neurotransmitters and their receptors, mitochondrial dysfunction, metabolic disturbances, transcriptional dysregulation and disruption of microtubule based transport, among others [7].

Histone deacetylases (HDACs) have been proposed as possible therapeutic targets for HD [8]. There are altogether 18 mammalian HDAC's, divided into four classes depending on their homology to yeast enzymes. Class I and II enzymes have Zn^{2+} dependent catalytic domains and are homologous to yeast Rpd3 and Hda1, respectively. HDAC11 is also Zn^{2+} dependent but has been placed in a separate category (class IV) due to a lack of sufficient sequence similarity to any other group [9]. Sirtuins (class III) are homologous to yeast Sir2 and use a different mechanism requiring NAD^+ as a co-factor [10]. Studies on HDAC inhibition have shown promising results in fly, worm and mouse models of HD [11,12,13,14].

HDAC6 is a target of some of the broad range HDAC inhibitors including suberoyl anilide hydroxamic acid (SAHA) and trichostatin A (TSA) [15]. It is a particularly interesting protein, in that it is the only known HDAC with two catalytically active deacetylase domains and a ubiquitin interacting domain [16,17]. Moreover, its main activity appears to be in the cytoplasm, where it has been shown to deacetylate α-tubulin, HSP90 and cortactin, among others [18,19,20,21]. HDAC6 is also of particular interest in HD. In cell models, HDAC6 has been shown to act against protein misfolding toxicity by taking part in the formation of a juxtanuclear structure termed the aggresome, a microtubule dependent inclusion body to which dispersed aggregates are targeted and transported by the dynein motor [22]. HDAC6 is required for the targeting of ubiquitinated aggregates to the aggresome, thought to serve as an adaptor protein by binding both poly-ubiquitin chains and the dynein motor. Interestingly, deacetylase activity and intact microtubules are essential to this process implying that aggresome formation depends on tubulin acetylation status [23]. Similarly, it has been shown that HDAC6 is critical for the formation of stress granules [24]. In addition, it has recently been shown that in the case of proteasome overload, aggresome formation might provide the means by which the cell removes accumulated misfolded proteins by autophagy and that HDAC6 is essential for this pathway [25]. In a *Drosophila melanogaster* model of spinal and bulbar muscular atrophy (SBMA) HDAC6 expression rescued neurodegeneration in an autophagy-dependent manner [26]. In fact, HDAC6 has also recently been shown to be involved in ubiquitin selective quality control autophagy by regulating the lysosome to autophagosome fusion [27]. On the other hand, a study in an HD cell model has indicated that increasing tubulin acetylation by HDAC6 inhibition could rescue the brain-derived neurotrophic factor (BDNF) transport deficit from the cortex to the striatum [28]. Taken together, these findings strongly suggest that HDAC6 inhibition should modify HD progression.

Based on the previous studies in cell culture models of HD, we might expect that loss of HDAC6 would increase aggregate load and exacerbate the phenotype in a mouse model of HD. On the other hand, an increase in cortico-striatal BDNF transport might be expected to improve some HD-related phenotypes. To determine whether HDAC6 regulates aggregate formation and turnover and/or plays a role in BDNF transport in a mouse model of HD, we crossed the R6/2 transgene onto an *Hdac6* knock-out background. As *Hdac6* is located on the X-chromosome, hemizygous male mice are nullizygous for *Hdac6* [29]. The R6/2 mouse has an early onset and rapid phenotype progression [30] and at late stage disease expresses HD-related phenotypes that are extremely similar to those that develop in the *Hdh*Q150 knock-in model of HD [31,32,33,34,35]. We showed that in the absence of HDAC6, levels of tubulin acetylation were increased throughout the brain. However, this had no effect on R6/2 readouts in a battery of physiological and behavioural assessments. We also found no difference in levels of soluble or aggregated huntingtin trans-protein upon ablation of HDAC6. Our data thus suggest that HDAC6 is not important for aggregate clearance in a mouse model of HD. Finally, we established that increased tubulin acetylation did not affect levels of BDNF in the striatum. We conclude that inhibition of HDAC6 should not be pursued as a high priority therapeutic target for HD.

Results

Hdac6 knock-out mice (*Hdac6*KO) are viable and fertile, and do not show any overt phenotypes [36]. Before analysing the effect of the genetic depletion of HDAC6 on phenotype progression in the R6/2 mice, we wanted to verify that these mice do not express HDAC6 at the mRNA or protein level. cDNA was prepared from cortex, striatum, cerebellum, muscle and liver from 4 week old wild type (WT) and *Hdac6*KO mice and analysed by real-time quantitative RT-PCR (qPCR). *Hdac6* was not expressed in tissue from *Hdac6*KO mice (Fig. 1A). HDAC6 protein could not be detected in brain or testes by western blot analysis (Fig. 1B). Consistent with previous reports, HDAC6 levels were higher in testes than in brain [36]. R6/2 mice in our colony reach end-stage disease at 15 weeks of age. In order to determine whether *Hdac6* is stably expressed during this disease time-frame, we compared the levels of *Hdac6* mRNA in WT mice at 4, 9 and 15 weeks of age. We established that *Hdac6* is expressed at relatively stable levels in WT mice from 4 to 15 weeks of age, with only a 15% reduction being detected in the cortex at 9 weeks as compared to 4 weeks of age (Fig. 1C). Transcriptional dysregulation is a hallmark of the molecular pathogenesis of HD and is recapitulated by the R6/2 mouse model [37]. Thus, to ensure that *Hdac6* is not dysregulated in R6/2 mice, we measured *Hdac6* expression levels in R6/2 mice at 4, 9 and 15 weeks of age in cortex, striatum and cerebellum and compared them to those observed in WT mice. *Hdac6* levels were unchanged between WT and R6/2 mice (Fig. 1D) indicating that there was no effect of disease progression on the expression of *Hdac6*.

Tubulin is hyperacetylated upon genetic depletion of HDAC6 but is not altered by the presence of the R6/2 transgene

As HDAC6 is an α-tubulin deacetylase, depletion of HDAC6 should result in tubulin hyper-acetylation. It has been previously reported that the *Hdac6*KO line of mice used in this study, has elevated levels of acetylated tubulin in peripheral tissue but not in brain [36]. However, increased tubulin acetylation has been shown to occur in brain as a consequence of HDAC6 depletion in an alternative *Hdac6* knock-out mouse [38]. To resolve this discrepancy, we analysed tubulin acetylation in our *Hdac6*KO mice by western blotting, normalising levels of acetylated tubulin to those of total α–tubulin. We found that tubulin is hyperacetylated in the cortex, striatum and cerebellum of *Hdac6*KO mice at 4, 9 and 15 weeks of age as compared to WT littermates (Fig. 2A and C). The extent of hyperacetylation in *Hdac6*KO mice became less pronounced with age in the cortex and cerebellum, perhaps explaining the earlier results.

Acetylation of lysine 40 on α-tubulin has been demonstrated to increase the binding of certain molecular motor proteins to microtubules, thus modulating intracellular transport dynamics [39]. Impairment of intracellular transport has been suggested to contribute to the molecular pathology of HD [40]. Therefore, we investigated whether tubulin acetylation is altered by the presence of the R6/2 transgene. Our results indicate that there is no difference in tubulin acetylation between R6/2 and WT mice in cortex, striatum and cerebellum at 4, 9 or 15 weeks of age (Fig. 2B and D). This is consistent with the fact that there is no difference in the expression of *Hdac6* between WT and R6/2 mice in the same tissues throughout disease progression (Fig. 1D).

Genetic Depletion of HDAC6 does not modify HD physiological and behavioural phenotypes in R6/2 mice

Previous studies have indicated that both over-expression and depletion of HDAC6 could ameliorate HD phenotypes in cell culture [25,28]. Here, we investigate whether HD-related phenotypes are modulated by the genetic depletion of HDAC6 in an HD mouse model. R6/2 males were bred to *Hdac6*KO heterozygous females and a longitudinal phenotyping study was performed to compare *Hdac6*KOxR6/2 double mutant (Dble) mice to WT, *Hdac6*KO and R6/2 littermates. As *Hdac6* is an X-linked gene [29], males carrying the mutant allele are effectively nullizygous for *Hdac6* (Fig. 1A–B). We obtained at least 16 males for each genotype and the R6/2 and Dble groups were well matched for their CAG repeat size ($p = 0.338$) (Fig. 3A).

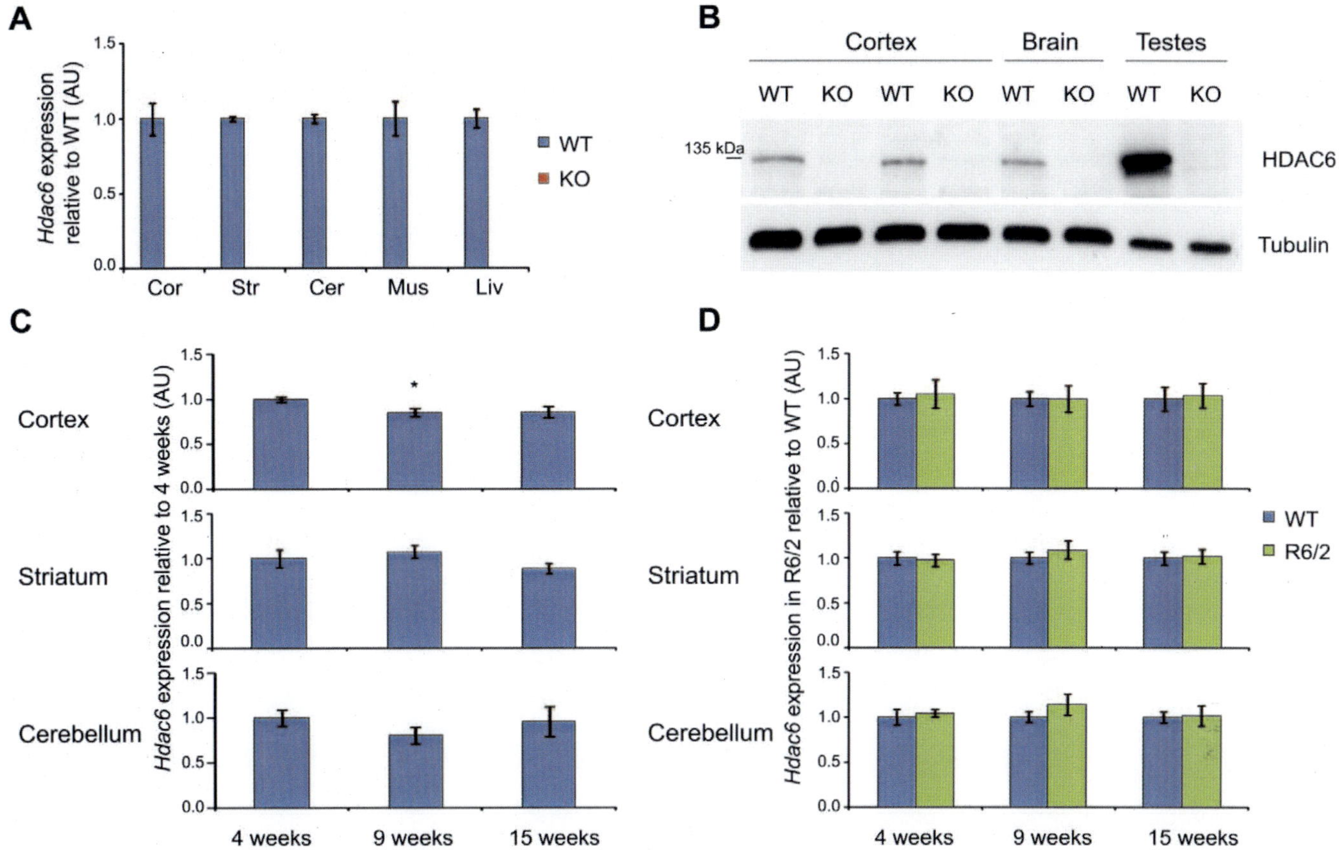

Figure 1. HDAC6 expression in *Hdac6*KO, WT and R6/2 mice. (**A**) Taqman qPCR assay showing absence of *Hdac6* mRNA expression in *Hdac6*KO mice as compared to WT; n = 3/genotype. Data normalised to *Atp5b* and expressed as fold change of WT for each tissue. (**B**) Western blot showing absence of HDAC6 protein expression in *Hdac6*KO mice as compared to WT. (**C**) Taqman qPCR assay showing that *Hdac6* mRNA expression does not change with age in WT mice in cortex, striatum and cerebellum; n = 8/genotype, data normalised to *Atp5b and Rpl13a* (cortex), *Gapdh* (striatum) and 18S RNA (cerebellum) and expressed as fold change of 4 weeks. (**D**) Taqman qPCR assay showing no difference in *Hdac6* mRNA expression between WT and R6/2 mice in cortex, striatum and cerebellum at 4, 9 and 15 weeks; n≥6/genotype, data normalised to WT for each time point and brain region. Error bars represent SEM. * $p<0.05$ as compared to 4 weeks. KO – *Hdac6* knock out, WT – wild type, Cor - cortex, Str - striatum, Cer - cerebellum, Mus - muscle, Liv - liver.

Mice were weighed weekly to the nearest 0.1 g from 4 weeks of age onwards (Fig. 3B). R6/2 mice weighed significantly less than WT mice overall ($F_{(1,64)} = 14.28$, $p<0.001$) and gained weight at a significantly slower rate ($F_{(2,640)} = 55.99$, $p<0.001$). HDAC6 depletion by itself had no impact on the weight ($F_{(1,64)} = 0.567$, $p = 0.454$) and weight gain ($F_{(2,640)} = 0.247$, $p = 0.741$) when compared to WT mice. Absence of HDAC6 did not affect the loss of weight in R6/2 ($F_{(1,64)} = 0.007$, $p = 0.931$) or the decreased rate in weight gain ($F_{(2,640)} = 0.512$, $p = 0.567$). These data indicate that depletion of HDAC6 does not affect weight loss in the R6/2 mice (Fig. 3B).

RotaRod measures motor coordination and balance, both of which become significantly impaired in R6/2 mice. Here the animals were subjected to RotaRod analysis at 4, 8, 10, 12 and 14 weeks of age (Fig. 3C). As expected, R6/2 mice performed worse than WT mice ($F_{(1,71)} = 39.74$, $p<0.001$) and that performance deteriorated over the course of the study ($F_{(3,1420)} = 18.23$, $p<0.001$). The performance of *Hdac6*KO mice was similar to WT ($F_{(1,71)} = 0.32$, $p = 0.573$) but the variability in their performance over time was significantly different to that of WT mice ($F_{(3,1420)} = 3.53$, $p = 0.020$). Nevertheless, the *Hdac6* knock-out genotype did not modify the performance of R6/2 mice overall ($F_{(1,71)} = 0.40$, $p = 0.529$) or with age ($F_{(3,1420)} = 1.09$, $p = 0.352$).

Forelimb grip strength was measured at 4 weeks of age and weekly from 11 to 14 weeks of age (Fig. 3D). As expected, the overall grip strength of R6/2 mice was worse than that of WT ($F_{(1,67)} = 142.41$, $p<0.001$) and deteriorated over time ($F_{(3,536)} = 50.69$, $p<0.001$). The grip strength of *Hdac6*KO mice was no different from WT mice either overall ($F_{(1,67)} = 0.621$, $p = 0.434$) or with time ($F_{(3,536)} = 1.97$, $p = 0.121$). Nullizygosity for *Hdac6* did not have an effect on the overall grip strength of R6/2 mice ($F_{(1,67)} = 3.17$, $p = 0.081$) nor did it influence the deterioration in grip strength over the course of the experiment ($F_{(3,536)} = 0.856$, $p = 0.463$). Therefore, genetic depletion of HDAC6 does not modify loss of forelimb muscle strength in R6/2 mice.

Spontaneous motor activity was recorded for each mouse for 30 min in an infrared activity monitoring cage bi-weekly from 5 weeks of age onwards (Fig. 3E and Fig. S1). Data were analysed by repeated measures general linear model ANOVA and *p*-values are presented in Table S1. At 5 weeks of age, levels of activity between mice of all genotypes were comparable (Fig. 3E and Table S1: R6/2 Genotype and *Hdac6*KO Genotype), but a significant difference in the pattern of activity over time was already evident for activity ($p = 0.011$) and rearing ($p = 0.016$) for mice carrying the R6/2 transgene. At 7 weeks of age the R6/2 genotype significantly affected the activity and mobility ($p<0.001$) of the mice. A clear

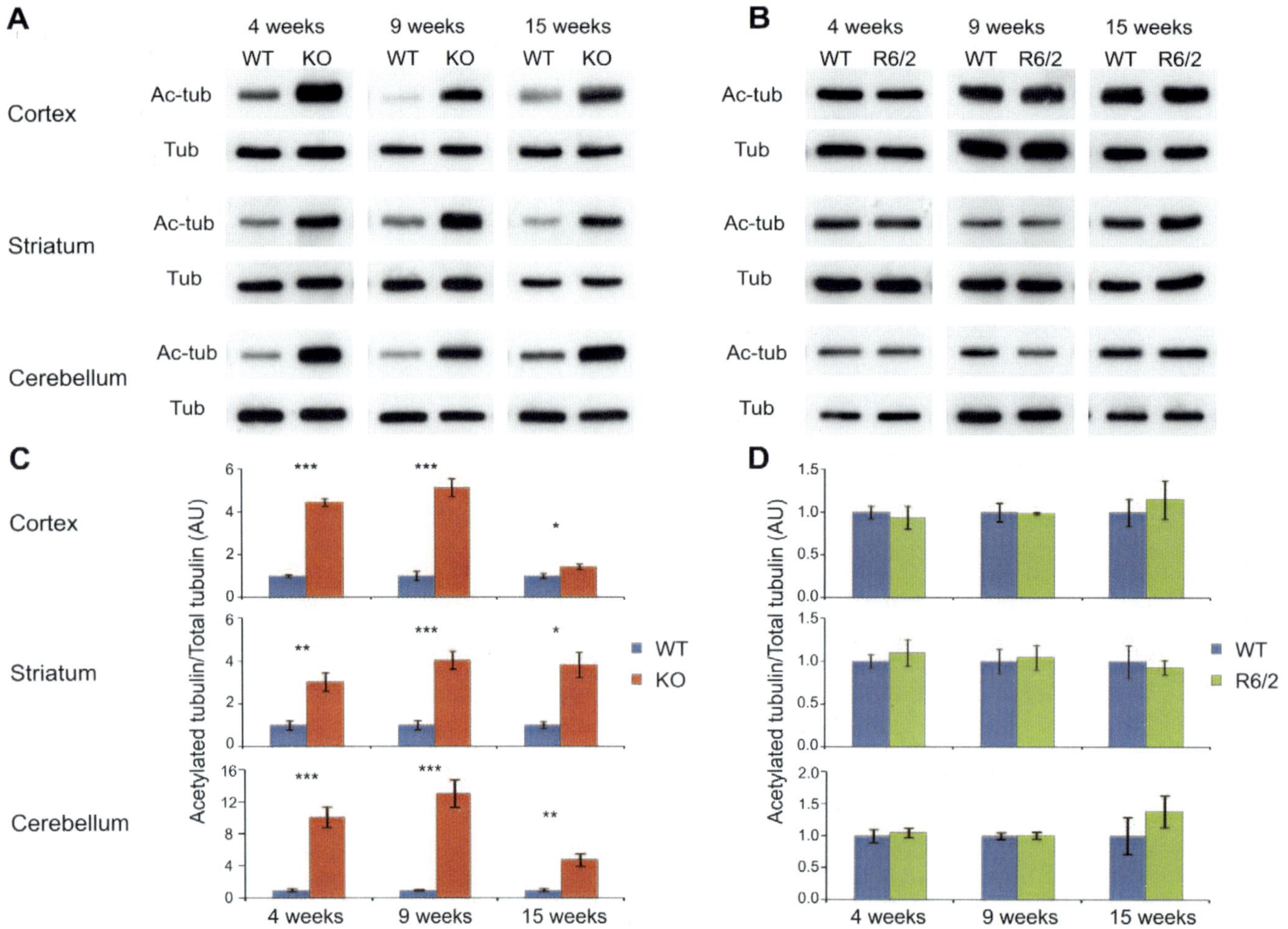

Figure 2. Tubulin acetylation in the brains of *Hdac6*KO and R6/2 mice compared to WT. (A–B) Representative western blots showing acetylated tubulin (Ac-tub) between *Hdac6*KO and WT mice (A) and R6/2 and WT mice (B) at 4, 9 and 15 weeks in cortex, striatum and cerebellum with tubulin (Tub) as a loading control. **(C–D)** Densitometric quantification of western blots represented in (A–B). Acetylated tubulin was normalised to α-tubulin and the relative signal for *Hdac6*KO (C) or R6/2 (D) expressed as fold change compared to WT. Error bars represent SEM. * $p<0.05$, ** $p<0.01$, *** $p<0.001$; n≥4/genotype. KO – *Hdac6* knock out, WT – wild type.

hypoactivity was evident in both the R6/2 and Dble mice at 9, 11 and 13 weeks of age (Fig. 3E and Table S1, R6/2 Genotype). *Hdac6*KO mice were comparable to WT and the Dble mutant mice to R6/2 at almost all time points indicating that depletion of HDAC6 had no influence on the R6/2 hypoactivity phenotype.

Mice were sacrificed at 15 weeks of age and brains weighed to the nearest 0.001 g (Fig. 3F). As expected, R6/2 mice had a significantly lower brain weight than WT mice ($p<0.001$). The weight of *Hdac6*KO brains was similar to WT ($p<0.057$) and that of the Dble mutant mice was similar to R6/2 ($p=0.784$). Thus, absence of HDAC6 does not modify the loss in brain weight exhibited by the R6/2 mice at end-stage disease.

Genetic Depletion of HDAC6 does not modify huntingtin aggregation

Aggregation of mutant huntingtin is a prominent feature of HD neuropathology and occurs in all of the HD rodent models that have thus far been developed. Aggregates in the R6/2 mouse appear prior to the onset of behavioural symptoms and continue to accumulate throughout the course of the disease. At the same time, a steady decrease in the levels of soluble transprotein can be observed. In cells, HDAC6 acts as a linker between ubiquitinated protein and/or aggregates and the dynein/dynactin motor complex enabling their transport to the aggresome for autophagic degradation [23]. If this phenomenon is relevant to the mammalian brain, an absence of HDAC6 should result in an increase in aggregate load [25].

We measured the amount of SDS insoluble aggregates by the Seprion ligand ELISA [34] and found no difference in aggregate load between R6/2 and Dble mice at 4, 9 and 15 weeks of age in cortex, hippocampus and brain stem (Fig. 4A and Fig. S2A), or at 9 and 15 weeks in quadriceps muscle (Fig. S2E). The corresponding levels of soluble transprotein were measured in these tissues by means of TR-FRET (Fig. 4B and Fig. S2D–E), similarly, no difference between R6/2 and Dble mice was detected. These results were confirmed by a TR-FRET aggregation assay (Fig. S2D) and by western blotting of SDS-PAGE resolved lysates with an antibody that detects soluble and aggregated huntingtin (S830) (Fig. 4C and Fig. S2B).

Our data show that HDAC6 ablation does not influence aggregate load or levels of soluble mutant huntingtin in the cortex, hippocampus or brain stem at 4, 9 or 15 weeks of age (Fig. 4, Fig. S2A–C) or in quadriceps muscle at 9 and 15 weeks of age (Fig. S2E). In support of this, we did not detect any obvious differences in the level or distribution of aggregates between R6/2 and Dble

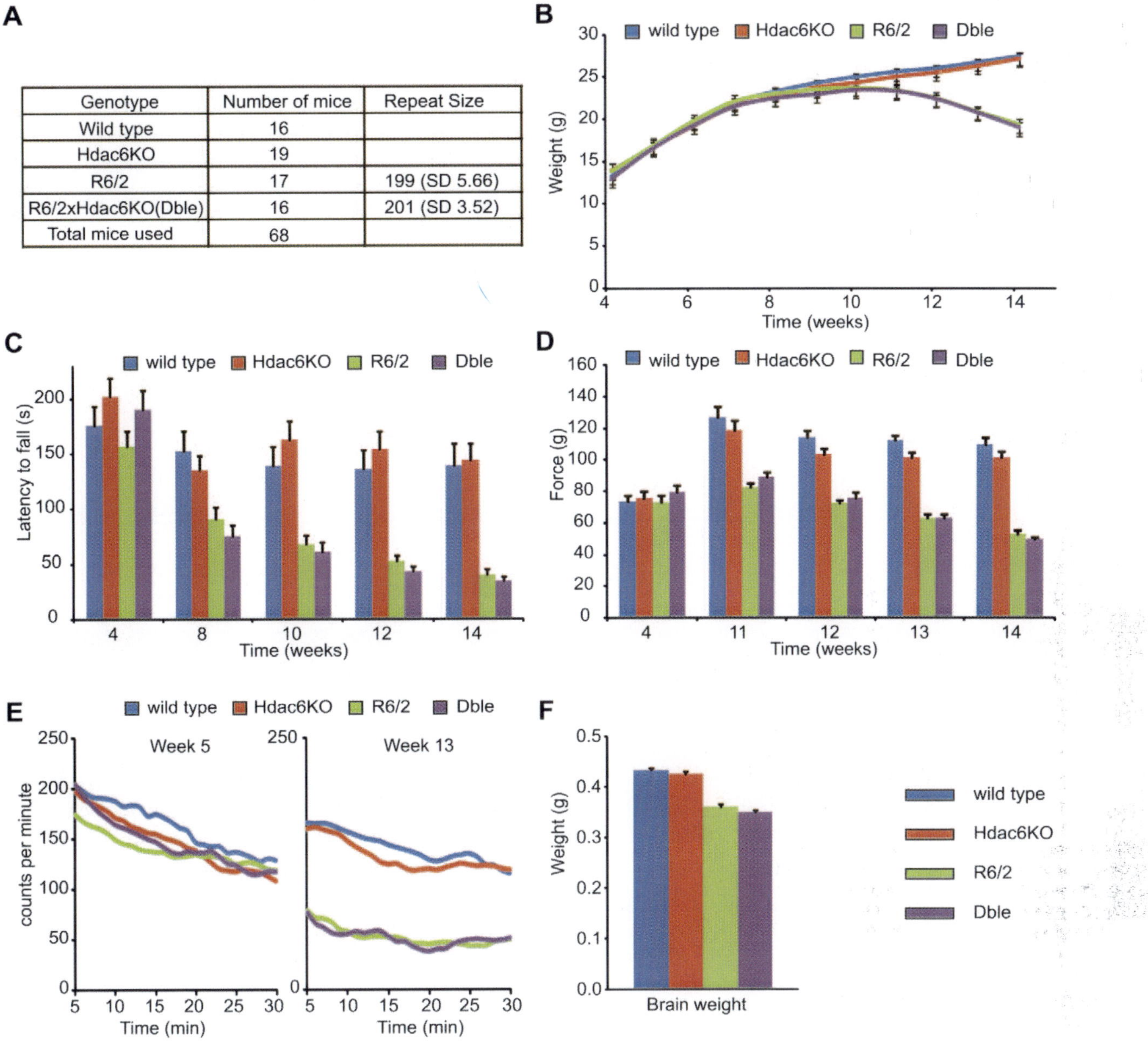

Genotype	Number of mice	Repeat Size
Wild type	16	
Hdac6KO	19	
R6/2	17	199 (SD 5.66)
R6/2xHdac6KO(Dble)	16	201 (SD 3.52)
Total mice used	68	

Figure 3. Behavioural and physiological phenotypes in the absence of HDAC6. (**A**) The number of male mice analysed per genotype with the mean CAG repeat size for the groups carrying the R6/2 transgene (SD-standard deviation). (**B**) Body weight (**C**) Time spent on RotaRod (**D**) Forelimb grip strength (**E**) Spontaneous motor activity recorded at the beginning (week 5) and end (week 13) of the study. Graphs were created by plotting 5 min moving averages (**F**) Brain weight measured at week 15. Error bars represent SEM.

striata at 9 weeks of age by immunohistochemistry (Fig. 4D). Although a significant decrease in soluble cortical transprotein levels was detected by TR-FRET in the Dble as compared to the R6/2 mice at 9 weeks of age, further analysis by western blot has shown that this difference, if real, is not large (Fig. 4B–C). At the same age, there was no difference in the cortical aggregate load measured by either Seprion ELISA or TR-FRET (Fig. 4A and Fig. S2D).

Genetic Depletion of HDAC6 results in tubulin hyperacetylation in the brains of R6/2 mice

We have found that the absence of HDAC6 has no effect on R6/2 behavioural phenotypes or on the accumulation of aggregated transprotein in these animals. It is possible that the presence of the R6/2 transgene prevented the hyperacetylation of tubulin from occurring in response to HDAC6 depletion. Therefore, we compared the levels of acetylated tubulin between R6/2 and Dble mice at 4, 9 and 15 weeks of age in the cortex, striatum and cerebellum. We found that HDAC6 depletion resulted in a pronounced increase in tubulin acetylation in R6/2 mice in all brain regions and at all time-points studied (Fig. 5). The increase in tubulin acetylation was comparable between *Hdac6*KO and Dble mutant mice (Fig. S3). We conclude that the substantial increase in tubulin acetylation levels throughout the brain has no consequence on HD-related phenotypes in the R6/2 mouse.

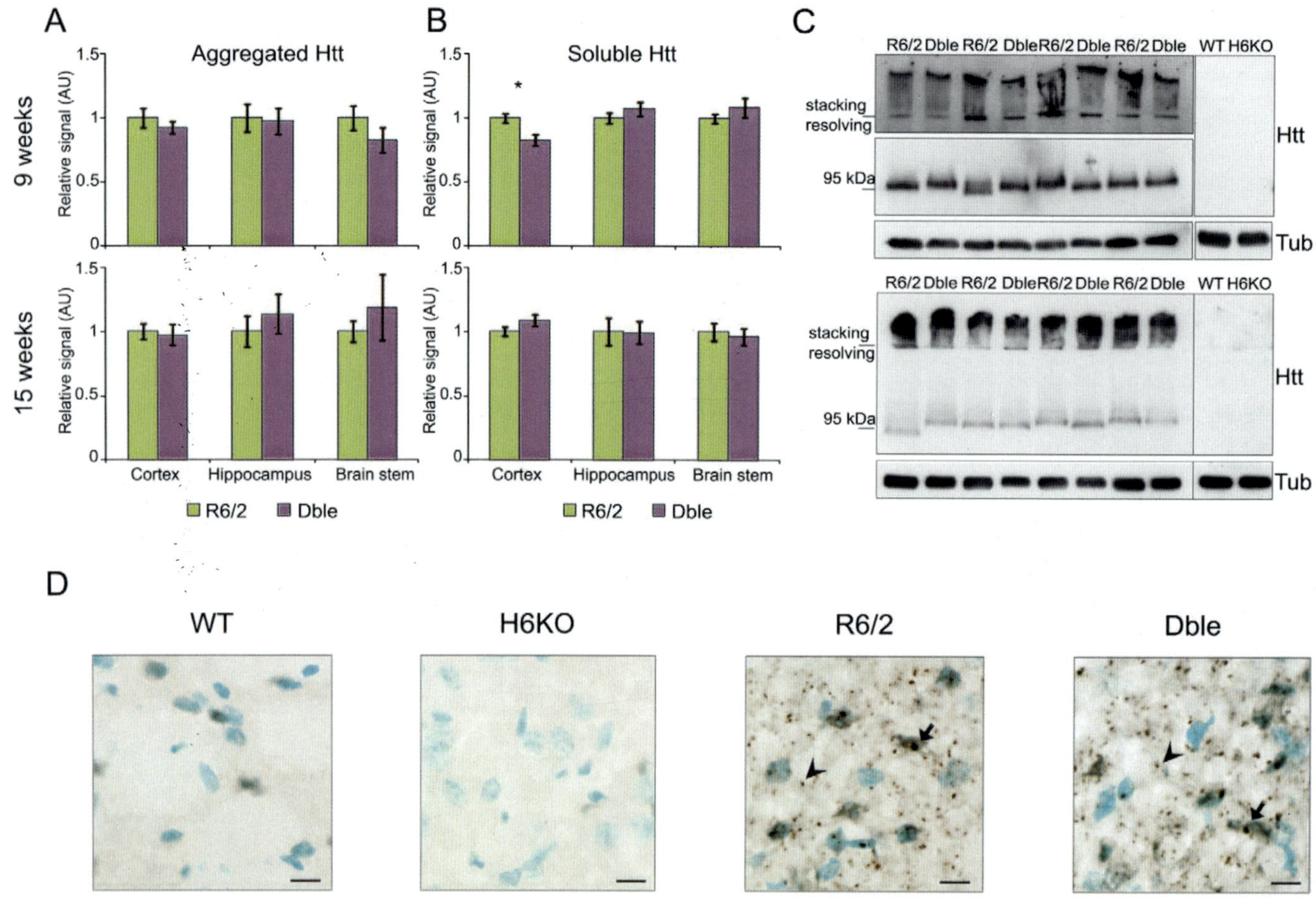

Figure 4. No effect of *Hdac6* knock-out on aggregate load or soluble transprotein levels. (**A**) Aggregate load was measured by Seprion ligand ELISA (MW8 antibody) and (**B**) soluble transprotein levels were measured by TR-FRET (2B7-MW1 antibodies) in the cortex, hippocampus and brain stem of R6/2 and Dble mice at 9 and 15 weeks. The average of the WT and *Hdac6*KO background signal was subtracted from both R6/2 and Dble signals. The Dble signal is expressed as fold change of the R6/2 signal. * $p<0.05$; $n\geq8$/genotype. (**C**) Representative western blots with S830 anti-huntingtin antibody showing aggregated and soluble transprotein (Htt) in the cortex at 9 (upper panel) and 15 (lower panel) weeks. α-tubulin (Tub) was used as a loading control. Specificity of S830 staining is confirmed by lack of signal in WT and *Hdac6*KO cortices. (**D**) Representative sagittal sections from 9 week old mice showing the striatum immunostained with S830 antibody. Nuclei are counterstained with methyl green. Scale bar = 10 µm. Arrow = nuclear inclusion, arrowhead = cytoplasmic aggregate. Error bars represent SEM.

Genetic Depletion of HDAC6 does not modify BDNF content in the striatum

Cell culture studies have shown that an increase in tubulin acetylation increases the transport of BDNF from the cortex to the striatum in the context of both WT and HD [28]. In accordance with previous data [41], we found that *Bdnf* mRNA expression is lower in the cortex of R6/2 mice at 9 weeks of age and that this phenotype is not altered by HDAC6 depletion (Fig. 6A). However, at the same age, levels of BDNF protein in the cortex as measured by ELISA were comparable between mice of all four genotypes (Fig. 6B). Equally, BDNF protein levels in the striatum of *Hdac6*KO, R6/2 and Dble mice were not different from those of WT mice (Fig. 6C). Therefore, the decrease in *Bdnf* mRNA did not translate to a reduction in BDNF protein. As *Bdnf* is expressed in the striatum at a very low level (Fig. S4A) and it has been published that most striatal BDNF protein originates in the cortex [42], we conclude that there is no effect of HDAC6 ablation on the transport efficiency of BDNF from the cortex to the striatum in either WT or R6/2 mice.

Discussion

Previous studies in cell culture models of HD have shown that modulation of HDAC6 levels alters HD-related phenotypes [25,28]. To extend this analysis to a mouse model, we investigated the effects of HDAC6 genetic depletion in the R6/2 mouse. We showed that *Hdac6* knock-out mice (*Hdac6*KO) do not express HDAC6 at the mRNA or protein levels and have hyperacetylated tubulin in the cortex, striatum and cerebellum from 4 to 15 weeks of age. We show that in the presence of the polyQ expanded R6/2 transprotein, levels of acetylated tubulin do not differ from that in wild type animals and similarly, the HD mutation does not interfere with the effect that HDAC6 ablation has on tubulin hyperacetylation. We found that depletion of HDAC6 had no effect on the aggregate load or BDNF levels in the R6/2 brain and did not modify physiological or behavioural HD-related phenotypes in R6/2 mice.

In this study, we have used mice in which the endogenous *Hdac6* gene has been disrupted [36]. One possible concern with using mice that do not express HDAC6 throughout development is that

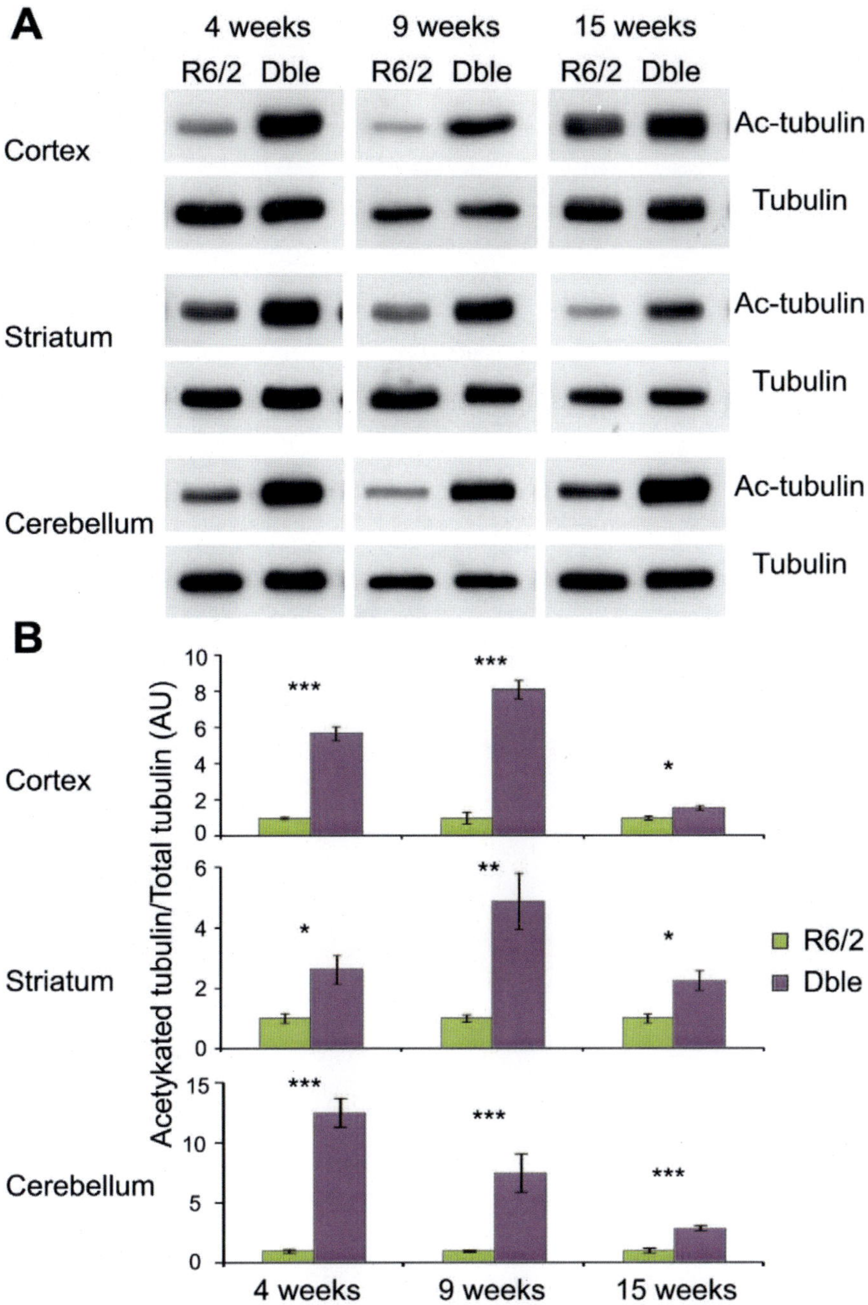

Figure 5. Tubulin acetylation in the brains of Dble as compared to R6/2 mice. (**A**) Representative western blots showing acetylated tubulin in Dble and R6/2 mice at 4, 9 and 15 weeks in cortex, striatum and cerebellum with α-tubulin as a loading control. (**B**) Densitometric quantification of western blots presented in (A). Acetylated tubulin was normalised to α-tubulin and the relative signal for Dble mice expressed as fold change to R6/2. Error bars represent SEM. * $p<0.05$, ** $p<0.01$, ***$p<0.001$; n≥4/genotype.

the expression of other genes will adjust to compensate for the deficit. The HDAC6 mechanisms of action under investigation here are based on HDAC6-tubulin interactions. Our demonstration that tubulin acetylation is increased in the brain from 4 to 15 weeks of age indicates that compensation has not occurred for the HDAC6 target in which we are primarily interested and that the constitutive *Hdac6* knock-out mice used here are a suitable model. There are numerous mouse models of HD, which include mice transgenic for an N-terminal fragment of *HTT*, YAC and BAC mice that are transgenic for full-length *HTT* gene and knock-in mice in which an expanded CAG repeat has been introduced into the mouse *Hdh* gene [43]. The HD cell culture model used by Iwata and colleagues [25] to show that HDAC6 is required for aggresome formation expressed an exon 1 huntingtin transprotein. The R6/2 mice express an exon 1 N-terminal fragment of mutant huntingtin [30] and therefore, they represent an appropriate model with which to first follow-up on their findings. Also, recent analysis has shown that the R6/2 mice develop HD-related phenotypes that are highly comparable to a genetically accurate knock-in mouse model of HD [31,33,34,35] and that, in these knock-in mice, mutant huntingtin is processed to generate N-terminal fragments [32]. Despite this, analysing the effects of the

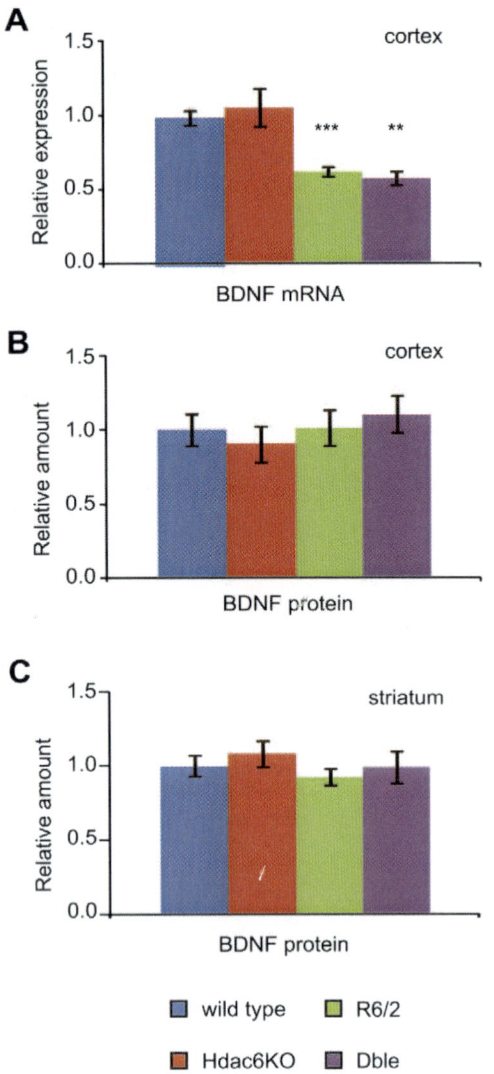

Figure 6. Influence of *Hdac6* knock-out on *Bdnf* mRNA and protein levels. (**A**) Taqman qPCR assay showing a significant down-regulation of *Bdnf* coding region mRNA expression in cortex of mice carrying the R6/2 transgene. Data normalised to WT. ** $p<0.01$ (to *Hdac6KO*), *** $p<0.001$ (to WT); $n\geq4$/genotype. (**B–C**) BDNF protein content in the cortex (B) and striatum (C) measured by ELISA. Data normalised to WT. $n\geq3$/genotype in (B) and $n\geq4$/genotype in (C). Error bars represent SEM.

modulation of *Hdac6* levels on HD phenotypes in these more genetically precise models might be considered important. However, before embarking on such a project, it would be wise to determine whether a reduction in HDAC6 levels has an effect in cell culture models expressing a mutant version of full-length huntingtin.

HDAC6 has been extensively characterised as being required for the formation and subsequent autophagic degradation of the aggresome [23,25,27]. In an HD cell culture model, HDAC6 was required for aggresome formation and an increase in aggregate load was observed upon HDAC6 knock-down [25]. Proteasome inhibition resulted in an increase in ubiquitin positive aggregates in *Hdac6*KO mouse embryonic fibroblasts as compared to wild type cells indicating that HDAC6 is important for autophagy [44]. HDAC6 knock-down in a *Drosophila melanogaster* model of SBMA exacerbated retinal degeneration and overexpression of HDAC6 decreased aggregate load and ameliorated retinal degeneration, effects that required HDAC6 catalytic activity [26]. In keeping with a role for HDAC6 in protein homeostasis, ubiquitin positive aggregates have been reported to accumulate in the brains of another strain of *Hdac6*KO mice by 6 months of age [27]. Given that an increase in aggregation was not detected in R6/2 mice that lack HDAC6, we conclude that either quality-control autophagy is not important for the clearance of polyQ aggregates or that HDAC6 is not essential for this process in the R6/2 mouse brain. It is possible that the mechanism of aggregate handling could differ between lower organisms/cell culture models and HD mice.

In cultured cells, an increase in tubulin acetylation has been shown to enhance kinesin-1 binding and microtubule-based transport [39]. BDNF is a kinesin-1 cargoe [28], which is actively transported from the cortex to the striatum [42]. A recent study in cells has shown that by increasing tubulin acetylation one can increase BDNF cortico-striatal transport and that this is an HDAC6 dependent process [28]. In HD there is a well documented decrease in cortical *BDNF* mRNA expression [41] and we have confirmed that R6/2 mice at 9 weeks of age recapitulate this phenotype, regardless of presence or absence of HDAC6. However, this did not translate into a reduction in BDNF in either the cortex or the striatum in accordance with some, but not all previously published data [45,46,47], suggesting that R6/2 mice at 9 weeks do not display a deficit in BDNF transport. If HDAC6 depletion increases BDNF transport independent of the presence of the huntingtin mutation, as has been reported [28], we would expect to see an increase in striatal BDNF protein levels in both *Hdac6*KO and double mutant mice. We did not observe any change in BDNF levels. Strategies that increase BDNF levels have been shown to be beneficial in R6/2 mice and other N-terminal fragment models [45,48,49,50]. If small changes had occurred, that were beyond the sensitivity of our detection method, they were not sufficient to improve the phenotype of R6/2 mice.

There has been an increased focus on HDAC6 in neurodegenerative disease. In addition to the polyglutamine diseases, over-expression of HDAC6 was protective in *Drosophila melanogaster* models of Parkinson's disease [51] and Alzheimer's disease [52]. HDAC6 has also been found to localise to Lewy bodies in Parkinson's disease patient brains [23] and there is also evidence supporting a role for HDAC6 in Alzheimer's disease via its association with tau [53]. Our finding that the knock-out of HDAC6 does not affect the phenotype, aggregate load or BDNF transport in R6/2 mice was very surprising. This study underlines the importance of validating pathogenic mechanisms and therapeutic targets in mammalian models. At the same time, our findings indicate that the protective effect of broad range HDAC inhibitors that has been observed in invertebrate and mouse HD models [8] is not predominantly mediated via inhibition of HDAC6. The current study is part of a wider project to investigate the effects of the genetic depletion (knock-out or knock-down) of specific HDACs on HD-related phenotypes in the R6/2 mouse. Genetic reduction of *Hdacs3, 5, 7* and *9* have not resulted in a phenotypic improvement ([54] and unpublished data) whereas knock-down of *Hdac4* has shown beneficial effects (unpublished data). Based on our data, we can conclude that HDAC6 inhibition would not be a valid therapeutic strategy for HD.

Materials and Methods

Ethics statement

All experimental procedures performed on mice were approved by the King's College London Ethical Review Process Committee and carried out under the UK Home Office License 70/6545.

Mouse strains and husbandry

Hemizygous R6/2 mice were maintained by backcrossing R6/2 males to CBAxC57BL/6 F1 (CBF) females (B6CBAF1/OlaHsd, Harlan Olac, UK) [30]. *Hdac6* knock-out (*Hdac6*KO) mice [36] on C57BL/6 background were backcrossed once to CBF. For the R6/2x*Hdac6*KO genetic cross, R6/2 males were bred to *Hdac6* heterozygous females. At 4 weeks of age, mice were weaned into cages of 5, each containing at least one representative of each genotype. Animals were housed under 12 h light/12 h dark cycle, with unlimited access to water and chow (Special Diet Services, Witham, UK). Cages were environmentally enriched as described [55]. Mice from the R6/2x*Hdac6*KO cross were given mash food consisting of powdered chow mixed with water during 4–6 and 12–15 weeks of age and sacrificed at 15 weeks.

Genotyping

Mice were genotyped by PCR of tail-tip DNA. R6/2 mice were genotyped and their repeat sizes determined as described [34]. For the *Hdac6* genotyping, the primers were forward: 5′-GTACAATGTGGCTCACAGAA, reverse wt: 5′-CAGGCACAGGAATATGAGTT and reverse KO: 5′-CAACTCTGCCTCTCCTGG each used 1 µL at 10 µM in one multiplex 10 µL reaction, containing also 1 µL of 100 ng/µL DNA, 0.8 µL 25 mM $MgCl_2$, 1 µL 2 mM dNTP, 1 µL Sigma 10×PCR buffer and 0.1 µL Sigma Taq Polymerase (D4545, Sigma). Cycling conditions were as follows: 94°C for 5 min, (94°C for 30 s, 64°C for 30 s and 72°C for 1 min)×40 followed by 10 min at 72°C.

Phenotypic assessment

The phenotypes of the mice from the R6/2x*Hdac6*KO cross were assessed blind to genotype. Mice were weighed weekly to the nearest 0.1 g. RotaRod performance was measured at 4 weeks of age for 4 consecutive days, 3 runs a day and after that at 8, 10, 12 and 14 weeks of age for 3 consecutive days, 3 runs a day, using an accelerating (4–44 rpm in 5 min) Ugo Basile 7650 Rotarod, (Linton Instrumentation, UK) modified as described [55]. Exploratory, spontaneous motor activity was recorded at 5, 7, 9, 11 and 13 weeks of age by placing mice in AM1053 activity cages for 30 min during the day, as described previously [56]. Activity was the total number of lower level beam breaks. Mobility was the number of at least two consecutive beam breaks occurring in the lower level. Rearing was the number of rearing beam breaks and centre rearing was the number of rearing beam breaks occurring away from the cage walls. Forelimb grip strength was assessed at 4 weeks of age and then weekly from 11 to 14 weeks, always prior to RotaRod measurements, with San Diego Instruments Grip Strength Meter (San Diego, CA, USA) as described previously [55]. Mice were sacrificed at 15 weeks of age and brains were weighed to the nearest 0.001 g.

Antibodies

The HDAC6 antibody was a kind gift from Dr. Tso-Pang Yao [38]. Acetylated α-tubulin (6-11B-1, T7451) and α-tubulin (DM1A, T9026) antibodies were purchased from Sigma. S830 is a sheep polyclonal antibody raised against a GST tagged huntingtin exon 1 with 53 glutamines, characterized elsewhere [57] and was generated at Scottish Antibody Production Unit. MW8, MW1 [58] and 2B7 [59] were obtained from Novartis, Basel. Secondary peroxidase coupled antibodies were purchased from Dako (anti-goat, anti-mouse), Pierce (anti-rabbit) or KPL (anti-mouse for Seprion).

Sample preparation

For tubulin acetylation analysis, tissues were homogenised using 1% Triton X-100 buffer with 50 mM Tris-HCl pH 7.5, 150 mM NaCl, 2 mM EDTA, 5 µM TSA (Trichostatin A, Sigma) and 10 mM nicotinamide (Sigma), supplemented with protease inhibitor cocktail (Roche). For HDAC6 immuno-detection, tissues were homogenised in RIPA buffer (1% NP-40, 0.5% Deoxycholate, 0.1% SDS, 50 mM Tris-HCl pH 8, 150 mM NaCl, 1 mM β-mercaptoethanol, 100 µM PMSF, 1 mM DTT) supplemented with protease inhibitor cocktail (Roche). Samples were sonicated on ice for 10 s at 80 Hz (Vibracell Sonicator). Lysates were cleared by centrifugation at 16 200 rcf for 15 min at 4°C. Protein concentration was measured with Pierce BCA assay kit (Thermo Scientific). Samples were diluted with 2× protein Laemmli buffer (1 M Tris-HCl pH 6.8, 2.3% SDS, 4.5% glycerol, 10% β-mercaptoethanol, 0.001 g/mL bromophenol blue) and denatured for 5 min at 95°C.

Western blotting

Equal amounts of protein were loaded onto SDS polyacrylamide gel with a size reference (Broad Range Protein Marker, Cell Signalling or Spectra Broad Range Protein Ladder, Fermentas). Proteins were transferred onto Protran nitrocellulose membrane (Whatman) at 120 V for 90 min by submerged transfer apparatus (Bio-Rad) in transfer buffer (20% v/v methanol, 25 mM Tris, 192 mM glycine). Membranes were blocked in 5% non-fat dried milk in PBS for at least 1 hour. Primary antibodies were applied in 0.02% PBS-Tween 20 (PBST) for 20 min (1:40000 acetylated α-tubulin; 1:30000 α-tubulin) or 1 hour (1:5000 S830) at room temperature or overnight (1:250 HDAC6) at 4°C. Blots were washed thrice for 5 min in 0.2% PBST and incubated with appropriate HRP coupled secondary antibody (all 1:5000 except anti-rabbit 1:20000). For signal detection, GE Healthcare Enhanced Chemiluminescence detection system and Amersham Hyperfilms (both GE Healthcare) were used according to the manufacturer's instructions. Signals were quantified using a GS-800 densitometer (Bio-Rad).

Aggregate detection with Seprion ligand ELISA

For aggregate detection 2.5% lysates (w/v) were prepared by homogenising tissue in RIPA. Aggregate capture and detection were performed in Seprion ligand coated plates (Microsens) as described [34].

TR-FRET

Time resolved - Förster resonance energy transfer experiments (TR-FRET) were performed as described [60].

BDNF ELISA

BDNF protein content was measured by the commercially available ELISA kit (Promega) according to manufacturer's instructions modified as described [61]. Lysates were prepared at 2.2% dilution (w/v) and were not acid treated.

Taqman real time quantitative PCR

RNA extraction, cDNA synthesis, Taqman RT-qPCR and ΔCt analysis were performed as described previously [62]. Housekeeping genes (primer and probe mix purchased from Primer Design) were chosen appropriate to the brain region analysed. For time-course or across tissue analysis, several housekeeping genes were tested and the most stable ones chosen. Primers for *Hdac6* expression analysis were forward: 5′ - GGAGACAACCCAGTACATGAATGAA; reverse: 5′ - CGGAGGACAGAGCCTGTAG and the probe was 5′-FAM-TATCTGCATCCGAACTCATATTCCTGTGCCTG-TAMRA. Primers for *Bdnf* coding region were forward: 5′ - GGGTCACAGCGGCAGATAAA; reverse: 5′ - GCCTTTGGATACCGGGACTT; and the probe was: 5′ - FAM - TCTGGCGGGACGGTCACAGTCC - TAMRA.

Immunohistochemistry

Whole brains were snap frozen in isopentane at −50°C. Immunohistochemistry was performed as described [31].

Statistical Analysis

Data from the R6/2x*Hdac6*KO cross were analysed with SPSS using one way ANOVA or General Linear Model ANOVA with Greenhouse-Geisser correction for non-sphericity. Data from qPCR and tubulin acetylation assay were analysed with Microsoft Excel using Student's *t*-test (two tailed).

Supporting Information

Figure S1 ***Hdac6*** **knock-out has no effect on spontaneous motor activity in WT or R6/2 mice.** Five minute moving averages for Activity, Mobility, Rearing and Centre rearing at 5, 7, 9, 11 and 13 weeks of age for WT, *Hdac6KO*, R6/2 and Dble mice. n≥16/genotype (as shown in Fig. 3A).

Figure S2 ***Hdac6*** **knock-out does not change aggregate load in the brain or muscle.** (**A**) Aggregate load was measured by Seprion ligand ELISA with the MW8 antibody in the cortex, hippocampus and brain stem of R6/2 and Dble mice at 4 weeks. n≥5/genotype. (**B**) Representative western blot with S830 anti-huntingtin antibody showing aggregated and soluble transprotein (Htt) in the cortex at 4 weeks. α-tubulin (Tub) was used as a loading control. Specificity of S830 staining is confirmed by lack of signal in WT and *Hdac6*KO cortices. (**C**) Densitometric quantification of soluble Htt from western blots shown in (A) and Fig. 4C. Htt signal was normalised to α-tubulin and the relative signal for Dble mice expressed as fold change to R6/2 for each time point. (**D**) Soluble (2B7-MW1 antibodies, upper panel) and aggregated (MW8-MW8 antibodies, lower panel) transprotein levels were measured by TR-FRET in the cortex at 9 and 15 weeks. Data normalised to R6/2 at 9 weeks. * $p<0.05$; n≥8/genotype. (**E**) Aggregate load was measured by Seprion ligand ELISA with the MW8 antibody and soluble transprotein levels were measured by TR-FRET (2B7-MW1 antibodies) in the quadriceps muscle at 9 and 15 weeks. Data normalised to R6/2 at each time point. n≥7/genotype. Error bars represent SEM.

Figure S3 **The increase in tubulin acetylation in brain is comparable between Hdac6KO and Dble mice.** (**A**) Representative western blots showing acetylated tubulin (Ac-tub) in Dble and *Hdac6*KO mice at 4, 9 and 15 weeks in cortex, striatum and cerebellum with α-tubulin (Tub) as a loading control. There was insufficient tissue to perform the analysis on striatum at 9 and 15 weeks. (**B**) Densitometric quantification of western blots presented in (A). Acetylated tubulin was normalised to α-tubulin and the relative signal for Dble mice expressed as fold change to *Hdac6*KO. Error bars represent SEM. KO - *Hdac6*KO, Dble - *Hdac6*KOxR6/2; n≥3/genotype.

Figure S4 **Similar levels of BDNF protein in striatum, cortex and hippocampus despite very low** ***Bdnf*** **mRNA striatal expression.** (**A**) *Bdnf* mRNA coding region expression in WT mice at 9 weeks between cortex, striatum and hippocampus. Data normalised to *Ubc* and expressed as fold change of cortex. n≥3/genotype. ** $p<0.01$ (to cortex) *** $p<0.001$ (to cortex and to hippocampus) (**B**) BDNF protein content measured by ELISA in cortex, striatum, hippocampus and liver in WT mice at 9 weeks of age. Data normalised to cortex. * $p<0.05$; n = 3/genotype. Error bars represent SEM.

Table S1 Statistical analysis of the influence of time (30 min duration) and genotype(s) on the spontaneous motor activity parameters: activity, mobility, rearing and centre rearing presented as *p* - values calculated via ANOVA General Linear Model with Greenhouse-Geisser correction.

Acknowledgments

We thank Tso-Pang Yao for the HDAC6 antibody, and members of the Neurogenetics Laboratory for the provision of R6/2 males for breeding.

Author Contributions

Conceived and designed the experiments: AB PP PM GPB. Performed the experiments: AB. Analyzed the data: AB GPB. Contributed reagents/materials/analysis tools: PP PM GPB. Wrote the paper: AB GPB. Proofread the manuscript: PP PM.

References

1. Bates G, Harper PS, Jones L (2002) Huntington's disease. Oxford: Oxford University Press. xvi558 p.
2. Novak MJ, Tabrizi SJ (2010) Huntington's disease. BMJ 340: c3109.
3. The Huntington's Disease Collaborative Research Group (1993) A novel gene containing a trinucleotide repeat that is expanded and unstable on Huntington's disease chromosomes. Cell 72: 971–983.
4. Tabrizi SJ, Langbehn DR, Leavitt BR, Roos RAC, Durr A, et al. (2009) Biological and clinical manifestations of Huntington's disease in the longitudinal TRACK-HD study: cross-sectional analysis of baseline data. The Lancet Neurology 8: 791–801.
5. Tabrizi SJ, Scahill RI, Durr A, Roos RAC, Leavitt BR, et al. (2011) Biological and clinical changes in premanifest and early stage Huntington's disease in the TRACK-HD study: the 12-month longitudinal analysis. The Lancet Neurology 10: 31–42.
6. DiFiglia M, Sapp E, Chase KO, Davies SW, Bates GP, et al. (1997) Aggregation of huntingtin in neuronal intranuclear inclusions and dystrophic neurites in brain. Science 277: 1990–1993.
7. Zuccato C, Valenza M, Cattaneo E (2010) Molecular mechanisms and potential therapeutical targets in Huntington's disease. Physiol Rev 90: 905–981.
8. Butler R, Bates GP (2006) Histone deacetylase inhibitors as therapeutics for polyglutamine disorders. Nat Rev Neurosci 7: 784–796.
9. de Ruijter AJ, van Gennip AH, Caron HN, Kemp S, van Kuilenburg AB (2003) Histone deacetylases (HDACs): characterization of the classical HDAC family. Biochem J 370: 737–749.
10. Finkel T, Deng CX, Mostoslavsky R (2009) Recent progress in the biology and physiology of sirtuins. Nature 460: 587–591.
11. Bates EA, Victor M, Jones AK, Shi Y, Hart AC (2006) Differential contributions of Caenorhabditis elegans histone deacetylases to Huntingtin polyglutamine toxicity. Journal of Neuroscience 26: 2830–2838.
12. Hockly E, Richon VM, Woodman B, Smith DL, Zhou X, et al. (2003) Suberoylanilide hydroxamic acid, a histone deacetylase inhibitor, ameliorates motor deficits in a mouse model of Huntington's disease. Proc Natl Acad Sci U S A 100: 2041–2046.
13. Steffan JS, Bodai L, Pallos J, Poelman M, McCampbell A, et al. (2001) Histone deacetylase inhibitors arrest polyglutamine-dependent neurodegeneration in Drosophila. Nature 413: 739–743.
14. Pallos J, Bodai L, Lukacsovich T, Purcell JM, Steffan JS, et al. (2008) Inhibition of specific HDACs and sirtuins suppresses pathogenesis in a Drosophila model of Huntington's disease. Hum Mol Genet 17: 3767–3775.
15. Khan N, Jeffers M, Kumar S, Hackett C, Boldog F, et al. (2008) Determination of the class and isoform selectivity of small-molecule histone deacetylase inhibitors. Biochem J 409: 581–589.
16. Grozinger CM, Hassig CA, Schreiber SL (1999) Three proteins define a class of human histone deacetylases related to yeast Hda1p. Proc Natl Acad Sci U S A 96: 4868–4873.
17. Seigneurin-Berny D, Verdel A, Curtet S, Lemercier C, Garin J, et al. (2001) Identification of components of the murine histone deacetylase 6 complex: link between acetylation and ubiquitination signaling pathways. Mol Cell Biol 21: 8035–8044.
18. Zhang Y, Li N, Caron C, Matthias G, Hess D, et al. (2003) HDAC-6 interacts with and deacetylates tubulin and microtubules in vivo. EMBO J 22: 1168–1179.
19. Hubbert C, Guardiola A, Shao R, Kawaguchi Y, Ito A, et al. (2002) HDAC6 is a microtubule-associated deacetylase. Nature 417: 455–458.
20. Kovacs JJ, Murphy PJ, Gaillard S, Zhao X, Wu JT, et al. (2005) HDAC6 regulates Hsp90 acetylation and chaperone-dependent activation of glucocorticoid receptor. Mol Cell 18: 601–607.

21. Zhang X, Yuan Z, Zhang Y, Yong S, Salas-Burgos A, et al. (2007) HDAC6 modulates cell motility by altering the acetylation level of cortactin. Mol Cell 27: 197–213.
22. Kopito RR (2000) Aggresomes, inclusion bodies and protein aggregation. Trends in Cell Biology 10: 524–530.
23. Kawaguchi Y, Kovacs JJ, McLaurin A, Vance JM, Ito A, et al. (2003) The deacetylase HDAC6 regulates aggresome formation and cell viability in response to misfolded protein stress. Cell 115: 727–738.
24. Kwon S, Zhang Y, Matthias P (2007) The deacetylase HDAC6 is a novel critical component of stress granules involved in the stress response. Genes Dev 21: 3381–3394.
25. Iwata A, Riley BE, Johnston JA, Kopito RR (2005) HDAC6 and microtubules are required for autophagic degradation of aggregated huntingtin. J Biol Chem 280: 40282–40292.
26. Pandey UB, Nie Z, Batlevi Y, McCray BA, Ritson GP, et al. (2007) HDAC6 rescues neurodegeneration and provides an essential link between autophagy and the UPS. Nature 447: 859–863.
27. Lee JY, Koga H, Kawaguchi Y, Tang W, Wong E, et al. (2010) HDAC6 controls autophagosome maturation essential for ubiquitin-selective quality-control autophagy. EMBO J 29: 969–980.
28. Dompierre JP, Godin JD, Charrin BC, Cordelieres FP, King SJ, et al. (2007) Histone deacetylase 6 inhibition compensates for the transport deficit in Huntington's disease by increasing tubulin acetylation. J Neurosci 27: 3571–3583.
29. Mahlknecht U, Schnittger S, Landgraf F, Schoch C, Ottmann OG, et al. (2001) Assignment of the human histone deacetylase 6 gene (HDAC6) to X chromosome p11.23 by in situ hybridization. Cytogenet Cell Genet 93: 135–136.
30. Mangiarini L, Sathasivam K, Seller M, Cozens B, Harper A, et al. (1996) Exon 1 of the HD gene with an expanded CAG repeat is sufficient to cause a progressive neurological phenotype in transgenic mice. Cell 87: 493–506.
31. Moffitt H, McPhail GD, Woodman B, Hobbs C, Bates GP (2009) Formation of polyglutamine inclusions in a wide range of non-CNS tissues in the HdhQ150 knock-in mouse model of Huntington's disease. PLoS One 4: e8025.
32. Landles C, Sathasivam K, Weiss A, Woodman B, Moffitt H, et al. (2010) Proteolysis of Mutant Huntingtin Produces an Exon 1 Fragment That Accumulates as an Aggregated Protein in Neuronal Nuclei in Huntington Disease. Journal of Biological Chemistry 285: 8808–8823.
33. Woodman B, Butler R, Landles C, Lupton MK, Tse J, et al. (2007) The Hdh(Q150/Q150) knock-in mouse model of HD and the R6/2 exon 1 model develop comparable and widespread molecular phenotypes. Brain Res Bull 72: 83–97.
34. Sathasivam K, Lane A, Legleiter J, Warley A, Woodman B, et al. (2010) Identical oligomeric and fibrillar structures captured from the brains of R6/2 and knock-in mouse models of Huntington's disease. Hum Mol Genet 19: 65–78.
35. Kuhn A, Goldstein DR, Hodges A, Strand AD, Sengstag T, et al. (2007) Mutant huntingtin's effects on striatal gene expression in mice recapitulate changes observed in human Huntington's disease brain and do not differ with mutant huntingtin length or wild-type huntingtin dosage. Human Molecular Genetics 16: 1845–1861.
36. Zhang Y, Kwon S, Yamaguchi T, Cubizolles F, Rousseaux S, et al. (2008) Mice lacking histone deacetylase 6 have hyperacetylated tubulin but are viable and develop normally. Mol Cell Biol 28: 1688–1701.
37. Luthi-Carter R, Hanson SA, Strand AD, Bergstrom DA, Chun W, et al. (2002) Dysregulation of gene expression in the R6/2 model of polyglutamine disease: parallel changes in muscle and brain. Human Molecular Genetics 11: 1911–1926.
38. Gao YS, Hubbert CC, Lu J, Lee YS, Lee JY, et al. (2007) Histone deacetylase 6 regulates growth factor-induced actin remodeling and endocytosis. Mol Cell Biol 27: 8637–8647.
39. Reed NA, Cai D, Blasius TL, Jih GT, Meyhofer E, et al. (2006) Microtubule acetylation promotes kinesin-1 binding and transport. Curr Biol 16: 2166–2172.
40. Gauthier LR, Charrin BC, Borrell-Pages M, Dompierre JP, Rangone H, et al. (2004) Huntingtin controls neurotrophic support and survival of neurons by enhancing BDNF vesicular transport along microtubules. Cell 118: 127–138.
41. Zuccato C, Cattaneo E (2009) Brain-derived neurotrophic factor in neurodegenerative diseases. Nat Rev Neurol 5: 311–322.
42. Altar CA, Cai N, Bliven T, Juhasz M, Conner JM, et al. (1997) Anterograde transport of brain-derived neurotrophic factor and its role in the brain. Nature 389: 856–860.
43. Crook ZR, Housman D (2011) Huntington's Disease: Can Mice Lead the Way to Treatment? Neuron 69: 423–435.
44. Martin EJ, Kim M, Velier J, Sapp E, Lee HS, et al. (1999) Analysis of Huntingtin-associated protein 1 in mouse brain and immortalized striatal neurons. J Comp Neurol 403: 421–430.
45. Apostol BL, Simmons DA, Zuccato C, Illes K, Pallos J, et al. (2008) CEP-1347 reduces mutant huntingtin-associated neurotoxicity and restores BDNF levels in R6/2 mice. Mol Cell Neurosci 39: 8–20.
46. Cepeda C, Cummings DM, Hickey MA, Kleiman-Weiner M, Chen JY, et al. (2010) Rescuing the Corticostriatal Synaptic Disconnection in the R6/2 Mouse Model of Huntington's Disease: Exercise, Adenosine Receptors and Ampakines. PLoS Curr 2.
47. Seo H, Kim W, Isacson O (2008) Compensatory changes in the ubiquitin-proteasome system, brain-derived neurotrophic factor and mitochondrial complex II/III in YAC72 and R6/2 transgenic mice partially model Huntington's disease patients. Hum Mol Genet 17: 3144–3153.
48. Cho S-R, Benraiss A, Chmielnicki E, Samdani A, Economides A, et al. (2007) Induction of neostriatal neurogenesis slows disease progression in a transgenic murine model of Huntington disease. The Journal of Clinical Investigation 117: 2889–2902.
49. Canals JM, Pineda JR, Torres-Peraza JF, Bosch M, Martin-Ibanez R, et al. (2004) Brain-derived neurotrophic factor regulates the onset and severity of motor dysfunction associated with enkephalinergic neuronal degeneration in Huntington's disease. J Neurosci 24: 7727–7739.
50. Gharami K, Xie Y, An JJ, Tonegawa S, Xu B (2008) Brain-derived neurotrophic factor over-expression in the forebrain ameliorates Huntington's disease phenotypes in mice. J Neurochem 105: 369–379.
51. Du G, Liu X, Chen X, Song M, Yan Y, et al. (2010) Drosophila histone deacetylase 6 protects dopaminergic neurons against {alpha}-synuclein toxicity by promoting inclusion formation. Mol Biol Cell 21: 2128–2137.
52. Pandey UB, Batlevi Y, Baehrecke EH, Taylor JP (2007) HDAC6 at the intersection of autophagy, the ubiquitin-proteasome system and neurodegeneration. Autophagy 3: 643–645.
53. Ding H, Dolan PJ, Johnson GV (2008) Histone deacetylase 6 interacts with the microtubule-associated protein tau. J Neurochem 106: 2119–2130.
54. Benn CL, Butler R, Mariner L, Nixon J, Moffitt H, et al. (2009) Genetic knock-down of HDAC7 does not ameliorate disease pathogenesis in the R6/2 mouse model of Huntington's disease. PLoS One 4: e5747.
55. Hockly E, Woodman B, Mahal A, Lewis CM, Bates G (2003) Standardization and statistical approaches to therapeutic trials in the R6/2 mouse. Brain Res Bull 61: 469–479.
56. Hockly E, Tse J, Barker AL, Moolman DL, Beunard JL, et al. (2006) Evaluation of the benzothiazole aggregation inhibitors riluzole and PGL-135 as therapeutics for Huntington's disease. Neurobiol Dis 21: 228–236.
57. Sathasivam K, Woodman B, Mahal A, Bertaux F, Wanker EE, et al. (2001) Centrosome disorganization in fibroblast cultures derived from R6/2 Huntington's disease (HD) transgenic mice and HD patients. Hum Mol Genet 10: 2425–2435.
58. Ko J, Ou S, Patterson PH (2001) New anti-huntingtin monoclonal antibodies: implications for huntingtin conformation and its binding proteins. Brain Research Bulletin 56: 319–329.
59. Weiss A, Roscic A, Paganetti P (2009) Inducible mutant huntingtin expression in HN10 cells reproduces Huntington's disease-like neuronal dysfunction. Mol Neurodegener 4: 11.
60. Weiss A, Abramowski D, Bibel M, Bodner R, Chopra V, et al. (2009) Single-step detection of mutant huntingtin in animal and human tissues: a bioassay for Huntington's disease. Anal Biochem 395: 8–15.
61. Szapacs ME, Mathews TA, Tessarollo L, Ernest Lyons W, Mamounas LA, et al. (2004) Exploring the relationship between serotonin and brain-derived neurotrophic factor: analysis of BDNF protein and extraneuronal 5-HT in mice with reduced serotonin transporter or BDNF expression. Journal of Neuroscience Methods 140: 81–92.
62. Benn CL, Fox H, Bates GP (2008) Optimisation of region-specific reference gene selection and relative gene expression analysis methods for pre-clinical trials of Huntington's disease. Mol Neurodegener 3: 17.

15

Underlying Factors Associated with Anemia in Amazonian Children: A Population-Based, Cross-Sectional Study

Marly A. Cardoso[1]*, Kézia K.G. Scopel[2], Pascoal T. Muniz[3], Eduardo Villamor[4], Marcelo U. Ferreira[5]

1 Department of Nutrition, School of Public Health, University of São Paulo, São Paulo, Brazil, **2** Department of Parasitology, Immunology and Microbiology, Federal University of Juiz de Fora, Juiz de Fora, Minas Gerais, Brazil, **3** Department of Health Sciences, Federal University of Acre, Rio Branco, Acre, Brazil, **4** Departments of Environmental Health Sciences and Epidemiology, University of Michigan School of Public Health, Ann Arbor, Michigan, United States of America, **5** Department of Parasitology, Institute of Biomedical Sciences, University of São Paulo, São Paulo, Brazil

Abstract

Background: Although iron deficiency is considered to be the main cause of anemia in children worldwide, other contributors to childhood anemia remain little studied in developing countries. We estimated the relative contributions of different factors to anemia in a population-based, cross-sectional survey.

Methodology: We obtained venous blood samples from 1111 children aged 6 months to 10 years living in the frontier town of Acrelândia, northwest Brazil, to estimate the prevalence of anemia and iron deficiency by measuring hemoglobin, erythrocyte indices, ferritin, soluble transferrin receptor, and C-reactive protein concentrations. Children were simultaneously screened for vitamin A, vitamin B_{12}, and folate deficiencies; intestinal parasite infections; glucose-6-phosphate dehydrogenase deficiency; and sickle cell trait carriage. Multiple Poisson regression and adjusted prevalence ratios (aPR) were used to describe associations between anemia and the independent variables.

Principal Findings: The prevalence of anemia, iron deficiency, and iron-deficiency anemia were 13.6%, 45.4%, and 10.3%, respectively. Children whose families were in the highest income quartile, compared with the lowest, had a lower risk of anemia (aPR, 0.60; 95%CI, 0.37–0.98). Child age (<24 months, 2.90; 2.01–4.20) and maternal parity (>2 pregnancies, 2.01; 1.40–2.87) were positively associated with anemia. Other associated correlates were iron deficiency (2.1; 1.4–3.0), vitamin B_{12} (1.4; 1.0–2.2), and folate (2.0; 1.3–3.1) deficiencies, and C-reactive protein concentrations (>5 mg/L, 1.5; 1.1–2.2).

Conclusions: Addressing morbidities and multiple nutritional deficiencies in children and mothers and improving the purchasing power of poorer families are potentially important interventions to reduce the burden of anemia.

Editor: Alfredo Mayor, Barcelona Centre for International Health Research/Hospital Clinic/IDIBAPS/University of Barcelona, Spain

Funding: This work was supported by the São Paulo State Research Agency (FAPESP 07/53042-1) and the National Research Agency of Brazil (CNPq 470573/2007-4). The funders had no role in study design, data collection and analysis, decision to publish, or preparation of the manuscript.

Competing Interests: The authors have declared that no competing interests exist.

* E-mail: marlyac@usp.br

Introduction

Iron deficiency (ID) is the most common and widespread nutritional deficiency worldwide. Because global prevalence estimates are not available for ID, anemia is often used as a proxy of ID and iron-deficiency anemia (IDA). Globally, half of the burden of childhood anemia is thought to be caused by ID [1]. Dietary inadequacies during the first two years of life, a critical period when children switch from a predominantly milk-based diet to a diet based on solid foods and require more iron for growth [2], are major determinants of anemia in young children. As a consequence, the WHO guidelines for primary prevention of anemia in young children have focused on iron supplementation [3]. However, the relative contribution of ID to childhood anemia varies widely across populations and age groups [4,5]. Additional factors, such as infections, glucose-6-phosphate dehydrogenase (G6PD) deficiency, and hemoglobinopathies, are understudied contributors to anemia in tropical settings.

Recent socioeconomic development, with increased family income, wider access to education, and better income distribution, has led to a major decrease in the prevalence of child stunting in Brazil [6]. However, no clear downward trends have been observed for the prevalence of childhood anemia in this country [1]. Data from the most recent countrywide Demographic and Health Survey, carried out between 2006 and 2007, revealed that one-fifth of Brazilian children under the age of 5 years are anemic [7].

The prevalence of childhood anemia due to ID in Brazil remains largely unknown because hemoglobin (Hb) measurements used in nationwide representative surveys are neither sensitive nor specific as a screening test for ID. Lack of sensitivity occurs because a large proportion of total body iron must be lost before Hb concentrations fall below the conventional cut-off points to define anemia [8]. Low specificity is due to the presence of other causes of anemia, such as infection [9–11]. Many iron status indicators are affected by conditions commonly seen in children living in the tropics. Microcytosis, for example, may be caused by hemoglobinopathies [12]. Plasma ferritin (PF) concentration, the most specific biochemical correlate of total body iron stores, increases in infectious and inflammatory diseases, as do many other acute-phase proteins, including C-reactive protein (CRP) [8]. In contrast, concentrations of soluble transferrin receptor (sTfR), a sensitive indicator of ID at the tissue level, remain unaltered in inflammation and in most, although not all, infections [8].

In the present investigation, Hb, PF, sTfR, and CRP measurements were combined to determine the iron status of Amazonian children between 6 months and 10 years of age. In this population-based, cross-sectional study, children were simultaneously screened for vitamin A, vitamin B_{12}, and folate deficiencies; intestinal parasite infections; G6PD deficiency; and sickle cell trait carriage. The aim of the study was to estimate the relative contribution of ID and other nutritional and non-nutritional factors to anemia in this population to provide a basis for public health intervention.

Methods

Ethical Statement

This study protocol was approved by the institutional review board of the School of Public Health, University of São Paulo, Brazil (No. 1681/07). Written informed consent was obtained from the parents or guardians of children who participated in the study. Data were analyzed anonymously.

Study Design and Population

A population-based, cross-sectional study of children's nutrition and health was carried out in December 2007 in Acrelândia, a frontier town situated 112 km east of Rio Branco, the capital of the state of Acre, western Brazilian Amazonia. The adult inhabitants of Acrelândia (urban population, 6000) are mainly migrants from southeast and south Brazil who are currently engaged in commercial agriculture and cattle raising. Infant mortality in Acrelândia, estimated at 70.7 per thousand live births in 2000, is substantially higher than the country average (27.7 per thousand live births) [13].

Sampling strategies, questionnaires, and field procedures were similar to those of a previous survey carried out in the same area in 2003 [14]. Briefly, a census of all households in the urban area of Acrelândia was performed, and 749 households with children younger than 10 years of age were identified. A total of 1225 children living in 734 households (98.0% of those identified in the census) were enrolled; mothers or guardians declined participation in 13 households, and two additional houses were closed. A questionnaire was administered through a face-to-face interview to the mothers or guardians of 1151 children (94.0% of those eligible). The interview, carried out during home visits by trained fieldworkers, addressed the following topics: (a) demographic characteristics (child's sex, age, and race/ethnicity, classified as white, black, "pardo" [brown], yellow, or indigenous according to skin color as used in the Brazilian census) [15]; (b) socioeconomic status (ownership of household assets, paternal schooling, presence of the father in the household, maternal occupation, and number of inhabitants in the household) and environmental conditions (water supply, sewage disposal, and garbage disposal); (c) reproductive health variables (maternal age, child's gestational age at birth, and birth weight); (d) nutritional history (duration of total and exclusive breastfeeding and age at introduction of weaning foods); and (e) morbidity (diarrhea, cough, or fever up to 15 days prior to the interview; episodes of malaria and wheezing in the past 12 months; and past hospitalization). The questionnaire was pilot-tested for clarity in a sample of the target population and revised accordingly before use in the study. After the interview, mothers and children were invited to visit the local family health clinic, where research clinicians carried out a physical examination and trained phlebotomists obtained a venous blood sample. During the interview, the fieldworker also provided participants with a plastic container, labeled with each child's name and study code, and asked the mothers and guardians to collect a stool sample to be examined for intestinal parasites.

Anthropometric Measurements

Length/height and weight were measured during the clinic visit by trained research assistants following standardized procedures and using calibrated equipment [16]. Among children <24 months of age, recumbent length was measured to the nearest millimeter with a locally made infant measuring board; weight was measured to the nearest 10 g with an electronic pediatric scale (model 1583; Tanita, Tokyo, Japan). Children 2 years or older were measured to the nearest 0.1 cm with a stadiometer (model 208; SECA, Hamburg, Germany) affixed to a flat surface on a wall, without a baseboard and perpendicular to the floor. The children were placed barefoot in a standing position in the middle of the stadiometer, with head, shoulders, buttocks, and heels pressed back against the wall; weight readings were taken on an electronic scale (model HS-302; Tanita, Tokyo, Japan) and recorded to the nearest 100 g. Each measurement was repeated and the mean value calculated. Birth date was recorded directly from birth certificates or child health cards. Z-scores for length/height-for-age (HAZ) were calculated according to the WHO child growth standards [17] for children aged 0 to 5 years and the WHO Growth Reference Data [18] for children >5 years. Stunting was defined as a HAZ of <−2.0 [16].

Laboratory Analysis

A sample (approximately 5 mL) of fasting venous blood was collected from 1111 children aged between 6 months and 10 years (90.7% of those enrolled). Because limited sample volumes were available, not all laboratory analyses were performed for all children. At the field laboratory in Acrelândia, whole blood aliquots collected in EDTA-containing vacuum tubes were used to carry out full blood cell counts and measure Hb concentrations on an automated cell counter (ABX Micro 60; Horiba, Montpellier, France). A separate blood sample was protected from light and centrifuged within 1 h of collection; serum and plasma samples were shipped to São Paulo on dry ice and frozen at −70°C until further analysis. In São Paulo, PF and sTfR concentrations were measured using commercially available enzyme immunoassays (Ramco, Houston, TX); CRP concentrations were measured using a high-sensitivity chemiluminescent assay (Immulite; DPC, Los Angeles, CA). Anemia, ID, and IDA were defined according to Hb, PF, sTfR, and CRP concentrations as follows [3]: Anemia was defined as an Hb concentration of <110.0 g/L (children 6–59 months of age) or <115.0 g/L (children >60 months of age). ID was defined when PF concentrations were low (<12 μg/L for children <5 years of age or <15 μg/L for those >5 years of age) or when sTfR concentrations were high (>8.3 mg/L). IDA was defined when ID occurred in anemic children. Because inflammation or infection may increase PF concentrations in iron-deficient children, concentrations of the acute-phase protein CRP were employed to estimate the CRP-containing index, defined as

(0.34+0.0043×PF – [2.7×sTfR]/PF+0.00696×CRP+0.05×sTfR). Children with a CRP-containing index below zero were also considered to have ID [19,20]. The cut-off CRP level of >5 mg/L was considered to be associated with inflammation as described in a recent meta-analysis [21]. Serum folate and vitamin B_{12} concentrations were measured using commercial fluoroimmunoassays (Perkin Elmer, Wallac Oy, Turku, Finland); values <10 nmol/L and <150 pmol/L were considered diagnostic of folate and vitamin B_{12} deficiency, respectively [22]. Serum concentrations of vitamin A (retinol) were measured by standard HPLC methods [23]; concentrations of <0.70 μmol/L were considered diagnostic of vitamin A deficiency [24]. Frozen samples were analyzed within 6 months of collection. Children with anemia or nutrient deficiencies detected during the survey received adequate treatment prescribed by the medical team involved in the project in accordance with WHO guidelines [2,22,24].

DNA-based tests were used to screen for G6PD deficiency and sickle cell trait carriage. DNA was extracted from EDTA-containing whole blood samples using DNA kits (Qiagen, Hilden, Germany). The G6PD202A mutation (rs1050828) was genotyped, constituting the most frequent diagnostic single-nucleotide polymorphism associated with G6PD deficiency found in the Amazon Basin of Brazil [25]. Boys who were hemizygous and girls that were homozygous for the G6PD202A allele were considered to be G6PD-deficient. The sickle mutation (HbS, rs334) in the β-globin gene was also genotyped to detect carriers of the sickle cell trait (heterozygotes for HbS) and sickle cell disease (homozygotes for HbS). Genotyping was carried out by allele-specific PCR with molecular beacons, under contract, by Prevention Genetics (Marshfield, MA). The internal quality of genotypic data was assessed by typing 10% of blinded samples in duplicate; agreement was >99%.

Stool samples were collected in plastic containers containing a preservative solution (10% formalin) from 989 children aged between 6 months and 10 years (80.7% of those enrolled). Logistic limitations prevented the collection of more than one stool sample from each participant, but prevalence estimates derived from examination of a single sample have been shown to be accurate for most infections with soil-transmitted helminths (geohelminths) associated with anemia [26]. Because variable volumes of feces were mixed with formalin for preservation, no attempt was made to perform egg counts. The stool samples were examined for parasite ova, cysts, and larvae as described elsewhere [14]. Geohelminths found in this population included *Ascaris lumbricoides*, *Trichuris trichiura*, and *Strongyloides stercoralis*. Children with intestinal parasitic infections received free treatment prescribed by research clinicians.

Statistical Analysis

Principal component analysis was used to derive a wealth index, a proxy of household income [27], from information on ownership of 12 household assets as described elsewhere [14]. In most of the analyses, children were grouped into three age categories: infants and toddlers (6–23 months of age), preschool children (24–59 months of age), or school children (5–10 years of age). Multiple Poisson regression was used with robust variance to estimate adjusted prevalence ratios (PR) for independent associations with anemia according to demographic, socioeconomic, environmental, and morbidity covariates. To this end, a hierarchical model with three concentrations of determination was used [28]: (i) socioeconomic and demographic variables (wealth index, race/ethnicity, maternal schooling, maternal age, and parity); (ii) birth and perinatal variables (birth weight and gestational age) and breastfeeding practices; and (iii) reported morbidity and conditions diagnosed by laboratory analysis. At each level of determination, covariates were retained in the model if they were associated with the outcome at $P<0.10$ and for ordinal variables when they followed a dose-response pattern or if their inclusion in the model changed the PR by 10% or more. Missing observations were included in the multiple models by creating missing-value categories. Potential correlations among siblings within the same household were assessed in multilevel regression models using the STATA "xtmepoisson" procedure. Estimates of the population attributable fraction for dichotomous exposures were calculated using the following formula: attributable fraction = p (PR-1)/PR, where p is the proportion of cases exposed, and PR is the adjusted PR [29]. In supplemental analyses, we carried out multiple linear regression to describe independent associations between concentrations of Hb, PF, and sTfR (dependent variables) and demographic, socioeconomic, and morbidity covariates; natural log transformations of PF, sTfR, and CRP were used to fit the models. All p-values reported are two-tailed. Statistical analyses were performed using STATA version 11.0 (College Station, TX).

Results

Of the 1151 participants, 1111 children (97%) >6 months of age provided blood samples and constituted the analytic sample. On average, there were 1.7 participants per household, ranging from 1 to 5 children. No sanitation system was available in the town. Among those identified as either head of the household or the primary caregiver, 38.1% had studied for <5 years. The race/ethnicity of the majority of the participants was classified as brown (86%); a high proportion of mothers with only primary school education (38%) and a history of more than two pregnancies (64%) was observed (Table 1).

Median values and interquartile ranges for iron status indicators and prevalence of anemia and other conditions are shown in Table 2. The overall prevalence of anemia was 13.6%; the highest rates were found in infants and toddlers (40%), and no significant differences were found between sexes. No cases of severe anemia (Hb <70 g/L) were diagnosed, and only 1.5% of the study subjects had Hb ≤100 g/L. Evidence for ID (altered PF, sTfR, or both) was found in 45% of subjects, with the highest prevalence among children under the age of 2 years. A total of 76% of all anemic children had evidence of ID, whereas the proportion was 94% among infants and toddlers. The overall prevalence of IDA was 10.3%, and only 23% of subjects with ID were anemic. The overall prevalence rates of stunting and deficiencies of retinol, vitamin B_{12}, and folate were 5.5%, 14.2%, 3.7%, and 2.5%, respectively. Only one case of sickle cell disease was observed. Of the 1034 children for whom plasma CRP information was available, only 41 (4%) had CRP values of ≥10 mg/L. The CRP index yielded similar percentage estimates of ID in all age groups.

Infants and toddlers had the highest prevalence of anemic children with coexistence of two or more nutrient deficiencies (17.5%) compared with preschool and school children (2.4 and 1.4, respectively; $P<0.05$, χ^2 test). Microcytosis (low mean corpuscular volume as defined in Table 2) was observed in 56%, 31% and 15% of children with IDA, folate and vitamin B12 deficiency, respectively. Anemia was uniformly prevalent according to race/ethnicity, birth conditions, and breastfeeding practices. The most common reported morbidities over the preceding 15 days were diarrhea (overall, 23.4%; <2 years, 46.0%) and wheezing (overall, 10.7%; <2 years, 22.3%). Twelve cases of malaria and one case of dengue fever over the previous year were reported. The use of antihelminthics over the past 6 months was

Table 1. General characteristics of children aged 6 months to 10 years (N = 1111).

Variable	Value[a]
	n (%)
Sex	
Female	559 (50.3)
Male	552 (49.7)
Race/ethnicity	
White	98 (9.5)
Black	52 (5.0)
Brown	882 (85.5)
Maternal schooling	
≤4 years	423 (38.1)
5–8 years	319 (28.7)
≥9 years	331 (29.8)
Maternal pregnancies	
≤2	378 (34.0)
≥3	712 (64.1)
Maternal age	
10–21 years	106 (9.5)
22–35 years	743 (66.9)
>35 years	262 (23.6)
Age at introduction of cow milk	
<90 d	300 (27.0)
≥90 d	655 (64.1)
Diarrhea in the last 15 d	
No	840 (75.6)
Yes, 1–3 d	178 (16.0)
Yes, ≥4 d	89 (8.0)

[a]Totals differ from the total number of study children because of missing values.

reported by the caregivers for 35.4% of the participants, with a higher frequency of use among preschool children (43.5%) (data not shown in Tables).

The relative contribution of each risk factor to anemia was estimated from adjusted prevalence ratios (aPR) derived from multiple Poisson regression models with anemia as the outcome. Children living in families that belonged to a higher wealth index quartile were at lower risk for anemia (adjusted PR, 0.60; 95%CI, 0.37–0.98). In contrast, children <2 years of age (2.90; 2.01–4.20) and children whose mothers had more than two pregnancies (2.01; 1.40–2.87) were at higher risk for anemia. Other associated risk factors were ID, deficiency of folate or vitamin B_{12}, and high CRP concentrations (>5 mg/L). Attributable fractions were estimated for factors other than age, sex, wealth index, maternal schooling, and maternal age (Table 3). Overall, 5.3% and 4.8% of all cases of anemia were attributable to ID and to high parity of mothers (more than two pregnancies), respectively. The corresponding figures among children <2 years of age were 16.8% and 7.9%, respectively (Table 3). Similar results from multiple models were found with additional adjustment for household on multilevel analysis (data not shown).

In addition to age and wealth index, circulating concentrations of sTfR, retinol, vitamin B_{12}, and CRP were strong independent predictors of Hb concentrations. The final model explained 37.6% of the variance of Hb concentration in the children studied. On average, (a) increases of 1 mg/L of sTfR and 2.72 mg/L of CRP (1 log unit) were associated with 1.21 and 0.31 g/L decreases in Hb, respectively; (b) decreases of 1 μmol/L of retinol and 1 pmol/L of vitamin B_{12} were associated with 1.71 and 0.01 g/L decreases in Hb, respectively (Table 4). In separate analysis, the predictors of sTfR were examined in linear models (results not shown in Tables). In addition to age and sex, log CRP concentrations were positively associated with plasma sTfR ($\beta = 0.021$; 95%CI, 0.013–0.028; $P = 0.000$).

Discussion

Anemia in the Amazonian children studied was twice as prevalent as that in comparable population groups from industrialized countries [1,30], but remained less frequent than that in most of the developing world [4,31]. In line with rates reported by previous studies (31,32), more than 50% of anemic young children had evidence of ID, but only 5% of all cases of anemia in the overall population were attributable to ID. Among children under 2 years of age, 17% of all cases of anemia were attributable to ID along with deficiencies in vitamin B_{12} and folate and high plasma CRP (approximately 3% for each risk factor).

Although the overall prevalence of vitamin B_{12} and folate deficiency found in this study (3.7% and 2.5%, respectively) was low, vitamin B_{12} deficiency was observed in 12% of examined children under the age of 2 years and was associated with anemia. Comparisons with available data within and between countries are difficult because the majority of data on the prevalence of folate and vitamin B_{12} deficiencies are derived from relatively small surveys with different nutritional status indicators. Anemia due to folate and vitamin B_{12} deficiency has been considered uncommon worldwide. This is probably due to limitations in diagnosis because iron deficiency tends to lower the mean corpuscular volume (MCV) in the complete blood count more readily than it is raised by folate or vitamin B12 deficiency while the use of other biochemical indicators is expensive [22]. A study of 2800 children aged 5 to 12 years from Bogota's public schools in Colombia found vitamin B_{12} deficiency (<148 pmol/L) in 1.6% of children. Plasma vitamin B_{12} concentrations were inversely related to the mother's parity and positively associated with socioeconomic status and a dietary pattern that included frequent intake of beef, chicken, and dairy products in a dose-response manner [33]. An earlier study of 12- to 23-month-old toddlers who lived in rural India found that 2.3% of children had vitamin B_{12} deficiency alone (<150 pmol/L) and 66% had at least one micronutrient deficiency (vitamin B_{12}, folate, iron, or vitamin A) [34]. One explanation for the higher prevalence of vitamin B_{12} deficiency among toddlers in the present study might be related to low daily intakes of vitamin B_{12} as described in a previous study in the Amazon area [35]. The diet of young Amazonian children tends to comprise few foods in small amounts. The dietary pattern reflects a high intake of carbohydrate-rich foods and cow milk, with irregular intakes of fruit, vegetables, and meat. Compulsory fortification of flours with iron and folate, in place in Brazil since 2003, has been shown to be less effective in children under 2 years of age because their flour consumption may not be sufficient to meet the required intake of key micronutrients [36].

The high prevalence (14.2%) of vitamin A deficiency observed in our population of a similar magnitude across all age groups is of particular concern. Although this vitamin A deficiency was not found to be associated with anemia, a positive association between serum retinol and Hb concentration was observed, as reported by other authors in studies of children in Latin America and

Table 2. Iron status indicators and prevalence of anemia and other nutritional and non-nutritional conditions in urban Amazonian children[a].

	Infants and toddlers, 6–24 mo (n = 190)	Pre-school children, 25–59 mo (n = 336)	School children, 5–10 y (n = 585)	Overall (n = 1111)
Hb (g/L)				
Median (IQR)	112.0 (104.0; 120.0)	122.0 (115.0; 128.0)	127.0 (122.0; 133.0)	123.0 (115.0; 131.0)
% (95% CI) below cut-off[b]	40.0 (33.0 – 47.3)	10.4 (7.4–14.2)	6.8 (4.9–9.2)	13.6 (11.6–15.7)
Mean corpuscular volume (fl)				
Median (IQR)	72 (67; 76)	79 (75; 81)	82 (80; 84)	80 (76; 83)
% (95% CI) below cut-off[c]	22.5 (16.7 – 29.1)	15.0(11.3 – 19.3)	3.8(2.4 – 5.6)	10.3(8.6 – 12.3)
Plasma ferritin (PF, μg/L)	[183]	[294]	[582]	[1094]
Median	12.2 (5.9; 20.2)	26.9 (13.7; 46.8)	45.3 (30.9; 65.7)	34.5 (17.8; 54.8)
% (95% CI) below cut-off[d]	48.9 (41.5–56.4)	22.5 (18.1–27.4)	5.0 (3.4 – 7.1)	17.6 (15.4 – 20.0)
Soluble transferrin receptor (sTfR, mg/L)	[183]	[294]	[582]	[1094]
Median (IQR)	10.8 (8.6; 14.0)	8.1 (6.8; 9.6)	7.1 (6.1; 8.2)	7.7 (6.5; 9.4)
% (95% CI) above cut-off[e]	79.9 (73.3 – 85.4)	47.1 (41.6 – 52.7)	23.1 (19.7 – 26.7)	39.9 (36.9 – 42.8)
CRP (mg/L)	[170]	[305]	[559]	[1034]
Median (IQR)	0.70 (0.21; 3.00)	0.39 (0.01; 1.21)	0.39 (0.01; 1.05)	0.43 (0.01; 1.31)
% (95% CI) above cut-off[f]	28.1 (21.5 – 35.4)	17.0 (13.0 – 21.7)	13.3 (10.6 – 16.4)	16.8 (14.6 – 19.2)
CRP-index <0[g]	86.0 (79.8–90.8) [170]	44.9 (39.2 – 50.7) [294]	14.9 (12.0–18.1) [559]	35.5 (32.6–38.5) [1023]
Vitamin A (μmol/L)	[165]	[302]	[561]	[1028]
Median (IQR)	1.13 (0.88; 1.50)	1.17 (0.88; 1.52)	1.14 (0.87; 1.46)	1.15 (0.87 ; 1.50)
% (95% CI) below cut-off[h]	13.3 (8.5–19.5)	13.9 (10.2–18.3)	14.6 (11.8–17.8)	14.2 (12.1–16.5)
Vitamin B-12 (pmol/L)	[159]	[291]	[517]	[967]
Median (IQR)	244 (181; 308)	279 (225; 364)	250 (208; 306)	258 (209; 320)
% (95% CI) below cut-off[i]	12.0 (7.4–18.0)	2.8 (1.2–5.3)	1.7 (0.8–3.3)	3.7 (2.6–5.1)
Folate (nmol/L)	[167]	[305]	[560]	[1032]
Median (IQR)	22.1 (17.0; 32.2)	23.0 (17.4; 30.0)	23.6 (18.1; 29.8)	23.3 (17.7; 30.3)
% (95% CI) below cut-off[j]	4.2 (1.7–8.4)	2.3 (0.9–4.7)	2.1 (1.1–3.7)	2.5 (1.7–3.7)
Prevalence of selected conditions, % (95% CI)				
Iron deficiency[k]	84.8 (78.8–89.6) [183]	55.0 (49.5–60.5) [294]	26.7 (23.1 – 30.5) [582]	45.0 (42.0–48.0) [1094]
Iron deficiency anemia	37.5 (30.5–45.0) [183]	8.5 (5.7–12.1) [294]	2.8 (1.6 – 4.4) [582]	10.3 (8.6–12.2) [1094]
Stunting	11.8 (7.5–17.3)	4.5 (2.5–7.3)	3.8 (2.4–5.7)	5.4 (4.1–6.9)
Geohelminth infection[l]	2.4 (0.6–5.9) [169]	2.4 (0.9–4.8) [297]	5.2 (3.4–7.4) [523]	3.8 (2.7–5.2) [989]
G6PD deficiency	7.0 (3.7–11.9) [170]	10.4 (7.2–14.3) [308]	8.6 (6.4–11.3) [536]	8.9 (7.2–10.8) [1104]
Sickle cell trait carriage	3.9 (1.6–7.9) [178]	5.3 (3.1–8.3) [321]	3.9 (2.5–5.8) [565]	4.3 (3.2–5.7) [1064]

IQR, interquartile ranges.
[a]Totals in brackets differ from the total number of study children by age group because of missing values.
[b]Cut-offs for anemia: <110.0 and <115.0 g/L for 6–59 months and ≥60 months, respectively;
[c]Cut-offs for microcytosis by age: <67, <73, <74, and <76 fl for <24 months, 24–59 months, 5–7.9 years, and 8–11.9 years, respectively;
[d]PF: <12 and <15 μg/L for <59 and ≥60 months, respectively;
[e]sTfR: >8.3 mg/L;
[f]Cut-off for high CRP: >5 mg/L;
[g]CRP index defined as (0.34+0.0043×PF – [2.7×sTfR]/PF+0.00696×CRP+0.05×sTfR);
[h]Serum retinol <0.70μmol/L;
[i]Serum vitamin B_{12}<150 pmol/L;
[j]Serum folate <10 nmol/L;
[k]According to cut-offs for PF or sTfR.
[l]Geohelminths in this population included *Ascaris lumbricoides* (overall prevalence, 2.4%), *Strongyloides stercoralis* (0.5%), and *Trichuris trichiura* (0.8%) - the same subject may be co-infected with more than one species.

elsewhere [4,37]. Although the role of vitamin A in iron status has been described in the literature [38,39], the effect of suboptimal vitamin A status on the prevalence of anemia has not been considered in public health programs to prevent and control anemia in children. Several lines of evidence indicate that vitamin A metabolism is altered in situations of iron deficiency, with low serum retinol concentrations and increased hepatic retinyl ester or retinol stores. These changes probably result from a reduction in

Table 3. Attributable fractions (AF) of anemia according to age group in urban Amazonian children.

	Infants and toddlers, 6–24mo (n = 190)		Pre-school children, 25–59 mo (n = 336)		School children, 5–10 y (n = 585)		Overall (n = 1111)	
Risk factors	**p[a] aPR(95%CI)[b]**	**AF[c] %**	**p[a] aPR(95%CI)[b]**	**AF[c] %**	**p[a] aPR(95%CI)[b]**	**AF[c]%**	**p[a] aPR(95%CI)[b]**	**AF[c] %**
High parity (≥3 pregnancies)	22.2 1.55 (1.03–2.33)	7.9	7.7 3.24 (1.48–7.08)	5.3	–	–	9.5 2.01 (1.40–2.87)	4.8
Iron deficiency	37.2 1.82 (0.93–3.59)	16.8	8.5 3.41 (1.54–7.51)	6.0	2.9 1.96 (1.08–3.53)	1.4	10.3 2.06 (1.40–3.04)	5.3
Folate deficiency	4.2 2.46 (1.62–3.72)	2.5	0.7 3.63 (1.34–9.82)	0.5	–	–	0.9 2.00 (1.27–3.13)	0.5
Vitamin B-12 deficiency	7.6 1.75 (1.13–2.71)	3.3	–	–	–	–	1.4 1.44 (0.95–2.19)	0.4
High plasma CRP (>5 mg/L)	10.0 1.42 (0.90–2.23)	3.0	–	–	–	–	3.1 1.53 (1.08–2.17)	1.1

[a]Prevalence (%) of cases exposed in each risk factors.
[b]Adjusted prevalence ratio (aPR) estimated from multiple Poisson regression models with additional adjustment for age (in overall analysis), sex, wealth index (quartile), maternal schooling (≤4, 5–8, and ≥9 years), and maternal age (10–21, 22–35, and >35 years).
[c]Attributable fraction defined as p(aPR −1)/aPR.

the activity of retinyl ester hydrolases with a consequent decrease in vitamin A mobilization, or from an increase in retinol sequestration to the liver [39]. It seems that restricted access to diverse micronutrient-rich diets can exacerbate nutritional anemias. Thus, multiple deficiencies and frequent exposure to endemic disease tend to cluster within individuals, and the synergistic effect of these deficiencies is important in the development of anemia [40].

As expected, the high frequency of morbidities observed in this study population increased the concentrations of both PF and sTfR [11,41]; the effect on sTfR may be due to true infection-associated ID or increased erythropoiesis following hemolysis [8]. These effects on PF and sTfR complicated the analysis of the contribution of morbidities to ID in our population, despite its relatively high attributable fraction. Geohelminth infection was infrequent (overall prevalence, 3.8%), and the impact of geohelminth control on the iron status of our population, although not negligible, is likely to be less pronounced than that in African [11] or Asian [4,9] populations. Previous surveys of risk factors for anemia have implicated ID and malaria as strong predictors of anemia (prevalence, 9%–30%) in rural Amazonian communities, with no significant contribution of geohelminth infection [42,43]. The estimated prevalence of G6PD deficiency is <10% in this and other Amazonian populations [44]. G6PD-deficient subjects are prone to hemolysis induced by primaquine, an antimalarial drug used in this area without screening, further aggravating malaria-related anemia [45]. However, because malaria infection was uncommon in the present study, G6PD deficiency was not associated with anemia risk. Sickle-cell disease is unlikely to represent a major cause of anemia in our area; low HbS allele frequencies (<5%) were found in this and other Amazonian populations with a similar ethnic composition [46].

Previous studies have demonstrated that the role of anemia of inflammation in the pathogenesis of anemia within the developing world plays a central role in the context of infectious diseases prevalent in these regions [47,48]. Both IDA and anemia of chronic or acute disease is difficult to distinguish because increased circulating hepcidin seen during inflammation blocks iron release from enterocytes and the reticuloendothelial system, resulting in iron-deficient erythropoiesis [40]. In the present study population, children under 2 years of age showed higher median values of CRP with frequent exposure to comorbidities (mainly diarrhea and respiratory tract infections), conditions that may distort estimates of iron status. In age-adjusted models, CRP was inversely associated with Hb concentrations, suggesting inflammation as a predictor of Hb levels independent of the child's age.

A body of evidence reinforces the concept that anemia is a marker of socioeconomic disadvantage, with the poorest and least educated being at greatest risk of exposure to risk factors for anemia and its sequelae [40]. In the present study, anemia was predicted by socioeconomic factors: the risk of anemia among children living in a household belonging to the lowest wealth quartile was 40% higher than among those in the highest wealth quartile. Higher wealth index values predicted higher Hb concentrations. In Brazil, child health has improved in recent decades, but this improvement has been less marked in the

Table 4. Multiple linear regression analysis of factors associated with hemoglobin in urban Amazonian children.

Dependent variable	Independent variable	β	95% CI	*P*	R^2	n[a]
Hemoglobin (g/L)					0.376	943
	Age (months)	0.114	0.095; 0.133	0.000		
	Wealth index (continuous)	0.238	0.079; 0.397	0.003		
	sTfR (mg/L)	−1.209	−1.419; −0.998	0.000		
	Serum Vitamin B-12 (pmol/L)	0.013	0.007; 0.019	0.000		
	Serum retinol (μmol/L)	1.713	0.552; 2.875	0.004		
	Log CRP (mg/L)	−0.310	−0.574; −0.045	0.022		

[a]Total differs from total number of study children because of missing values.

northern region, which encompasses the Amazon. Brazilian national household surveys carried out over a 33-year period have shown a steep decline in the overall prevalence of stunting among children under 5 years of age because of economic growth coupled with equity-oriented public policies and improvements in the population's purchasing power, maternal education, sanitation, and access to health care [6]. However, declines of a similar magnitude have not been confirmed for the prevalence of anemia in Brazilian children. Trend data from selected Latin American countries with nationally representative data show that reductions in anemia are generally occurring slowly [32].

In our study, high maternal parity (more than 2 pregnancies) was positively associated with anemia. In developing countries this factor can be considered as a marker of early onset of childbearing, short intervals between births, and poor access to antenatal care and supplementation [49]. The intergenerational transfer of poor iron status from mother to child has been proposed as an additional factor to explain the vulnerability of infants to ID and anemia [40]. Thus, in addition to socioeconomic progress, strategies to lower the risk of anemia in early infancy should include optimization of maternal nutritional status and antenatal care, delayed cord clamping at delivery, improvement of complementary feeding practices, and prevention and treatment of infectious disease [40,50].

Certain limitations in the present study should be noted. The principal constraint of our study is its cross-sectional design. Therefore, the temporal relation between exposures and outcomes (anemia or Hb concentrations) could not be established to ensure that micronutrient deficiencies and elevations in CRP concentrations precede the outcomes. Despite this limitation, we have identified a comprehensive set of associated factors with anemia and Hb concentrations in Amazonian children aged 6 months to 10 years. No other population-based surveys of anemia and ID in Brazil have used a wide-ranging combination of biochemical indicators; available national estimates of ID prevalence have mostly been based on Hb determination.

In conclusion, approximately 5% of all cases of anemia in our study population were attributable to ID; a similar attributable fraction was estimated for high parity (more than two pregnancies) among mothers. Among infants and toddlers, almost one in five cases of anemia was attributable to ID; purchasing power, serum concentrations of vitamin B_{12} and retinol, and elevated CRP concentrations as a measure of recent infection were additional factors shown to affect Hb concentrations. Strategies to control anemia based exclusively on iron supplementation are likely to have only a limited impact on the overall prevalence of anemia. Controlling morbidities and multiple nutritional deficiencies and improving maternal nutritional status and the purchasing power of poorer families represent potentially important interventions.

Acknowledgments

We are profoundly grateful to all children and their families who participated in the study, to the Municipality Health Service of Acrelândia, and to our fieldwork research team for valuable assistance.

Author Contributions

Conceived and designed the experiments: MAC. Performed the experiments: MAC KKGS PTM MUF. Analyzed the data: MAC. Contributed reagents/materials/analysis tools: MAC. Wrote the paper: MAC EV MUF.

References

1. World Health Organization (2008) Worldwide prevalence of anaemia 1993–2005. Geneva: WHO.
2. World Health Organization (2001) Iron deficiency anaemia. Assessment, ed. prevention and control. A guide for programme managers. Geneva: WHO.
3. World Health Organization (2007) Assessing the iron status of populations. 2nd ed. Geneva: WHO.
4. Thurlow RA, Winichagoon P, Green T, Wasantwisut W, Pongcharoen T, et al. (2005) Only a small proportion of anemia in northeast Thai schoolchildren is associated with iron deficiency. Am J Clin Nutr 82: 380–387.
5. Cogswell ME, Looker AC, Pfeiffer CM, Cook JD, Lacher DA, et al. (2009) Assessment of iron deficiency in US preschool children and nonpregnant females of childbearing age: National Health and Nutrition Examination Survey 2003–2006. Am J Clin Nutr 89: 1334–1342.
6. Monteiro CA, Benicio MHD, Conde WL, Konno S, Lovadino AL, et al. (2010) Narrowing socioeconomic inequality in child stunting: the Brazilian experience, 1974–2007. Bull World Health Organ 88: 305–311.
7. Ministério da Saúde (2008) Pesquisa Nacional de Demografia e Saúde da Criança e da Mulher – relatório final. Brasília, Brasil: Ministério da Saúde.
8. Cook JD (2005) Diagnosis and management of iron-deficiency anaemia. Best Pract Res Clin Haematol 18: 319–332.
9. Dreyfuss ML, Stoltzfus RJ, Shrestha JB, Pradhan EK, LeClerq SC, et al. (2000) Hookworms, malaria and vitamin A deficiency contribute to anemia and iron deficiency among pregnant women in the plains of Nepal. J Nutr 130: 2527–2536.
10. Lewis DK, Whitty CJM, Walsh AL, Epino H, van den Broek NR, et al. (2005) Treatable factors associated with severe anaemia in adults admitted to medical wards in Blantyre, Malawi, an area of high HIV seroprevalence. Trans R Soc Trop Med Hyg 99: 561–567.
11. Stoltzfus RJ, Chwaya HM, Montresor A, Albonico M, Savioli L, et al. (2000) Malaria, hookworms and recent fever are related to anemia and iron status indicators in 0- to 5-y old Zanzibari children and these relationships change with age. J Nutr 130: 1724–1733.
12. Bowden DK, Hill AVS, Higgs DR, Weatherall DJ, Clegg JB (1985) Relative roles of genetic factors, dietary deficiency and infections in anaemia in Vanuatu, South-West Pacific. Lancet 2: 1025–1028.
13. Instituto Brasileiro de Geografia e Estatística (2000) Resultados da amostra do censo demográfico 2000. Available http://www.ibge.gov.br/home/estatistica/populacao/censo2000/populacao/pop_Censo2000.pdf. Accessed 2006 May 9.
14. Muniz PT, Castro TG, Araujo TS, Nunes NB, da Silva-Nunes M, et al. (2007) Child health and nutrition in the Western Brazilian Amazon: population-based surveys in two counties in Acre State. Cad Saúde Públ 23: 1283–1293.
15. Travassos C, Williams DR (2004) The concept and measurement of race and their relationship to public health: a review focused on Brazil and the United States. Cad Saude Publica 20: 660–678.
16. WHO Expert Committee on Physical Status (1995) Physical status: the use and interpretation of anthropometry: report of a WHO Expert Committee. Geneva: WHO.
17. World Health Organization (2006) WHO child growth standards based on length/height, weight and age. Acta Paediatric 450: S76–85.
18. de Onis M, Onyango AW, Borghi E, Siyam A, Nishida C, et al. (2007) Development of a WHO growth reference for school-aged children and adolescents. Bull World Health Organ 85: 660–667.
19. van den Broek NR, Letsky EA, White SA, Shenkin A (1998) Iron status in pregnant women: which measurements are valid? Br J Haematol 103: 817–824.
20. Calis JCJ, Phiri KS, Faragher EB, Brabin BJ, Bates I, et al. (2008) Severe anemia in Malawian children. N Engl J Med 358: 888–899.
21. Thurnham DI, McCabe LD, Haldar S, Wieringa FT, Northrop-Clewes CA, et al (2010) Adjusting plasma ferritin concentrations to remove the effects of subclinical inflammation in the assessment of iron deficiency: a meta-analysis. Am J Clin Nutr 92: 546–555.
22. World Health Organization (2008) Conclusions of a WHO Technical Consultation on folate and vitamin B-12 deficiencies. Food Nutr Bull 29(Suppl): S238–S244.
23. Gomes LF, Alves AF, Sevanian A, Peres Cde A, Cendoroglo MS, et al. (2004) Role of beta2-glycoprotein I, LDL-, and antioxidant concentrations in hypercholesterolemic elderly subjects. Antioxid Redox Signal 6: 237–244.
24. World Health Organization (2009) Global prevalence of vitamin A deficiency in populations at risk 1995–2005. WHO Global database on vitamin A deficiency. Geneva: WHO.
25. Hamel AR, Cabral IR, Sales TS, Costa FF, Olalla Saad ST (2002) Molecular heterogeneity of G6PD deficiency in an Amazonian population and description of four new variants. Blood Cells 28: 399–406.
26. Gyorkos TW, McLean JD, Law CG (1989) Absence of significant differences in intestinal parasite estimates after examination of either one or two stool specimens. Am J Epidemiol 130: 976–980.
27. Filmer D, Pritchett LH (2001) Estimating wealth effects without expenditure data-or tear: an application to educational enrolments in states of India. Demography 38: 115–132.

28. Victora CG, Huttly SR, Fuchs SC, Olinto MTA (1997) The role of conceptual frameworks in epidemiological analysis: a hierarchical approach. Int J Epidemiol 26: 224–227.
29. Darrow L, Steenland NK (2011) Confounding and bias in the attributable fraction. Epidemiology 22: 53–58.
30. Cusick SE, Mei Z, Freedman DS, Looker AC, Ogden CL, et al. (2008) Unexplained decline in the prevalence of anemia among US children and women between 1988–1994 and 1999–2002. Am J Clin Nutr 88: 1611–1617.
31. Pasricha S-R, Black J, Muthayya S, Shet A, Bhat V, et al. (2010) Determinants of anemia among young children in rural India. Pediatrics 126: e140–149.
32. Lutter CK (2008) Iron deficiency in young children in low-income countries and new approaches for its prevention. J Nutr 138: 2523–2528.
33. Villamor E, Mora-Plazas M, Forero Y, Lopez-Arana S, Baylin A (2008) Vitamin B-12 status is associated with socioeconomic level and adherence to an animal food dietary pattern in Colombian school children. J Nutr 138: 1391–1398.
34. Paricha S-R, Shet AS, Black JF, Sudarshan H, Prashanth NS, et al. (2011) Vitamin B-12, folate, iron, and vitamin A concentrations in rural Indian children are associated with continued breastfeeding, complementary diet, and maternal nutrition. Am J Clin Nutr 94: 1358–1370.
35. Castro TG, Baraldi L, Muniz PT, Cardoso MA (2009) Dietary practices and nutritional status of 0–24-month-old children from Brazilian Amazonia. Publ Health Nutr 12: 2335–2342.
36. Stoltzfus RJ (2008) Research needed to strengthen science and programs for the control of iron deficiency and its consequences in young children. J Nutr 138: 2542–2546.
37. Maslova E, Mora-Plazas M, Forero Y, López-Arana S, Baylin A, et al. (2009) Are vitamin A and iron deficiencies re-emerging in urban Latin America? A Survey of schoolchildren in Bogota, Colombia. Food Nutr Bull 30: 103–111.
38. Semba RD, Bloem MW (2002) The anemia of vitamin A deficiency: epidemiology and pathogenesis. Eur J Clin Nutr 56: 271–281.
39. Oliveira JM, Michelazzo FB, Stefanello J, Rondó PHC (2008) Influence of iron on vitamin A nutritional status. Nutr Rev 66: 141–147.
40. Balarajan Y, Ramakrishnan, Özaltin E, Shankar AH, Subramanian SV (2012) Anaemia in low-income and middle-income countries. Lancet 378: 2123–2135.
41. Menendez C, Quinto LL, Kahigwa E, Alvarez L, Fernandez R, et al. (2001) Effect of malaria on soluble transferrin receptor levels in Tanzanian infants. Am J Trop Med Hyg 65: 138–142.
42. Cardoso MA, Ferreira MU, Camargo LMA, Szarfarc SC (1994) Anaemia, iron deficiency and malaria in a rural community in Brazilian Amazon. Eur J Clin Nutr 48: 326–332.
43. Ferreira MU, Silva-Nunes M, Bertolino CN, Malafronte RS, Muniz PT, et al. (2007) Anemia and iron deficiency in school children, adolescents and adults: a community-based study in rural Amazonia. Am J Public Health 97: 237–239.
44. Katsuragawa TH, Gil LHS, Stábile RG, Pires MG, Bonini-Domingos CR (2004) Evaluation of the prevalence of glucose-6-phospate dehydrogenase and hematologic profile of a population from Rondônia. Rev Bras Hematol Hemoter 26: 268–273.
45. López-Antuñano FJ (1999) Is primaquine useful and safe as true exo-erythrocytic merontocidal, hypnozoitocidal and gametocidal antimalarial drug? Salud Publica Mex 41: 410–419.
46. Ferreira RG, Moura MM, Engracia V, Pagotto RC, Alves FP, et al. (2002) Ethnic admixture composition of two Western Amazonian populations. Hum Biol 74: 607–613.
47. Levy A, Fraser D, Rosen SD, Dagan R, Deckelbaum RJ, et al. (2005) Anemia as a risk factor for infectious diseases in infants and toddlers: results from a prospective study. Eur J Epidemiol 20: 277–284.
48. Agho KE, Dibley MJ, D'Este C, Gibberd R (2008) Factors associated with haemoglobin concentration among Timor-Leste children aged 6–59 months. J Health Popul Nutr 26: 200–209.
49. Kalaivani K (2009) Prevalence and consequences of anaemia in pregnancy. Indian J Med Res 130: 627–633.
50. Chaparro CM (2008) Setting the stage for child health and development: prevention of iron deficiency in early infancy. J Nutr 138: 2529–2533.

16

A New Drug Design Targeting the Adenosinergic System for Huntington's Disease

Nai-Kuei Huang[1]⁹, Jung-Hsin Lin[2,3,4]⁹, Jiun-Tsai Lin[3], Chia-I Lin[5], Eric Minwei Liu[4], Chun-Jung Lin[4], Wan-Ping Chen[1], Yuh-Chiang Shen[1], Hui-Mei Chen[3], Jhih-Bin Chen[5], Hsing-Lin Lai[3], Chieh-Wen Yang[5], Ming-Chang Chiang[7], Yu-Shuo Wu[3], Chen Chang[3], Jiang-Fan Chen[8], Jim-Min Fang[5,6]*, Yun-Lian Lin[1]*, Yijuang Chern[3]*

1 National Research Institute of Chinese Medicine, Taipei, Taiwan, **2** Division of Mechanics, Research Center for Applied Sciences, Academia Sinica, Taipei, Taiwan, **3** Institute of Biomedical Sciences, Academia Sinica, Taipei, Taiwan, **4** School of Pharmacy, National Taiwan University, Taipei, Taiwan, **5** Department of Chemistry, National Taiwan University, Taipei, Taiwan, **6** The Genomics Research Center, Academia Sinica, Taipei, Taiwan, **7** Graduate Institute of Biotechnology, Chinese Culture University, Taipei, Taiwan, **8** Department of Neurology, Boston University School of Medicine, Boston, Massachusetts, United States of America

Abstract

Background: Huntington's disease (HD) is a neurodegenerative disease caused by a CAG trinucleotide expansion in the Huntingtin (Htt) gene. The expanded CAG repeats are translated into polyglutamine (polyQ), causing aberrant functions as well as aggregate formation of mutant Htt. Effective treatments for HD are yet to be developed.

Methodology/Principal Findings: Here, we report a novel dual-function compound, N^6-(4-hydroxybenzyl)adenine riboside (designated T1-11) which activates the $A_{2A}R$ and a major adenosine transporter (ENT1). T1-11 was originally isolated from a Chinese medicinal herb. Molecular modeling analyses showed that T1-11 binds to the adenosine pockets of the $A_{2A}R$ and ENT1. Introduction of T1-11 into the striatum significantly enhanced the level of striatal adenosine as determined by a microdialysis technique, demonstrating that T1-11 inhibited adenosine uptake *in vivo*. A single intraperitoneal injection of T1-11 in wildtype mice, but not in $A_{2A}R$ knockout mice, increased cAMP level in the brain. Thus, T1-11 enters the brain and elevates cAMP via activation of the $A_{2A}R$ *in vivo*. Most importantly, addition of T1-11 (0.05 mg/ml) to the drinking water of a transgenic mouse model of HD (R6/2) ameliorated the progressive deterioration in motor coordination, reduced the formation of striatal Htt aggregates, elevated proteasome activity, and increased the level of an important neurotrophic factor (brain derived neurotrophic factor) in the brain. These results demonstrate the therapeutic potential of T1-11 for treating HD.

Conclusions/Significance: The dual functions of T1-11 enable T1-11 to effectively activate the adenosinergic system and subsequently delay the progression of HD. This is a novel therapeutic strategy for HD. Similar dual-function drugs aimed at a particular neurotransmitter system as proposed herein may be applicable to other neurotransmitter systems (e.g., the dopamine receptor/dopamine transporter and the serotonin receptor/serotonin transporter) and may facilitate the development of new drugs for other neurodegenerative diseases.

Editor: Olivier Jacques Manzoni, Institut National de la Santé et de la Recherche Médicale, France

Funding: This work was supported by the National Science Council for financial support (NRICM 94-DMC-2, NRICM 95-DMC-2, NSC95-2323-B-077-002, NSC96-2323-B-077-001, NSC96-2628-M-002-003, and NSC 97-2323-B-077-001). The funders had no role in study design, data collection and analyses, decision to publish, or preparation of the manuscript.

Competing Interests: The authors have read the journal's policy and have the following conflicts: based on results of the present study, two pending patent applications regarding the possible therapeutic use of T1-11 in patients with HD were submitted to patent offices in the US, China, and Taiwan. This does not alter the authors' adherence to all the PLoS ONE policies on sharing data and materials.

* E-mail: bmychern@ibms.sinica.edu.tw (YC); yllin@nricm.edu.tw (YLL); jmfang@ntu.edu.tw (JMF)

⁹ These authors contributed equally to this work.

Introduction

Huntington's disease (HD) is an autosomal dominant neurodegenerative disease characterized by chorea, dementia, and psychiatric symptoms. As the disease progresses, concentration and short-term memory diminish and involuntary movements of the head, trunk, and limbs increase. Walking, speaking, and swallowing abilities deteriorate. Eventually, death results from complications such as choking, infection, or heart failure. The causative mutation is a CAG trinucleotide expansion in exon 1 of the Huntingtin gene (Htt) [1]. The normal Htt gene has 35 or fewer CAG repeats in its N-terminal region, whereas that of HD patients is associated with 36 or more repeats. The expanded CAG repeats are translated into polyglutamine residues (polyQ) in the Htt protein. When the number of CAG repeats exceeds 35, degeneration of several brain areas (particularly the striatum) occurs. Formation of Htt aggregates and alteration of overall gene expression profiles have also been reported in peripheral tissues, including blood cells, the liver, and the kidney [2,3]. Drugs currently available for treating HD patients are mostly for symptom relief, and some have unfavorable side effects [4]. Effective treatments for HD are yet to be developed.

Adenosine is an important neuromodulator that links neuronal activity with energy metabolism [5]. Conditions that drain energy reserves or cause an energy imbalance, such as intensive exercise and ischemia, elevate adenosine levels [6]. There are four adenosine receptors (A_1, A_{2A}, A_{2B}, and A_3) and several adenosine transporters. Because of their expression profiles and affinities toward adenosine, the A_1R and $A_{2A}R$ are believed to regulate important physiological functions in the brain. In particular, the $A_{2A}R$ has attracted attention as a potential drug target in HD because it is highly prevalent in the striatum, where mutant Htt causes early damage. In addition, evidence from various laboratories has clearly shown that tonic activation of the $A_{2A}R$ is required for the function of several important neurotrophic factors (including brain-derived neurotrophic factor, fibroblast growth factor, and glial cell line-derived neurotrophic factor) [7–9]. A_{2A}-related drugs therefore have been implicated in the treatment of HD [10–16]. We previously reported that an A_{2A} agonist (CGS21680, CGS) significantly ameliorates several symptoms of HD (viz, brain atrophy, striatal aggregates, deteriorated motor coordination, and urea cycle deficiency) in a transgenic mouse model of HD [12,13]. Nevertheless, certain adverse effects of currently available A_{2A} drugs (e.g., CGS) that exhibit high $A_{2A}R$ affinity prevent their clinical application [17]. In the present study, we describe a novel agonist [N^6-(4-hydroxybenzyl)adenine riboside (designated T1-11)] of the $A_{2A}R$ that also inhibits the adenosine transporter, and which may be used to treat HD without evident side effects because of its moderate affinity to its target molecules.

T1-11 was originally purified from *Gastrodia elata* (GE), a Chinese medicinal herb that has been used extensively in Asia for at least 1500 years. It is traditionally used to treat headaches, dizziness, limb numbness, and spasms, especially those of convulsive illnesses such as epilepsy and tetanus. Because of its efficacy in treating epileptic diseases, many studies have been performed to investigate its role in preventing neuronal damage. For example, gastrodin, a component of GE, was shown to alter GABA metabolism in the gerbil hippocampus [18]. The ether fraction of GE also significantly reduced neuronal cell death induced by β-amyloid [19]. We previously reported that two active components [T1-11 and bis(4-hydroxybenzyl)sulfide] purified from an aqueous methanolic extract of GE prevented apoptosis of serum-deprived PC12 cells by suppressing JNK activity [20,21]. Herein, we demonstrate that T1-11 protects PC12 cells *in vitro* and also exerts a beneficial effect on symptom progression in a mouse model of HD via targeting two components of the adenosinergic mechanism.

Results

Purification of T1-11 from a Chinese herb

We previously reported that a fraction of GE prevents apoptosis in PC12 cells by activating the $A_{2A}R$ [20]. In the present study, we further purified the active component of this GE extract. The aqueous ethanolic extract of GE (~15% yield based on dried weight) was subjected to Diaion HP-20 column chromatography using elution from H_2O to MeOH gradients. As shown in Figure 1A, several fractions of the aqueous methanolic extract conferred protection against PC12 cell death induced by serum withdrawal. The most effective dosage was the 75% MeOH fraction, which was subjected to further fractionation and purification using Sephadex LH-20 column chromatography (Fig. 1B). Sixteen known compounds (including gastrodin, 4-hydroxybenzaldehyde, and parishin) and one previously uncharacterized component (T1-11) were identified [22–24]. Of these compounds, T1-11 was considered the most promising because it is an adenosine analogue (Fig. 1B). HPLC was used to monitor the chemical profiles of various batches based on their ability to prevent cell death induced by serum withdrawal. Chromatograms of the active fractions showed that the retention time for T1-11 was 22.03 min (Fig. 1B; Supplementary Figs. S1, S2). T1-11 is a colorless amorphous powder with a molecular formula of $C_{17}H_{20}O_5N_5$. Spectral methods (HR-FAB-MS, IR, ^1H, and ^{13}C NMR) determined that the structure of T1-11 is N^6-(4-hydroxybenzyl)adenine riboside [21], which we subsequently confirmed by synthesis (Supplementary Fig. S3). T1-11 constitutes about 0.3% of the 75% MeOH fraction of GE. To the best of our knowledge, the clinical use of T1-11 has not previously been investigated. In PC12 cells, T1-11 protected against serum withdrawal-induced cell death in a dose-dependent manner (Fig. 1C). Staining with annexin V-FITC confirmed that T1-11 rescued serum-deprived PC12 cells from apoptosis (Fig. 1D).

T1-11 is an agonist of the $A_{2A}R$ and an inhibitor of the adenosine transporter

We further characterized the pharmacological properties of T1-11 using radioligand binding assays. Of the 208 receptors/transporters tested, 10 μM T1-11 bound to only three molecules of the adenosinergic system including the $A_{2A}R$, A_3R, and an adenosine transporter - equilibrative nucleoside transporter 1 (ENT1; Table 1, Supplementary Table S1). Of these molecules, T1-11 bound to the A_3R with the highest affinity ($K_i = 0.1$ μM, Table 1). However, at a concentration (100 μM) approximately 1000-fold higher than its K_i value, T1-11 induced less than 50% GTP binding compared to a well-characterized A_3 agonist (2-Cl-IB-MECA, 3 μM, Supplementary Fig. S4). This low level of GTP binding is considered insufficient to trigger the G protein-dependent signaling of the A_3R, suggesting that despite its strong binding affinity, T1-11 may not be a functional ligand for the A_3R.

In contrast, T1-11 appeared to activate the $A_{2A}R$ (Table 1). We assessed the effect of two $A_{2A}R$ antagonists (ZM241385 and SCH58216) on T1-11's ability to prevent serum deprivation-induced death in PC12 cells and found that treatment with either antagonist blocked the effect of T1-11, indicating that T1-11's anti-apoptotic function is mediated at least in part by its role as a ligand for the $A_{2A}R$ (Fig. 1E). Treatment of PC12 cells with T1-11 dose-dependently elevated the cellular cAMP levels (Fig. 2A), and the EC_{50} value (~2.2 μM) was similar to its binding property toward the $A_{2A}R$ (Table 1). The $A_{2A}R$-selective antagonist (SCH58216, SCH) effectively blocked the T1-11-induced elevation in the cAMP level (Fig. 2B), further supporting the hypothesis that T1-11 activates a cAMP-dependent pathway by stimulating $A_{2A}R$. Importantly, a single intraperitoneal injection of T1-11 (5 mg/kg body weight) increased cAMP levels in the brains of wildtype, but not $A_{2A}R$ knockout [25], mice (Fig. 2C). In addition, T1-11 was detected in the brain 30 min after the intraperitoneal injection (0.12±0.01 ng/g brain lysate, $n = 4$; mean ± s.e.m.). These data indicate that T1-11 enters the brain and elevates cAMP via activation of the $A_{2A}R$ *in vivo*.

T1-11 also bound to an adenosine transporter ENT1 (Table 1, $K_i = 0.54$ μM). T1-11 inhibited adenosine uptake by PC12 cells in a dose-dependent manner (Fig. 3A). The maximal inhibition of adenosine transport evoked by T1-11 at a concentration of 30 μM (~55-fold its K_i value, Table 1) was similar to that caused by a well-characterized ENT1 inhibitor [nitrobenzylthioinosine, NBTI; 100 nM, 118-fold its K_i value (0.85 nM)] (Fig. 3B). Most importantly, introduction of T1-11 into the striatum of wildtype

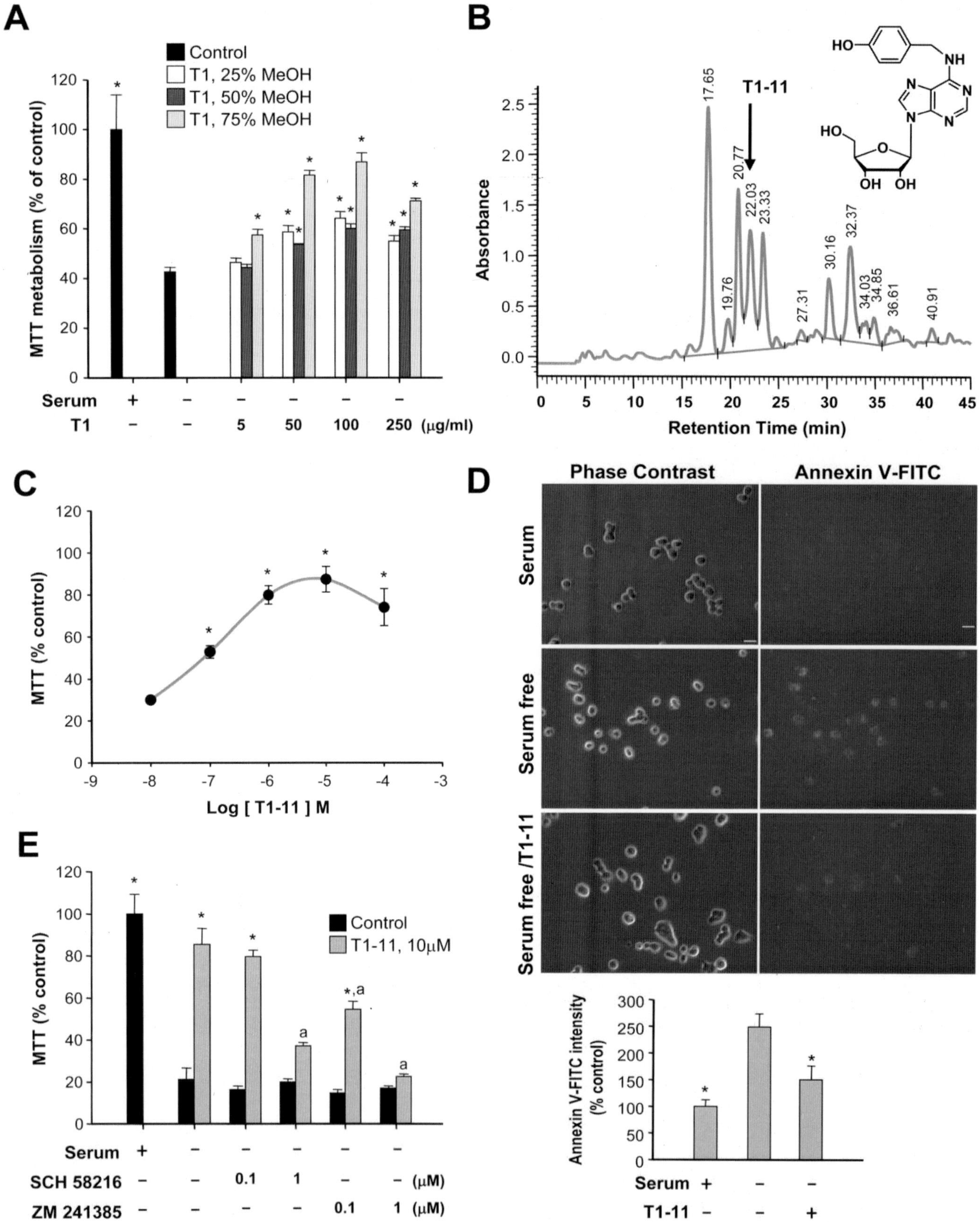

Figure 1. A fraction of the GE extract prevents serum-deprived PC12 cell apoptosis. (A, C, E) Serum-deprived PC12 cells were treated with or without the indicated reagent(s) for 24 h. Cell viability was expressed as a percentage of the MTT activity measured in the serum-containing group. Data points represent the mean ± s.e.m. of at least three independent experiments. *$p<0.05$, versus the corresponding serum-deprived group. [a] $p<0.05$, versus the corresponding serum-deprived/T1-11 treated group. (B) Chromatogram of active fractions of GE conducted by HPLC on a Merck

RP-18e (250×4.6 mm) column. The position of T1-11 is indicated by an arrow. The structure of T1-11 is shown in the upper right corner. (D) Serum-deprived PC12 cells were treated with serum or T1-11 (10 μM) as indicated for 24 h, stained with annexin V-FITC, and analyzed using microscope and flow cytometry. The median values of FITC fluorescence intensities were collected using an FL-1 channel (bottom panel). Representative pictures of cells in each condition are shown. Bars:10 μm. Data points represent the mean ± s.e.m. of at least three independent experiments.

mice significantly enhanced the level of striatal adenosine as determined by microdialysis (Fig. 3C), demonstrating that T1-11 inhibited adenosine uptake *in vivo*. Thus, in addition to its ability to activate the $A_{2A}R$, administration of T1-11 increases adenosinergic tone *in vivo*.

T1-11 binds to the adenosine pockets of the $A_{2A}R$ and of the ENT1

We next analyzed whether T1-11 fits into the ligand binding sites of activated $A_{2A}R$ (Fig. 4) and ENT1 (Fig. 5). From the newly resolved structure of human $A_{2A}R$ bound to the antagonist, ZM241385, in the inactive state [26] and previous mutagenesis experiments [17,27], it was evident that the -NH_2 interaction of the adenine core in CGS has the same binding interaction motifs as the antagonist, ZM241385 [26]. As shown in Figure 4A, the predicted binding of CGS to the structural model of the activated state of the human $A_{2A}R$ involves many hydrogen bonds with residues Thr88 [27], Asn253 [28], Glu169 [29], Ser277 [28], and His278 [30], which were identified by previous mutagenesis experiments. T1-11 docked to the same $A_{2A}R$ structural model, and was also involved in interactions with residues Asn253, Ser277, and His278, but with fewer hydrogen bonds (Fig. 4B). This analysis indicates that T1-11 fits into the ligand-binding site of the $A_{2A}R$ with a weaker affinity than CGS.

Because of the lack of a suitable structural template for homologous modeling of human ENT1 (hENT1), we conducted threading-based *ab inito* modeling of this transporter. The structural model of hENT1 resembles the structure of lactose permease (GlpT) [31], even though the number of transmembrane helices is different (11 for hENT1 vs. 12 for GlpT). This structure was further refined by a molecular-dynamics simulation in the fully solvated lipid bilayer, as detailed in "Materials and Methods". Docking the well-known hENT1 inhibitor, NBTI, and T1-11 to the refined structure generated the binding modes depicted in Figure 5A and 5B, respectively. NBTI and T1-11 bound to the transporter in the substrate translocation channel with similar orientations at similar binding sites.

Table 1. Pharmacological properties of T1-11.

Target Molecules	IC_{50} (μM)	K_i (μM)	Function
A_1 adenosine receptor	n.s.	n.s.	n.d.
A_{2A} adenosine receptor	4.66	2.62	agonist
A_{2B} adenosine receptor	n.s.	n.s.	n.d.
A_3 adenosine receptor	0.11	0.10	n.s.
Adenosine transporter (ENT1)	1.57	0.54	inhibitor

Binding properties of T1-11 toward four adenosine receptors (A_1, A_{2A}, A_{2B}, and A_3 receptors) and one adenosine transporter (ENT1) were conducted and characterized using standard binding protocols. T1-11 is an agonist of the $A_{2A}R$ to activate adenylyl cyclases and subsequently elevate cellular cAMP levels (Fig. 2). T1-11 also suppressed the uptake of adenosine (Fig. 3), and therefore was considered an inhibitor of ENT1. No significant binding of T1-11 toward the A_1R or $A_{2B}R$ at 10 μM was found. Although T1-11 also bound to the A_3R, it evoked no significant GTPγS binding at a concentration (10 μM) 1000-fold of its 1000-fold of its K_i value. n.d., not determined. n.s., not significant.

Chronic treatment with T1-11 has beneficial effects on several major symptoms of HD in a transgenic mouse model of HD

As the $A_{2A}R$ and ENT1 are located in the striatum and have been implicated in striatal function [32], we hypothesized that chronic treatment with T1-11 would modulate the progression of HD. We first tested the effect of T1-11 in a transgenic mouse model (R6/2) of HD in which $A_{2A}R$ agonists have beneficial effects [12,13]. The addition of T1-11 (0.05 mg/ml) to the drinking water of mice from the age of 7 weeks counteracted the progressive deterioration in motor coordination as assessed by rotarod performance (Fig. 6A). The mean survival times of control and T1-11-treated R6/2 mice were 99.0±2.1 d ($n=22$) and 103.3±3.9 d ($n=11$), respectively (Supplementary Fig. S5A). Using *in vivo* 3D MRI imaging, we found that T1-11 slightly ameliorated the brain atrophy of R6/2 mice but the improvement did not reach statistic significance (Supplementary Fig. S5B). Importantly, chronic treatment with T1-11 markedly reduced the formation of striatal Htt aggregates, a hallmark of HD, as assessed by filtered retardation assays (Fig. 6B) and immunofluorescence analyses (Fig. 6C). We recently reported that activation of the $A_{2A}R$ enhances mHtt-induced suppression of proteasome activity via a PKA-dependent pathway in the liver [12]. Therefore, we determined whether T1-11 decreases aggregate formation by elevating proteasome activity. As shown in Figure 6D, chymotrypsin-like activity in the striatal synaptosome fractions was lower in HD mice than in wildtype mice. Chronic treatment with T1-11 significantly enhanced chymotrypsin-like activity in the HD striatum (Fig. 6D). We also assessed whether T1-11 modulates other changes in brains of R6/2 mice. A previous study showed that the level of brain derived neurotrophic factor (BDNF) was decreased in the brains of HD mice [33]. Consistent with the beneficial effects of T1-11 on motor coordination, we found that T1-11-treated R6/2 mice contained more cortical BDNF than R6/2 mice that received no treatment (Fig. 6E). These results demonstrate the therapeutic potential of T1-11 for treating HD.

Discussion

We identified a novel adenosine analogue, T1-11, that possesses a dual function - both activating adenosine receptors and blocking the adenosine transporter ENT-1. Our data suggest that by simultaneously activating the $A_{2A}R$ and inhibiting adenosine uptake, T1-11 produces beneficial effects on HD by selectively elevating the adenosinergic tone of the brain, a novel protective mechanism.

Adenosine is an important endogenous neuroprotective substance and is a metabolite of many biosynthetic pathways. The endogenous adenosine level is known to be associated with the status of energy homeostasis in the brain [5]. Certain psychopharmacological agents (e.g., caffeine and ethanol) function by modulating the endogenous adenosine tone of the brain [34]. Our finding that T1-11-mediated elevation of adenosine tone had beneficial effects in R6/2 mice is consistent with a previous report showing that an increase in the adenosine tone of the brain exerts a protective effect on cerebral ischemia [35]. Modulation of the adenosine tone by pharmacological means may be useful in developing therapies for neurodegenerative diseases and/or

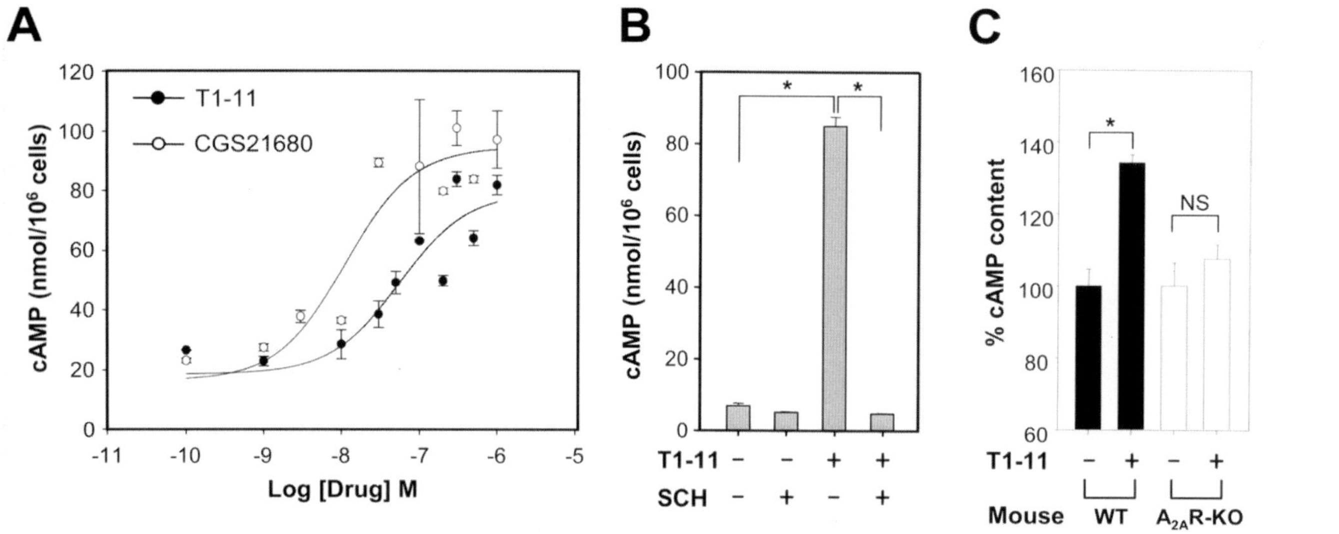

Figure 2. T1-11 is an agonist of the $A_{2A}R$. (A) PC12 cells were treated with T1-11 (closed circles) and CGS21680 (open circles) at the indicated concentration for 20 min at room temperature (RT). (B) PC12 cells were stimulated with T1-11 (10 μM) in the absence or presence of an $A_{2A}R$ antagonist (SCH, 1 μM) for 20 min at RT. (C) Wildtype and $A_{2A}R$ knockout (KO) mice were intraperitoneally administrated with T1-11 (5 mg/kg body weight, $n=4$) or vehicle for 60 min to measure the cAMP level in the brain.

traumas of the CNS. Several interesting adenosine drugs have been developed. For example, propentofylline, a weak inhibitor of three adenosine receptors (with a preference for the A_1R) and adenosine transporters, can be used to treat dementia and ischemic brain damage [36]. The action of propentofylline is intriguing and complex as it indirectly enhances functions of adenosine receptors via inhibition of adenosine transporters which elevate extracellular adenosine concentrations, and directly suppresses adenosine receptors, limiting its former action [36]. Although the binding affinities of T1-11 were not as strong as those of the best adenosine drugs currently available (Table 1, Figs. 2, 3, 6), the dual functions of these compounds in activating adenosine receptors and inhibiting adenosine transporters is likely to enable T1-11 to effectively activate the adenosinergic system in synapses where both adenosine receptors and transporters are located.

Despite the significant interest in $A_{2A}R$-related drugs for HD, earlier studies using different mouse models of HD showed complex and even conflicting conclusions on the neuroprotective *versus* neurodegenerative roles of the $A_{2A}R$ in HD. We earlier published a review in which we evaluated whether the $A_{2A}R$ is a feasible drug target for HD, and concluded that more studies are needed to clarify the application of $A_{2A}R$ drugs to HD [37]. Because stimulation of the $A_{2A}R$ triggers glutamate release, it was proposed that the presynaptic $A_{2A}R$ on the glutminergic terminals would be harmful, while that on the postsynaptic GABAergic

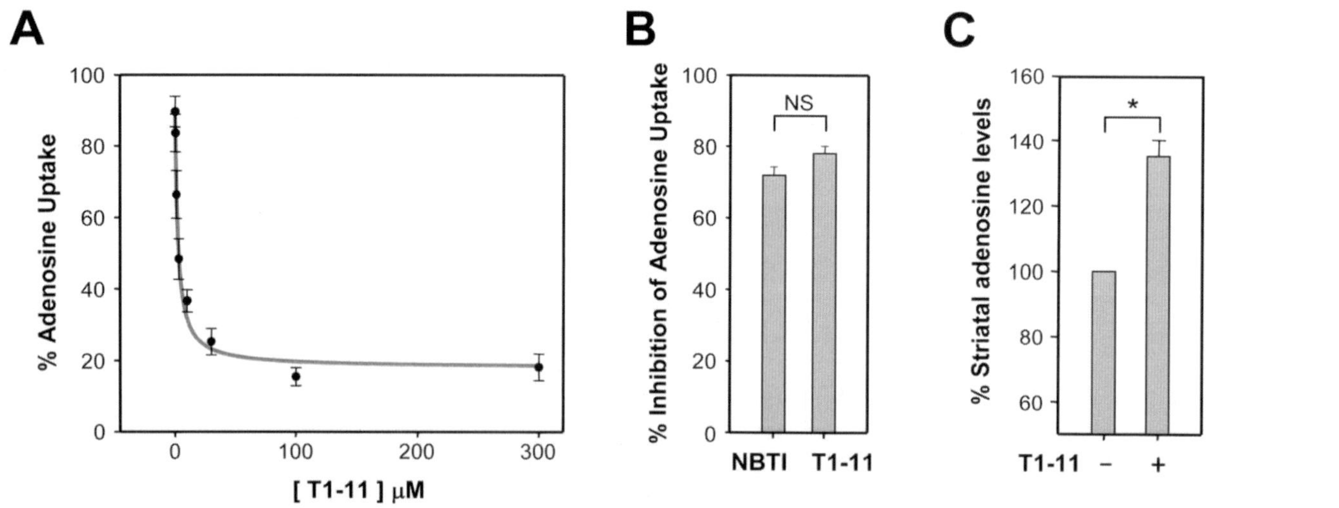

Figure 3. T1-11 inhibited the uptake of adenosine. (A) Adenosine uptake by PC12 cells was analyzed in the presence of T1-11 at the indicated concentration. (B) Adenosine uptake by PC12 cells was evaluated in the presence of T1-11 (30 μM) or NBTI (0.1 μM) as indicated for 10 min. (C) T1-11 (100 μM) was perfused throughout the dialysis probe. The collected perfusates were analyzed for striatal adenosine levels. Data points represent the mean ± s.e.m.. * $p<0.05$, compared to the basal level.

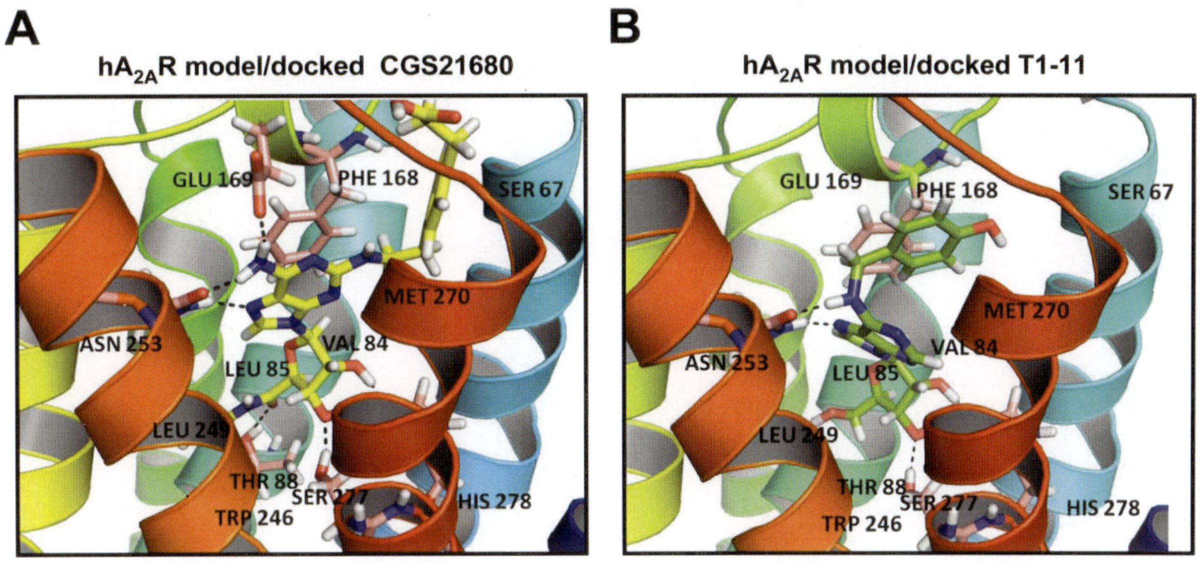

Figure 4. Interactions of the agonists with the ligand binding sites of the $A_{2A}R$. (A) The binding pose of CGS21680 (a selective agonist) on the human $A_{2A}R$, as predicted by combined homology modeling and docking analysis. The three-dimensional structure of the activated-state $A_{2A}R$ was constructed based on the inactive-state structure of the $A_{2A}R$ and the opsin structure. (B) Similar to (A), the binding pose of T1-11 on the human $A_{2A}R$.

terminals would be protective [10,15,16]. On the contrary, the $A_{2A}R$ is closely linked to BDNF which is markedly impaired in HD [7,33,38,39]. Activation of the $A_{2A}R$ enhances the signal of BDNF by facilitating localization of its receptor (TrkB) in lipid rafts through a cAMP/PKA-dependent pathway, transactivates TrkB, and increases the synthesis of TrkB [40,41,42]. Stimulation of the $A_{2A}R$ also facilitates the functions of other neurotrophic factors [such as the glial cell line-derived neurotrophic factor (GDNF) and fibroblast growth factor (FGF)]. These findings are important because supplementation with BDNF, GDNF, or FGF in HD mice all led to beneficial effects on disease progression [43,44]. Small molecules which activate the $A_{2A}R$ thus might provide a unique means to elicit trophic responses in HD. It is important to note that the expression and signaling of the $A_{2A}R$ as well as other receptors (e.g., D2 dopamine receptor and metabotropic glutamate receptor) are altered in both HD mice and patients [13,45–49]. The roles of the $A_{2A}R$ revealed by studies conducted in wildtype animals therefore need to be re-evaluated in genetic models of HD. Indeed, studies from several laboratories showed that activation of the $A_{2A}R$ produces opposite effects in the striatum of WT and HD (R6/2) mice [11,50]. In R6/2 mice, treatment with an $A_{2A}R$ antagonist (SCH58261) for 1 week worsened motor coordination [51]. Genetic removal of the $A_{2A}R$ in another HD mouse model (N171-82Q) also exacerbated motor

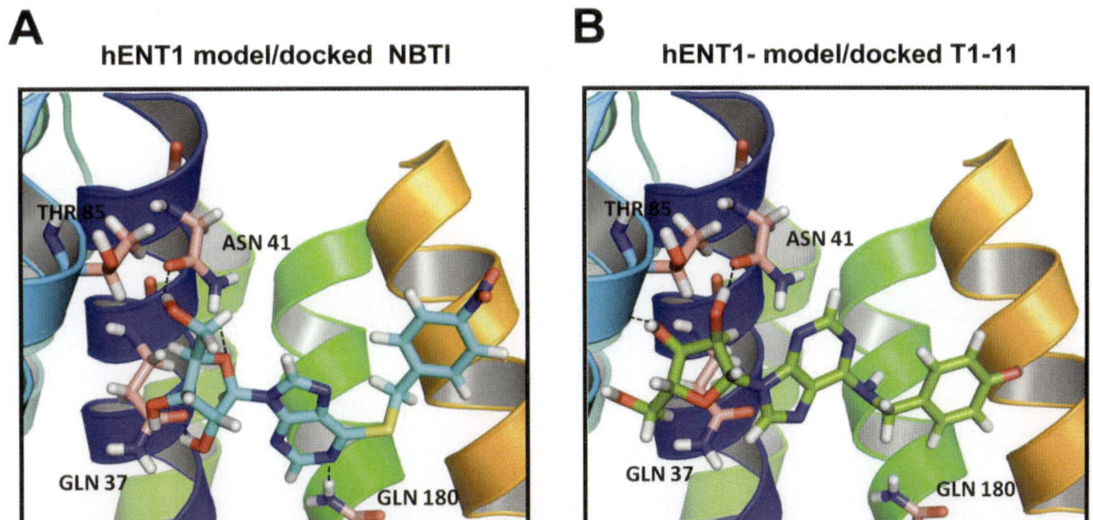

Figure 5. Interactions of inhibitors with ligand binding sites of ENT1. (A) The binding pose of NBTI (a selective inhibitor of ENT1) on human ENT1, as predicted using threading-based *ab inito* modeling of this transporter. The three-dimensional structure of ENT1 was constructed based on the lactose permease (GlpT) structure. (B) Similar to (A), the binding pose of T1-11 on human ENT1.

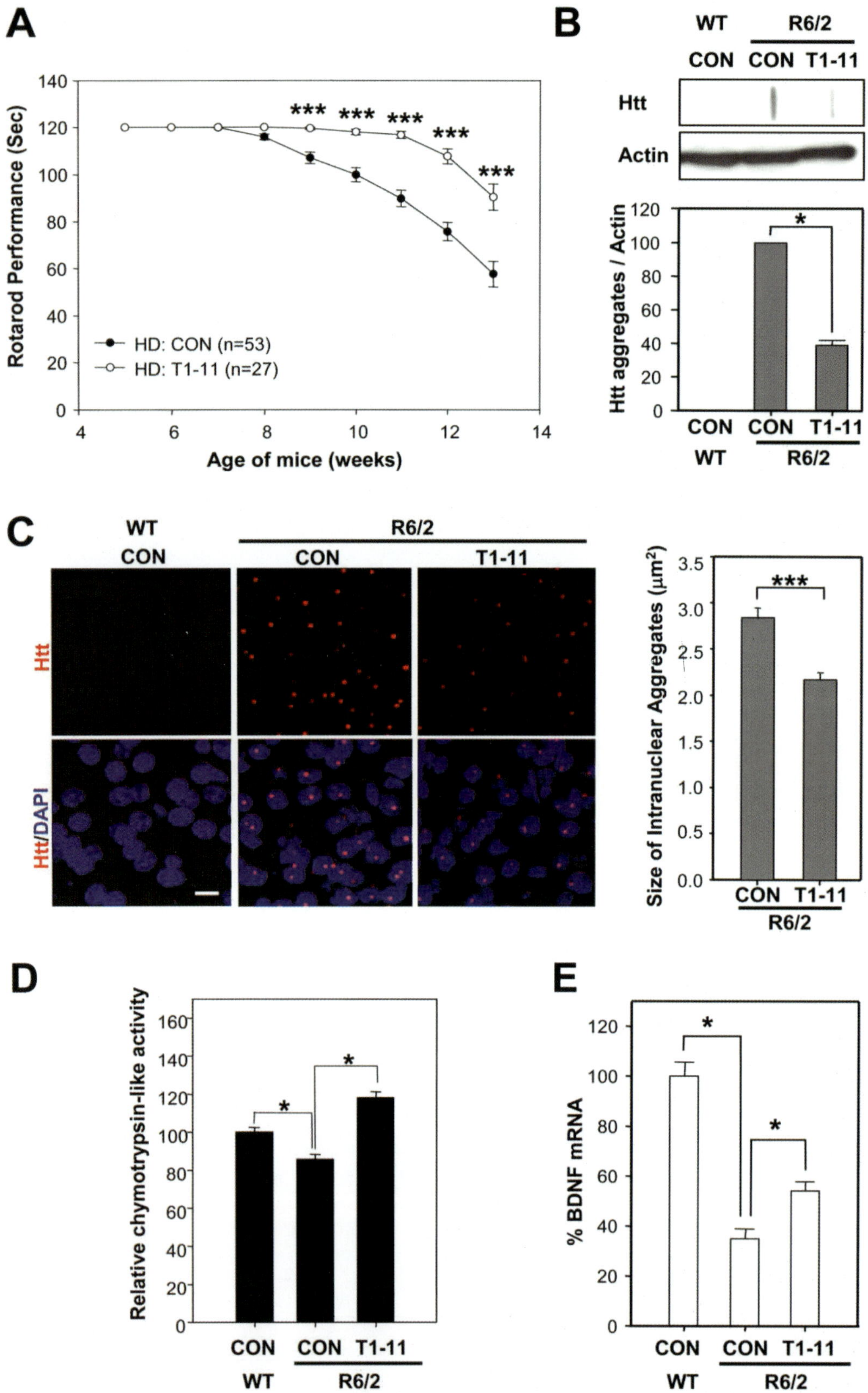

Figure 6. T1-11 exhibited beneficial effects in a mouse model of HD. R6/2 mice were given the vehicle (1% DMSO; CON, $n=53$) or T1-11 (0.05 mg/ml, $n=27$)-containing drinking water from the age of 7 weeks. (A) Rotarod performance was conducted as described in "Methods". (B) Striatal lysates (50~100 μg) collected from the indicated mice at the age of 12 weeks old were subjected to a filter retardation assay. The insoluble Htt aggregates retained on the filter were detected using an anti-Htt antibody (upper panel). The amount of protein in each corresponding lysate was independently assessed by Western blot analyses using an anti-actin antibody (middle panel). The relative aggregate formation was quantified by

dividing the Htt signals in filter assays with those of the corresponding actin signals in Western blots (bottom panel). Data are presented as the mean ± s.e.m. values from three independent experiments. * $p<0.05$, versus R6/2 mice with no treatment (CON, Student's *t* test). (C) Brain sections of 12-week-old animals [vehicle (CON)-treated WT mice ($n=5$), vehicle-treated R6/2 mice ($n=5$), and T1-11-treated R6/2 mice ($n=5$)] were stained with an anti-Htt antibody. Mutant Htt aggregates were visualized using Alexa Flour 568 (red). Nuclei were visualized using H33258 (blue). Representative pictures are shown. The scale bar is 10 μm. Data are presented as the mean ± SEM in each group. *** $p<0.001$, versus R6/2 mice treated with vehicle (CON, Student's *t* test). (D) The chymotrypsin-like activity of proteasomes in striatal synaptosomes of the indicated 12-week-old mice ($n=3$) was assessed as described in "Methods". (E) Cortical tissues (n = 3) were collected to determine the transcript level of BDNF using a quantitative RT-PCR technique. The expression levels of BDNF were normalized to that of GAPDH. * $P<0.05$, versus R6/2 mice with no treatment (CON, Student's *t* test).

degeneration and shortened the lifespan [14]. However, the abovementioned 1-week treatment with SCH58261 in the presymptomatic stage of R6/2 mice was associated with a reduction in NMDA-induced toxicity, indicating a potential protective effect [51]. Because the glutamate release was dynamically altered from an enhancement at the presymptomatic stage to a decrease at the symptomatic stage during disease progression of HD mice [49], and since local glutamate level was recently shown to dictate the effect of $A_{2A}R$ on neuronal death in an animal model of traumatic brain injury [52], it is possible that the stage of disease progression might contribute to the complex role of $A_{2A}R$ in HD. Further investigations using both pharmacological and genetic approaches are necessary to verify whether early and/or chronic blockage of the $A_{2A}R$ is detrimental during HD progression. Conversely, activation of the $A_{2A}R$ using CGS provides beneficial effects on several major HD symptoms (including brain atrophy, striatal aggregates, and deteriorated motor coordination) in R6/2 mice [12,13]. In line with our studies, Cepeda and colleagues also demonstrated that CGS ameliorates the corticostriatal synaptic disconnection in R6/2 mice [11]. Agonists of the $A_{2A}R$ therefore might be used to treat HD. Unfortunately, full A_{2A} agonists (e.g., CGS) have unfavorable acute side effects, including low food intake, sedation/drowsiness, an increased heart rate, and systematic hypotension [17,53,54]. A modest agonist such as T1-11 may have fewer side effects in peripheral tissues and may thus be superior to full A_{2A} agonists for therapeutic uses such as those of other classes of adenosine drugs [55]. We tested this hypothesis by treating R6/2 mice with T1-11 using a subcutaneous Alzet minipump for 48 h. At a dose that improved motor deterioration, T1-11 did not change the blood pressure of R6/2 mice (Supplementary Materials, Figure S6). The rapid entry of T1-11 into the brain suggests that it may have great potential for treating brain diseases. Collectively, T1-11 possesses key features of an ideal A_{2A} drug for HD. In the present study, T1-11 was delivered via the drinking water because it is one of the most common routes for drug delivery in human patients and it causes much less stress on mice than intraperitoneal injection or oral gavage. Nonetheless, such mode of drug delivery did not permit an accurate assessment of the actual doses taken by the animals. In addition, HD mice at late stage of the disease drink less water because of impaired motor function, and thus receive less T1-11. Such reduced intake of T1-11 by mice with late stage HD might compromise the beneficial effect of T1-11 and account for the inability of T1-11 to rescue certain symptoms of HD (e.g., shorten lifespan and brain atrophy, Supplementary Figure S5). For potential clinical application of T1-11 in the future, it is critical to further optimize its effective dose, formulation, and administration protocol to maximize its beneficial effect.

The protective effects of the GE extract and T1-11 are consistent with a previously implied neuroprotective effect of GE [18,19]. By targeting multiple components in the adenosinergic system, T1-11 is expected to elevate the adenosine tone and is a potential candidate for treating HD. In addition to the role of the $A_{2A}R$ as discussed above, the functions of other adenosine receptors (particularly, the A_1R and A_3R) in HD also warrant further studies. In an earlier report, an A_1R-specific agonist (adenosine amine congener) showed neuroprotective effects in a rat HD model created by the systemic administration of 3-nitropropionic acid which caused striatal lesions [56]. The functions of the A_3R have not been evaluated in HD before. Nonetheless, agonists of the A_3R provide neuroprotective effects against subarachnoid hemorrhage-induced brain damage [57]. The contributions of the A_1R and A_3R to the beneficial effects of T1-11 on HD mice require further experimental evaluation.

The concept of a small molecule that targets multiple components in the same regulatory system to optimize its function at a specific location (such as synapses) is a novel strategy for developing therapeutic methods for HD, for which there is currently no effective treatment [58]. This approach is particularly critical for the design of neurotransmitter-based drugs for CNS diseases in which side effects from peripheral tissues are a major obstacle. Dual-action drugs have recently attracted much attention [59]. A drug (tapentadol) recently approved by the US FDA, also a dual-action molecule, acts on molecules of two different neurotransmitter systems (a μ-opioid receptor agonist and a norepinephrine transporter) [60]. Another interesting example is 8-(3-chlorostyryl)caffeine, a well-characterized A_{2A}-selective antagonist which ameliorates MPTP neurotoxicity by simultaneously inhibiting monoamine oxidase and the $A_{2A}R$ [61]. A similar design as for dual-function drugs may be applicable to other neurotransmitter systems (e.g., dopamine receptor/transporter and serotonin receptor/transporter) and may facilitate the development of new drugs for other neurodegenerative diseases.

Materials and Methods

Preparation of the GE extract and T1-11

The rhizome of *G. elata* (GE) was purchased from a local herbal store in Taipei. Slices of GE were extracted at 60°C using 80% ethanol/H_2O overnight (3 times). The crude extract was concentrated using a vacuum rotary evaporator (Büchi) under reduced pressure. The dried sample (about 15% yield based on the dried herbal weight) was subjected to Diaion HP-20 column chromatography using elution from a H_2O/MeOH gradient. Fractions were examined for their abilities to prevent apoptosis induced by serum withdrawal in PC12 cells. The active fractions of 50%~75% MeOH/H_2O were combined and purified on a Sephadex LH-20 column by repeated elution with MeOH to give T1-11. High-pressure liquid chromatography was performed on a Merck RP-18e (250×4.6 mm) column using a mobile phase gradient from 70% to 40% H_2O/MeOH for 40 min and from 40% to 20% H_2O/MeOH for 5 min at a flow rate of 0.8 ml/min. A UV 270-nm detector was used to monitor the chemical profiles of different batches.

Synthesis of T1-11

Compound T1-11 was synthesized in a high yield by the substitution reaction of 6-chloropurine ribonucleoside with 4-hydroxybenzylamine (as hydrochloric acid) in the presence of a base diisopropylethylamine [62,63]. Because the hydrochloric salt of 4-hydroxybenzylamine is not commercially available, it was prepared by hydrogenation of the corresponding 4-hydroxybenzaldehyde oxime.

Cell culture

PC12 cells purchased from ATCC (Manassas, VA, USA) were maintained in Dulbecco's modified Eagle's medium (DMEM) supplemented with 10% horse serum and 5% fetal bovine serum and incubated in a CO_2 incubator (5%) at 37°C.

MTT metabolism assay

Survival was assessed by the 3-(4,5-dimethylthiazol-2-yl)-2,5-diphenyltetrazolium bromide (MTT) metabolism assay as described elsewhere [64,65]. In brief, cells grown on 150-mm plates were washed three times with PBS and resuspended in DMEM. Suspended cells (1×10^4 cells) were plated on 96-well plates and treated with or without the indicated reagent. After incubation for 24 h, MTT (0.5 mg/ml) was added to the medium and incubated for 3 h. After discarding the medium, DMSO (100 μl) was then applied to the well to dissolve the formazan crystals derived from the mitochondrial cleavage of the tetrazolium ring by live cells. The absorbance at 570/630 nm in each well was measured on a micro-enzyme-linked immunosorbent assay reader.

Annexin V-FITC staining

An annexin V (FITC-conjugated) apoptosis kit (K101-400; BioVision, Mountain View, CA, USA) was used to analyze apoptotic cells. The experimental protocol followed the manufacturer's instructions and a previous article [66]. In brief, after treatment with serum, serum-free medium, or serum-free medium plus T1-11 of the indicated concentration for 24 h, cells growing on 12-well plates at $(3\sim4)\times10^5$ cells/well were loaded with 0.5 ml binding buffer and 5 μl annexin V-FITC. After incubation for 5 min in the dark, cells were washed once with 1 ml of culture medium (without phenol red) for fluorescent imaging analyses (Axiovert-200M, Carl Zeiss, Gôttingen, Germany) or a flow cytometric analysis (Beckton Dickinson, Franklin Lakes, NJ, USA). Median values of the FITC fluorescent intensities were determined using an FL-1 channel (488/530Ex/Em nm). Five thousand live cells were analyzed per sample.

Radioligand binding assays

Radioligand binding assays were performed by MDS Pharma Services Taiwan (Taipei, Taiwan) using standard binding protocols. For the binding assay of the $A_{2A}R$ [67], membrane proteins collected from HEK293 cells overexpressing the human $A_{2A}R$ were incubated in reaction buffer [50 mM Tris-HCl (pH 7.4), 10 mM $MgCl_2$, 1 mM EDTA, and 2 U/mL adenosine deaminase] containing ^{3}H-CGS21680 (50 nM) for 90 min at 25°C. Nonspecific binding was assessed in the presence of 50 μM adenosine- 5′-*N*-ethylcarboxamide. To measure the binding affinity of T1-11 to the A_3R [68,69], membrane proteins collected from CHO-K1 cells overexpressing the human A_3R were incubated with ^{3}H-AB-MECA (0.5 nM) for 60 min at 25°C in a reaction buffer containing 25 mM HEPES (pH 7.4), 5 mM MgC_2, 1 mM CaCl., and 0.1% bovine serum albumin. Nonspecific binding was assessed in the presence of 1 μM IB-MECA (Tocris Bioscience, Ellisville, MS, USA). Binding assays for adenosine transporters were conducted as described earlier ([70]. Membrane fractions collected from the cerebral cortex of Duncan Hartley derived guinea pigs were incubated with ^{3}H-labeled 6-[(4-nitrobenzyl)thio]-9-β-D-ribofuranosylpurine (NBTI, 0.5 nM) for 30 min at 25°C in an incubation buffer containing 50 mM Tris-HCl (pH 7.4). Nonspecific binding was assessed in the presence of 5 μM NBTI, an effective inhibitor of equilibrative nucleoside transporters. Note that NBTI is a high-affinity inhibitor of ENT1, and inhibits only human (h)ENT1 at 0.5 nM [71]. Reactions were terminated by filtration over GF/B glass fibers and washing with the corresponding reaction buffer.

cAMP assay

PC12 cells were plated at the density of 5×10^5 cells/well (on 12-well plates) and incubated with the indicated reagent(s) for the desired period of time. Cells were washed twice with ice-cold Locke's solution (150 mM NaCl, 5.6 mM KCl, 5 mM glucose, 1 mM $MgCl_2$, and 10 mM HEPES, adjusted to pH 7.4). Cellular cAMP was extracted by adding 0.3 ml of 0.1 M HCl to each well and incubating this for 10 min on ice. The cAMP content was assayed using the ^{125}I-cAMP assay system (GE Healthcare, Little Chalfont, Buckinghamshire, UK).

C57BL6 mice (8 weeks old) were intraperitoneally (i.p.) administrated with T1-11 (5 mg/kg body weight, $n=4$) or vehicle for 60 min. Brain tissues were carefully removed, and homogenized in 1 ml of assay buffer (25 mM Tris (pH 8), 1 mM EGTA, 1 mM $MgCl_2$, 40 mM leupeptin, 100 mM PMSF, 10 nM okadaic acid, 1 × EDTA free proteinase inhibitor cocktail (Roche), 0.5 mM IBMX, and 20 mM papaverine). Trichloroacetic acid (6%, final concentration) was then added to the lysate to precipitate proteins. The cAMP level in the supernatant was analyzed as previously described.

GTPγS binding assay

The GTPγS binding assay was conducted by MDS Pharma Services Taiwan using a previously described protocol [55] with slight modifications. In brief, membrane proteins collected from Chinese hamster ovary (CHO-K1) cells expressing the human A_3R (5~10 μg per reaction) were incubated with the indicated drug and ^{35}S-GTPγS (0.1 nM) in a total volume of 500 μl for 30 min at 30°C. The reaction buffer was composed of 20 mM HEPES (pH 7.4), 100 mM NaCl, 10 mM $MgCl_2$, 1 mM DTT, and 1 mM EDTA. The reaction was terminated by filtration over GF/B glass fibers and washed with the same reaction buffer. Relative GTPγS binding was defined as the percentage of ^{35}S-GTPγS binding when compared to that of a selective agonist of the A_3R (2-Cl-IB-MECA, 3 μM) under the same binding conditions.

Adenosine transport

For adenosine uptake of PC12, cells were seeded approximately 16 h before each uptake assay at $\sim2\times10^5$ cells per well in 24-well plates coated with poly-L-lysine. To perform adenosine uptake assays, cells were washed with Krebs Ringer-Henseleit buffer [125 mM NaCl, 4.8 mM KCl, 1.3 mM $CaCl_2$, 1.2 mM $MgSO_4$, 1.2 mM KH_2PO_4, 5.6 mM glucose, 10 μM pargyline, and 10 mM HEPES (pH 7.2)] and incubated in the same buffer for 10 min at 37°C in the presence or absence of the indicated reagent(s). Adenosine uptake was initiated by adding [^{3}H]adenosine at the indicated concentration (0.5 μCi/mmol) at 37°C. At the end of the incubation, cells were placed on ice, washed twice with ice-cold Krebs Ringer-Henseleit buffer to remove free [^{3}H]adenosine, lysed with 1% Triton X-100, and added to scintillation vials to count the radioactivity. Non-specific uptake was determined as the uptake performed in the presence of 100 μM adenosine, and was subtracted from the total adenosine uptake.

In vivo brain dialysis and adenosine measurement

The level of adenosine in the brain was determined using microdialysis as previously described [72,73]. In brief, concentrated dialysis probes with 4-mm dialysis membranes (CMA, Stockholm, Sweden) were used to monitor the extracellular adenosine in the striatum of rats. After inducing anesthesia with chloral hydrate (400 mg/ml, IP), rats were implanted with the probe, and the coordinates for implantation were AP +1.0 mm, LM +2.8 mm, and VD −6.5 mm. Ringer's solution (140 mM NaCl, 1.2 mM $CaCl_2$, 3.0 mM KCl, 1.0 mM $MgCl_2$, and 0.04 mM ascorbic acid) was continuously perfused (0.5 µl/min) via probes throughout the experiments. After implantation and perfusion for 1.5 h, the perfusate was collected for 1 h as a baseline and then Ringer's solution containing T1-11 (100 µM) was perfused for another 1 h. The perfusate was analyzed by high-performance liquid chromatography (HPLC; Agilent 1100 series, Germany) coupled with a photo diode array detector (Agilent G1315B,) at 260 nm. Separations were obtained with a reversed-phase column (Cosmosil 5C18-AR-II, 250×4.6 mm, Kyoto, Japan) eluted at a flow rate of 1.0 ml/min with a linear solvent gradient elution system composed of eluents A and B (A: 0.0085% H_3PO_4 in H_2O; B: 100% acetonitrile) according to the following profile: 0~15 min, 100%~90% A, 0%~10% B.

Animals and drug administration

Male R6/2 mice [74] and littermate controls were originally obtained from Jackson Laboratories (Bar Harbor, ME, USA), and mated to female control mice (B6CBAFI/J). Offspring were identified by a polymerase chain reaction (PCR) genotyping technique of genomic DNA extracted from tail tissues using primers located in the transgene (5′-CCGCTCAGGTTCT-GCTTTTA-3′ and 5′-GGCTGAGGAAGCTG- AGGAG-3′) to ensure that the number of CAG repeats remained approximately 150. In total, 211 R6/2 transgenic mice were used in this study. Animals were housed at the Institute of Biomedical Sciences Animal Care Facility under a 12-h light/dark cycle. Body weights of mice were recorded once daily. Animal experiments were performed under protocols approved by the Academia Sinica Institutional Animal Care and Utilization Committee, Taipei, Taiwan.

Rotarod performance

Motor coordination was assessed using a rotarod apparatus (UGO BASILE, Comerio, Italy) at a constant speed (12 rpm) over the period of 2 min [75]. All mice were trained for 2 days at the age of 4 weeks to allow them to become acquainted with the rotarod apparatus. Animals were then tested three times per week from the ages of 4~12 weeks. For each test, animals were placed in the apparatus before initiation of rotation. Latency to falling was automatically recorded. Each mouse was given three trials for a maximum of 2 min for each trial.

Hemodynamic Examination

Heart rates and blood pressure of conscious and anesthetized mice were measured using a blood pressure monitor (model MK-2000; Muromachi Kikai, Tokyo, Japan) between 10 AM to 6 PM. Values of 12–18 successful readings per mouse were used to determine the blood pressure.

Filter retardation assay

SDS-insoluble mutant Htt aggregates were detected and quantified as described [76]. A filter retardation assay was performed as described previously [2]. Blots were blocked with 5% skim milk in phosphate-buffered saline (PBS) and incubated with an anti-Htt antibody (EM48, 1:500; Chemicon International, Temecula, CA, USA) at 4°C overnight followed by the corresponding secondary antibody for 1 h at room temperature. Immunoreactive bands were detected by enhanced chemiluminescence (Pierce) and recorded using Kodak XAR-5 film.

Immunohistochemistry and quantitation

Coronal serial sections (20 µm) containing the striatum (interaural 5.34 mm/bregma 1.54 mm to interaural 3.7 mm/ bregma −0.1 mm) were immunohistochemically stained as described previously [77]. Brain sections were blocked with normal goat serum and incubated overnight with an anti-Htt antibody (EM48, 1:500) at 4°C, followed by a 2 h-incubation with a goat anti-mouse IgG conjugated to Alexa Fluor® 568 at room temperature. The nuclei were stained with Hoechst 33258. The patterns of immunostaining were analyzed with a laser confocal microscope (LSM510, Carl Zeiss MicroImaging Inc, Germany). Five different brain sections of each animal were analyzed. At least 2000 cells from each animal were used to quantify the sizes of mHtt aggregates using ImageJ software (http://rsbweb.nih.gov/ij/; Research Services Branch of the National Institute of Mental Health, Bethesda, MD, USA).

Proteasome activity assay

The chymotrypsin-like activity of the proteasome was determined using a specific proteasome substrate [succinyl (suc)-Leu-Leu-Val-Tyr-7-amino-4-methyl coumarin (AMC)] (Sigma-Aldrich, St Louis, MO, USA) as described earlier [12]. In brief, the synaptosome-enriched fraction (10 µg) were incubated with the substrate (40 µM) in 100 µl of proteasome assay buffer [0.05 M Tris-HCl (pH 8.0), 0.5 mM EDTA, 1 mM ATP, and 1 mM DTT] at 37°C for 60 min where the relationship between the incubation time and product formation remained linear. The fluorescence of the released AMC was detected using a Fluorescence Microplate Reader System (Device, Sunnyvale, CA, USA) at 380-nm excitation and 460-nm emission wavelengths.

Western blot assays

Equal amounts of protein were separated by sodium dodecyl-sulfate polyacrylamide gel electrophoresis (SDS-PAGE) using 10% polyacrylamide gels according to the method of Laemmli [78]. The resolved proteins were electroblotted onto Immobilon polyvinylidene difluoride membranes (Millipore, Bedford, MA, USA). Membranes were blocked with 5% skim milk in PBS and incubated with an anti-actin antibody (1:2500; Chemicon International) at 4°C overnight followed by the corresponding secondary antibody for 1 h at room temperature. Immunoreactive bands were detected by enhanced chemiluminescence (Pierce) and recorded using Kodak XAR-5 film.

RNA isolation and quantitative real-time PCR

Total RNA was isolated from the cortex of the indicated mice using the TriReagent kit (Molecular Research Center, Cincinnati, OH, USA), treated with RNase-free DNase (RQ1; Promega) to remove potential contamination by genomic DNA, and transcribed into complementary (c)DNA using Superscript* II reverse transcriptase. A real-time quantitative PCR was performed using a TaqMan kit (PE Applied Biosystems, Foster City, CA, USA) on a TaqMan ABI 7700 Sequence Detection System (PE Applied Biosystems) using heat-activated TaqDNA polymerase (Amplitaq Gold; PE Applied Biosystems). The PCR mixtures were incubated at 50°C for 2 min and 95°C for 10 min, and then 40 PCR cycles were conducted (95°C for 15 s and 65°C for 1 min). The sequences of primers are listed below: for BDNF (the target gene), 5′-GGCTTCACAGGAGACATCAG-3′ and 5′-CAGAACCA-GAACGAACAGAAAC-3′; and for GAPDH (the reference gene), 5′TATCCGTTGTGGATCTGACAT-3′ and 5′-ACAACCTG-GTCCTCAGTGTA-3′. Independent reverse-transcription PCRs were performed using the same cDNA for both the indicated target gene and reference gene (GAPDH). A melting curve was created at the end of the PCR cycle to confirm that a single product had been amplified. Data were analyzed using ABI 7700 operating software to determine the threshold cycle (CT) above the background for each reaction. The relative transcript amount of the target gene, which was calculated using standard curves of serial RNA dilutions, was normalized to that of GAPDH of the same RNA.

Structure modeling of the activated human adenosine A_{2A} receptor

Multiple sequence alignment was performed with ClustalW [79] for bovine rhodopsin, and the human adenosine A_1, A_{2A}, A_{2B}, and A_3 receptors, where the BLOSUM scoring matrix, a gap open penalty of 10, and a gap extension penalty of 0.05 were used. Sequences were retrieved from Swiss-Prot [80]. To model the active state of the human adenosine $A_{2A}R$ (residues 1~310), residues 1~172 (except for the unresolved residues, 1 and 2, and 148~156) were taken from the recently solved inactivated structure (PDB ID: 3EML) [26], because it was found that these residues probably remained intact during the transition between the active and inactive states [81]. The extracellular loop 2, which should contribute to the binding of ligands to the receptor, is therefore based on the inactive structure of the $A_{2A}R$. The unsolved residues, 1 and 2 and 148~156 were patched with the program loopy [82]. TM5, TM6, TM7, and helix 8, i.e., residues 175~310, were modeled based on the opsin structure [81]. MODELLER9v5 [83] was used for the chimerical modeling, and 100 models were generated. Finally, the model with the lowest DOPE energy [84] was selected. The hydrogen atoms were added by the PDB2PQR web server [85] at pH 7, but the N_δ atom of His278 was manually assigned to be protonated and the N_ε atom was not protonated, because the binding mode of this protonation assignment would be in better agreement with the mutation experiment. During the revision of the manuscript, the structure of $A_{2A}R$ bound with the agonist UK-432097 has been published [86]. We compared the model we constructed in this work with the newly released structure and found that these two structures are very similar, especially at the binding pocket of the receptor.

Structure modeling of hENT1

The sequence of hENT1 was retrieved from Swiss-Port [80]. The initial models of hENT1 were constructed by iTASSER [87], which is the iterative implementation of the Threading ASSEmbly Refinement (TASSER) program [88]. One model was selected based on the spatial distribution of the transmembrane regions annotated by Swiss-Prot, to see whether the all the transmembrane helices can be packed into the hydrophobic slab of a membrane. All other models generated by iTASSER failed to meet this criterion. This hENT1 model was inserted into the POPC bilayer equilibrated in a previous study [89], where all the lipids and water molecules having van der Waals contacts with the transporter were removed. The system was energy-minimized by the steepest descent method for 500 cycles, with all transporter atoms restrained. The system was then equilibrated by conventional molecular dynamics at 300 K and 1 bar for 1 ns. The self-guided molecular dynamics simulation [90] was then conducted for 40 ns to refine the hENT1 structure. The lipid force field parameters were adopted from a previous study [89], and the AMBER parm99SB force field [91] was used for the transporter. The sander module of AMBER 9 [92] was employed for the simulations.

Docking protocols

The partial charges of atoms on the ligand and the receptor molecules were determined by the Gasteiger method [93], aided by AutoDockTools. The number of chromosomes was set to 100, and the number of generations was set to 5000. The Solis-Wet local search iteration was set to 600. The binding pose of CGS21680 was predicted with the program AutoDock 4 [94].

Supporting Information

Figure S1 ^{1}H NMR spectrum of T1-11 (DMSO-d_6, 400 MHz).

Figure S2 ^{13}C NMR spectrum of T1-11 (DMSO-d_6, 100 MHz).

Figure S3 HPLC diagram of a synthetic sample of T1-11.

Figure S4 T1-11 binds to the A_3 adenosine receptor (A_3R) without evoking a significant binding of GTP. Membrane fractions collected from CHO-K1 cells expressing the human A_3R were incubated with T1-11 at the indicated concentration and ^{35}S-GTPγS (0.1 nM) for 30 min at 30°C. Relative GTPγS binding was defined as the percentage of ^{35}S-GTPγS binding when compared with a selective agonist of the A_3R (2-Cl-IB-MECA, 3 μM).

Figure S5 Effect of T1-11 on the shorten lifespan and enlarged ventricle of R6/2 mice. Animals were given the vehicle (1% DMSO; CON) or T1-11 (0.05 mg/ml)-containing drinking water from the age of 7 weeks. (A) Survival was assessed. Specific comparison to R6/2 mice treated with the vehicle ($p = 0.306$; Mantel-Cox test). (B) Five weeks after T1-11 treatment, 3D-lMRI was performed to determine the ventricle-to-brain ratio of the indicated animals as described. * $p<0.05$.

Figure S6 Treatment of R6/2 mice with T1-11 did not affect their heart rate and blood pressure. (A) T1-11 (125 μg/mouse/day) or vehicle (CON) was administrated subcutaneously to the indicated mice of 7 weeks old using ALZET osmotic minipumps for 6 weeks. Rotarod performance was assessed. (B, C) T1-11 (125 μg/mouse/day) was administrated subcutaneously to the indicated mice of 9 weeks old using ALZET osmotic minipumps for 48 h. Heart rate (B) and blood pressure (C) were determined by a tail-cuff method. * $p<0.05$. *** $p<0.005$.

Table S1 Binding properties of T1-11 toward 208 proteins.

Acknowledgments

We thank Dr. Susan E. Lewis and Mr. Dan Chamberlin for reading and editing the manuscript.

Author Contributions

Conceived and designed the experiments: N-KH J-HL J-MF Y-LL YC. Performed the experiments: J-TL C-IL EML C-JL W-PC Y-CS H-MC J-BC H-LL C-WY M-CC Y-SW CC. Analyzed the data: N-KH J-HL CC J-MF Y-LL YC. Contributed reagents/materials/analysis tools: J-FC. Wrote the paper: J-HL J-MF YC.

References

1. The Huntington's Disease Collaborative Research Group (1993) A novel gene containing a trinucleotide repeat that is expanded and unstable on Huntington's disease chromosomes. Cell 72: 971–983.
2. Chiang MC, Chen HM, Lee YH, Chang HH, Wu YC, et al. (2007) Dysregulation of C/EBPalpha by mutant Huntingtin causes the urea cycle deficiency in Huntington's disease. Hum Mol Genet 16: 483–498.
3. Panov AV, Lund S, Greenamyre JT (2005) Ca^{2+}-induced permeability transition in human lymphoblastoid cell mitochondria from normal and Huntington's disease individuals. Mol Cell Biochem 269: 143–152.
4. Brusa L, Orlacchio A, Moschella V, Iani C, Bernardi G, et al. (2009) Treatment of the symptoms of Huntington's disease: preliminary results comparing aripiprazole and tetrabenazine. Mov Disord 24: 126–129.
5. Fredholm BB, Chen JF, Cunha RA, Svenningsson P, Vaugeois JM (2005) Adenosine and brain function. Int Rev Neurobiol 63: 191–270.
6. Dworak M, Diel P, Voss S, Hollmann W, Struder HK (2007) Intense exercise increases adenosine concentrations in rat brain: implications for a homeostatic sleep drive. Neurosci 150: 789–795.
7. Lee FS, Chao MV (2001) Activation of Trk neurotrophin receptors in the absence of neurotrophins. Proc Natl Acad Sci U S A 98: 3555–3560.
8. Flajolet M, Wang Z, Futter M, Shen W, Nuangchamnong N, et al. (2008) FGF acts as a co-transmitter through adenosine A_{2A} receptor to regulate synaptic plasticity. Nat Neurosci 11: 1402–1409.
9. Gomes CA, Vaz SH, Ribeiro JA, Sebastiao AM (2006) Glial cell line-derived neurotrophic factor (GDNF) enhances dopamine release from striatal nerve endings in an adenosine A_{2A} receptor-dependent manner. Brain Res 1113: 129–136.
10. Blum D, Galas MC, Pintor A, Brouillet E, Ledent C, et al. (2003) A dual role of adenosine A_{2A} receptors in 3-nitropropionic acid-induced striatal lesions: implications for the neuroprotective potential of A_{2A} antagonists. J Neurosci 23: 5361–5369.
11. Cepeda C, Cummings DM, Hickey MA, Kleiman-Weiner M, Chen JY, et al. (2010) Rescuing the Corticostriatal Synaptic Disconnection in the R6/2 Mouse Model of Huntington's Disease: Exercise, Adenosine Receptors and Ampakines. PLoS Curr 2.
12. Chiang MC, Chen HM, Lai HL, Chen HW, Chou SY, et al. (2009) The A_{2A} adenosine receptor rescues the urea cycle deficiency of Huntington's disease by enhancing the activity of the ubiquitin-proteasome system. Hum Mol Genet 18: 2929–2942.
13. Chou SY, Lee YC, Chen HM, Chiang MC, Lai HL, et al. (2005) CGS21680 attenuates symptoms of Huntington's disease in a transgenic mouse model. J Neurochem 93: 310–320.
14. Mievis S, Blum D, Ledent C (2011) A_{2A} receptor knockout worsens survival and motor behaviour in a transgenic mouse model of Huntington's disease. Neurobiol Dis 41: 570–576.
15. Orru M, Bakesova J, Brugarolas M, Quiroz C, Beaumont V, et al. (2011) Striatal Pre- and Postsynaptic Profile of Adenosine A_{2A} Receptor Antagonists. PloS One 6: e16088.
16. Fink JS, Kalda A, Ryu H, Stack EC, Schwarzschild MA, et al. (2004) Genetic and pharmacological inactivation of the adenosine A_{2A} receptor attenuates 3-nitropropionic acid-induced striatal damage. J Neurochem 88: 538–544.
17. Gordi T, Frohna P, Sun HL, Wolff A, Belardinelli L, et al. (2006) A population pharmacokinetic/pharmacodynamic analysis of regadenoson, an adenosine A_{2A}-receptor agonist, in healthy male volunteers. Clin Pharmacokinet 45: 1201–1212.
18. An SJ, Park SK, Hwang IK, Choi SY, Kim SK, et al. (2003) Gastrodin decreases immunoreactivities of gamma-aminobutyric acid shunt enzymes in the hippocampus of seizure-sensitive gerbils. J Neurosci Res 71: 534–543.
19. Kim HJ, Moon KD, Lee DS, Lee SH (2003) Ethyl ether fraction of Gastrodia elata Blume protects amyloid beta peptide-induced cell death. J Ethnopharmacol 84: 95–98.
20. Huang NK, Lin YL, Cheng JJ, Lai WL (2004) Gastrodia elata prevents rat pheochromocytoma cells from serum-deprived apoptosis: the role of the MAPK family. Life Sci 75: 1649–1657.
21. Huang NK, Chern Y, Fang JM, Lin CI, Chen WP, et al. (2007) Neuroprotective principles from Gastrodia elata. J Nat Prod 70: 571–574.
22. Hayashi J, Sekine T, Deguchi S, Lin Q, Horie S, et al. (2002) Phenolic compounds from Gastrodia rhizome and relaxant effects of related compounds on isolated smooth muscle preparation. Phytochem 59: 513–519.
23. Lin JH, Liu YC, Hau JP, Wen KC (1996) Parishins B and C from rhizomes of *Gastrodia elata*. Phytochem 42: 549–551.
24. Taguchi H, Yosioka I, Yamasaki K, Kim IH (1981) Studies on the Constituents of *Gastrodia elata* Blume. Chem Pharm Bull 29: 55–62.
25. Chen JF, Huang Z, Ma J, Zhu J, Moratalla R, et al. (1999) A_{2A} adenosine receptor deficiency attenuates brain injury induced by transient focal ischemia in mice. J Neurosci 19: 9192–9200.
26. Jaakola VP, Griffith MT, Hanson MA, Cherezov V, Chien EYT, et al. (2008) The 2.6 Angstrom Crystal Structure of a Human A_{2A} Adenosine Receptor Bound to an Antagonist. Science 322: 1211–1217.
27. Jiang QL, VanRhee AM, Kim JH, Yehle S, Wess J, et al. (1996) Hydrophilic side chains in the third and seventh transmembrane helical domains of human A_{2A} adenosine receptors are required for ligand recognition. Mol Pharm 50: 512–521.
28. Kim J, Wess J, van Rhee AM, Schoneberg T, Jacobson KA (1995) Site-directed mutagenesis identifies residues involved in ligand recognition in the human A_{2a} adenosine receptor. J Biol Chem 270: 13987–13997.
29. Kim JH, Jiang QL, Glashofer M, Yehle S, Wess J, et al. (1996) Glutamate residues in the second extracellular loop of the human A_{2a} adenosine receptor are required for ligand recognition. Mol Pharm 49: 683–691.
30. Gao ZG, Jiang QL, Jacobson KA, Ijzerman AP (2000) Site-directed mutagenesis studies of human A_{2A} adenosine receptors - Involvement of Glu(13) and His(278) in ligand binding and sodium modulation. Biochem Pharm 60: 661–668.
31. Abramson J, Smirnova I, Kasho V, Verner G, Kaback HR, et al. (2003) Structure and mechanism of the lactose permease of Escherichia coli. Science 301: 610–615.
32. Jennings LL, Hao C, Cabrita MA, Vickers MF, Baldwin SA, et al. (2001) Distinct regional distribution of human equilibrative nucleoside transporter proteins 1 and 2 (hENT1 and hENT2) in the central nervous system. Neuropharmcol 40: 722–731.
33. Zuccato C, Ciammola A, Rigamonti D, Leavitt BR, Goffredo D, et al. (2001) Loss of Huntingtin-Mediated BDNF Gene Transcription in Huntington's Disease. Science 293: 493–498.
34. Parkinson FE, Xiong W, Zamzow CR, Chestley T, Mizuno T, et al. (2009) Transgenic expression of human equilibrative nucleoside transporter 1 in mouse neurons. J Neurochem 109: 562–572.
35. Gidday JM, Kim YB, Shah AR, Gonzales ER, Park TS (1996) Adenosine transport inhibition ameliorates postischemic hypoperfusion in pigs. Brain Res 734: 261–268.
36. Fredholm BB, Fastbom J, Kvanta A, Gerwins P, Parkinson F (1992) Further evidence that propentofylline (HWA 285) influences both adenosine receptors and adenosine transport. Fundam Clin Pharmacol 6: 99–111.
37. Popoli P, Blum D, Domenici MR, Burnouf S, Chern Y (2008) A critical evaluation of adenosine A_{2A} receptors as potentially "druggable" targets in Huntington's disease. Curr Pharm Des 14: 1500–1511.
38. Tebano MT, Martire A, Chiodi V, Ferrante A, Popoli P (2010) Role of adenosine A_{2A} receptors in modulating synaptic functions and brain levels of BDNF: a possible key mechanism in the pathophysiology of Huntington's disease. Scientific World Journal 10: 1768–1782.
39. Wiese S, Jablonka S, Holtmann B, Orel N, Rajagopal R, et al. (2007) Adenosine receptor A_{2A}-R contributes to motoneuron survival by transactivating the tyrosine kinase receptor TrkB. Proc Natl Acad Sci U S A 104: 17210–17215.
40. Assaife-Lopes N, Sousa VC, Pereira DB, Ribeiro JA, Chao MV, et al. (2010) Activation of adenosine A_{2A} receptors induces TrkB translocation and increases BDNF-mediated phospho-TrkB localization in lipid rafts: implications for neuromodulation. J Neurosci 30: 8468–8480.
41. Fontinha BM, Diogenes MJ, Ribeiro JA, Sebastiao AM (2008) Enhancement of long-term potentiation by brain-derived neurotrophic factor requires adenosine A_{2A} receptor activation by endogenous adenosine. Neuropharmacol 54: 924–933.
42. Golder FJ, Ranganathan L, Satriotomo I, Hoffman M, Lovett-Barr MR, et al. (2008) Spinal adenosine A_{2a} receptor activation elicits long-lasting phrenic motor facilitation. J Neurosci 28: 2033–2042.
43. Jin K, LaFevre-Bernt M, Sun Y, Chen S, Gafni J, et al. (2005) FGF-2 promotes neurogenesis and neuroprotection and prolongs survival in a transgenic mouse model of Huntington's disease. Proc Natl Acad Sci U S A 102: 18189–18194.
44. Kells AP, Fong DM, Dragunow M, During MJ, Young D, et al. (2004) AAV-mediated gene delivery of BDNF or GDNF is neuroprotective in a model of Huntington disease. Mol Ther 9: 682–688.
45. Chiang MC, Lee YC, Huang CL, Chern Y (2005) cAMP-response element-binding protein contributes to suppression of the A_{2A} adenosine receptor promoter by mutant Huntingtin with expanded polyglutamine residues. J Biol Chem 280: 14331–14340.
46. Tarditi A, Camurri A, Varani K, Borea PA, Woodman B, et al. (2006) Early and transient alteration of adenosine A_{2A} receptor signaling in a mouse model of Huntington disease. Neurobiol Dis 23: 44–53.
47. Varani K, Abbracchio MP, Cannella M, Cislaghi G, Giallonardo P, et al. (2003) Aberrant A_{2A} receptor function in peripheral blood cells in Huntington's disease. FASEB J 17: 2148–2150.
48. Ribeiro FM, Paquet M, Ferreira LT, Cregan T, Swan P, et al. (2010) Metabotropic glutamate receptor-mediated cell signaling pathways are altered in a mouse model of Huntington's disease. J Neurosci 30: 316–324.

49. Joshi PR, Wu NP, Andre VM, Cummings DM, Cepeda C, et al. (2009) Age-dependent alterations of corticostriatal activity in the YAC128 mouse model of Huntington disease. J Neurosci 29: 2414–2427.
50. Martire A, Calamandrei G, Felici F, Scattoni ML, Lastoria G, et al. (2007) Opposite effects of the A2A receptor agonist CGS21680 in the striatum of Huntington's disease versus wild-type mice. Neurosci Lett 417: 78–83.
51. Domenici MR, Scattoni ML, Martire A, Lastoria G, Potenza RL, et al. (2007) Behavioral and electrophysiological effects of the adenosine A_{2A} receptor antagonist SCH 58261 in R6/2 Huntington's disease mice. Neurobiol Dis 28: 197–205.
52. Dai SS, Zhou YG, Li W, An JH, Li P, et al. (2010) Local glutamate level dictates adenosine A_{2A} receptor regulation of neuroinflammation and traumatic brain injury. J Neurosci 30: 5802–5810.
53. He ZX, Cwajg E, Hwang W, Hartley CJ, Funk E, et al. (2000) Myocardial blood flow and myocardial uptake of (201)Tl and (99m)Tc-sestamibi during coronary vasodilation induced by CGS-21680, a selective adenosine A_{2A} receptor agonist. Circulation 102: 438–444.
54. Mingote S, Pereira M, Farrar AM, McLaughlin PJ, Salamone JD (2008) Systemic administration of the adenosine A_{2A} agonist CGS 21680 induces sedation at doses that suppress lever pressing and food intake. Pharmacol Biochem Behav 89: 345–351.
55. Jacobson KA, Park KS, Jiang JL, Kim YC, Olah ME, et al. (1997) Pharmacological characterization of novel A3 adenosine receptor-selective antagonists. Neuropharmacol 36: 1157–1165.
56. Blum D, Gall D, Galas MC, d'Alcantara P, Bantubungi K, et al. (2002) The adenosine A1 receptor agonist adenosine amine congener exerts a neuroprotective effect against the development of striatal lesions and motor impairments in the 3-nitropropionic acid model of neurotoxicity. J Neurosci 22: 9122–9133.
57. Luo C, Yi B, Tao G, Li M, Chen Z, et al. (2010) Adenosine A3 receptor agonist reduces early brain injury in subarachnoid haemorrhage. Neuroreport 21: 892–896.
58. Mestre T, Ferreira J, Coelho MM, Rosa M, Sampaio C (2009) Therapeutic interventions for disease progression in Huntington's disease. Cochrane Database Syst Rev. pp CD006455.
59. Day JW, Ottaway N, Patterson JT, Gelfanov V, Smiley D, et al. (2009) A new glucagon and GLP-1 co-agonist eliminates obesity in rodents. Nat Chem Biol 5: 749–757.
60. Tzschentke TM, Christoph T, Koegel B, Schiene K, Hennies HH, et al. (2007) (-)-(1R,2R)-3-(3-Dimethylamino-1-ethyl-2-methyl-propyl)- phenol hydrochloride (Tapentadol HCl): a novel mu-opioid receptor agonist norepinephrine Reuptake inhibitor with broad-spectrum analgesic properties. J Pharmacol Exp Ther 323: 265–276.
61. Chen JF, Steyn S, Staal R, Petzer JP, Xu K, et al. (2002) 8-(3-Chlorostyryl)caffeine may attenuate MPTP neurotoxicity through dual actions of monoamine oxidase inhibition and A2A receptor antagonism. J Biol Chem 277: 36040–36044.
62. Rooseboom M, Commandeur JN, Vermeulen NP (2004) Enzyme-catalyzed activation of anticancer prodrugs. Pharmacol Rev 56: 53–102.
63. Too K, Brown DM, Bongard E, Yardley V, Vivas L, et al. (2007) Anti-malarial activity of N6-modified purine analogues. Bioorg Med Chem 15: 5551–5562.
64. Mosmann T (1983) Rapid colorimetric assay for cellular growth and survival: application to proliferation and cytotoxicity assays. J Immunol Methods 65: 55–63.
65. Huang NK, Lin YW, Huang CL, Messing RO, Chern Y (2001) Activation of protein kinase A and atypical protein kinase C by A_{2A} adenosine receptors antagonizes apoptosis due to serum deprivation in PC12 cells. J Biol Chem 276: 13838–13846.
66. Huang NK, Cheng JJ, Lai WL, Lu MK (2005) Antrodia camphorata prevents rat pheochromocytoma cells from serum deprivation-induced apoptosis. FEMS Microbiol Lett 244: 213–219.
67. Varani K, Gessi S, Dalpiaz A, Borea PA (1996) Pharmacological and biochemical characterization of purified A_{2a} adenosine receptors in human platelet membranes by [^{3}H]-CGS 21680 binding. Br J Pharmacol 117: 1693–1701.
68. Olah ME, Gallo-Rodriguez C, Jacobson KA, Stiles GL (1994) 125I-4-aminobenzyl-5′-N-methylcarboxamidoadenosine, a high affinity radioligand for the rat A3 adenosine receptor. Mol Pharmacol 45: 978–982.
69. Salvatore CA, Jacobson MA, Taylor HE, Linden J, Johnson RG (1993) Molecular cloning and characterization of the human A3 adenosine receptor. Proc Natl Acad Sci U S A 90: 10365–10369.
70. Verma A, Marangos PJ (1985) Nitrobenzylthioinosine binding in brain: an interspecies study. Life Sci 36: 283–290.
71. Ward JL, Sherali A, Mo ZP, Tse CM (2000) Kinetic and pharmacological properties of cloned human equilibrative nucleoside transporters, ENT1 and ENT2, stably expressed in nucleoside transporter-deficient PK15 cells. Ent2 exhibits a low affinity for guanosine and cytidine but a high affinity for inosine. J Biol Chem 275: 8375–8381.
72. Huang NK, Tseng CJ, Wong CS, Tung CS (1997) Effects of acute and chronic morphine on DOPAC and glutamate at subcortical DA terminals in awake rats. Pharmacol Biochem Behav 56: 363–371.
73. Lu MK, Cheng JJ, Lai WL, Lin YR, Huang NK (2006) Adenosine as an active component of Antrodia cinnamomea that prevents rat PC12 cells from serum deprivation-induced apoptosis through the activation of adenosine A(2A) receptors. Life Sci 79: 252–258.
74. Mangiarini L, Sathasivam K, Seller M, Cozens B, Harper A, et al. (1996) Exon 1 of the HD gene with an expanded CAG repeat is sufficient to cause a progressive neurological phenotype in transgenic mice. Cell 87: 493–506.
75. Carter RJ, Lione LA, Humby T, Mangiarini L, Mahal A, et al. (1999) Characterization of progressive motor deficits in mice transgenic for the human Huntington's disease mutation. J Neurosci 19: 3248–3257.
76. Sathasivam K, Hobbs C, Turmaine M, Mangiarini L, Mahal A, et al. (1999) Formation of polyglutamine inclusions in non-CNS tissue. Hum Mol Genet 8: 813–822.
77. Liu FC, Wu GC, Hsieh ST, Lai HL, Wang HF, et al. (1998) Expression of type VI adenylyl cyclase in the central nervous system: implication for a potential regulator of multiple signals in different neurotransmitter systems. FEBS Lett 436: 92–98.
78. Laemmli UK (1970) Cleavage of structural proteins during the assembly of the head of bacteriophage T4. Nature 227: 680–685.
79. Thompson JD, Higgins DG, Gibson TJ (1994) Clustal-W - Improving the Sensitivity of Progressive Multiple Sequence Alignment through Sequence Weighting, Position-Specific Gap Penalties and Weight Matrix Choice. Nucl Acids Res 22: 4673–4680.
80. Boeckmann B, Bairoch A, Apweiler R, Blatter MC, Estreicher A, et al. (2003) The SWISS-PROT protein knowledgebase and its supplement TrEMBL in 2003. Nucl Acids Res 31: 365–370.
81. Scheerer P, Park JH, Hildebrand PW, Kim YJ, Krauss N, et al. (2008) Crystal structure of opsin in its G-protein-interacting conformation. Nature 455: 497-U430.
82. Xiang ZX, Soto CS, Honig B (2002) Evaluating conformational free energies: The colony energy and its application to the problem of loop prediction. Proc Natl Acad Sci U S A 99: 7432–7437.
83. Sali A, Blundell TL (1993) Comparative Protein Modeling by Satisfaction of Spatial Restraints. J Mol Biol 234: 779–815.
84. Shen MY, Sali A (2006) Statistical potential for assessment and prediction of protein structures. Prot Sci 15: 2507–2524.
85. Dolinsky TJ, Czodrowski P, Li H, Nielsen JE, Jensen JH, et al. (2007) PDB2PQR: expanding and upgrading automated preparation of biomolecular structures for molecular simulations. Nucl Acids Res 35: W522–W525.
86. Xu F, Wu H, Katritch V, Han GW, Jacobson KA, et al. (2011) Structure of an agonist-bound human A_{2A} adenosine receptor. Science 332: 322–327.
87. Zhang Y (2008) I-TASSER server for protein 3D structure prediction. Bmc Bioinformatics 9.
88. Zhang Y, Skolnick J (2004) Automated structure prediction of weakly homologous proteins on a genomic scale'. Proc Natl Acad Sci U S A 101: 7594–7599.
89. Lin JH, Baker NA, McCammon JA (2002) Bridging implicit and explicit solvent approaches for membrane electrostatics. Biophys J 83: 1374–1379.
90. Wu XW, Brooks BR (2003) Self-guided Langevin dynamics simulation method. Chem Phys Lett 381: 512–518.
91. Simmerling C, Strockbine B, Roitberg AE (2002) All-atom structure prediction and folding simulations of a stable protein. J Am Chem Soc 124: 11258–11259.
92. Case DA, Darden TA, Cheatham ITE, Simmerling CL, Wang RE, et al. (2006) AMBER 9. University of California, San Diego.
93. Gasteiger J, Marsili M (1980) Iterative Partial Equalization of Orbital Electronegativity - a Rapid Access to Atomic Charges. Tetrahedron 36: 3219–3228.
94. Huey R, Morris GM, Olson AJ, Goodsell DS (2007) A semiempirical free energy force field with charge-based desolvation. Journal of Computational Chemistry 28: 1145–1152.

Replication Study in Chinese Population and Meta-Analysis Supports Association of the 11q23 Locus with Colorectal Cancer

Li Zou[1,2], Rong Zhong[2], Jiao Lou[2], Xuzai Lu[2], Qi Wang[1], Yang Yang[1], Jiahong Xia[3], Juntao Ke[2], Ti Zhang[2], Yu Sun[2], Li Liu[4], Yongping Cui[5], Haibing Xiao[1], Lei Chang[1], Ding Xia[1], Hua Xu[1]*

1 Department of Urology, Tongji Hospital, Tongji Medical College, Huazhong University of Science and Technology, Wuhan, China, **2** Department of Epidemiology and Biostatistics and MOE Key Lab of Environment and Health, School of Public Health, Tongji Medical College, Huazhong University of Science and Technology, Wuhan, China, **3** Department of Cardiovascular Surgery, Union Hospital, Huazhong University of Science and Technology, Wuhan, China, **4** Department of Epidemiology and Biostatistics, School of Public Health, Guangdong Pharmaceutical University, Guangzhou, China, **5** Key Laboratory of Cellular Physiology, Ministry of Education, Shanxi Medical University, Taiyuan, Shanxi, China

Abstract

Background: A common single nucleotide polymorphism (SNP), rs3802842, located at 11q23, was identified by genome-wide association studies (GWAS) to be significantly associated with the risk of colorectal cancer (CRC); however, the results of following replication studies were not always concordant. Thus, a case-control study and a meta-analysis were performed to clearly discern the effect of this variant in CRC.

Method and Findings: We determined the genotypes of rs3802842 in 641 unrelated Chinese patients with CRC and 1037 cancer-free controls. Additionally, a meta-analysis comprising current and previously published studies was conducted. In our case-control study, significant associations between the polymorphism and CRC risk were observed in all genetic models, with an additive OR being 1.45 (95% CI = 1.26–1.67). The meta-analysis of 38534 cases and 39446 controls further confirmed the significant associations in all genetic models but with obvious between-study heterogeneity. Nevertheless, ethnicity, study type and whether subjects affected by Lynch syndrome could synthetically accounted for the heterogeneity. Besides, the cumulative and sensitivity analyses indicated the robust stability of the results.

Conclusion: The results from our case-control study and meta-analysis provided convincing evidence that rs3802842 significantly contributed to CRC risk.

Editor: Xiao-Ping Miao, Tongji Medical College, Huazhong University of Science and Technology, China

Funding: This work was supported by the National Natural Science Foundation of China (31072238, 31172441, 81170650). The funders had no role in study design, data collection and analysis, decision to publish, or preparation of the manuscript.

Competing Interests: The authors have declared that no competing interests exist.

* E-mail: xuhuawhu@163.com

Introduction

Colorectal cancer (CRC), as one of the most common malignancies, accounted for an estimated 1,230,000 new cases and 680,000 deaths worldwide in 2008 [1]. In United States, CRC was the second most commonly diagnosed cancer and the second leading cause of cancer death, with an incidence of 51.6 and a mortality of 19.7 per 100,000 population in 2008 [2]. In China, epidemiology studies indicate that the incidence rate of CRC has grown rapidly, especially in urban areas. The number of affected people increased as much as 4.2% every year from 1973 to 1993 in Shanghai, which was even higher than the global level (2%) [3]. Additionally, the data from 56 cancer registries in China showed that the incidence and mortality rates of CRC respectively ranked the third (31.4/100,000) and fifth (14.8/100,000) among the cancers that affected men and women in 2008 [4]. Among the risk factors for the disease, inherited susceptibility plays a role in the development of CRC, which is responsible for about 35% of variance in CRC risk [5]. However, high-penetrance germline mutations account for only 6% of CRC cases [6], suggesting that the remaining inheritance is likely to be a consequence of many common variants with low penetrance.

Genome-wide association studies (GWAS), efficiently applied to identify common genetic variants for complex diseases without prior knowledge of gene function, have so far uncovered multiple novel single nucleotide polymorphisms (SNPs) to CRC susceptibility [7–12]. Among these SNPs, rs3802842 (11q23.1), located in the intron region of *C11orf93*, was firstly identified in a GWA set of 3004 cases and 3094 controls and 8 replication sets of 14453 cases and 13259 controls [7]. Pittman AM et al. immediately validated the positive finding in the pooling data from 8 independent case-control series comprising a total of 10638 cases and 10457 controls [13]. Besides, rs3802842 is the first locus reported to exhibit a population difference between the Japanese and Caucasian populations [7]. Although there is much statistical evidence of this SNP for CRC, the results from replication studies are not always concordant [14–16], which is probably due to the so-called "winner's curse" phenomenon that initial studies generally overestimate the effect sizes, replication studies are likely to be underpowered and so more likely to fail if the sample size calculations are based on the overestimated effect sizes [17]. Additionally, the modest effect of this variant may be also one of the important reasons for the failure of replication. Nevertheless, meta-analysis is a powerful technique to clarify the inconsistent findings in genetic association studies by increasing the sample size [18]. Notably, although the individual associated variants identified through GWAS confer only modest risks for CRC, the population attributable risk proportions have been considered to be significant because of substantial minor allele frequencies [19]. Thus, we conducted a replication study to examine the association between rs3802842 and CRC risk in a Chinese population using a case-control design, after that, a meta-analysis combining current and previously published studies about rs3802842 was further performed to provide a more precise estimate of this association. Then, the population attributable risk (PAR) was calculated in order to evaluate the effect of rs3802842 for CRC occurrence in general population.

Materials and Methods

Study Population

A total of 641 CRC cases were inpatients consecutively enrolled through the Tongji Hospital of Huazhong University of Science and Technology between 2009 and 2011, which is a top integrated hospital absorbing majority of cancer patients in Wuhan and nearby region. All cases were newly diagnosed and histopathologically confirmed without any treatment prior to blood samples collection. And 1037 cancer-free controls were selected randomly among the individuals who participated in health check-up programs at the same hospital in the same time period as the cases were enrolled. The health check up programs also primarily involved residents living in Wuhan and nearby region. The selection criteria for controls were no individual history of cancer and frequency matched to CRC cases on sex and age (±5 years). If a person was suspected to have CRC through the health check up programs and then histopathologically confirmed, he/she was selected as a case, whereas no case was ascertained through the health check up programs in this case-control study. All subjects were unrelated ethnic Han Chinese. At recruitment, epidemiologic data were collected by personal interview or a review of medical records, and 5-ml peripheral venous blood was drawn from each participant. Participants provided their written informed consent to participate in this study and this study was approved by ethnics committee of Tongji Hospital of Huazhong University of Science and Technology.

Genotyping

Genomic DNA was extracted from 5-ml blood sample using the RelaxGene Blood System DP319-02 (Tiangen, Beijing, China) by reference to the manufacturer's instructions. The rs3802842 was genotyped using the TaqMan SNP Genotyping Assay (Applied Biosystems, Fostercity, CA) on a 7900HT Fast Real-Time PCR System (Applied Biosystems, Fostercity, CA). To ensure quality control, 5% duplicated samples were randomly selected to assess the reproducibility, with a concordance rate of 100%.

Statistical Analysis

Deviation of the genotype frequencies in controls from those expected under Hardy-Weinberg equilibrium was calculated using goodness-of-fit χ^2 test. Differences in demographic variables and distribution of genotypes between cases and controls were examined by χ^2 test or *t* test when appropriate. The association between rs3802842 and CRC risk was estimated as odds ratio (OR) with 95% confidence interval (95% CI), which was computed by unconditional multivariate logistic regression with adjustment for sex and age. ORs and 95% CIs as the metrics of effect size were recalculated for the allele C versus A, genotypes AC versus AA and CC versus AA. In order to avoid the assumption of genetic models, dominant, recessive and additive models were also analyzed. To adjust for multiple comparisons, the Bonferroni method was applied. Additionally, stratified analyses by tumor site and tumor differentiation were carried out to further evaluate the role of rs3802842 in CRC. All statistical analyses were performed in the SPSS 18.0 and all *P* values are two-tailed with a significant level at 0.05.

Meta-analysis of rs3802842 in Association with CRC Risk

To ensure the rigour of this current meta-analysis, we designed and reported it according to the Preferred Reporting Items for Systematic Reviews and Meta-analyses (PRISMA) statement (http://www.prisma-statement.org) and the checklist is shown in Checklist S1.

We searched PubMed, EMBASE, and ISI Web of Science databases for studies published in any language up to April 2012 using the search terms *rs3802842*, *C11orf53*, or *11q23.1* combined with *colorectal cancer*, *colorectal neoplasia*, *colorectal adenoma*, *colon cancer*, or *rectal cancer*. To expand the coverage of our searches, we further performed searches in Chinese Biomedical (CBM) database [20] based on the above searching strategy. References of retrieved articles and reviews were also checked for additional studies. Searching was performed in duplicate by two independent reviewers (L. Zou and R. Zhong). The following criteria were applied for literature selection: (1) case-control study assessing the association between rs3802842 and CRC risk; (2) presentation of crude/adjusted OR with 95% CI or sufficient data to calculate crude/adjusted OR with 95% CI; (3) studies of humans. When there were multiple published reports from the same study population, the one with complete design or larger sample size was finally selected. If more than one ethnic population were included in one report, each population was considered separately. All data were extracted independently by two reviewers (L. Zou and R. Zhong) and any disagreement was adjudicated by a third author (Q. Wang). For each study, we summarized first author, year of publication, geographic location, ethnicity of study population, study type, genotyping method, numbers of cases and controls, male/female rate, mean age, family history of cancer, source of control group and frequencies of genotypes in cases and controls. The allele C versus A, genotypes AC versus AA and CC versus AA were all calculated and dominant, recessive and additive models were also assumed for rs3802842 respectively. The Bonferroni correction was also applied to counteract the problem of multiple comparisons. The between-study heterogeneity was assessed by χ^2-based Cochran's *Q* statistic (heterogeneity was considered significant at $P<0.10$). The I^2 statistic was then utilized to estimate heterogeneity quantitatively ($I^2<30\%$, no between-study heterogeneity or marginal between-study heterogeneity; $I^2=30\%–75\%$, mild heterogeneity; $I^2>75\%$, notable heterogeneity) [21]. A fixed-effects model, using Mantel-Haenszel method, was adopted to compute the pooled OR when no significant heterogeneity was detected [22]; otherwise, a random-effects model, using DerSimonian and Laird method, was applied [23]. Overall meta-analysis for rs3802842 was initially performed. Then we conducted stratification analyses if data permitted (the number of studies obtained in each subgroup is not less than 3), according to ethnicity (European, Asian and African), study type (GWAS and replication studies), tumor site (colon and rectum cancers) and whether subjects affected by Lynch syndrome. Additionally, sensitivity analysis was carried out, in which the pooled ORs were calculated after omission of each study in turn [24]. Cumulative meta-analysis was also applied through assortment of studies with publication time [25]. An estimation of potential publication bias was executed by Egger's test [26]. If there was an significant association between the polymorphism and CRC risk detected in the overall meta-analysis for any genetic model, bioinformatics analyses were further carried out to predict the function of rs3802842 using three integrated bioinformatics tools "SNP Info" (http://manticore.niehs.nih.gov/snpfunc.htm), "FastSNP" (http://fastsnp.ibms.sinica.edu.tw/pages/input_CandidateGeneSearch.jsp) and "F-SNP" (http://compbio.cs.queensu.ca/F-SNP/). To examine the contribution of this polymorphism to the occurrence of CRC in general population, the PAR was computed using the following formula: Pr (RR-1)/[1+Pr (RR-1)], where *Pr*, the proportion of control subjects exposed to the allele of interest, can be calculated by minor allele frequency (MAF) reported in dbSNP database and the relative risk (RR) is estimated using the pooled OR produced by the meta-analysis [27]. All statistical analyses were performed with Stata 11.0 software and *P* values less than 0.05 are considered statistically significant for all tests except for *Q* test for heterogeneity.

Results

Results of Case-control Study

Population characteristics. The characteristics of cases and controls are listed in Table 1. No significant differences were found between cases and controls for sex and age. Males were 59.9% among cases compared with 59.1% among controls ($P = 0.748$). The mean age (±standard deviation) was 56.31 (±12.59) years for cases and 57.24 (±10.86) years for controls ($P = 0.119$). Of the cases, 250 had colon cancer and 391 had rectal cancer. For tumor differentiation, 80, 445 and 116 cases were classified as poorly, moderately and well differentiated respectively.

Association analysis. The genotype data of rs3802842 for cases and controls are shown in Table 2. The genotype distribution in controls complied with Hardy-Weinberg equilibrium ($P = 0.323$). The genotype frequencies for this polymorphism in the case group differed from those in the control group ($P = 0.000$). In the multivariate logistic regression model adjusted for age and sex, individuals who carried the C allele, AC or CC genotype had significantly elevated risks of CRC compared with those carried the A allele or AA genotype (C versus A: OR = 1.44, 95% CI = 1.25–1.66; AC versus AA: OR = 1.76, 95% CI = 1.40–2.21; CC versus AA: OR = 1.99, 95% CI = 1.48–2.67). Likewise, significant associations between this polymorphism and CRC risk were found in dominant, recessive and additive models (dominant model: OR = 1.82, 95% CI = 1.46–2.26; recessive model: OR = 1.41, 95% CI = 1.09–1.82; additive model: OR = 1.45, 95% CI = 1.26–1.67). The association between rs3802842 and risk of CRC for all comparisons and genetic models remained significant after correction for multiple testing.

We then stratified data according to the pathological factors (Table 2). The polymorphism was associated with increased risk of colon cancer in all genetic models except the recessive model. Significant associations between the polymorphism and rectum cancer for all genetic models were also observed. However, the adjustment for multiple testing resulted in null-significant association in recessive model for colon or rectum cancer. Regarding tumor differentiation, the variant in all genetic models presented significantly elevated risk of CRC with poorly or moderated differentiated. For well differentiated cancer, apart from the recessive model, significant associations between the polymorphism and CRC risk were detected. After correction for multiple testing, the association was observed to be null significant in recessive model for poorly, moderated or well differentiated cancer.

Results of Meta-analysis

Study characteristics. Figure S1 shows the literature search and study selection procedures. After comprehensive searching, 31 potentially relevant publications were identified and screened for retrieval, of which, 15 publications met the inclusion criteria. However, the publications respectively reported by Hutter CM et al. [28], Mates IN et al. [29], Niittymäki I et al. [30], and Lubbe SJ et al. [31] were excluded since the cases largely overlapped with the samples of previous studies. Therefore, 11 publications plus

Table 1. The characteristics of the study population.

Variables	Case (N = 641) No. (%)	Control (N = 1037) No. (%)	*P*
Sex			0.748[b]
Male	384 (59.9)	613 (59.1)	
Female	257 (40.1)	424 (40.9)	
Age	56.31±12.59[a]	57.24±10.86[a]	0.119[c]
Tumor site			
Colon	250 (39.0)		
Rectum	391 (61.0)		
Tumor differentiation			
Poorly	80 (12.5)		
Moderately	445 (69.4)		
Well	116 (18.1)		

[a]Age was represented as mean±standard deviation.
[b]*P* value was calculated by the x^2 test.
[c]*P* value was calculated by the *t* test.

Table 2. Association between rs3802842 and colorectal cancer risk in a Chinese population[a].

	Case	Control	OR (95% CI)					
	AA/AC/CC	AA/AC/CC	C VS. A	AC VS. AA	CC VS. AA	Dominant model	Recessive model	Additive model
Total	163/345/133	397/477/163	1.44 (1.25–1.66)	1.76 (1.40–2.21)	1.99 (1.48–2.67)	1.82 (1.46–2.26)	1.41 (1.09–1.82)	1.45 (1.26–1.67)
Tumor site								
Colon	52/148/50	397/477/163	1.56 (1.28–1.89)	2.37 (1.68–3.34)	2.34 (1.52–3.59)	2.36 (1.70–3.28)	1.34 (0.94–1.91)[b]	1.57 (1.28–1.91)
Rectum	111/197/83	397/477/163	1.38 (1.17–1.63)	1.47 (1.12–1.92)	1.85 (1.32–2.59)	1.57 (1.22–2.02)	1.47 (1.09–1.98)[b]	1.37 (1.16–1.62)
Tumor differentiation								
Poorly+Moderately	137/280/108	397/477/163	1.42 (1.22–1.65)	1.70 (1.33–2.17)	1.92 (1.41–2.63)	1.76 (1.39–2.21)	1.39 (1.06–1.82)[b]	1.42 (1.22–1.65)
Well	26/65/25	397/477/163	1.56 (1.18–2.05)	2.03 (1.26–3.26)	2.39 (1.33–4.27)	2.12 (1.34–3.34)	1.53 (0.95–2.46)[b]	1.56 (1.18–2.05)

Abbreviations: OR, Odds ratio; 95% CI, 95% confidence interval.
[a]ORs and their corresponding 95% CIs were calculated by multivariate logistic regression model after adjusting for age and sex.
[b]The association between rs3802842 and colorectal cancer risk turned to be null significant after Bonferroni correction for multiple testing was applied.

current study comprising 32 case-control studies of 38534 cases and 39446 controls contributed data for this meta-analysis [7,13–16,32–37]. Among these, the publications respectively reported by Kupfer SS et al. [15] and He J et al. [16] just provided adjusted additive ORs, thus were merely included in the pooled analysis for additive model. Besides, there was only an allelic OR obtained in the publication by Middeldorp A et al. [32], hence the study merely participated in the pooled analysis for allelic model. In addition, 3 studies included some Lynch syndrome patients [32,33,35]. Table 3 shows the characteristics of the included studies.

Overall meta-analysis of rs3802842 in associated with CRC. As shown in Table 4, significant evidence of heterogeneity was detected in all genetic models (all P for heterogeneity <0.10), therefore ORs for all genetic models were pooled under random-effects model. Compared to the A allele, the C allele conferred a pooled OR of 1.15 (95% CI = 1.11–1.19) in the allelic model. Genotypic ORs of the AC versus AA and CC versus AA were 1.18 (95% CI = 1.12–1.24) and 1.31 (95% CI = 1.20–1.42), respectively. Similarly, significant associations between this polymorphism and CRC risk were found in dominant, recessive and additive models (dominant model: OR = 1.20, 95% CI = 1.15–1.26; recessive model: OR = 1.20, 95% CI = 1.12–1.29; additive model: OR = 1.15, 95% CI = 1.11–1.19). The additive OR and corresponding 95% CI did not change after both crude and adjusted ORs were combined (OR = 1.15, 95% CI = 1.11–1.19). The positive results remained significant after adjusted by multiple testing.

Stratified analysis. The stratified analysis was firstly conducted by ethnicity (Table 4). Because of less than 3 studies regarding African, the specific data for rs3802842 were only stratified into two subgroups: European and Asian. After stratifying by ethnicity, significant between-study heterogeneity was effectively reduced in European, whereas the heterogeneity in Asian was still detected. In European population, the polymorphism presented significantly increased risks of CRC in all genetic models. In Asian population, all genetic models except the recessive model exhibited significant associations with CRC risk. However, no significant association was found for the genotype AC versus AA, CC versus AA, dominant model and recessive model when the Bonferroni correction was performed. The data were further stratified by study type into GWAS and replication studies (Table 4). Heterogeneity for all genetic models was not detected in the subgroup of GWAS, however, there was significant heterogeneity in the subgroup of replication studies. Statistically significant findings for all genetic were seen either in the GWAS or in the replication studies. The data were additionally stratified into subgroup of subjects affected or not affected by Lynch syndrome (Table 4). All pooled ORs except the allelic OR could not be appraised in the subjects affected by Lynch syndrome due to limited number of studies. Significant association between the variant and CRC risk was observed without heterogeneity in the allelic model. In terms of subjects not affected by Lynch syndrome, there was evidence of heterogeneity in all genetic models and significant associations of CRC risk with the polymorphism were found. The stratified analysis by tumor site could not be performed owing to lack of data.

Sensitivity analysis. Since significant between-heterogeneity for the overall meta-analyses was observed in all genetic models, we performed sensitivity analyses in an attempt to assess the effects of each individual study on the pooled OR under random-effects model. As shown in Table S1, S2, S3, S4, S5, S6, all of the results were not materially altered and did not draw different conclusion, suggesting that our results were robust.

Cumulative meta-analysis. Cumulative meta-analyses were also conducted in all genetic models via assortment of studies in chronologic order. As shown in Figure S2, the plots made it clear that although the studies reduced the 95% CI for the summary estimates, they did not change the inclinations toward significant associations.

Publication bias. The results of Egger's test indicated that no evidence of publication bias was observed in all genetic models (all $P>0.05$).

The bioinformatics analysis and PAR of rs3802842. All of the three bioinformatics tools conformably predicted that the SNP might change the transcription factor binding sites of *C11orf93*. In order to evaluate the percent of the incidence of a disease in the population that is due to exposure, the PAR was calculated. The MAF of rs3802842 (C allele) was 31.3% and the pooled OR of overall meta-analysis in additive model was 1.15, so the PAR for C allele was estimated to be 4.5%.

Discussion

The present study demonstrated an association between rs3802842 and increased risk of CRC in a Chinese population. Then, the following meta-analysis based on 32 case-control studies of 38534 cases and 39446 controls also suggested that the SNP was

Table 3. The characteristics of included studies.

First author	Year	Country	Ethnicity	Study type	Genotyping method	Case/control	Cases' characteristics			Controls' characteristics		
							Male/female ratio	Mean age (SD)	Family history of cancer	Male/female ratio	Mean age (SD)	Control source
Tenesa A (Scotland 1)	2008	Scotland	European	GWAS	Illumina	3004/3094	–	–	–	–	–	Population based
Tenesa A (Scotland 2)	2008	Scotland	European	Replication	TaqMan	937/941	–	–	–	–	–	Population based
Tenesa A (Canada)	2008	Canada	European	Replication	TaqMan, Sequenom	1175/1184	–	–	–	–	–	Population based
Tenesa A (DACHS)	2008	German	European	Replication	TaqMan	1373/1480	–	–	–	–	–	Population based
Tenesa A (England)	2008	England	European	Replication	TaqMan	2253/2262	–	–	–	–	–	Population based
Tenesa A (Israel)	2008	Israel	European	Replication	TaqMan	1789/1771	–	–	–	–	–	Population based
Tenesa A (Japan)	2008	Japan	Asian	Replication	Invader assay	4400/3179	–	–	–	–	–	–
Tenesa A (Kiel)	2008	German	European	Replication	TaqMan	2169/2145	–	–	–	–	–	Population based
Tenesa A (Spain)	2008	Spain	European	Replication	TaqMan	357/297	–	–	–	–	–	Hospital based
Pittman AM (CORGI)	2008	England	European	GWAS	Illumina	619/932	0.82	–	Yes	0.87	–	Population based
Pittman AM (DFCCS)	2008	Netherlands	European	Replication	KASPar	783/664	0.90	53.4 (13.4)	Yes	0.61	51.1 (11.3)	Population based
Pittman AM (EPICOLON)	2008	Spain	European	Replication	Sequenom iPLEX	515/515	1.45	70.6 (11.3)	No	1.29	69.8 (11.7)	Hospital based
Pittman AM (FCCPS)	2008	Finland	European	Replication	KASPar	1001/1034	1.03	67.4 (11.8)	–	–	–	Population based
Pittman AM (MCCS)	2008	Australia	European	Replication	HRM	515/709	1.10	66.2 (7.7)	–	0.99	57.9 (7.0)	Population based
Pittman AM (NSCCG1)	2008	England	European	GWAS	Illumina	2863/2838	0.72	59.3 (8.7)	–	0.67	59.8 (10.8)	Population based
Pittman AM (NSCCG2)	2008	England	European	Replication	KASPar	3036/2944	1.16	59.4 (8.2)	–	0.67	55.2 (12.3)	Population based
Pittman AM (VCQ)	2008	England	European	Replication	KASPar,	1251/799	0.89	–	–	0.73	–	Population based
Middeldorp A[ac]	2009	Netherlands	European	Replication	KASPar	995/1340	0.92	–	Yes	0.90	–	Population based
Wijnen JT[a]	2009	Netherlands	European	Replication	KASPar	131/544	1.43	–	–	0.70	–	Population based

Table 3. Cont.

First author	Year	Country	Ethnicity	Study type	Genotyping method	Case/control	Cases' characteristics			Controls' characteristics		
							Male/female ratio	Mean age (SD)	Family history of cancer	Male/female ratio	Mean age (SD)	Control source
Kupfer SS (Combined African-American)[b]	2010	America	African	Replication	MassARRAY	795/985	0.88	64.5 (11.7)	–	0.72	62.3 (13.2)	Population based
Kupfer SS (European-American)[b]	2010	America	European	Replication	MassARRAY	399/367	1.35	64.6 (13.1)	–	1.01	61.1 (12.7)	Population based
Von Holst S	2010	Sweden	European	Replication	DeCode test	1786/1749	1.13	68.6	22%[d]	–	66.3	Population based
Xiong F	2010	China	Asian	Replication	PCR-RFLP	2124/2124	1.48	56.9 (11.8)	–	1.4	56.4 (11.3)	Population based
Talseth-Palmer BA[a]	2010	Australia, Poland	European	Replication	Real-Time PCR	262/314	–	–	–	–	–	Hospital based
He J (European American)[b]	2011	America	European	Replication	TaqMan	1171/1534	–	–	–	–	–	–
He J (African American)[b]	2011	America	African	Replication	TaqMan	382/510	–	–	–	–	–	–
He J (Native Hawaiian)[b]	2011	America	European	Replication	TaqMan	323/472	–	–	–	–	–	–
He J (Japanese American)[b]	2011	America	Asian	Replication	TaqMan	1042/1426	–	–	–	–	–	–
He J (Latinos)[b]	2011	America	European	Replication	TaqMan	393/524	–	–	–	–	–	–
Ho JW	2011	HK, China	Asian	Replication	Sequenom	892/890	1.64	66.75 (12.25)	–	–	–	Hospital based
Mates IN	2012	Romania	European	Replication	DeCode test	153/182	0.99	67.9 (11.2)	15.7% [d]	3.92	60.8 (14.7)	Hospital based
Current study	2012	China	Asian	Replication	TaqMan	641/1037	1.49	56.31 (12.59)	–	1.45	57.24 (10.86)	Population based

Abbreviations: GWAS, genome-wide association studies; SD, standard deviation; HRM, high resolution melt curve analysis.
[a]The study included some Lynch syndrome patients.
[b]The study only provided an adjusted additive OR.
[c]The study only provided an allelic OR.
[d]The percentage of patients having a family history of cancer.

Table 4. Meta-analysis of the rs3802842 in association with colorectal cancer risk[a].

	Genetic model	OR (95% CI)	P	I^2 (%)	$P_{heterogeneity}$	P for Egger's test
Overall						
Overall (n = 25)	C VS. A	1.15 (1.11–1.19)	0.000	49.6%	0.003	0.533
Overall (n = 24)	AC VS. AA	1.18 (1.12–1.24)	0.000	46.3%	0.007	0.216
	CC VS. AA	1.31 (1.20–1.42)	0.000	51.3%	0.002	0.968
	Dominant model	1.20 (1.15–1.26)	0.000	54.0%	0.001	0.283
	Recessive model	1.20 (1.12–1.29)	0.000	37.2%	0.036	0.818
	Additive model	1.15 (1.11–1.19)	0.000	47.2%	0.006	0.568
Overall (n = 31)	Additive model[b]	1.15 (1.11–1.19)	0.000	43.2%	0.006	0.499
Ethnicity						
European (n = 21)	C VS. A	1.14 (1.11–1.18)	0.000	8.4%	0.349	0.934
European (n = 20)	AC VS. AA	1.15 (1.11–1.20)	0.000	0.0%	0.457	0.665
	CC VS. AA	1.30 (1.20–1.40)	0.000	20.9%	0.195	0.482
	Dominant model	1.18 (1.14–1.22)	0.000	0.0%	0.467	0.841
	Recessive model	1.21 (1.12–1.31)	0.000	24.5%	0.155	0.432
	Additive model	1.13 (1.09–1.17)	0.000	29.3%	0.108	0.890
Asian (n = 4)	C VS. A	1.20 (1.02–1.38)	0.000	88.1%	0.000	0.443
	AC VS. AA	1.33 (1.07–1.66)[c]	0.011	86.6%	0.000	0.210
	CC VS. AA	1.39 (1.03–1.87)[c]	0.033	87.1%	0.000	0.518
	Dominant model	1.35 (1.06–1.71)[c]	0.014	90%	0.000	0.272
	Recessive model	1.16 (0.97–1.39)[c]	0.100	71%	0.016	0.801
	Additive model	1.22 (1.09–1.36)	0.000	73.2%	0.011	0.428
Study type						
GWAS (n = 3)	C VS. A	1.20 (1.14–1.27)	0.000	0.0%	0.948	0.204
	AC VS. AA	1.17 (1.09–1.26)	0.000	0.0%	0.571	0.535
	CC VS. AA	1.49 (1.33–1.68)	0.000	0.0%	0.463	0.428
	Dominant model	1.22 (1.14–1.31)	0.000	0.0%	0.882	0.607
	Recessive model	1.40 (1.23–1.59)	0.000	21.3%	0.281	0.453
	Additive model	1.20 (1.14–1.26)	0.000	0.0%	0.903	0.275
Replication (n = 22)	C VS. A	1.14 (1.10–1.19)	0.000	50.2%	0.004	0.376
Replication (n = 21)	AC VS. AA	1.18 (1.13–1.24)	0.000	52.1%	0.003	0.163
	CC VS. AA	1.27 (1.16–1.39)	0.000	48.5%	0.007	0.798
	Dominant model	1.20 (1.13–1.28)	0.000	59.0%	0.000	0.190
	Recessive model	1.15 (1.08–1.24)	0.000	21.0%	0.190	0.936
	Additive model	1.14 (1.09–1.19)	0.000	48%	0.008	0.380
Subjects with/without Lynch syndrome						
With Lynch syndrome (n = 3)	C VS. A	1.22 (1.08–1.35)	0.000	0.0%	0.589	0.355
Without Lynch syndrome (n = 22)	C VS. A	1.16 (1.11–1.20)	0.000	56.2%	0.001	0.525
	AC VS. AA	1.18 (1.12–1.24)	0.000	50.3%	0.004	0.167
	CC VS. AA	1.31 (1.20–1.43)	0.000	55.5%	0.001	0.957
	Dominant model	1.21 (1.15–1.27)	0.000	57.6%	0.000	0.224
	Recessive model	1.20 (1.12–1.29)	0.000	42.5%	0.019	0.860
	Additive model	1.15 (1.11–1.19)	0.000	51.5%	0.003	0.492

[a]Crude ORs were combined in a fixed- or random- effects model.
[b]Both crude and adjusted ORs were combined.
[c]The association between rs3802842 and colorectal cancer risk turned to be null significant after Bonferroni correction for multiple testing was applied.

significantly associated with CRC risk, with an additive OR being 1.15. Accordingly, PAR which takes into account both magnitude of the risk and risk allele frequency in the general population was 4.5%. Cumulative analysis in chronologic order further confirmed the positive findings, exhibiting that the effect of this variant progressively significant with more precise estimation. In addition, sensitivity analyses indicated the stability of the result. To the best of our knowledge, this is the first meta-analysis seeking to clarify the association between rs3802842 and risk of CRC and the results strongly emphasize the role of this polymorphism in CRC susceptibility.

rs3802842 is located at 11q23 and there are four ORFs (*LOC120376*, *FLJ45803*, *C11orf53* and *POU2AF1*) and a SNP (rs12296076) recognized as polymorphic binding site target for miRNAs in high linkage disequilibrium around rs3802842 within a range of 100 kb [7]. Moreover, rs3802842 is near the genes encoding POU transcription factors [7]. Thus it can be seen that the region where rs3802842 is located doubtlessly adds difficulty and complexity to discern the role of this polymorphism in CRC. Little is known about the function of rs3802842, but our bioinformatics analyses indicated that it was likely to alter the transcription factor binding sites of *C11orf93* and further affected the expression of the gene, whereas the function of *C11orf93* also remains elusive. Besides, albeit the important role of the region 11q23 in the pathogenesis of CRC has been confirmed [38], Pittman AM et al. inferred that the potential genomic sequence change caused by rs3802842 might affect the expression of genes mapping outside 11q23.1 through *cis*- or *trans*- regulatory [13]. Alternatively, most of the variants identified by GWAS cannot be *per se* causal but imply the probability of being in linkage with the "real" causal variants [19], so it is possible that the polymorphism is in linkage disequilibrium with "real" causal loci which are hitherto uncharacterized. However, the achievements of fine-mapping the causal variants responsible for GWAS signals which have been largely predicated on common disease common variant theory remain limited, one reason for this may be that a number of rare variants which are not identified by GWAS account for much of the remaining heritability of diseases, reflecting the important role of rare variants in the risk of disease occurrence [39]. Moreover, understanding the biological function of risk loci, with a focus on non-coding variants, is the greatest challenge in the post-GWAS era [40].

After the first GWAS with respect to rs3802842, multiple replication studies were carried out in succession with inconsistent results. Our case-control study found a significant association between the polymorphism and CRC risk in all genetic models, which was consistent with the GWAS and some replication studies [7,13,34]. Stratified analyses by tumor site or differentiation showed similar results, but not statistically significant in recessive model, which may be due to the sample size or inheritance pattern. Despite positive findings corroborated in our meta-analysis, obvious between-study heterogeneity cannot be ignored; hence stratified analyses were conducted to dig out the source of heterogeneity. When stratified by ethnicity, heterogeneity was greatly reduced in European but not in Asian, implying that there might be varied manners of action and different allele frequencies of rs3802842 between the two populations. Besides, it was noted that Tenesa A et al. observed significantly different allelic effects of rs3802842 between the Japanese and Europeans and further discovered that the population difference was site-specific, that is, the Japanese population showed the variant only associated with the increased risk of rectal cancer, but not associated with the risk of colon cancer that was detected in European population [7]. However, whether colon or rectal cancer risk was related to the polymorphism in our case-control study, suggesting that notwithstanding the same ethnicity the Chinese and Japanese both belong to, the two populations may differ in the causes of CRC to some extent. Regarding study type, heterogeneity disappeared in GWS studies but still remained in replication studies, which was resulted from the diverse genotyping methods. After stratifying by whether subjects affected by Lynch syndrome, heterogeneity was almost removed in the subgroup of subjects affected by Lynch syndrome but did not change in the other subgroup, naturally reflecting the different attributes of research subjects. Taken together, ethnicity, study type and whether subjects affected by Lynch syndrome were likely to be the sources of heterogeneity in this meta-analysis.

Despite the clear strengthen of this study that conducted a case-control study and a meta-analysis at the same time to substantiate the association between rs3802842 and CRC risk, some limitations should be acknowledged. First, the sample size of our case-control study was relatively small. Second, we merely performed bioinformatics analyses rather than functional experiments, so whether this variant is causal remained uncertain. Third, CRC is a complex disease related to environmental and genetic factors. However, in this study, only genetic factor was taken into consideration which restricted to explore the gene-environment interaction.

In conclusion, our case-control study and the following meta-analysis provided convincing evidence for the genetic involvement of rs3802842 polymorphism in CRC susceptibility. However, it is needed to carry out fine-mapping of 11q23 region and functional experiments to identify causal loci.

Supporting Information

Figure S1 Flow diagram of the study selection procedure.

Figure S2 Forest plots of cumulative meta-analysis of rs3802842 in association with colorectal cancer by published year under different genetic models. (A) the C versus A; (B) the AC versus AA; (C) the CC versus AA; (D) the dominant model; (E) the recessive model; (F) the additive model.

Table S1 Sensitivity analysis of allelic model.

Table S2 Sensitivity analysis of the genotypic model of AC versus AA.

Table S3 Sensitivity analysis of the genotypic model of CC versus AA.

Table S4 Sensitivity analysis of dominant model.

Table S5 Sensitivity analysis of recessive model.

Table S6 Sensitivity analysis of additive model.

Checklist S1 The PRISMA 2009 Checklist.

Author Contributions

Conceived and designed the experiments: LZ HX. Performed the experiments: LZ RZ JL XL QW YY. Analyzed the data: JX JK TZ YS LL YC. Contributed reagents/materials/analysis tools: HX LC DX. Wrote the paper: LZ HX.

References

1. Ferlay J, Shin HR, Bray F, Forman D, Mathers C, et al. (2010) Estimates of worldwide burden of cancer in 2008: GLOBOCAN 2008. Int J Cancer 127: 2893–2917.
2. US Cancer Statistics Working Group (2010) United States Cancer Statistics (USCS): 1999–2007 incidence and mortality data. Atlanta, GA: U.S. Department of Health and Human Services, CDC, National Cancer Institute.
3. Wan DS (2009) Epidemiologic trend of and strategies for colorectal cancer. ChineseJournal of Cancer 28: 897–902.
4. Zheng R, Zhang S, Wu L, Li G, Zhao P, et al. (2012) Report of incidence and mortality from China cancer registries in 2008. China Cancer 21: 1–12.
5. Lichtenstein P, Holm NV, Verkasalo PK, Iliadou A, Kaprio J, et al. (2000) Environmental and heritable factors in the causation of cancer–analyses of cohorts of twins from Sweden, Denmark, and Finland. N Engl J Med 343: 78–85.
6. Aaltonen L, Johns L, Jarvinen H, Mecklin JP, Houlston R (2007) Explaining the familial colorectal cancer risk associated with mismatch repair (MMR)-deficient and MMR-stable tumors. Clin Cancer Res 13: 356–361.
7. Tenesa A, Farrington SM, Prendergast JG, Porteous ME, Walker M, et al. (2008) Genome-wide association scan identifies a colorectal cancer susceptibility locus on 11q23 and replicates risk loci at 8q24 and 18q21. Nat Genet 40: 631–637.
8. Houlston RS, Webb E, Broderick P, Pittman AM, Di Bernardo MC, et al. (2008) Meta-analysis of genome-wide association data identifies four new susceptibility loci for colorectal cancer. Nat Genet 40: 1426–1435.
9. Zanke BW, Greenwood CM, Rangrej J, Kustra R, Tenesa A, et al. (2007) Genome-wide association scan identifies a colorectal cancer susceptibility locus on chromosome 8q24. Nat Genet 39: 989–994.
10. Tomlinson IP, Webb E, Carvajal-Carmona L, Broderick P, Howarth K, et al. (2008) A genome-wide association study identifies colorectal cancer susceptibility loci on chromosomes 10p14 and 8q23.3. Nat Genet 40: 623–630.
11. Lascorz J, Forsti A, Chen B, Buch S, Steinke V, et al. (2010) Genome-wide association study for colorectal cancer identifies risk polymorphisms in German familial cases and implicates MAPK signalling pathways in disease susceptibility. Carcinogenesis 31: 1612–1619.
12. Tomlinson I, Webb E, Carvajal-Carmona L, Broderick P, Kemp Z, et al. (2007) A genome-wide association scan of tag SNPs identifies a susceptibility variant for colorectal cancer at 8q24.21. Nat Genet 39: 984–988.
13. Pittman AM, Webb E, Carvajal-Carmona L, Howarth K, Di Bernardo MC, et al. (2008) Refinement of the basis and impact of common 11q23.1 variation to the risk of developing colorectal cancer. Hum Mol Genet 17: 3720–3727.
14. Von Holst S, Picelli S, Edler D, Lenander C, Dalen J, et al. (2010) Association studies on 11 published colorectal cancer risk loci. Br J Cancer 103: 575–580.
15. Kupfer SS, Anderson JR, Hooker S, Skol A, Kittles RA, et al. (2010) Genetic heterogeneity in colorectal cancer associations between African and European americans. Gastroenterology 139: 1677–1685, 1685 e1671–1678.
16. Marino C, Mascheretti S, Riva V, Cattaneo F, Rigoletto C, et al. (2011) Pleiotropic effects of DCDC2 and DYX1C1 genes on language and mathematics traits in nuclear families of developmental dyslexia. Behav Genet 41: 67–76.
17. Zhong H, Prentice RL (2010) Correcting "winner's curse" in odds ratios from genomewide association findings for major complex human diseases. Genet Epidemiol 34: 78–91.
18. Pabalan NA (2010) Meta-analysis in cancer genetics. Asian Pac J Cancer Prev 11: 33–38.
19. Pardini B, Naccarati A, Vodicka P, Kumar R (2012) Gene expression variations: potentialities of master regulator polymorphisms in colorectal cancer risk. Mutagenesis 27: 161–167.
20. Xia J, Wright J, Adams CE (2008) Five large Chinese biomedical bibliographic databases: accessibility and coverage. Health Info Libr J 25: 55–61.
21. Higgins JP, Thompson SG (2002) Quantifying heterogeneity in a meta-analysis. Stat Med 21: 1539–1558.
22. Mantel N, Haenszel W (1959) Statistical aspects of the analysis of data from retrospective studies of disease. J Natl Cancer Inst 22: 719–748.
23. DerSimonian R, Laird N (1986) Meta-analysis in clinical trials. Control Clin Trials 7: 177–188.
24. Thakkinstian A, McElduff P, D'Este C, Duffy D, Attia J (2005) A method for meta-analysis of molecular association studies. Stat Med 24: 1291–1306.
25. Mullen B, Muellerleile P, Bryant B (2001) Cumulative meta-analysis: a consideration of indicators of sufficiency and stability. PSPB 27: 1450–1462.
26. Egger M, Davey Smith G, Schneider M, Minder C (1997) Bias in meta-analysis detected by a simple, graphical test. BMJ 315: 629–634.
27. Mocellin S, Verdi D, Pooley KA, Landi MT, Egan KM, et al. (2012) Telomerase Reverse Transcriptase Locus Polymorphisms and Cancer Risk: A Field Synopsis and Meta-Analysis. J Natl Cancer Inst.
28. Hutter CM, Chang-Claude J, Slattery ML, Pflugeisen BM, Lin Y, et al. (2012) Characterization of gene-environment interactions for colorectal cancer susceptibility loci. Cancer Res 72: 2036–2044.
29. Mates IN, Csiki I, Mates D, Constantinescu V, Badea P, et al. (2010) Association of common genetic variants with colorectal cancer risk in a Romanian sample. Chirurgia (Bucur) 105: 749–757.
30. Niittymaki I, Tuupanen S, Li Y, Jarvinen H, Mecklin JP, et al. (2011) Systematic search for enhancer elements and somatic allelic imbalance at seven low-penetrance colorectal cancer predisposition loci. BMC Med Genet 12: 23.
31. Lubbe SJ, Di Bernardo MC, Broderick P, Chandler I, Houlston RS (2012) Comprehensive evaluation of the impact of 14 genetic variants on colorectal cancer phenotype and risk. Am J Epidemiol 175: 1–10.
32. Middeldorp A, Jagmohan-Changur S, van Eijk R, Tops C, Devilee P, et al. (2009) Enrichment of low penetrance susceptibility loci in a Dutch familial colorectal cancer cohort. Cancer Epidemiol Biomarkers Prev 18: 3062–3067.
33. Wijnen JT, Brohet RM, van Eijk R, Jagmohan-Changur S, Middeldorp A, et al. (2009) Chromosome 8q23.3 and 11q23.1 variants modify colorectal cancer risk in Lynch syndrome. Gastroenterology 136: 131–137.
34. Xiong F, Wu C, Bi X, Yu D, Huang L, et al. (2010) Risk of genome-wide association study-identified genetic variants for colorectal cancer in a Chinese population. Cancer Epidemiol Biomarkers Prev 19: 1855–1861.
35. Talseth-Palmer BA, Brenne IS, Ashton KA, Evans TJ, McPhillips M, et al. (2011) Colorectal cancer susceptibility loci on chromosome 8q23.3 and 11q23.1 as modifiers for disease expression in Lynch syndrome. J Med Genet 48: 279–284.
36. Mates IN, Jinga V, Csiki IE, Mates D, Dinu D, et al. (2012) Single nucleotide polymorphisms in colorectal cancer: associations with tumor site and TNM stage. J Gastrointestin Liver Dis 21: 45–52.
37. Ho JW, Choi SC, Lee YF, Hui TC, Cherny SS, et al. (2011) Replication study of SNP associations for colorectal cancer in Hong Kong Chinese. Br J Cancer 104: 369–375.
38. Lee AS, Seo YC, Chang A, Tohari S, Eu KW, et al. (2000) Detailed deletion mapping at chromosome 11q23 in colorectal carcinoma. Br J Cancer 83: 750–755.
39. Dickson SP, Wang K, Krantz I, Hakonarson H, Goldstein DB (2010) Rare variants create synthetic genome-wide associations. PLoS Biol 8: e1000294.
40. Freedman ML, Monteiro AN, Gayther SA, Coetzee GA, Risch A, et al. (2011) Principles for the post-GWAS functional characterization of cancer risk loci. Nat Genet 43: 513–518.

18

Clinical Characteristics and Disease Predictors of a Large Chinese Cohort of Patients with Autosomal Dominant Polycystic Kidney Disease

Dongping Chen[1¶], Yiyi Ma[1¶], Xueqi Wang[1], Shengqiang Yu[1], Lin Li[1], Bing Dai[1], Zhiguo Mao[1], Lijun Sun[1], Chenggang Xu[1], Shu Rong[1], Mengjun Tang[1], Hongbo Zhao[2], Hongchao Liu[2], Andreas L. Serra[3], Nicole Graf[4], Shiyuan Liu[2], Rudolf P. Wüthrich[3]*, Changlin Mei[1]*

1 Kidney Institute, Department of Nephrology, Shanghai Changzheng Hospital, Second Military Medical University, Shanghai, P. R. China, **2** Department of Radiology, Shanghai Changzheng Hospital, Second Military Medical University, Shanghai, P. R. China, **3** Division of Nephrology, University Hospital, Zürich, Switzerland, **4** Graf biostatistics, Winterthur, Switzerland

Abstract

Objective: Autosomal dominant polycystic kidney disease (ADPKD) is a relentlessly progressing form of chronic kidney disease for which there is no cure. The aim of this study was to characterize Chinese patients with ADPKD and to identify the factors which predict cyst growth and renal functional deterioration.

Methods: To analyze disease predicting factors we performed a prospective longitudinal observational study in a cohort of 541 Chinese patients with ADPKD and an eGFR $\geq$30 ml/min/1.73 m^2. Patients were followed clinically and radiologically with sequential abdominal magnetic resonance imaging (MRI). Clinical characteristics and laboratory data were related to changes in estimated glomerular filtration rate (eGFR) and total kidney volume (TKV). A linear regression model was developed to analyze the factors which determine eGFR and TKV changes.

Results: The age range of this unselected cohort ranged from 4 to 77 years. Median follow-up time was 14.3$\pm$10.6 months. Although inter-individual differences in eGFR and TKV were large, there was a consistent link between these two parameters. Baseline $\log_{10}$-transformed TKV and urinary protein/creatinine ratio were identified as the major predictors for a faster eGFR decline and were associated with a higher TKV growth rate. Interestingly, a lower thrombocyte count correlated significantly with lower eGFR ($r = 0.222$) and higher TKV ($r = 0.134$).

Conclusions: This large cohort of Chinese patients with ADPKD provides unique epidemiological data for comparison with other cohorts of different ethnicity. In Chinese patients we identified a lower thrombocyte count as a significant predictor of disease progression. These results are important for the design of future clinical trials to retard polycystic kidney disease progression.

Editor: Partha Mukhopadhyay, National Institutes of Health, United States of America

Funding: This work was supported by an Institutional Partnership Grant from the Sino Swiss Science & Technology Cooperation (SSSTC) Program, National High Technology Reseach Development (863) Project of China (2007AA02Z3Z1), National Natural Science Foundation of China (30570867, 30771016, 30971368), National Natural Science Foundation of China for Young Scientists (81000281, 81100482), Shanghai Key Clinical Disciplines Construction Project, Key Scientific and Technological Project of Shanghai Committee of Science and Technology (11431920800). The funders had no role in study design, data collection and analysis, decision to publish, or preparation of the manuscript.

Competing Interests: NG is the founder and owner of graf biostatistics. This does not alter the authors' adherence to all the PLOS ONE policies on sharing data and materials.

* E-mail: chlmei1954@126.com (CLM); rudolf.wuethrich@usz.ch (RPW)

¶ These authors contributed equally to this work.

Introduction

Autosomal dominant polycystic kidney disease (ADPKD) is a distinct genetic disease which occurs with variable frequency in all parts of the world [1,2]. Its prevalence is estimated to average 100 cases per 100'000 population, although recent studies concluded that the prevalence is closer to orphan diseases, i.e., in the range of 50 per 100'000 [3]. Mutations in two different genes (*PKD1* and *PKD2*) are known to cause ADPKD [4,5]. Numerous different mutations in the *PKD1* gene which encodes the ciliary protein polycystin-1 are responsible for 85% of the cases, and mutations in *PKD2* encoding polycystin-2 are responsible for the remaining 15% of the cases [6]. Mutations in both genes cause significant phenotypic variability, and *PKD2* gene mutations generally lead to milder disease than *PKD1* gene mutations [6,7].

Although the clinical description of ADPKD is well known, it remains difficult to predict the clinical course and the occurrence of complications. Therefore longitudinal cohorts have been established to document the long-term clinical course of the disease and to identify parameters which predict progression. The

Table 1. Baseline demographics and clinical characteristics of Chinese ADPKD cohort.

Characteristics	N	Female	Male	Total
Age (years)	541	39.2±12.3	40.0±12.0	39.7±12.1
Weight (kg)	539	56.5±9.7	70.8±11.6	64.2±12.9
Height (cm)	539	160.6±8.1	173.4±6.5	167.5±9.7
BMI (kg/m^2)	539	21.8±3.0	23.5±3.2	22.7±3.2
SBP (mm Hg)	403	129.8±17.4	132.8±16.0	131.4±16.7
DBP (mm Hg)	403	86.6±11.4	88.1±10.1	87.4±10.7
History of hypertension	531	56.6%	76.3%	67.2%
Number of antihyper-tensive drugs	522	0.9±1.1	1.2±1.0	1.1±1.0
- ACE or ARB		45.2%	61.1%	53.8%
- CCB		22.6%	26.5%	24.7%
Previous or current smokers	513	1.7%	30.6%	17.3%
Family history for ADPKD	509	74.2%	76.4%	75.4%
Presence of liver cysts	541	73.7%	70.7%	72.1%
Presence of regular pain	509	39.5%	34.8%	36.9%
History of macro-hematuria	517	18.7%	27.5%	23.4%

Baseline demographics and clinical characteristics for female (n = 251) and male (n = 290) patients with ADPKD are reported separately, and for both sexes combined (n = 541). Data show mean ± standard deviation or relative frequency (%), respectively.

Table 2. Baseline renal parameters and eGFR data stratified by age categories.

Age category	years	≤18	19–30	31–40	41–50	51–60	>60	All
Blood								
Creatinine (n = 502)	μmol/l	84.4±81.2	81.2±44.1	90.7±60.3	103.1±46.9	113.2±44.1	140.6±88.1	98.1±56.0
eGFR (n = 502)	ml/min/1.73 m^2	130.9±50.2	116.4±13.0	105.9±13.1	94.2±11.8	84.2±10.1	75.7±14.6	100.4±20.1
Yearly eGFR change (n = 416)	ml/min/1.73 m^2	+7.0±26.8	+1.3±8.0	−0.7±7.9	−1.8±7.1	−3.5±10.6	−1.3±2.2	−0.9±9.6
Cystatin C (n = 331)	mg/l	0.92±0.31	0.92±0.56	1.00±0.55	1.23±0.57	1.49±0.66	1.75±0.81	1.17±0.63
BUN (n = 503)	mmol/l	6.8±5.4	5.7±3.2	5.8±2.4	6.5±2.4	7.1±2.6	8.2±4.0	6.3±2.9
Uric acid (n = 488)	μmol/l	340±109	318±86	322±91	363±104	386±101	385±88	347±100
β_2-micro-globulin (n = 383)	mg/l	1.69±1.21	1.64±1.06	1.95±1.64	2.35±1.27	4.19±4.69	3.80±2.80	2.45±2.56
Urine								
Protein/ creatinine ratio (n = 324)	g/g	0.33±0.67	0.14±0.20	0.19±0.34	0.22±0.27	0.26±0.25	0.38±0.30	0.21±0.32
Specific gravity (n = 253)	g/cm^3	1.018±0.007	1.020±0.007	1.016±0.007	1.015±0.007	1.016±0.007	1.019±0.007	1.016±0.007
pH (n = 257)		5.50±0.37	5.72±0.54	5.70±0.48	5.70±0.55	5.70±0.46	5.70±0.46	5.69±0.50

Baseline laboratory data and eGFR for age categories ≤18 years (n = 20), 19–30 years (n = 74), 31–40 years (n = 171), 41–50 years (n = 128), 51–60 years (n = 90), and >60 years (n = 19) are reported. To reduce the number of missing values, baseline cystatin C, β_2-microglobulin and the protein/creatinine ratio were replaced by the mean of all measured values from all visits. Data show mean ± standard deviation.

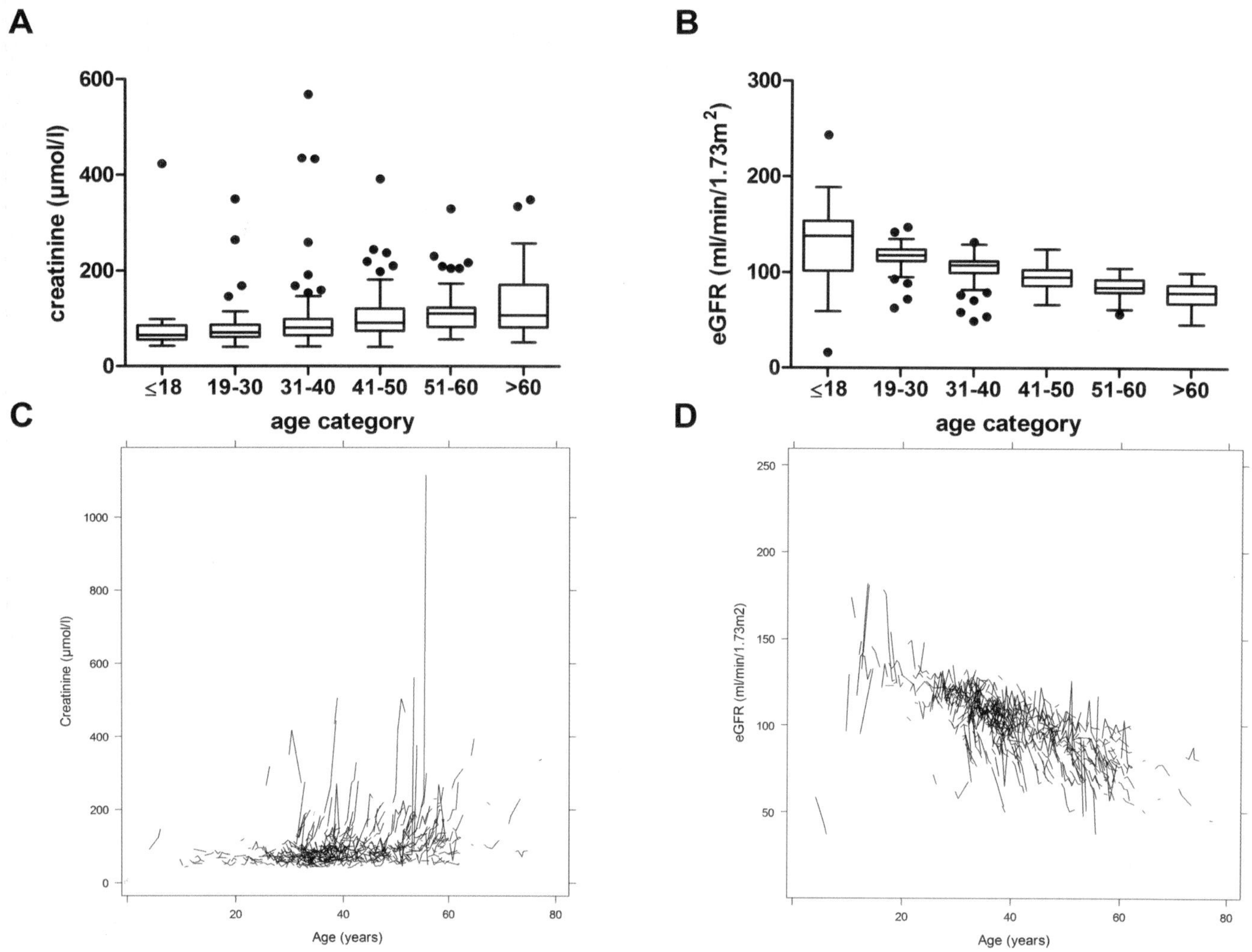

Figure 1. Renal function in different age categories of ADPKD patients. A) Creatinine (μmol/l) for age categories ≤18 years (n = 20), 19–30 years (n = 74), 31–40 years (n = 171), 41–50 years (n = 128), 51–60 years (n = 90), and >60 years (n = 19). B) eGFR (ml/min/1.73 m^2) for age categories ≤18 years (n = 20), 19–30 years (n = 74), 31–40 years (n = 171), 41–50 years (n = 128), 51–60 years (n = 90), and >60 years (n = 19). Boxes show the median and the 25th and 75th percentile. Whiskers extend to the farthest points that are not outliers (i.e., that are within 3/2 times the interquartile range) and dots indicate outliers. C) Spaghetti plots for course of creatinine and D) eGFR over entire observation time in individual patients.

best characterized cohort (n = 241) with the longest follow-up is the cohort of the Consortium for Radiologic Imaging Studies of Polycystic Kidney Disease (CRISP) in the United States which has provided important information regarding the main predictors of renal disease progression [8–10]. Other well characterized longitudinal cohorts have been set up, including the Swiss ADPKD (n = 100) [11] and the recently established global OVERTURE (n of ca. 3000) [12] cohorts, which will continue to provide important information regarding major determinants of disease progression. Data generated from these cohorts will also be essential to define the clinically relevant parameters which are needed to evaluate the efficacy of novel treatments.

Here we describe the clinical characteristics and the factors which predict disease progression in a unique longitudinal cohort of Chinese patients (n = 541) with ADPKD. These data will be useful to design future clinical trials which endeavor to define therapies which retard disease progression in ADPKD.

Subjects and Methods

Patient recruitment

The study protocol and consent form were developed, reviewed and approved by the Kidney Institute of PLA. The study was approved by the Ethics Committee of the Second Military Medical University (Shanghai, China). Chinese patients with an established diagnosis of polycystic kidney disease were identified by a nationwide search in mainland China. All patients were recruited at a single nephrology center at Changzheng Hospital (Shanghai, China). Recruitment started in June 2009, and is ongoing. Informed written consent was obtained from each potentially eligible subject or his legal representative prior to enrollment.

Inclusion and exclusion criteria

Patients had to have an established diagnosis of autosomal dominant polycystic kidney disease (ADPKD) as defined by the criteria of Pei [13]. There were no age limits, but the eGFR had to be ≥30 ml/min/1.73 m^2 according to the CKD-EPI formula for

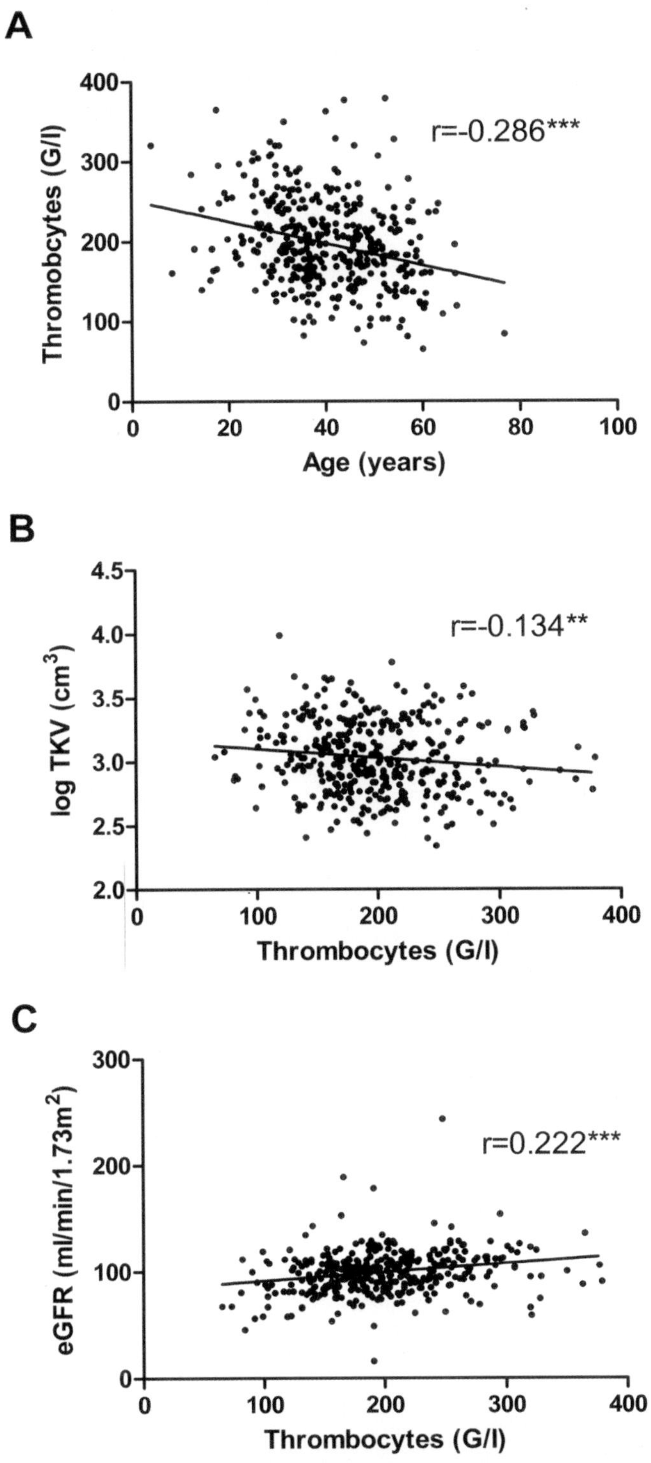

Figure 2. Thrombocytes were correlated to age, TKV and eGFR in ADPKD patients. A) Scatter plot between age and thrombocytes (n = 399). Pearson correlation coefficient is −0.286 ($P<0.001$). B) Scatter plot between thrombocytes and $\log_{10}$ TKV (n = 394). Pearson correlation coefficient is −0.134 ($P=0.008$). C) Scatter plot between thrombocytes and eGFR (n = 391). Pearson correlation coefficient is 0.222 ($P<0.001$).

adults or the Schwarz equation for children. Patients on dialysis treatment or having received a kidney transplant were excluded.

Subjects were ineligible to participate if they were unable to undergo breath-held magnetic resonance imaging (MRI), or had contraindications for MRI such as having a cardiac pacemaker, metallic foreign bodies or aneurysmal clips. Patients were also excluded if they had systemic diseases other than hypertension that could potentially affect renal function. Female patients who were pregnant, lactating or less than 6 months postpartum were also excluded.

Schedule of examinations

Medical histories were taken and physical examinations were performed at the time of screening and enrollment at Changzheng Hospital in Shanghai. Enrolled subjects were scheduled for a 2-day evaluation visit, and were then seen at 6 months intervals. Blood and urine samples were collected at each visit. Abdominal MRI scans were obtained at baseline and at each follow-up visit, using a previously described protocol [11]. Total kidney volumes (TKV) and total renal cyst volumes (TCV) were measured twice by two independent observers on an interactive workstation (Advantage Windows Workstation; GE Medical Systems Europe, Buc, France).

Statistical analyses

All medical data were anonymized and transferred to a spreadsheet. Descriptive analyses were performed for all baseline data (mean±SD, median, range). Female and male patients were compared with a two-tailed Fisher's exact test for nominal variables and with a two-tailed Mann-Whitney U test for quantitative variables. For the correlation analyses, the Pearson product-moment correlation coefficient or Spearman's rho was calculated.

A multiple linear regression was run with yearly eGFR change or yearly TKV growth (%) as dependent variable, and the following independent variables: age, sex, observation time, history of hypertension, intake of antihypertensive drugs, SBP, DBP, episodes of macrohematuria, baseline eGFR, protein/creatinine ratio, baseline TKV and baseline thrombocyte count. A total of 279 patients aged >18 years and ≤60 years with valid data for all variables of the model were included. For the variables SBP, DBP, episodes of macrohematuria and thrombocyte count, missing values were imputed by data from the next following visit. Overall, the missingness of data was dependent on observation time, i.e., patients with fewer visits and thus shorter observation time had more missing data. Except for observation time, Little's test indicated that data were missing completely at random ($P=0.105$).

For predictor selection, a stepwise forward and backward selection using the exact Akaike Information Criterion (AIC) was performed. In the model with yearly eGFR change as dependent variable, baseline eGFR was also included as additional controlling variable. Nonlinearity was evaluated with component plus residual plots, normality was checked with a Q-Q plot for studentized residuals. Homoscedasticity was evaluated with a studentized residuals versus fitted values plot and with the non-constant error variance test. The outlier test and Cook's D plot were used to check for outliers and influential points. Several measures had to be taken to meet the assumptions of linear regression. A normal distribution of the residuals was achieved by windsorizing the dependent variable. Linearity was reached by $\log_{10}$-transforming baseline TKV and protein/creatinine ratio. For the model with yearly TKV change as dependent variable, heterogeneity of variance could be reduced considerably by introducing observation time into the model. However, as the non-constant variance score test was still of borderline significance ($P=0.059$), a regression with robust standard errors was run.

All analyses were done using SPSS Version 20 except for the regression, which was performed in R version 2.15.2.

Table 3. Baseline kidney and cyst volumes and yearly volume growth rates stratified by age.

Age category	years	≤18	19–30	31–40	41–50	51–60	>60	All
Baseline TKV								
	N	23	81	180	134	95	19	532
	cm^3	458±385	842±646	1126±739	1495±909	1575±948	2180±2774	1265±1002
Yearly TKV growth								
	N	15	61	157	99	76	13	421
	cm^3/yr	40±174	65±153	71±185	83±193	61±154	130±328	72±183
	%/yr	2.3±24.3	4.9±10.8	5.4±9.6	4.8±9.3	3.6±7.3	1.1±11.5	4.6±10.2
Baseline TCV								
	N	23	81	180	134	95	19	532
	cm^3	187±359	464±602	719±652	1072±857	1189±858	1811±2613	869±929
Yearly TCV growth								
	N	15	61	157	99	76	13	421
	cm^3/yr	34±180	61±132	70±177	67±201	52±180	159±395	66±188
	%/yr	17.8±59.3	10.6±18.4	11.2±19.6	6.8±14.9	4.5±11.9	2.9±19.0	8.9±20.1

Baseline kidney volumes (TKV and TCV) and yearly volume growth rates for age categories ≤18 years, 19–30 years, 31–40 years, 41–50 years, 51–60 years, and >60 years are reported. Data show mean ± standard deviation.

Results

General characteristics of the cohort

The Chinese ADPKD cohort represents an ongoing longitudinal study. In the present interim report, we analyzed 541 patients who were enrolled between June 2009 and December 2011. Patients were followed up every six months. The mean follow-up duration was 14.3±10.6 months (median 16 months, range 0–38 months).

The recruitment strategy of the cohort subjects was designed to allow for the inclusion of a broad age range of patients with ADPKD, including children. Table 1 shows the baseline demographic and clinical characteristics of the cohort, stratified for male and female patients. The mean age was 40 years (range 4 to 77 years). Seventy-five percent of the patients had a positive family history for ADPKD. The average disease burden was important. Two thirds of the patients were hypertensive, taking on average 1.1±1.0 antihypertensive drugs (range 0–5). Approximately half of the patients used angiotensin converting enzyme inhibitors (ACEI) or angiotensin receptor blockers (ARB) and a quarter of the patients used calcium channel blockers (CCB) to treat hypertension. Approximately three quarters of the patients had liver cysts, 37% complained of chronic pain, and 23% have had episodes of macrohematuria. Compared to male patients, female patients had a lower BMI ($P<0.001$), were less often hypertensive ($P<0.001$), had slightly more often liver cysts ($P=0.444$) and more pain ($P=0.311$), but less often macrohematuria ($P=0.035$). Frequency distributions for age, antihypertensive drugs, diastolic blood pressure (DBP), systolic blood pressure (SBP), eGFR, and TKV are shown in the Figures S1A to S1F.

Characteristics of renal function in the cohort

Table 2 displays the baseline renal parameters (blood and urine), stratified for six different age categories. In the age range between 19 and 60, a gradual rise in the serum levels of creatinine, cystatin C, BUN, uric acid and β_2-microglobulin was found with increasing age. Likewise, the eGFR (creatinine-based CKD-EPI formula) showed a steady decrease in these four age categories. Correlation analysis confirmed that age was negatively correlated with eGFR (see below). Of note, the yearly eGFR decline became more pronounced with increasing age, amounting to –3.5 ml/min/1.73 m^2 per year in the age category of 51 to 60. Furthermore, the urine protein/creatinine ratio also increased with age, whereas the urine specific gravity (1.016±0.007 g/cm^3) and the urine pH (5.69±0.50) did not change substantially in the different age groups. Table S1 in File S1 provides additional eGFR data for reference.

Figure 1 graphically depicts the distribution of serum creatinine and eGFR in the different age categories (Fig. 1A and 1B), and the change over time in serum creatinine and eGFR in individual patients (Fig. 1C and 1D). Overall, there was a wide spectrum of eGFR in all age categories. Of note, a pronounced creatinine rise and eGFR decline was apparent in many patients in all age categories.

Regarding other laboratory data such as electrolytes, lipids and hematological parameters, no apparent differences could be detected among the different age categories, except for the hemoglobin level and more importantly the thrombocyte count which were both lower in the advanced age groups (Table S2 in File S1). The correlation analysis confirmed that the thrombocyte count was negatively correlated with age (Fig. 2A). Moreover, the thrombocyte count was found to be negatively correlated with $\log_{10}$-transformed TKV and positively with eGFR (Fig. 2B and 2C). Out of 399 patients, 60 (15.0%) had a baseline thrombocyte count below 145 G/l and were thus clearly thrombocytopenic.

Characteristics of renal volume growth in the cohort

The mean TKV for the entire cohort amounted to 1265±1002 cm^3 at baseline, and the mean TCV was 869±929 cm^3, corresponding on average to 58±21% of the TKV. The mean yearly increase of TKV amounted to 72±183 cm^3, representing 4.6±10.2% TKV growth per year (Table 3). The large standard deviations are noticeable, illustrating the large inter-individual differences of the renal volume in the cohort. On average, female patients had a lower TKV than males

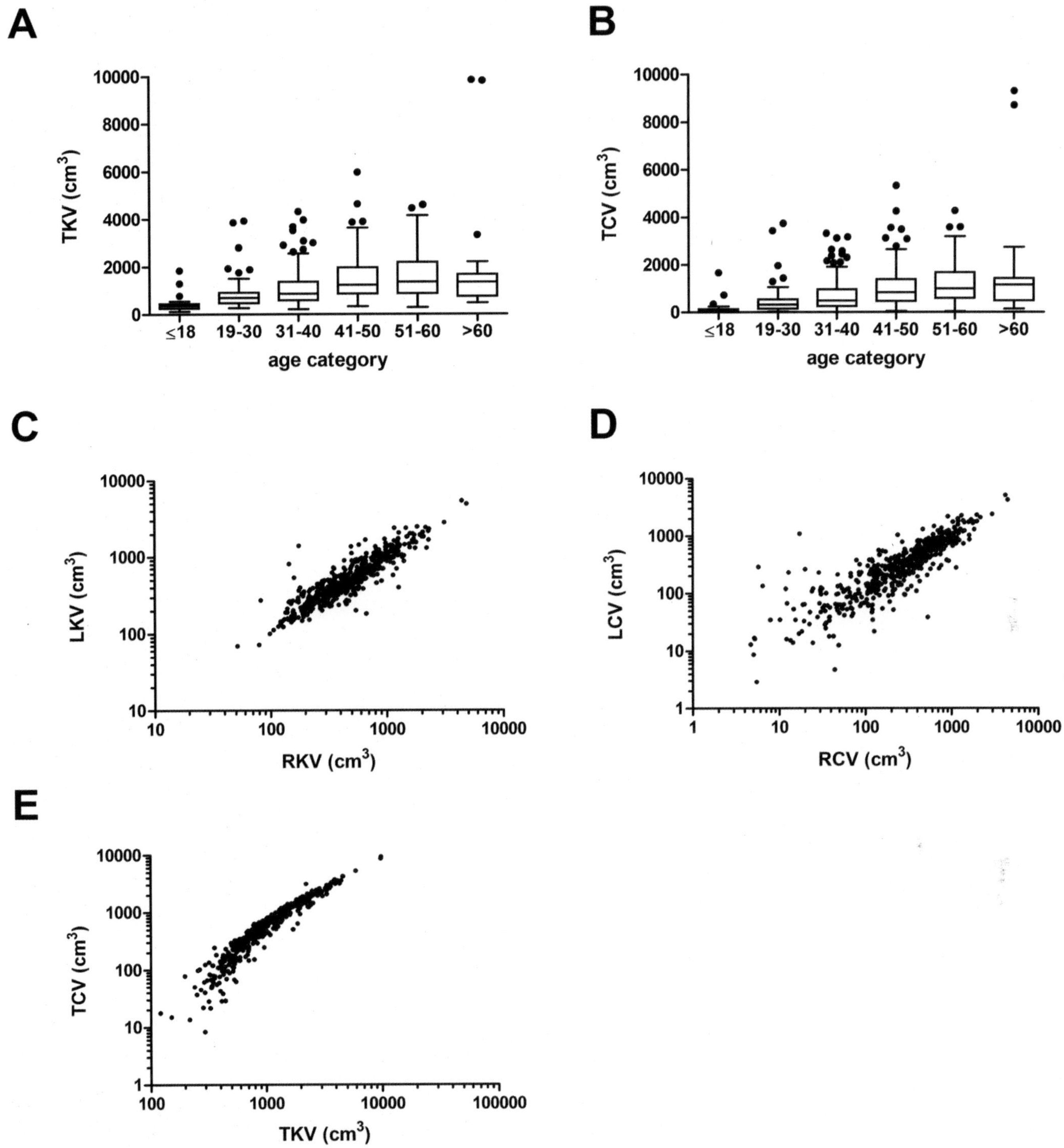

Figure 3. TKV and TCV in different age categories, and the correlations between kidney volumes (KV) and cyst volumes (CV). A) TKV and B) TCV for age categories ≤18 years (n = 23), 19–30 years (n = 81), 31–40 years (n = 180), 41–50 years (n = 134), 51–60 years (n = 95), and >60 years (n = 19). Boxes show the median and the 25th and 75th percentile. Whiskers extend to the farthest points that are not outliers (i.e., that are within 3/2 times the interquartile range) and dots indicate outliers. C) Scatter plot between RKV and LKV (n = 532). The regression line is defined by LKV = 0.337+0.889*RKV. Pearson correlation coefficient is 0.902 (P<0.001). D) Scatter plot between RCV and LCV (n = 530). Pearson correlation coefficient is 0.857 (P<0.001). E) Scatter plot between baseline TKV and baseline TCV (n = 532). Pearson correlation coefficient is 0.951 (P<0.001).

(1081±891 vs. 1427±1065 cm^3, P<0.001), and a lower yearly TKV growth rate (3.3±11.3 vs. 5.7±9.2%, P = 0.003).

Figure 3A and 3B graphically depict the TKV and the TCV in the different age categories, revealing that TKV and TCV increased up to the age of 60. TKV was indeed positively correlated with age (see below). Figures 3C, 3D and 3E illustrate that there was a tight correlation between RKV and LKV (r = 0.902), between RCV and LCV (r = 0.857), and between TKV

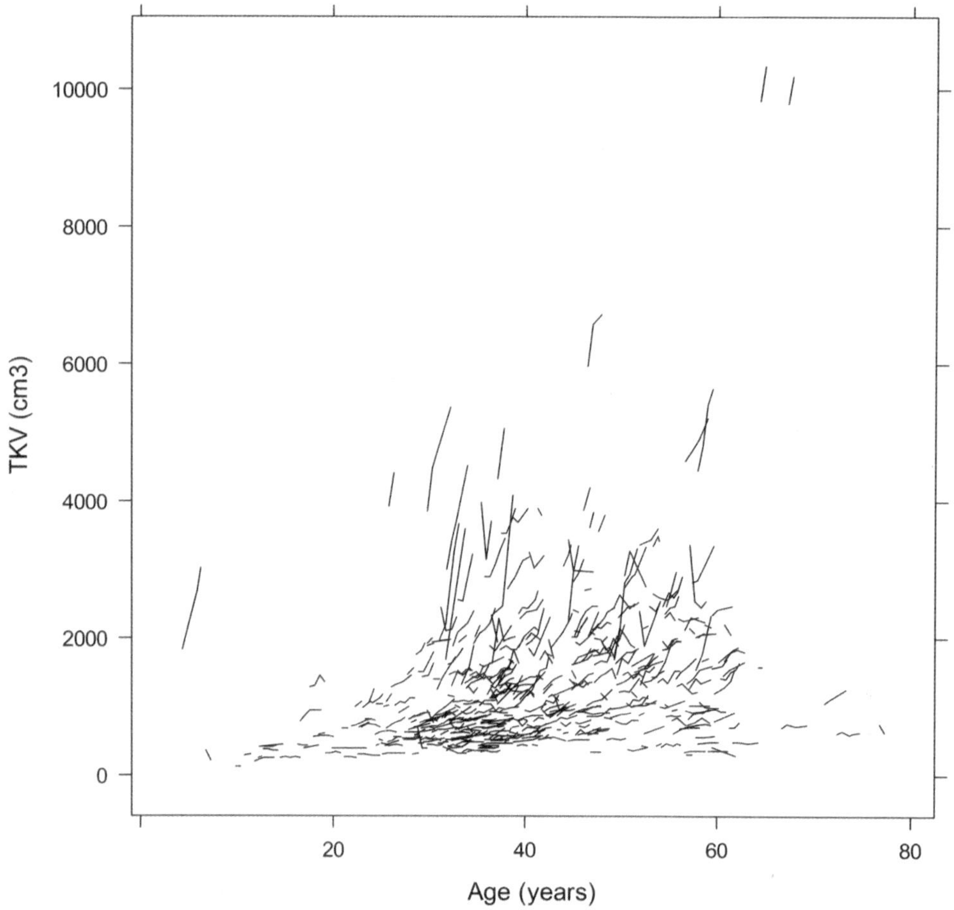

Figure 4. Spaghetti plot for TKV over entire observation time in individual patients (n = 421).

and TCV ($r = 0.951$). The Tables S3 and S4 in File S1 show additional kidney volume data for reference.

Figure 4 shows the TKV change over time in individual patients. Overall, the range of TKV increased with advancing age, reflecting large inter-individual differences. Of note, steep increases in TKV were found in all age categories and especially in patients with baseline TKV greater than 1500 cm^3. In Figure S2, baseline TKV and the yearly TKV growth rate are lined up in ascending order, with the corresponding yearly TKV growth rate and baseline TKV being displayed in the graph above, illustrating that the growth rate appeared to increase with increasing baseline TKV.

Correlations between TKV and eGFR

There was a significant negative correlation between baseline TKV and eGFR for the different age categories between age 19 and 60 (Fig. 5A). For all patients between age 19 and 60 the r amounted to -0.596 ($p<0.001$). TKV correlated best with eGFR in the age group 19–30 ($r = -0.622$) and was least in the age group 51–60 ($r = -0.382$). As mentioned above, age correlated positively with $\log_{10}$-transformed TKV ($r = 0.439$) and negatively with eGFR ($r = -0.645$) (Fig. 5B). However, there was only a very weak correlation between the yearly eGFR change and the yearly TKV volume growth (Fig. 6A and 6B).

Analysis of predictors of progression

Table 4 shows the results of the linear regression with yearly eGFR change as the dependent variable. The model explains only 19% of the total variance. We identified a highly significant association of $\log_{10}$ protein/creatinine ratio and also baseline $\log_{10}$ TKV with the yearly decrease of eGFR. Age and thrombocyte count were also significantly associated. At first sight the influence of history of hypertension and intake of antihypertensive drugs on eGFR change seems complicated. When developing the model we found that the association between the unadjusted estimate of history of hypertension and the yearly eGFR change was negative. When controlling for intake of antihypertensive drugs the association turned into a positive one. Since the intake of antihypertensive drugs may reflect a higher disease severity, the addition of this latter parameter to the model seems to be justified.

Table 5 shows the results of the linear regression with percental yearly TKV change as dependent variable. This model explains only 16% of the variance. Interestingly, age was identified as a highly significant predictor for reduction in the percentage rate of TKV, possibly as a reflection of a higher probability of cyst ruptures. In addition, the intake of antihypertensive drugs, male sex, lower thrombocyte count and $\log_{10}$ protein/creatinine were significant predictors for yearly TKV change. Although the dependent variable already accounted for baseline TKV insofar it represents the percental increase, baseline TKV was also retained in the regression model. Paradoxically, a lower diastolic blood pressure was associated with a higher yearly TKV change. It is however difficult to estimate the true effect of blood pressure on TKV change since in most hypertensive patients, blood pressure is controlled by antihypertensive drugs. The regression model for TKV change was hampered by heterogeneity of variance, which

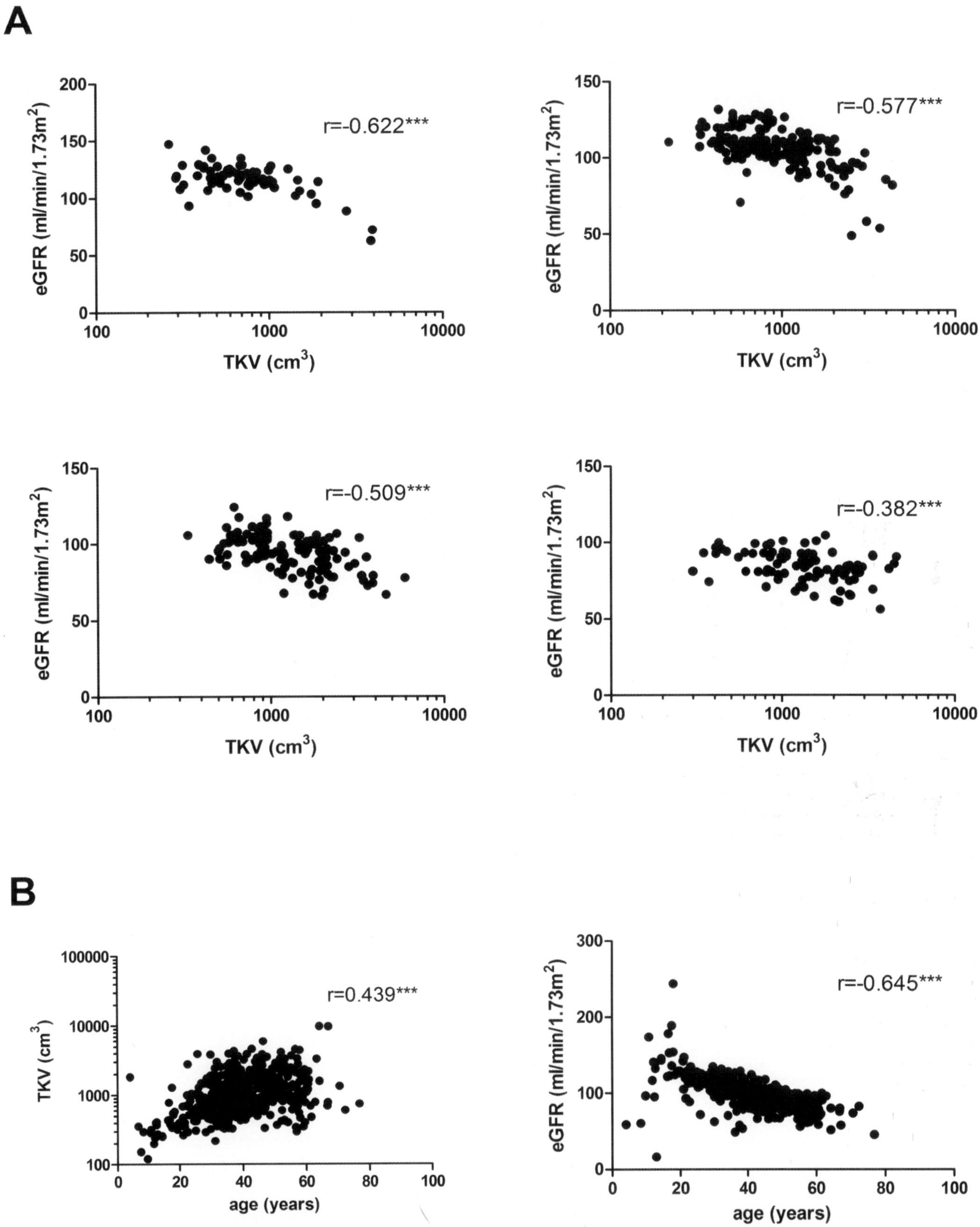

Figure 5. Correlations among TKV, eGFR and age in ADPKD patients. A) Scatter plots between baseline TKV and eGFR. The upper left panel shows patients of age 19–30 years (n = 72), the upper right panel patients of age 31–40 years (n = 171), the lower left panel patients of age 41–50 years (n = 127), and the lower right panel patients of age 51–60 years (n = 90). B) Scatter plots between age and baseline TKV (n = 532) (left panel), and between age and eGFR (n = 502) (right panel).

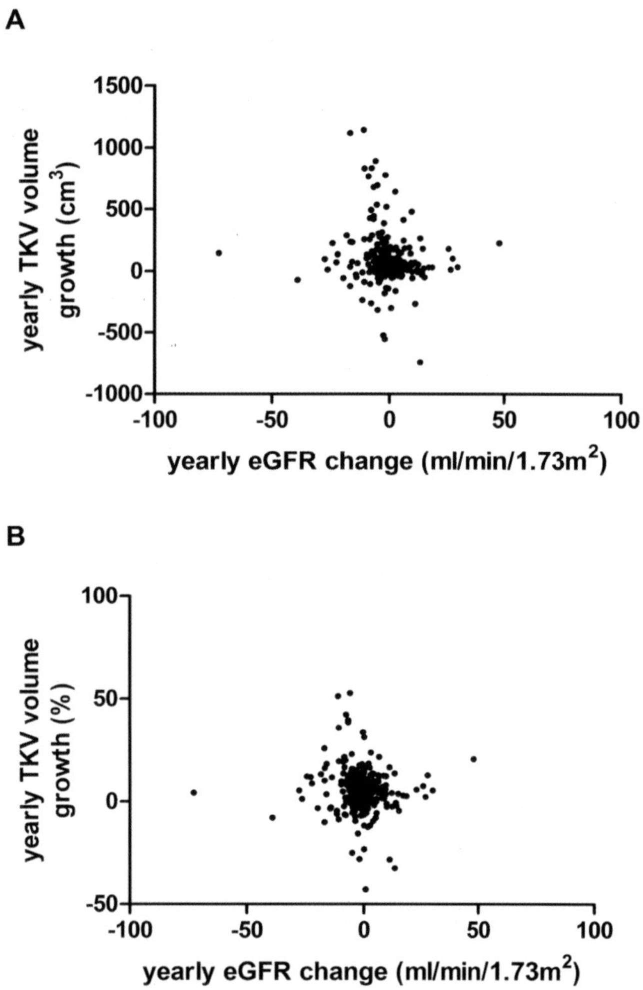

Figure 6. Correlations between yearly TKV growth and eGFR change in ADPKD patients. A) Scatter plot between yearly eGFR change and yearly TKV volume growth (cm^3) (n = 372). Spearman's rho is −0.119 (P = 0.022). Only patients >18 years and ≤60 years are included. B) Scatter plot between yearly eGFR change and yearly TKV volume growth (%) (n = 372). Spearman's rho is −0.055 (P = 0.288). Only patients >18 years and ≤60 years are included.

could be reduced considerably by introducing observation time into the model.

Discussion

A majority of patients with ADPKD reach end-stage renal disease (ESRD) in the 5th or 6th decade of life [14,15], but renal insufficiency may occur much earlier or later. While years ago it was felt that the course of polycystic kidney disease was totally unpredictable [16], more recent studies have shown that mutations in *PKD1*, male sex, early onset hypertension and macrohematuria, baseline GFR, albuminuria, renal cyst volume and uric acid are among the most important factors which predict more severe disease progression and an earlier onset of ESRD [8–11,17–23].

Large cross-sectional and retrospective studies of ADPKD cohorts have provided fundamental information on the clinical course and the predictive factors, but their value has been limited by the lack of prospective data for GFR decline and cyst growth. Thus it is only recently – and particularly in association with the advent of CT- and MRI-based radiological techniques that allow precise measurement of renal volume changes – that truly prospective cohorts have been set-up to elucidate the characteristics of polycystic kidney disease progression. The invaluable CRISP cohort has been established between 2001 and 2005 and represents the most detailed cohort of 241 patients with ADPKD [8,24]. Recently, 6- and 8-year follow-up data have been reported, providing important insight regarding the factors which determine the decline in GFR and TKV growth [10,25].

Here we describe a large longitudinal clinical cohort of 541 Chinese patients with ADPKD. Our data allow not only verification but also extension of the data from CRISP [8-10] and other cohorts [11,12,26]. The Chinese cohort is as detailed as the CRISP cohort, yet more than twice the size and specific for the Chinese population, but with only a short observation time. Contrasting with CRISP [8] and the smaller SUISSE ADPKD cohort [11], the Chinese cohort spans a broader age range which includes pediatric and older patients, with a majority of patients (n = 497) in a wider adult age range (19–60 years). This has the advantage to provide prospective data for additional age categories, but introduces some heterogeneity of the data, wherefore we have limited the analysis of the progression data to the age range between 19 and 60. Limitations of the cohort are its short follow-up time, the reliance on estimated rather than measured GFR, the lack of mutational analyses, and the fact that the study population is confined to China.

Table 4. Linear regression model with 97% windsorized yearly eGFR change as dependent variable.

Coefficients	Estimate	Standard error	*P*-value	Change of coefficient by	Adjustment in yearly eGFR change (ml/min/1.73m²/year)
Log_{10} protein/ creatinine	−4.572024	0.941120	<0.001	1%	−0.020
Log_{10} baseline TKV	−4.992699	1.478459	<0.001	1%	−0.022
Thrombocyte count	−0.012648	0.005818	0.031	1 G/l	−0.013
Age	−0.113218	0.046569	0.016	1 year	−0.113
History of hypertension	2.350887	1.223246	0.056	Presence vs. absence	2.350
Intake of antihypertensive drugs	−1.970294	1.199285	0.102	Presence vs. absence	−1.970
Baseline eGFR	−0.036897	0.034818	0.290	1 ml/min/1.73 m²	−0.037
Intercept	20.274693	7.778006	0.010		

Adjusted R^2 was 0.1943, F-statistic was 10.58 on 7 and 271 DF (P<0.001).

Table 5. Linear regression model with 96.4% windsorized yearly TKV change as dependent variable.

Coefficients	Estimate	Standard error	*P*-value	Change of coefficient by	Adjustment in yearly TKV change (%/year)
Log_{10} protein/creatinine	2.552477	1.295340	0.050	1%	0.011
Log_{10} baseline TKV	3.315135	1.961758	0.092	1%	0.014
Thrombocyte count	−0.014728	0.007203	0.042	−1 G/l	0.015
Male sex	1.846426	0.806099	0.023	male vs. female	1. 846
Intake of anti-hypertensive drugs	2.157377	0.884859	0.015	presence vs. absence	2.157
Age	−0.235288	0.065427	<0.001	1 year	−0.235
Diastolic blood pressure	−0.083163	0.040440	0.041	1 mm Hg	−0.083
Baseline eGFR	−0.072392	0.053032	0.173	1 ml/min/1.73 m^2	−0.072
Observation time	1.634095	0.905810	0.072	1 year	1.634
Intercept	18.597347	11.763321	0.115		

Adjusted R^2 was 0.1612, F-statistic was 6.935 on 9 and 269 DF ($P<0.001$).

In agreement with the CRISP and the SUISSE ADPKD results, our data confirm that ADPKD is more severe in male than in female patients, and that there is an age-dependent decrease of eGFR and increase in TKV which extends to older patients. Consistent with the two other cohorts we found similar values for eGFR and TKV and the yearly changes thereof in their respective age range. Thus at a mean age of 32.4±8.9 years, CRISP reported a baseline TKV of 1076±670 cm^3 and a 5.3±3.9% yearly increase of TKV [8]. At a mean age of 31.2±6.4 years, SUISSE ADPKD reported a TKV of 1003±568 cm^3 and an extrapolated yearly TKV growth of 5.4±9.5% [11]. Although not precisely comparable we also found a mean TKV around 1000 cm^3 and an average yearly TKV growth of approximately 5.2% in the age category between 19 and 40 years. Furthermore the baseline eGFR and the yearly eGFR changes seen in CRISP and SUISSE ADPKD were similar to the Chinese patients in the respective age categories. Taken together this suggests that the impact of the Chinese ethnicity on ADPKD is negligible. As a consequence, clinical trials in Chinese ADPKD patients might rely on similar assumptions regarding the definition of clinical endpoints.

Earlier prospective studies in patients with ADPKD have shown that GFR and kidney volume correlate [8,10,26–28]. Although the follow-up time in our cohort was short (14.6±10.6 months in the adult population of 19–60 years) we could compute the yearly changes in TKV and eGFR in an extended number of age categories. An important finding was that many patients displayed a pronounced and unpredictable creatinine rise and eGFR decline, and this was apparent in all age categories. This suggests that it remains difficult to predict the course of the renal function in individual patients. Furthermore, steep increases in TKV were also found in all age categories and especially in patients with baseline TKV greater than 1500 cm^3. For reasons not yet well understood it appears that the predictability of the change in TKV is as difficult as the predictability of changes in eGFR. This is also illustrated by the poor correlation between the yearly eGFR and TKV changes in our cohort, and by the data in Figure S2 which show that there are large excursions (increases and decreases) of TKV growth which do not correlate well with increasing baseline TKV. As longer follow-up times become available in our cohort the sudden volume changes - which could be due to hemorrhage or cyst rupture – might become less obvious, and the average TKV growth rate should become more reliable.

The linear regression analysis revealed that the yearly decrease of eGFR was significantly associated with higher $\log_{10}$ protein/creatinine ratio, $\log_{10}$ baseline TKV and age. On the other hand the linear regression analysis with percental yearly TKV change as dependent variable revealed that the intake of antihypertensive drugs, male sex, lower thrombocyte count and higher $\log_{10}$ protein/creatinine were associated with this variable. The fact that the TKV change was dependent on observation time implicates that the variance is larger for patients with short observation periods and decreases with longer observation periods. This might possibly be explained by the fact that bursting cysts lead to lower TKV at shorter observation periods but less so when the observation time is longer. With increasing observation time, the trend towards a steady TKV growth might get clearer. Consequentially and as stated above, it is essential for the study of TKV growth to maximize follow-up times in order to reduce the "noise" caused by ruptured cysts.

An important finding which has not been described in other cohorts was the identification of a reduced thrombocyte count in older age groups. Although there is a small decrease of the thrombocyte count with increasing age in the normal population, we found a 32% lower thrombocyte count (−71 G/l) in the oldest age group when compared with the youngest cohort patients. Furthermore we found a positive correlation between thrombocyte count and eGFR, and a negative correlation with TKV. Bath et al. also described a reduced number of thrombocytes in ADPKD patients (average age 31 years) in comparison with matched control subjects (−63 G/l), in addition to an increased platelet volume (median 8.4 vs 8.0 fl), suggesting that there is enhanced platelet consumption in ADPKD [29]. Our regression analysis showed that the TKV growth rate was significantly influenced by the thrombocyte count, suggesting that platelets might be implicated in the pathogenesis of cyst growth. Further studies need to be performed to define the pathogenic role of thrombocytes in ADPKD.

In conclusion, we describe the clinical characteristics and the factors that predict disease progression in a large cohort of Chinese patients with ADPKD. Among the progression factors we found that $\log_{10}$-transformed TKV and protein/creatinine ratio significantly predicted eGFR loss and were associated with TKV growth. Furthermore we identified the decreased thrombocyte count as a novel parameter which is associated with more advanced renal impairment, higher TKV and higher TKV growth. The Chinese cohort provides an important data source for the understanding of ADPKD disease progression and the design of future clinical trials in China.

Supporting Information

Figure S1 Frequency distributions for different categories. A) frequency distributions for age (years) (n = 541); B) frequency distributions for number of prescribed antihypertensive drugs (n = 522); C) frequency distributions for diastolic blood pressure (DBP) in mm Hg (n = 403); D) frequency distributions for systolic blood pressure (SBP) in mm Hg (n = 403); E) frequency distributions for estimated glomerular filtration rate (eGFR) in ml/min/1.73 m2 (n = 502); F) frequency distributions for total kidney volume (TKV) <5000 in cm3 (n = 529).

Figure S2 Correlations between baseline TKV and yearly TKV growth. A) Baseline TKV (cm^3) lined up in ascending order, with corresponding yearly TKV growth (cm^3) depicted in the graph above. B) Yearly TKV growth (cm^3) lined up in ascending order with corresponding baseline TKV (cm^3) depicted in the graph above. Only patients >18 years and ≤60 years are included (n = 393).

File S1 Supporting Tables. Table S1: Table shows the eGFR and the yearly changes of the eGFR, stratified by age categories. The eGFR was calculated according to the CKD-EPI formula in adults and according to the Schwarz formula in children. Table S2: Data show mean ± standard deviation. Table S3: Table reports baseline kidney volumes in cm3. RKV, right kidney volume; LKV, left kidney volume; TKV, total kidney volume. Table S4: Table reports baseline cyst volumes in cm3. RCV, right cyst volume; LCV, left cyst volume; TCV, total cyst volume.

Acknowledgments

The authors thank all the patients who contributed to this study. The authors thank Dr. Andreas L. Serra for instructions on MRI measurement techniques and cohort data organization.

Author Contributions

Conceived and designed the experiments: RPW CLM XQW. Performed the experiments: DPC YYM CLM SQY LL BD ZGM LJS CGX SR. Analyzed the data: NG DPC YYM. Contributed reagents/materials/analysis tools: MJT HBZ HCL. Wrote the paper: RPW CLM DPC YYM. MRI technique instruction and data sorting of the cohort: ALS. Instructed the whole imaging examinations: SYL.

References

1. Torres VE, Harris PC, Pirson Y (2007) Autosomal dominant polycystic kidney disease. Lancet 369: 1287–1301.
2. Orskov B, Sorensen VR, Feldt-Rasmussen B, Strandgaard S (2012) Changes in causes of death and risk of cancer in Danish patients with autosomal dominant polycystic kidney disease and end-stage renal disease. Nephrol Dial Transplant 27: 1607–1613.
3. Neumann HP, Jilg C, Bacher J, Nabulsi Z, Malinoc A, et al. (2013) Epidemiology of autosomal-dominant polycystic kidney disease: an in-depth clinical study for south-western Germany. Nephrol Dial Transplant 28: 1472–1487.
4. Rossetti S, Hopp K, Sikkink RA, Sundsbak JL, Lee YK, et al. (2012) Identification of gene mutations in autosomal dominant polycystic kidney disease through targeted resequencing. J Am Soc Nephrol 23: 915–933.
5. Audrézet MP, Cornec-Le Gall E, Chen JM, Redon S, Quéré I, et al. (2012) Autosomal dominant polycystic kidney disease: Comprehensive mutation analysis of *PKD1* and *PKD2* in 700 unrelated patients. Hum Mutat 33: 1239–1250.
6. Cornec-Le Gall E, Audrézet MP, Chen JM, Hourmant M, Morin MP, et al. (2013) Type of *PKD1* mutation influences renal outcome in ADPKD. J Am Soc Nephrol 24: 1006–1013.
7. Hateboer N, v Dijk MA, Bogdanova N, Coto E, Saggar-Malik AK, et al. (1999) Comparison of phenotypes of polycystic kidney disease types 1 and 2. Lancet 353: 103–107.
8. Grantham JJ, Torres VE, Chapman AB, Guay-Woodford LM, Bae KT, et al. (2006) Volume progression in polycystic kidney disease. N Engl J Med 354: 2122–30.
9. Grantham JJ, Cook LT, Torres VE, Bost JE, Chapman AB, et al. (2008) Determinants of renal volume in autosomal-dominant polycystic kidney disease. Kidney Int 73: 108–116.
10. Chapman AB, Bost JE, Torres VE, Guay-Woodford L, Bae KT, et al. (2012) Kidney volume and functional outcomes in autosomal dominant polycystic kidney disease. Clin J Am Soc Nephrol 7: 479–86
11. Kistler AD, Poster D, Krauer F, Weishaupt D, Raina S, et al. (2009) Increases in kidney volume in autosomal dominant polycystic kidney disease can be detected within 6 months. Kidney Int 75: 235–241.
12. Clinical trials webstie. Available: http://clinicaltrials.gov/ct2/show/NCT01430494 Accessed 2014 February 20.
13. Pei Y, Obaji J, Dupuis A, Paterson AD, Magistroni R, et al. (2009) Unified criteria for ultrasonographic diagnosis of ADPKD. J Am Soc Nephrol 20: 205–212.
14. Wilson PD (2004) Polycystic kidney disease. N Engl J Med 350:151–64.
15. Thong KM, Ong AC (2013) The natural history of autosomal dominant polycystic kidney disease: 30-year experience from a single centre. QJ Med 106: 639–646.
16. Simon HB, Thompson GJ (1955) Congenital renal polycystic disease, a clinical and therapeutic study of three hundred sixty-six cases. JAMA 159: 657–662.
17. Franz KA, Reubi FC (1983) Rate of functional deterioration in polycystic kidney disease. Kidney Int 23: 526–529.
18. Chapman AB, Johnson AM, Gabow PA, Schrier RW (1994) Overt proteinuria and microalbuminuria in autosomal dominant polycystic kidney disease. J Am Soc Nephrol 5: 1349–1354.
19. Choukroun G, Itakura Y, Albouze G, Christophe JL, Man NK, et al. (1995) Factors influencing progression of renal failure in autosomal dominant polycystic kidney disease. J Am Soc Nephrol 6: 1634–1642.
20. Johnson AM, Gabow PA (1997) Identification of patients with autosomal dominant polycystic kidney disease at highest risk for end-stage renal disease. J Am Soc Nephrol 8: 1560–1567.
21. Meijer E, Boertien WE, Nauta FL, Bakker SJ, van Oeveren W, et al. (2010) Association of urinary biomarkers with disease severity in patients with autosomal dominant polycystic kidney disease: a cross-sectional analysis. Am J Kidney Dis 56: 883–895.
22. Tokiwa S, Muto S, China T, Horie S (2011) The relationship between renal volume and renal function in autosomal dominant polycystic kidney disease. Clin Exp Nephrol 15: 539–545.
23. Helal I, McFann K, Reed B, Yan XD, Schrier RW, et al. (2013) Serum uric acid, kidney volume and progression in autosomal-dominant polycystic kidney disease. Nephrol Dial Transplant 28: 380–385.
24. Chapman AB, Guay-Woodford LM, Grantham JJ, Torres VE, Bae KT, et al. (2003) Renal structure in early autosomal-dominant polycystic kidney disease (ADPKD): The Consortium for Radiologic Imaging Studies of Polycystic Kidney Disease (CRISP) cohort. Kidney Int 64: 1035–1045.
25. Torres VE, Grantham JJ, Chapman AB, Mrug M, Bae KT, et al. (2011) Potentially modifiable factors affecting the progression of autosomal dominant polycystic kidney disease. Clin J Am Soc Nephrol 6: 640–647.
26. Ozkok A, Akpinar TS, Tufan F, Kanitez NA, Uysal M, et al. (2013) Clinical characteristics and predictors of progression of chronic kidney disease in autosomal dominant polycystic kidney disease: a single center experience. Clin Exp Nephrol 17: 345–351.
27. King BF, Reed JE, Bergstralh EJ, Sheedy PF 2nd, Torres VE (2000) Quantification and longitudinal trends of kidney, renal cyst, and renal parenchyma volumes in autosomal dominant polycystic kidney disease. J Am Soc Nephrol 11: 1505–1511.
28. Sise C, Kusaka M, Wetzel LH, Winklhofer F, Cowley BD, et al. (2000) Volumetric determination of progression in autosomal dominant polycystic kidney disease by computed tomography. Kidney Int 58: 2492–2501.
29. Bath PM, Saggar-Malik AK, Macdougall IC, Eastwood JB, Macgregor GA (1995) Increased platelet volume in patients with adult polycystic kidney disease. Platelets 6: 336–339.

19

Integration of SNP and mRNA Arrays with MicroRNA Profiling Reveals That MiR-370 Is Upregulated and Targets NF1 in Acute Myeloid Leukemia

Laura García-Ortí[1], Ion Cristóbal[1,2]**, Cristina Cirauqui[1], Elisabet Guruceaga[3], Nerea Marcotegui[1], María J. Calasanz[2], Remedios Castello-Cros[1], María D. Odero[1,2]***

1 Division of Oncology, Center for Applied Medical Research (CIMA), University of Navarra, Pamplona, Spain, **2** Department of Genetics, University of Navarra, Pamplona, Spain, **3** Unit of Proteomics, Genomics and Bioinformatics, Center for Applied Medical Research (CIMA), University of Navarra, Pamplona, Spain

Abstract

Background: Deregulated miRNA expression plays a crucial role in carcinogenesis. Recent studies show different mechanisms leading to miRNA deregulation in cancer; however, alterations affecting miRNAs by DNA copy number variations (CNV) remain poorly studied.

Results: Our integrative analysis including data from high resolution SNPs arrays, mRNA expression arrays, and miRNAs expression profiles in 16 myeloid cell lines highlights that CNV are alternative mechanisms to deregulate the expression of miRNAs in acute myeloid leukemia (AML), and represent a novel approach to identify novel candidate genes involved in AML. We found association between the expression levels of 19 miRNAs and CNVs affecting their loci. Functional analysis showed that NF1 is a direct target of miR-370, and that overexpression of miR-370 has similar effects that NF1 inactivation, increasing proliferation and colony formation in AML cells. Moreover, real time RT-PCR showed that *NF1* downregulation is a recurrent event in AML (30.8%), and western blot analysis confirmed this result. MiR-370 overexpression and deletions affecting the *NF1* locus were identified as alternative mechanisms to downregulate *NF1*.

Conclusions: *NF1* downregulation is a common event in AML, and both deletions in the *NF1* locus and overexpression of miR-370 are alternative mechanisms to downregulate *NF1* in this disease. Our results suggest a leukemogenic role of miR-370 through *NF1* downregulation in AML cells. Since NF1 deficiency leads to RAS activation, patients with AML and overexpression of miR-370 may potentially benefit from additional treatment with either RAS or mTOR inhibitors.

Editor: Kevin D. Bunting, Emory University, United States of America

Funding: This work was supported by Ministerio Educación y Ciencia [AP2006-03038], Ministerio Ciencia e Innovación [PI081687], Instituto de Salud Carlos III-Red Temática de investigación Cooperativa en Cáncer (ISCIII-RTICC)[RD06/0020/0078], and Fundación para la Investigación Médica Aplicada Unión (FIMA)(Spain). The funders had no role in study design, data collection and analysis, decision to publish, or preparation of the manuscript.

Competing Interests: The authors have declared that no competing interests exist.

* E-mail: modero@unav.es

• These authors contributed equally to this work.

Introduction

Acute myeloid leukemia (AML) is a heterogeneous clonal disease characterized by enhanced proliferation and impaired differentiation of early progenitors. Its heterogeneity is caused by a variety of genetic and epigenetic aberrations that, acting in combination, contribute to the initiation and progression of this disease. In addition, it has recently been reported the implication of specific microRNAs (miRNAs) in the pathogenesis of AML [1]. MiRNAs are small, non-coding RNAs that bind to the 3′-untranslated region of target genes, negatively regulating their expression levels by translation repression or mRNA degradation. MiRNAs are essential in key biological functions, such as cellular differentiation, development, stress response, apoptosis and cell growth [2]. In addition, miRNAs play important roles in normal hematopoiesis regulating hematopoietic differentiation, and their aberrant expression has been associated with hematological malignancies [1,3]. Several mechanisms are reported to lead to miRNA deregulation: mutations, chromosomal translocations, epigenetic alterations, or a defective miRNA biogenesis; however, little is known about the mechanisms of miRNA deregulation in AML [2].

MiRNA microarrays in large series of AML cases have identified miRNA signatures associated with several cytogenetic and molecular groups [1]. Furthermore, functional effects of some miRNA alterations have also been reported. For example, miR-155, which shows leukemogenic properties, has been found up-regulated in AML patients with *FLT3*-ITD [4]. In the same way, upregulation of miR-181a and miR-335 has been associated with *CEBPA* mutations and consequently, implicated in the regulation of several genes involved in erythroid differentiation in cytogenetically normal AML (CN-AML) [1]. Interestingly, higher miR-181a expression has been significantly associated with better outcome in CN-AML patients [5].

Analysis of human and mouse genomes reveals that miRNAs are frequently located at fragile sites and regions affected by copy number variations (CNVs) associated with cancer, suggesting that genomic instability could be an important mechanism of miRNA deregulation in cancer [6]. Recently, Starczynowsky et al. identified 18 miRNAs implicated in cellular processes relevant to AML, which map to common leukemia-associated genomic alterations in AML [7]. Here, we analyzed 16 myeloid cell lines using SNP and mRNA arrays, and quantified the expression of 250 mature miRNAs by real-time PCR (QRT-PCR). We identified 19 miRNAs with a significant association between their expression and the CNV of the corresponding genomic region in which the miRNAs were located. This integrative approach, together with bioinformatics and functional studies, allowed us to find that miR-370, located in a recurrent amplified region, was upregulated and that its target gene was the tumor suppressor *NF1*. Interestingly, functional analysis showed that overexpression of miR-370 has similar effects that NF1 inactivation, increasing proliferation and colony formation in AML cells. Finally, overexpression of miR-370 and deletions affecting the *NF1* locus were identified as contributing mechanisms to *NF1* downregulation in AML.

Results

Deregulation of miRNAs by gene copy number alterations in AML cell lines

To identify miRNAs deregulated by gene copy number alterations in AML cells, we first performed a SNP array analysis of 16 myeloid cell lines (Table S1 and Table S2). We next analyzed by QRT-PCR the expression profile of 250 miRNAs in these cell lines, evaluating whether the miRNAs located within the amplified or deleted regions identified by the genome-wide analysis were up- or downregulated. Of the 250 miRNAs, 19 showed a significant association between their expression and the CNV of the genomic region in which they were located, and were validated ($P<0.05$). Sixteen miRNAs were upregulated and located in two genomic regions of amplification (11q24.1 and 14q32.31), and 3 miRNAs were downregulated and located in regions with genomic deletions (9p21.32) (Figure S1 and Table 1). Altogether, these results indicate that CNVs are mechanisms that could lead to miRNA deregulation in AML cells.

Identification of the tumor suppressor NF1 as a target of miR-370

These results prompted us to determine the potential target genes for those 19 miRNAs whose expression were associated with CN alterations. For this purpose, we performed a whole genome expression analysis in the myeloid cell lines (Affymetrix Human Genome-U133 Plus-2.0). We observed that 4 out of these 19 miRNAs (miR-370, miR-379, miR-432 and miR-494) had *NF1* as a potential target gene (Table S3). Results were validated by QRT-PCR. Therefore, we decided to analyze whether these four miRNAs, all located on 14q32.31, could regulate *NF1*. The AML cell line HL-60, with low expression of the miRNAs and expression of *NF1*, was chosen as a cellular model for miRNA overexpression experiments. QRT-PCR confirmed overexpression of miR-370, miR-379, and miR-494 after transfection with the corresponding pre-miRNAs (Figure 1A). Transfection of premiR-432 could not be optimized. Western blot analysis showed that NF1 levels decreased after miR-370 overexpression (Figure 1B and Figure 2A). No changes in NF1 levels were observed after ectopic expression of miR-379 and miR-494 (data not shown). Transfection of pRL-NF1(3′UTR) in cells ectopically expressing miR-370 showed decreased luciferase reporter activity, indicating that miR-370 binds to the 3′UTR of *NF1*, negatively regulating its expression. Analysis using the same construct with the seed region of miR-370 mutated showed no changes in luciferase activity, confirming that miR-370 directly binds to *NF1* (Figure 1C).

MiR-370 enhances oncogenic potential of AML cells

It has been reported that *NF1* directly influences AML blast proliferation/growth [14]. Therefore, we first evaluated the functional effects of the transient downregulation of NF1. As expected, we found that NF1 knockdown by siRNA increased cell growth and number of colonies of TF-1 cells as compared to controls (Figure S2). To determine the effects of miR-370 in AML cells, we performed cell growth and colony formation analysis in TF-1 cells transfected with pre- and anti-miR-370. Downregulation of NF1 by miR-370 and upregulation by anti-miR-370 in these cells were confirmed by western blot (Figure 2A). We first analyzed the effects on cell growth of miR-370 and anti-miR-370 using a MTS assay. Consistent with the tumor suppressor activity of *NF1*, there was increased proliferation in TF-1 cells transfected with pre-miR-370 in comparison with control cells (Figure 2B). Overexpression of miR-370 was confirmed by QRT-PCR. Conversely, ectopic expression of anti-miR-370 significantly reduced cell growth of these cells (Figure 2B). To further confirm the importance of miR-370 as regulator of AML cell proliferation, we determined the effects on colony-forming ability of miR-370 in AML cells. Pre-miR-370-transfected TF-1 cells formed significantly higher number of colonies than controls, while anti-miR-370 reduced the number of colonies (Figure 2C). It was not possible to confirm these results in HL-60 because this cell line has an activating mutation in NRAS. Altogether, these results would suggest a leukemogenic role of miR-370 through *NF1* downregulation in AML cells.

NF1 downregulation is a recurrent event in AML

To further evaluate the clinical relevance of *NF1* in AML, we quantified *NF1* expression by QRT-PCR in a series of 68 patients with AML at diagnosis. Patient characteristics are shown in Table 2. *NF1* was downregulated in 30.8% cases (21/68). Levels of miR-370 could be determined in 50 out of these 68 patients, and we observed that miR-370 was overexpressed in 12% cases (6/50). *NF1* was downregulated in all the 6 cases with miR-370 overexpression, indicating a good association between both aberrations (Figure S3 and Table S4). To investigate other mechanisms involved in *NF1* downregulation, we analyzed the copy number at the *NF1* locus by Q-PCR in 55 out of the 68 cases. We found that 13 patient samples had deletions affecting *NF1* (13/55, 23.6%) (Table 2 and Table S4). These findings indicate that copy number changes involving the *NF1* locus represent a mechanism contributing to *NF1* deregulation in AML cells. Interestingly, 5 out of the 6 cases with overexpression of miR-370 had normal number of copies of *NF1* (Table S4), indicating that they are alternative mechanisms of *NF1* downregulation in AML. Altogether, these results suggest that *NF1* downregulation is a recurrent event in AML, and that both miR-370 overexpression and submicroscopic deletions of the *NF1* locus may represent important mechanisms to downregulate *NF1* expression in AML patients.

To confirm these results at protein level, we analyzed NF1 by western blot in 14 cases with AML at diagnosis: 9 had *NF1* downregulation and 5 normal mRNA levels of *NF1* (Figure 3). Patient characteristics are included in Table S5. NF1 protein was not detected in any of the 9 cases with *NF1* downregulation, including the 3 cases with miR-370 overexpression (P4, P7, and

Table 1. MicroRNA deregulated by copy number variations in 16 myeloid cell lines.

MicroRNA	Cytoband	Start	End	Copy number value (mean)	MicroRNA expression (QRT-PCR)	Myeloid cell lines
miR-7	9q21.32	85774483	85774592	0.9596	low	EOL-1, NOMO1, F36P, K562, KYO
miR-15a	13q14.2	50623255	50623337	1.071	low	F36P, K562
miR-16-1	13q14.2	50623109	50623197	1.071	low	F36P, K562
miR-192	11q13.1	64415185	64415294	3.365	high	KAS-1, OCI-AML2, F36P, HEL, K562, KU812, KYO, MEG01
miR-194	11q13.1	64415403	64415487	3.365	high	KAS-1, F36P, HEL, KG-1, K562, KU812, MEG01
miR-100	11q24.1	121528147	121528226	3.099	high	HEL, TF-1, KU812, KYO
miR-125b	11q24.1	121475675	121475762	3.099	high	HEL, TF-1, KU812, KYO, MEG01
miR-370	14q32.31	121528127	121528246	3.671	high	TF-1, KU812, K562, MEG01
miR-127	14q32.31	100419069	100419165	3.671	high	TF-1, KU812, K562, MEG01
miR-134	14q32.31	100590777	100590849	3.671	high	TF-1, KU812, MEG01
miR-154	14q32.31	100595845	100595928	3.671	high	TF-1, KU812, K562, MEG01
miR-376	14q32.31	100576872	100576939	3.671	high	KU812, MEG01
miR-379	14q32.31	100558156	100558222	3.671	high	KU812, MEG01
miR-382	14q32.31	100590396	100590471	3.671	high	TF-1, KU812, MEG01
miR-409-5p	14q32.31	100601390	100601468	3.671	high	TF-1, KU812, MEG01
miR-432	14q32.31	100420573	100590471	3.671	high	TF-1, KU812, K562, MEG01
miR-433	14q32.31	100417976	100418068	3.671	high	TF-1, KU812, K562, MEG01
miR-485-5p	14q32.31	100558156	100558222	3.671	high	TF-1, KU812, MEG01
miR-494	14q32.31	100565724	100565804	3.671	high	TF-1, KU812, MEG01

Amp: amplification; Del: deletion.

P14). Moreover, one of the five patients with normal mRNA levels of *NF1* had no protein (case P8), and other two cases had reduced expression of the NF1 protein (cases P9 and P10).

Discussion

Although the association of miRNA expression profiles with cytogenetic or molecular aberrations has been widely investigated in AML [1,20], the relevance of copy number changes affecting genomic regions that include miRNAs remains poorly explored. In this study, we show that CNVs are alternative mechanisms that regulate the levels of some miRNAs, which, in turn, modulate the expression of target genes with importance in AML development. Using an integrative analysis based in SNP, mRNA arrays and expression profile of 250 mature miRNAs, together with bioinformatics and functional studies, we found that miR-370, located in a recurrent amplified region, was upregulated and that its target gene was the tumor suppressor *NF1*. Interestingly, functional analysis showed that overexpression of miR-370 has similar effects that *NF1* inactivation, suggesting a leukemogenic role of miR-370 through *NF1* downregulation in AML cells. Besides, our results show that *NF1* downregulation is a common event in AML, and that both deletions in the *NF1* locus and overexpression of miR-370 are mechanisms involved in this downregulation.

Two recent studies in series of AML patients showed that microdeletions of *NF1* are common events in this disease, leading to reduction of *NF1* expression [14,21]. Importantly, we describe here a novel regulatory mechanism by which miR-370 modulates *NF1* expression by directly binding to its 3′-UTR. Germline loss-of-function mutations of *NF1* lead to neurofibromatosis type 1, a dominant autosomal genetic disorder clinically characterized by neurofibromas, cafe-au-lait spots, and a high risk to develop juvenile myelomonocytic leukemia (JMML) [22]. The *NF1* gene protein product, neurofibromin, is a GTPase-activating protein (GAP) that inhibits RAS signaling by hydrolysis of active RAS-GTP into inactive RAS-GDP; therefore, *NF1* deficiencies act as functional equivalents of activating mutations in *RAS*. The finding that the wild-type allele was lost in the bone marrow of children with JMML affected by neurofibromatosis type 1 established *NF1* as a tumor suppressor gene [23]. In fact, somatic inactivation of *NF1* in hematopoietic cells results in a progressive myeloproliferative disorder in mice, with elevated levels of RAS-GTP [24], although secondary genetic events are required to the development of AML. Recently it was shown that *NF1* downregulation in AML blasts caused a substantial and significant increase in AML blast colony formation in methylcellulose, confirming that *NF1* directly influences AML blast proliferation/growth [14]. Our functional studies confirmed these results and showed that

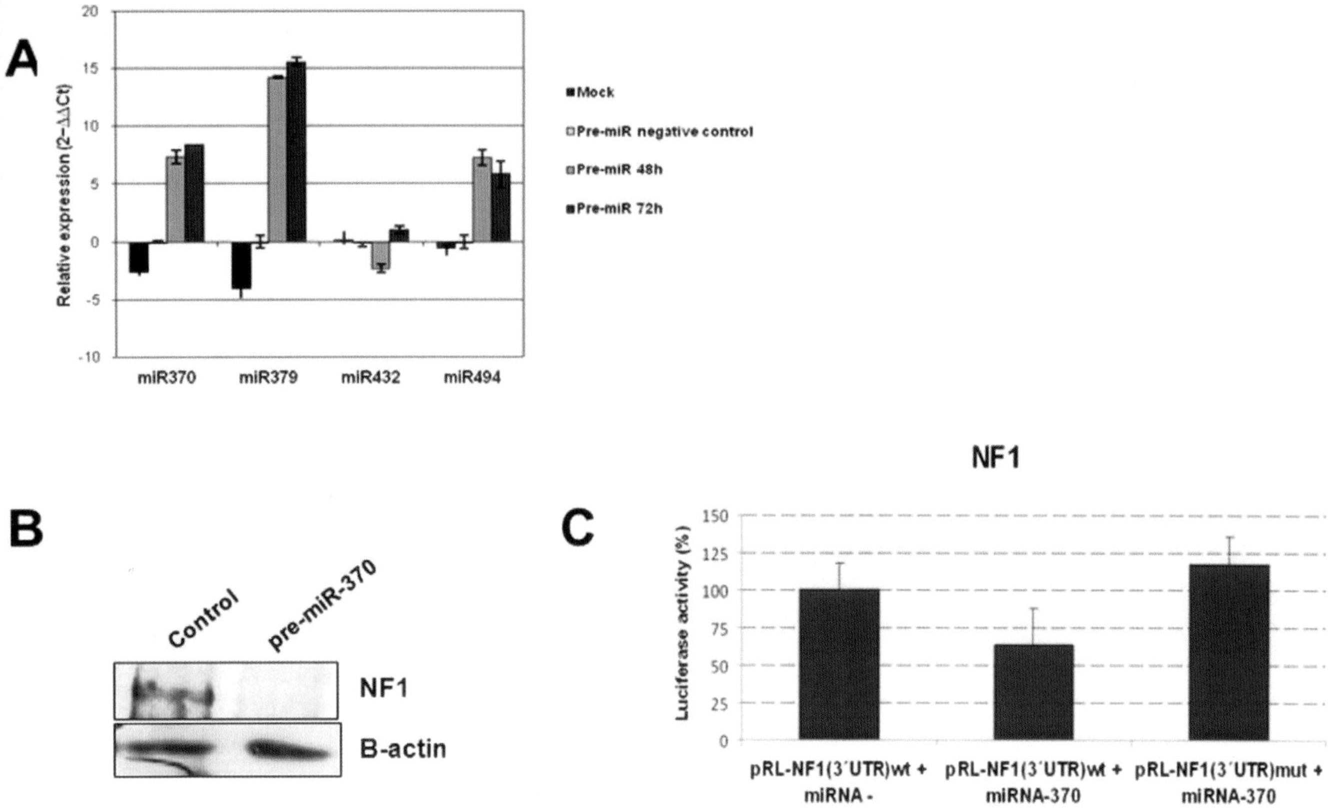

Figure 1. Functional analysis showing that miR-370 regulates *NF1*. (A) miRNAs expression analysis by real-time PCR after transfection with pre-miRs-370, −379, −432 and −494. (B) Western blot showing NF1 after transfection with pre-miR-370. (C) Luciferase assay showing changes in luciferase activity after transfection with pre-miR– (negative control) or pre-miR-370 in cells expressing the 3′UTR region of *NF1* that includes the miR-370 seed region [pRL-NF1(3′UTR)wt]. Transfection with the 3′UTR region of *NF1* including a mutated seed region for miR-370 was used as control.

overexpression of miR-370 promoted cell growth and colony forming potential of AML cells, the same effects that *NF1* downregulation. Altogether, these data strongly suggest that overexpression of miR-370 represents a novel mechanism of *NF1* inactivation in AML, and that this microRNA plays a relevant role in AML proliferation by downregulating *NF1* expression. It has been reported that miR-370 is overexpressed in acute promyelocitic leukemia [25] and gastric carcinomas [26]. However, contradictory results have been described about the functional role of this microRNA. Meng et al. found that miR-370 is a methylation-dependent miRNA regulated by interleukin-6 (IL-6), and that overexpression of miR-370 reduced the growth of cholagiocarcinoma cells by targeting the oncogene mitogen-activated protein kinase 8 (MAP3K8) [27]. In contrast, Lo et al. described that miR-370 enhanced the oncogenic potential of gastric carcinoma (GC) [26]. However, although they found that the increased in mobility induced by miR-370 in GC cells was via targeting transforming growth factor-β receptor II (TGFβ-RII), they did not observe any influence of the TGFβ pathway in the enhanced tumor cell growth elicited by miR-370 in GC cells. According to our results, it is possible that the enhanced growth after overexpressing miR-370 in GC cells observed by these authors was mediated by downregulation of *NF1*. The opposite roles of miRNA-370 in different malignancies could be explained considering that microRNAs are able to regulate the expression of multiple genes. Therefore, it is possible that miR-370 modulates the expression of all these targets; however, the dominant event may depend on cell type or cellular contexts [28]. Although miR-370 is likely to target other genes in addition to *NF1*, downregulation of *NF1* appears to play a critical role in enhanced tumorigenicity associated with overexpression of miR-370 in AML.

Quantification of the expression of *NF1* in our collection of 68 samples of patients with AML at diagnosis showed that *NF1* downregulation is a recurrent event in AML, accounting for 30.8% cases. Parkin et al. have also analyzed *NF1* expression by QRT-PCR in AML cases, and showed in their Figure 2 the high frequency of *NF1* downregulation in patients with one as well as with two copies of *NF1*; however, they did not indicate the number of cases with this downregulation [14]. Therefore, our results showed for the first time the prevalence of *NF1* downregulation in AML by QRT-PCR. Further studies in larger series of cases are needed to establish the prevalence of NF1 downregulation in AML. Deletions or/and mutations affecting *NF1* have been described as genetic aberrations responsible for *NF1* inactivation in adult AML, although inactivation mutations of *NF1* are rare events in de novo AML. Parkin et al. reported a detailed investigation in 95 AML patients and showed that 10 out of 95 (10.5%) had heterozygous deletions of the *NF1* locus, a lower percentage than our study (13/55, 26.5%)[14]. Since we used the same technique reported by this group, these results would indicate that additional studies are required to determine the real prevalence of *NF1* submicroscopic deletions in AML. In addition, in a recent study, Haferlach et al. showed that the prevalence of NF1 mutations in AML is 2% (19/889) [21]. In our study, we found 21 cases with reduced *NF1* at mRNA level: 5 had *NF1*

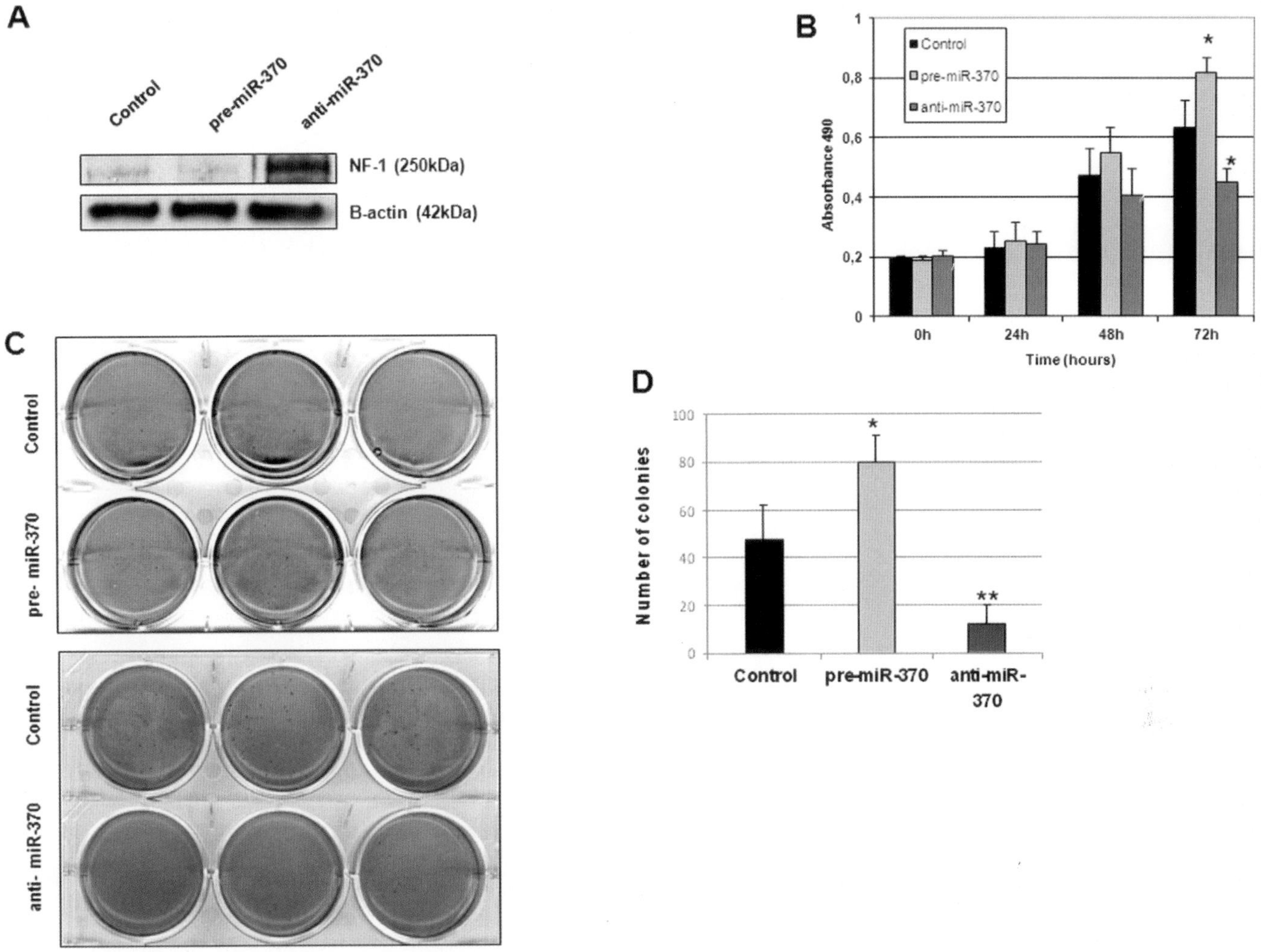

Figure 2. Effects of miR-370 on AML cell proliferation. (A) *NF1* expression after transfection with pre-miR-370 and anti-miR-370 in TF-1 cells. (B) Cell growth of TF1 cells after transfection with pre-miR-370, anti-miR-370 or miR-Control. Bars represent the mean ± SD of three independent experiments. **P*<0.05 determined using t-student test. (C) Colony forming ability of TF-1 cells transfected with miR-Control, pre-miR-370 or anti-miR-370. Bars represent the mean ± SD, experiments were done in triplicate. **P*<0.05 determined using t-student test.

deletions, 6 miR-370 overexpression, and 11 none of these aberrations (one case had both *NF1* deletion and overexpression of miR-370). Therefore, our results confirm the studies that showed that CNV could be one of the causes of *NF1* downregulation in AML [14,21], identify overexpression of miR-370 as a new mechanism of *NF1* downregulation in AML, and suggest that there are other unknown mechanisms involved in *NF1* downregulation. Therefore, it is possible that the altered expression of miR-370 could explain the 3 cases identified by Parkin et al. with normal copy number and null *NF1* expression [14].

Furthermore, in this study we have analyzed for the first time the status of NF1 protein in 14 AML patient samples, showing that the finding of null *NF1* is frequent in AML. Lu et al. (2003) had previously reported decreased bone marrow levels of the NF1 protein in 30% cases with AML (20/66) (24), a prevalence similar to that observed in this study at mRNA level (30.8%) (Table 2). The authors used solid-phase RIA to measure the NF1 protein because they were not able to detect NF1 by western blot in bone marrow samples from normal individuals. We could detect the NF1 protein in normal controls, suggesting that our results in AML cases with downregulation of Nf1 at protein level are reliable. Importantly, our results show that all patients with *NF1* downregulation, including 3 cases with overexpression of miR-370, have no protein at all. Moreover, we identified a case with normal levels of both *NF1* mRNA and miR-370 and no protein, confirming the complex regulation of *NF1*, and showing that there are other mechanisms of *NF1* regulation at post-transcriptional level. Parkin at al. have shown that complete *NF1* loss is required to Ras activation, and that heterozygous *NF1* states that preserve some *NF1* expression are not sufficient for robust Ras activation [14]. Of note, AML blasts without functional *NF1* were substantially and significantly more sensitive to mTOR inhibition than *NF1* wild-type blasts or blasts with one preserved *NF1* copy and retained *NF1* expression [14]. Therefore, our results would point out to a new group of patients susceptible of receiving these therapies.

In summary, our integrative analysis including data from high resolution SNPs arrays, mRNA expression arrays, and miRNAs expression profiles in 16 myeloid cell lines highlights that copy number alterations are alternative mechanisms to deregulate the expression of miRNAs in AML, and represent a novel approach to identify novel candidate genes involved in AML. Of note, functional studies identified *NF1* as a target of the miR-370 and,

Table 2. Clinical and molecular characteristics of the 70 patients with AML at diagnosis included in the study.

Sex		No.	(%)
	Male	49	(70)
	Female	21	(30)
Age			
	<60 years	24	(34.8)
	≥60 years	45	(65.2)
	No data	1	
Diagnosis			
	AML-M0	6	(8.6)
	AML-M1	19	(27.2)
	AML-M2	16	(22.8)
	AML-M4	6	(8.6)
	AML-M5	15	(21.4)
	AML-M6	2	(2.8)
	AML-NOS	6	(8.6)
Secondary AML			
	No	60	(87)
	Yes	9	(13)
	No data	1	
Cytogenetic group			
	good	4	(5.8)
	intermediate	59	(85.5)
	poor	6	(8.7)
	No data	1	
NF1 downregulation			
	No	47	(69.2)
	Yes	21	(30.8)
	No data	2	
Deletions affecting *NF1* locus			
	No	32	(76.4)
	Yes	13	(23.6)
	No data	15	
miR-370 overexpression			
	No	40	(87)
	Yes	6	(13)
	No data	24	
FLT3-ITD			
	No	40	(78.4)
	Yes	11	(21.6)
	No data	19	
NPM1 mutated			
	No	23	(54.8)
	Yes	19	(45.2)
	No data	28	

in agreement with the tumor suppressor activity of *NF1*, we found that overexpression of miR-370 enhanced the tumorigenic potential of AML cells. Finally, QRT-PCR and western blot analyses showed that *NF1* downregulation is a common event in AML, and that both deletions in the *NF1* locus and overexpression of miR-370 represent two alternative mechanisms to downregulate *NF1* in this disease. Since *NF1* deficiency leads to the activation of the RAS signaling pathway, patients with AML and overexpression of miR-370 may potentially benefit from additional treatment with either RAS or mTOR inhibitors. Further studies are required to identify other mechanisms leading to *NF1* deficiency and to decipher the prognostic impact of *NF1* inactivation in AML.

Materials and Methods

Cell culture and transfection

EOL-1, HL-60, Kasumi-1, OCI-AML2, MOLM13, MV4-11, HEL, KG-1, KYO-1, K562 and MEG-01 cells were maintained in RPMI-1640 (Invitrogen) with 10% fetal bovine serum (FBS); NOMO-1 and KU-812 in RPMI-1640 with 20% FBS; F-36P in RPMI-1640 with 20% FBS, and 10 ng/ml GM-CSF; MUTZ-3 in 80% alpha-MEM with 20% FBS and 10 ng/ml GM-CSF; and TF-1 in RPMI-1640 with 20% FBS and 5 ng/ml GM-CSF. Cell lines were grown at 37°C in a 5% CO2 atmosphere. Media were supplemented with penicillin G (100 U/ml), and streptomycin (0.1 mg/ml). Cell lines were obtained from the DSM Cell Culture Bank (Braunschweig, Germany). Characteristics of the 16 myeloid cell lines used in this study are summarized in Table S6. For transfection experiments HL-60 and TF-1 cells were seeded in culture flasks and transfected using the Nucleofector System (solution V and protocol T-019 for HL-60 cells; solution T and protocol T-001 for TF-1 cells) (Amaxa) with 5 nM of pre-miRNAs designed and synthesized by Ambion (Applied Biosystems) (hsa-miR-370 ID/PM12868; hsa-miR-432 ID/PM10838; hsa-miR-379 ID/PM10316; hsa-miR-494 ID/PM12409; anti-hsa-miR-370 ID/AM12868, hsa-miR-Control ID/AM17110), or with 100 pmol of NF-1 and scramble siRNA oligonucleotides (NF-1 siRNA: 5′-AAGGUUGCGCAGUUAGCAGUU-3′ and scramble siRNA: 5′-UUCUCCGAACGUGUCACGU-3′) synthesized by MGW Biotech (Ebersberg, Germany).

Patient samples

The study comprised bone marrow samples of 70 patients with AML at diagnosis. Bone marrow samples of normal healthy donors were used as controls.

Ethics Statement

The study has been approved by the Comisión de Ética de Investigación de la Facultad de Medicina de la Universidad de Navarra (037/2008). Informed consent for this study is not required because the samples are anonymous (anonymous samples have neither personal data nor individual clinical information that could allow the identity of the donor to be traced).

Single Nucleotide Polymorphism Array Analysis

Whole genome analyses were performed using the GeneChip Mapping 500 K Array Set (Affymetrix). Genomic DNA samples were isolated using QiAmpDNA MiniKit (Qiagen). Arrays were scanned individually using the GeneChip® Scanner 3000 7G under the GeneChip® CEL files were generated using Affymetrix GeneChip Command Console operating software and Genotyping Console 2.1 according to the manufacturer protocols (Affymetrix). We only analyzed samples which met the quality control (QC) thresholds recommended by Affymetrix in their Genotyping Console v2.1 software. The QC call rate of samples analyzed was at least 96%. Samples not meeting this specification were excluded from further analysis. CEL files were then imported into Partek Genomic Suite and analyzed using the Copy Number Analysis

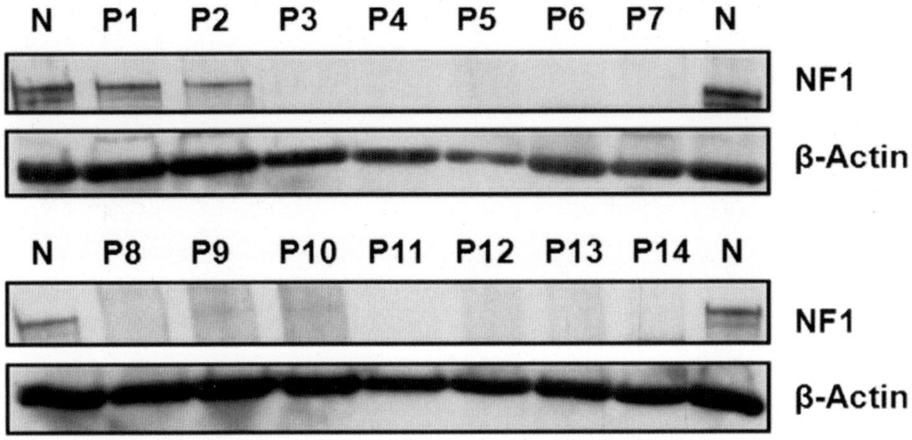

	Case	NF1 locus	NF1 downregulation	miR-370 overexpression
P1	32014	normal	no	no
P2	44581	normal	no	no
P3	27990	normal	yes	no
P4	24731	deleted	yes	yes
P5	27298	normal	yes	no
P6	23816	normal	yes	no data
P7	21507	normal	yes	yes
P8	44459	deleted	no	no
P9	29239	normal	no	no
P10	26499	normal	no	no
P11	43756	deleted	yes	no
P12	44325	normal	yes	no
P13	44214	deleted	yes	no
P14	24043	normal	yes	yes

Figure 3. Western blot analysis of NF1 in 14 samples of patients with AML at diagnosis. Data about NF1 status and expression of miR-370 are shown. N: normal control; P: patient sample.

workflow. Regions of CNVs were detected using an unpaired analysis and Genomic segmentation algorithm in the standard Partek. Genomic alterations identified by SNP array (SNPa) were compared with the 500K HapMap Genotype Data Set. We consider as amplification the regions whose copy number was over 3 copies, and as deletion, regions with copy number below 1.5 (homozygous deletion CN<0.5 and hemizygous deletions CN = 0.8–1.5) [8]. We considered the karyotype of each cell line to asses that results obtained in the SNPa analysis are not due to the presence of a previously described cytogenetic aberration.

Validation of copy number alterations

Genomic regions located within miRNAs genes were amplified with the primers included in Table S7. Glucose-6-Phosphate Dehydrogenase (*G6PDH*), Hydroxymethylbilane Synthase (*HEM3*) and Chloride channel 7 (*CLCN7*) genes were selected as internal controls for varying input DNA amounts as recommended by prior published guidelines [9,10]. Thus, any difference in the real time PCR obtained for test primers/markers would correspond to differences in the amount of the target sequence primers. SYBR Green I real time PCR assays were carried out in final reaction volumes of 15 µl with 7.5 µl of SYBR Green I Master mix (Applied Biosystems), 1 µM of forward and reverse primers and 10 ng of genomic DNA. Real time PCR reactions were performed using the 7500 Real Time PCR System (Applied Biosystems). The reaction profile was: initial step, 50°C for 2 min, denaturation, 95°C for 10 min, then 40 cycles of denaturing at 95°C for 15 sec, combined annealing and extension at 60°C for 30 sec and 72°C 30 sec, followed by the dissociation stage of 72°C 10 min. Data were analyzed as previously described [10].

Quantification of miRNA expression levels

Total RNA was isolated using TRIzol Reagent (Invitrogen) according to manufacturer's instructions. For quantification of miRNA expression levels, samples were reverse transcribed using the TaqManHMicroRNA Reverse Transcription Kit (P/N 4366597, Applied Biosystems) and mature miRNAs were quantified by quantitative real-time RT-PCR (QRT-PCR) using the TaqManH MicroRNA Assays - Human Panel Early Access Kit (P/N 4365409, Applied Biosystems). The kit contained assays for 250 miRNAs of the 733 currently listed in the Sanger miRBase database. Expression levels of miR-370, miR-379, miR-494, and miR-432 were confirmed using TaqMan MicroRNA Assays (Applied Biosystems) specific for each miRNA and U6B as internal control. Analysis of relative gene expression data was performed using the $2^{-\Delta\Delta C_T}$ method [11]where $\Delta\Delta C_T = (C_{T,\text{Target Gene}} - C_{T,\text{U6B}})_{\text{Cell Line}} - (C_{T,\text{Target Gene}} - C_{T,\text{U6B}})_{\text{Normal Control}}$.

Gene Expression Profiling

Total RNA was extracted from cell lines using miRNEasy Mini Kit (Qiagen) following manufacturer's protocol. The RNA integrity was assessed using Agilent 2100 Bioanalyzer (Agilent). Whole genome expression analysis was performed in the cell lines using the Affymetrix Human Genome-U133 Plus-2.0, which contains 54,676 probesets (47,000 transcripts). Microarray data analysis consisted in background correction and normalization using RMA algorithm [12] and a filtering process to eliminate low expression probesets. LIMMA (Linear Models for Microarray Data) [13] was used to identify the probesets with significant differential expression. Genes were selected as significant using a *B* statistic cut off ($B>0$) or a less stringent *P*-value cut off ($P<0.001$).

Quantification of NF1 by real-time RT-PCR and validation of copy number alterations

Total RNA was isolated using the RNeasy minikit (Qiagen). cDNA was synthesized with SuperScriptIII Reverse Transcriptase (Invitrogen). Quantification of the expression of *NF1* was performed by SYBR Green I real time PCR assays (Applied Biosystems), using specific primers for each gene (NF1_Fwd: AAGCCCTCACAACA-ACCAAC; NF1 Rv: GACAATACA-CAGCATCAATCT; HPRT Fwd: TGACAC-TGGCAAAA-CAATGCA; HPRT Rv: GGTCCTTTTCACCAGCAAGCT). *HPRT* was used as internal control. Analysis of relative gene expression data was performed using the $2^{-\Delta\Delta C_T}$ method [11]where $\Delta\Delta C_T = (C_{T,\text{Target Gene}} - C_{T,\text{HPRT}})_{\text{Cell Line}} - (C_{T,\text{Target Gene}} - C_{T,\text{HPRT}})_{\text{Normal Control}}$. A gene was considered deregulated if its expression value was higher or lower than the cut-off value established for each gene (mean+3SD), defined by the analysis of 10 normal BM samples.

Quantification of genomic copy number changes at the *NF1* locus (17q11) was performed using specific TaqMan-based probes for *NF1* (Hs06413068_cn) and *RAG2* (Hs01851142_s1) (Applied Biosystems) as previously described [14]. DNA was extracted using QuiAmp DNA Mini Kit (Qiagen). Analysis of relative gene copy number data for *NF1* was performed using the $\Delta\Delta C_T$ method. As indicated by Parkin et al. (2010), the C_T values for the *RAG2* locus were used as reference [14].

Integrative Genomic Analyses

Relationship between miRNA expression and the CN of the corresponding miRNA gene locus was measured by a parametric analysis. Data from SNP and miRNA analysis were crossed and analyzed using t-tests. A statistical hypothesis test was performed for each miRNA profile using the results of the CNV analysis (amplification/deletion) as sample labels. Associations were considered statistically significant when $P<0.05$. The set of differentially expressed genes were further studied using miRNA predicted targets stored in public databases to identify coherent targets [15,16,17,18,19].

Western blot analysis

Protein extracts were isolated using TRIzol Reagent (Invitrogen) following manufacturer's indications, clarified (12,000×g, 15 minutes, 4°C), denatured and subjected to sodium dodecyl sulfate-polyacrylamide gel electrophoresis and Western blot. Antibodies used were rabbit polyclonal anti-Nf1 (Santa Cruz) and mouse monoclonal anti-β-actin (Sigma-Aldrich). Proteins were detected with the appropriate secondary antibodies by chemiluminescence (ECL kit, GE Healthcare).

Luciferase assays

Luciferase assays were done using the Dual Luciferase System (Promega). One hundred nanograms of pRL-NF1(3′UTR) or pRL were transfected in the presence of 5 ng of pre-miR-370 or pre-miR-negative control, and 50 ng of pGL3-Promoter. A pRL-NF1(3′UTR) construct including a mutated miR-370 seed region was used to confirm *NF1* as a direct target of miR-370. Renilla luciferase activities were normalized to firefly luciferase activities.

Proliferation assays

TF-1 cells transfected with pre-miR-370, anti-miR-370, pre-miR-control, NF-1 siRNA or scramble siRNA, were seeded at 7.5×10^3 cells/well in 96-well plates. Cell growth was assessed by MTS assay using the CellTiter 96 Aqueous One Solution Cell Proliferation Assay (Promega) and following the manufacturer's indications. Experiments were performed in triplicate and repeated at least 3 times.

Colony-forming assay

Experiments were performed in 6-well plates were coated with 0.6% soft agarose (Sigma) in medium. 1×10^5 TF-1 transfected cells were suspended in 0.3% agarose in medium and plated in triplicated over the pre-coated wells. Fresh medium was supplied thrice a week. After 7 days, colonies were stained by adding 500 ul of 5 mg/mL MTT (Methylthiazolyldiphenyl-tetrazolium bromide, M-5655, Sigma) for 4 h at 37°C. Then, colonies were fixed by adding DMSO overnight at 37°C. Colony numbers were determined from triplicates.

Supporting Information

Figure S1 Boxplots of miRNAs whose expression significantly correlated with the inferred CN of the corresponding region. Cell lines are classified as carrying or not **A.** gain/amplification (inferred CN >3) or **B.** loss/deletion (inferred CN <1.5) of each specific miRNA gene.

Figure S2 Knockdown of NF1 reduces cell growth and colony-forming ability of TF-1 cells. A. Relative NF1 gene expression levels in TF-1 cells 48 h after transfection with scrambled and NF1 siRNA. Bars represent the fold change calculated by the 2−ΔCt method. Expression was normalized to the HPRT1 gene. **B.** Western blot showing NF1 expression levels from TF-1 cells transfected with NF1-targeting or scrambled siRNA, 48 h post-transfection. β-actin was used as a loading control. **C.** Growth curves of scrambled and NF1 siRNA-transfected TF-1 cells. *P<0.05 Student's t test. Data shown are mean ± SD of triplicate cultures and are representative of three independent experiments. **D.** Representative images of colonies formed by scramble and NF1 siRNA-transfected TF-1 cells after two weeks grown in soft agar. **E.** Number of colonies formed in the colony formation assay. **P<0.01, Student's t test. Data represented are mean ± SD.

Figure S3 Scatterplot showing the significant association between down expression of NF1 and high expression of miR-370.

Table S1 Genomic regions with amplifications or deletions found at least in 4 out of the 16 myeloid cell lines analyzed. Amplification was considered if CN >3, and deletion if CN <1.5.

Table S2 List of the high amplifications (CN>5) and homozygous deletions (CN<0.5) found in the copy number analysis of 16 myeloid cell lines.

Table S3 MicroRNAs located in amplified regions in myeloid cell lines, which were highly expressed, and had *NF1* as a potential target gene.

Table S4 NF1 status and miR-370 expression in the 68 samples of patients with AML at diagnosis included in the study.

Table S5 Clinical and molecular characteristics of 14 patients with AML at diagnosis included in the study of NF1 at protein level.

Table S6 Clinical and molecular characteristics of the 16 human myeloid cell lines.

Table S7 Oligonucleotide primers used for real-time Q-PCR.

Acknowledgments

We thank Victor Segura and Alberto Orta for bioinformatics analysis, and Marisol Gonzalez-Huarriz for technical assistance.

Author Contributions

Conceived and designed the experiments: LGO IC RCC MDO. Performed the experiments: LGO IC CC RCC NM. Analyzed the data: LGO IC CC RCC EG. Contributed reagents/materials/analysis tools: MJC. Wrote the paper: IC RCC MDO.

References

1. Marcucci G, Mrozek K, Radmacher MD, Garzon R, Bloomfield CD (2011) The prognostic and functional role of microRNAs in acute myeloid leukemia. Blood 117: 1121–1129.
2. Garzon R, Croce CM (2008) MicroRNAs in normal and malignant hematopoiesis. Curr Opin Hematol 15: 352–358.
3. Waldman SA, Terzic A (2009) A study of microRNAs in silico and in vivo: diagnostic and therapeutic applications in cancer. FEBS J 276: 2157–2164.
4. Garzon R, Volinia S, Liu CG, Fernandez-Cymering C, Palumbo T, et al. (2008) MicroRNA signatures associated with cytogenetics and prognosis in acute myeloid leukemia. Blood 111:3183–3189.
5. Schwind S, Maharry K, Radmacher MD, Mrozek K, Holland KB, et al. (2010) Prognostic significance of expression of a single microRNA, miR-181a, in cytogenetically normal acute myeloid leukemia: a Cancer and Leukemia Group B study. J Clin Oncol 28: 5257–5264.
6. Calin GA, Sevignani C, Dumitru CD, Hyslop T, Noch E, et al. (2004) Human microRNA genes are frequently located at fragile sites and genomic regions involved in cancers. Proc Natl Acad Sci U S A 101: 2999–3004.
7. Starczynowski DT, Morin R, McPherson A, Lam J, Chari R, et al. (2011) Genome-wide identification of human microRNAs located in leukemia-associated genomic alterations. Blood 117: 595–607.
8. Schiffman JD, Wang Y, McPherson LA, Welch K, Zhang N, et al. (2009) Molecular inversion probes reveal patterns of 9p21 deletion and copy number aberrations in childhood leukemia. Cancer Genet Cytogenet 193: 9–18.
9. Babashah S, Jamali S, Mahdian R, Nosaeid MH, Karimipoor M, et al. (2009) Detection of unknown deletions in beta-globin gene cluster using relative quantitative PCR methods. Eur J Haematol 83: 261–269.
10. Weksberg R, Hughes S, Moldovan L, Bassett AS, Chow EW, et al. (2005) A method for accurate detection of genomic microdeletions using real-time quantitative PCR. BMC Genomics 6: 180.
11. Livak KJ, Schmittgen TD (2001) Analysis of relative gene expression data using real-time quantitative PCR and the 2(-Delta Delta C(T)) Method. Methods 25: 402–408.
12. Irizarry RA, Bolstad BM, Collin F, Cope LM, Hobbs B, et al. (2003) Summaries of Affymetrix GeneChip probe level data. Nucleic Acids Res 31: e15.
13. Smyth GK (2004) Linear models and empirical bayes methods for assessing differential expression in microarray experiments. Stat Appl Genet Mol Biol 3: Article3.
14. Parkin B, Ouillette P, Wang Y, Liu Y, Wright W, et al. (2010) NF1 inactivation in adult acute myelogenous leukemia. Clin Cancer Res 16: 4135–4147.
15. Friedman RC, Farh KK, Burge CB, Bartel DP (2009) Most mammalian mRNAs are conserved targets of microRNAs. Genome Res 19: 92–105.
16. Lall S, Grun D, Krek A, Chen K, Wang YL, et al. (2006) A genome-wide map of conserved microRNA targets in C. elegans. Curr Biol 16: 460–471.
17. Kertesz M, Iovino N, Unnerstall U, Gaul U, Segal E (2007) The role of site accessibility in microRNA target recognition. Nat Genet 39: 1278–1284.
18. Betel D, Wilson M, Gabow A, Marks DS, Sander C (2008) The microRNA.org resource: targets and expression. Nucleic Acids Res 36: D149–153.
19. Griffiths-Jones S, Saini HK, van Dongen S, Enright AJ (2008) miRBase: tools for microRNA genomics. Nucleic Acids Res 36: D154–158.
20. Marcucci G, Radmacher MD, Mrozek K, Bloomfield CD (2009) MicroRNA expression in acute myeloid leukemia. Curr Hematol Malig Rep 4: 83–88.
21. Haferlach C, Grossmann V, Kohlmann A, Schindela S, Kern W, et al. (2012) Deletion of the tumor-suppressor gene NF1 occurs in 5% of myeloid malignancies and is accompanied by a mutation in the remaining allele in half of the cases. Leukemia 26:834–839.
22. Brems H, Beert E, de Ravel T, Legius E (2009) Mechanisms in the pathogenesis of malignant tumours in neurofibromatosis type 1. Lancet Oncol 10: 508–515.
23. Shannon KM, O'Connell P, Martin GA, Paderanga D, Olson K, et al. (1994) Loss of the normal NF1 allele from the bone marrow of children with type 1 neurofibromatosis and malignant myeloid disorders. N Engl J Med 330: 597–601.
24. Largaespada DA, Brannan CI, Jenkins NA, Copeland NG (1996) Nf1 deficiency causes Ras-mediated granulocyte/macrophage colony stimulating factor hypersensitivity and chronic myeloid leukaemia. Nat Genet 12: 137–143.
25. Dixon-McIver A, East P, Mein CA, Cazier JB, Molloy G, et al. (2008) Distinctive patterns of microRNA expression associated with karyotype in acute myeloid leukaemia. PLoS One 3: e2141.
26. Lo SS, Hung PS, Chen JH, Tu HF, Fang WL, et al. (2012) Overexpression of miR-370 and downregulation of its novel target TGFbeta-RII contribute to the progression of gastric carcinoma. Oncogene 31: 226–237.
27. Meng F, Wehbe-Janek H, Henson R, Smith H, Patel T (2008) Epigenetic regulation of microRNA-370 by interleukin-6 in malignant human cholangiocytes. Oncogene 27: 378–386.
28. Bartel DP (2009) MicroRNAs: target recognition and regulatory functions. Cell 136: 215–233.

Retinal Neurodegeneration in Wilson's Disease Revealed by Spectral Domain Optical Coherence Tomography

Philipp Albrecht[1]*, Ann-Kristin Müller[1], Marius Ringelstein[1], David Finis[2], Gerd Geerling[2], Eva Cohn[1], Orhan Aktas[1], Hans-Peter Hartung[1], Harald Hefter[1,9], Axel Methner[1,9]

1 Department of Neurology, Medical Faculty, Heinrich-Heine University, Düsseldorf, Germany, **2** Department of Ophthalmology, Medical Faculty, Heinrich-Heine University, Düsseldorf, Germany

Abstract

Background/Objective: In addition to cirrhosis of the liver, Wilson's disease leads to copper accumulation and widespread degeneration of the nervous system. Delayed visual evoked potentials (VEPs) suggest changes to the visual system and potential structural changes of the retina.

Methods: We used the latest generation of spectral domain optical coherence tomography to assess the retinal morphology of 42 patients with Wilson's disease and 76 age- and sex-matched controls. We measured peripapillary retinal nerve fiber layer (RNFL) thickness and total macular thickness and manually segmented all retinal layers in foveal scans of 42 patients with Wilson's disease and 76 age- and sex-matched controls. The results were compared with VEPs and clinical parameters.

Results: The mean thickness of the RNFL, paramacular region, retinal ganglion cell/inner plexiform layer and inner nuclear layer was reduced in Wilson's disease. VEPs were altered with delayed N75 and P100 latencies, but the N140 latency and amplitude was unchanged. An analysis of the laboratory parameters indicated that the serum concentrations of copper and caeruloplasmin positively correlated with the thickness of the outer plexiform layer and with N75 and P100 VEP latencies.

Conclusion: Neuronal degeneration in Wilson's disease involves the retina and changes can be quantified by optical coherence tomography. While the VEPs and the thickness of the outer plexiform layer appear to reflect the current copper metabolism, the thicknesses of the RNFL, ganglion cell/inner plexiform layer, inner nuclear layer and the total paramacular thickness may be the best indicators of chronic neuronal degeneration.

Editor: Pablo Villoslada, Institute Biomedical Research August Pi Sunyer (IDIBAPS) - Hospital Clinic of Barcelona, Spain

Funding: The Department of Neurology, Heinrich-Heine-Universität Düsseldorf, is supported in part by the Walter-and-Ilse-Rose-Stiftung (for OCT research, to OA and HPH) and in part by the "Deutsche Forschungsgemeinschaft" through Sonderforschungsbereich 974 "Kommunikation und Systemrelevanz bei Leberschädigung und Regeneration" (for research regarding CNS involvement upon liver damage, TP B7, to OA). The funders had no role in study design, data collection and analysis, decision to publish, or preparation of the manuscript.

Competing Interests: The authors have declared that no competing interests exist.

* E-mail: phil.albrecht@gmail.com

9 These authors contributed equally to this work.

Introduction

Wilson's disease is an autosomal recessively inherited disorder that leads to copper accumulation and, consequently, to hepatic damage and neuropsychological symptoms [1,2]. The causative mutations affect the copper-transporting P-type ATPase ATP7B, which regulates the hepatic copper metabolism, leading to impaired biliary excretion and the toxic accumulation of copper primarily in the brain and liver (reviewed in [3] and [4]). Intracellular copper deposits impede inhibitor of apoptosis proteins (IAPs), which eventually causes apoptotic cell death [5]. The clinical presentation varies from predominantly hepatic to predominantly neurologic and shows great heterogeneity regarding severity, age of onset and initial symptoms [6]. Wilson's disease results in severe disability and death if untreated. The key neurological features comprise extrapyramidal symptoms, ataxia, dystonia, seizures and psychiatric symptoms, such as personality changes, depression and psychosis (reviewed in [7]). Structural changes in the brain of Wilson's disease patients have been well documented by magnetic resonance imaging (MRI), which has revealed lesions of the basal ganglia, midbrain, pons and cerebellum and widespread cortical atrophy and white matter changes [8,9]. Histological studies have reported necrosis, gliosis and cystic changes in the brainstem, thalamus, cerebellum and cerebral cortex of Wilson's disease patients [4]. The functional consequences of these structural changes have been demonstrated in the acoustic, sensory, motor and visual systems and are reflected by disordered multimodality evoked potentials [10–13]. Visual evoked potentials (VEPs) have been reported to be abnormal in approximately 50% of symptomatic Wilson's disease patients [10,11,14–16]. Common ocular findings of Wilson's disease include the Kayser–Fleischer ring and sunflower cataracts. Both are due to copper deposition and do not cause visual impairment, suggesting that the observed pathologies in VEPs may be explained by retroocular changes. However, altered flash electroretinograms in Wilson's disease are indicative of a retinal pathology [12]. Optical coherence tomography is a fast and non-invasive technique and the latest generation of OCT devices is capable of depicting retinal changes at nearly the cellular level [17–25]. In this study, we used up-to-date OCT technology to analyze the retinal changes in Wilson's disease patients. We compared the morphological changes measured by a state-of-the-art spectral domain OCT device with VEPs as functional parameters and correlated these findings with laboratory parameters and a clinical Wilson's disease score [26].

Materials and Methods

Ethics Statement

The work was conducted in accordance with the declaration of Helsinki. Written informed consent was obtained from all patients and the study was approved by the local ethics committee, the "Ethikkommission der Heinrich Heine Universität, Düsseldorf".

Patients

We examined 42 patients with Wilson's disease and 76 control patients without ophthalmologic, inflammatory or degenerative neurological disease. All Wilson's disease patients were clinically diagnosed following the established criteria [27], underwent longterm follow-up examinations (mean follow up period 10±1 years) and were under therapy with D-penicillamine, trientine, tetrathiomolybdate and/or zinc. The copper and caeruloplasmin concentrations in serum and the 24 h urine copper excretion were measured at the time of the ocular exam and the patients were scored using an established clinical score [26]. All patients underwent formal ophthalmologic exams to rule out confounding ocular pathologies and three eyes were excluded due to central serous retinopathy, vitreomacular traction or paramacular scars.

Patients were consecutively recruited from the outpatient clinic of the department of neurology at the Heinrich-Heine University Düsseldorf, Germany.

Optical Coherence Tomography

The details of the principles of spectral-domain OCT have been described elsewhere [28]. Using a Spectralis OCT device (Heidelberg Engineering, Heidelberg, Germany) with image alignment eye tracking-software (TruTrack, Heidelberg Engineering, Heidelberg, Germany), we obtained perifoveal volumetric retinal scans consisting of 25 single vertical axial scans (scanning area: 6 × 6 mm, centered at the fovea). To assess the peripapillary RNFL, a circular scan with a diameter of approximately 3.4 mm was performed after manually positioning the center on the middle of the optic disc (figure 1 A). Furthermore, we performed high-resolution horizontal scans through the middle of the fovea. All of the scans were performed using the eye-tracking system. The RNFL measurements and high-resolution single horizontal scans were averaged from 100 images and measurements for volumetric calculations were averaged from 10 scans (Automatic Real Time, ART). All of the scans were of sufficient or good quality (>20 DB) and fulfilled OSCAR-IB quality control criteria for OCT scans [29].

While the results of the RNFL- and paramacular volumetric measurements were automatically analyzed by the Heidelberg Eye explorer software, the paramacular retinal layers were manually segmented as previously described [18,30]. In brief, the segmentation of the different retinal layers in the single horizontal foveal scans was performed manually by repositioning the measurement lines (the white dotted lines in figure 2 A) on

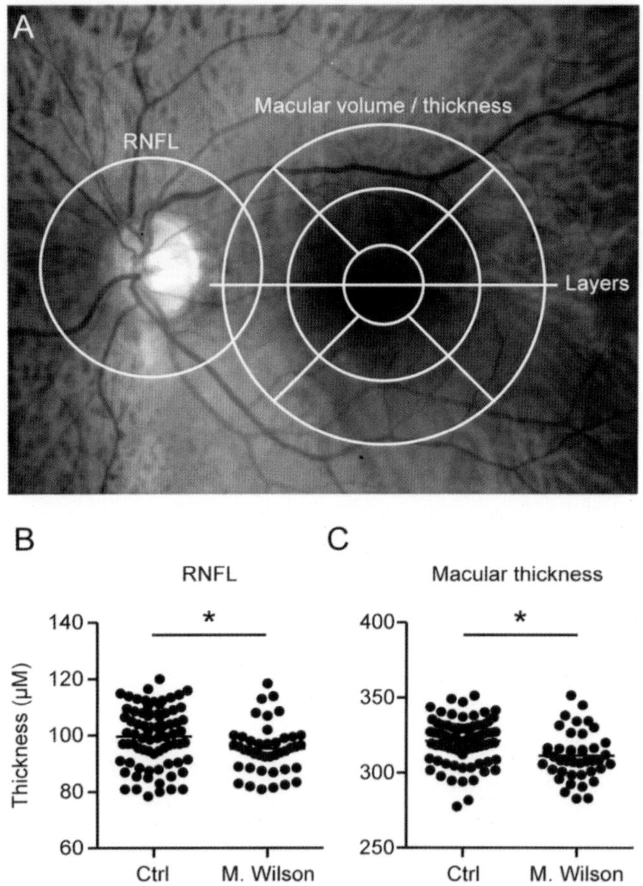

Figure 1. RNFL and mean macular thickness are reduced in Wilson's disease. A The areas of measurement are marked in an image of the fundus. The RNFL was measured in a circular scan centered on the optic disc and the macular thickness in scans around the fovea. The manual segmentation of the retinal layers was performed in a horizontal scan through the center of the fovea. The scatter plots display the thickness of the RNFL (**B**) and the total macular thickness (**C**). Each point represents the mean of the two eyes of one patient. The mean of all patients is indicated by a horizontal bar. Significant differences are indicated by asterisks ($p<0.05$, two-tailed t-test).

the borders between the different layers and measuring the layers at their thickest points nasally and temporally of the macula. In most subjects, the outer nuclear layer (ONL) presented only one central thickest point rather than nasal and temporal peaks as in the other layers. We therefore used the thickness at this point for analysis (the central vertical line in figure 2 A). In the few subjects with a nasal and temporal ONL thickness peaks, we used the higher value.

Visual Evoked Potentials (VEPs)

VEPs were recorded in 27 Wilson's disease patients and 26 control probands using monocular stimulation with a fullfield black and white checkerboard generated on a TV monitor and reversed in contrast at a rate of 3.1/s. The square size was 12 mm, which subtended a visual angle of 41 min at the subject's eyes. VEPs were recorded from the scalp using pin electrodes positioned at Oz (active) and Fz (reference) sites. A total of 150 responses were averaged in each recording and two trials were performed for each eye. The peak latencies of N75, P100 and N140 and peak-to-peak-amplitudes from P100 to N140 were measured.

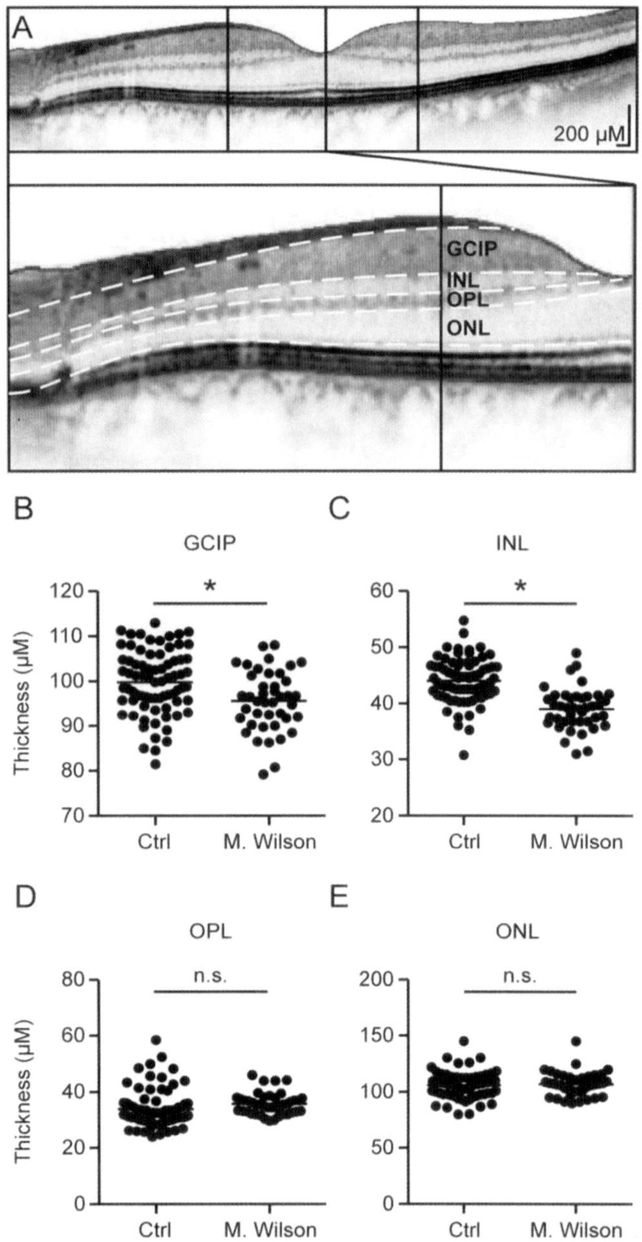

Figure 2. Manual segmentation: the thickness of GCIP and INL is reduced in Wilson's disease. A The different retinal layers were manually segmented in single horizontal foveal scans and the images are displayed as negatives to better differentiate the different layers. The thickness of the different layers was measured at the vertical lines indicating the thickest point, both nasally and temporally of the fovea, except for the ONL, which was measured centrally along the vertical line. **B–E** Scatter plots of the mean thickness of the different retinal layers. Each point represents the mean of the two eyes of one patient. The mean of all patients is indicated by a horizontal bar. Significant differences are indicated by asterisks ($p<0.05$, two-tailed t test); non-significant differences are indicated as n.s.

Statistical Evaluation

Statistical analyses were performed using Microsoft Excel and Prism 5.0 (GraphPad) and SPSS Statistics 20 (IBM). To compare Wilson's disease patients with controls, a two-tailed t-test was used and both eyes of each subject were included in the analysis as statistically dependent duplicates. ANOVA with Tukey's post hoc test was used to compare more than two groups in the subgroup analysis.

P-values below 0.05 were considered significant. Correlations between two eye parameters were evaluated using the values only from the left eyes of the patients, while laboratory parameters and clinical scores were correlated with the parameters of both eyes as statistically dependent duplicates. A Pearson correlation analysis was used for normally distributed parametric values and a Spearman correlation analysis was used for nonparametric or non-normally distributed values. SPSS partial correlation analysis was performed to calculate multivariate correlations of OCT- and VEP parameters, adjusting for age, sex, laboratory parameters and clinical disease score. Subjects with missing data were excluded from the respective analysis.

The means and standard deviations are reported in the results section.

Results

The patients and controls did not differ significantly in age or sex. The OCT findings, laboratory parameters and clinical data are shown in table 1.

Routine OCT Parameters, RNFL Thickness and Macular Thickness

The peripapillary RNFL thickness, paramacular thickness and the thickness of the different retinal layers were measured as illustrated in figure 1A. The patients' retinal parameters are shown in table 1. The mean peripapillary RNFL was significantly thinner compared to age and sex matched controls (Means ± standard deviation (M±SD): Wilson's disease 95.3±8.8 μm vs. controls 99.6±10.4 μm, figure 1 A) as was the mean total macular thickness (M±SD: Wilson's disease 311.2±15.79 μm vs. controls 321.0±14.8 μm, figure 1 B). The reduction of the macular thickness was most pronounced in the inferior quadrant and this was the only quadrant that was significantly reduced in Wilson's disease patients compared with controls. The RNFL of our Wilson's disease patients was more homogenously reduced and none of the quadrants alone was significantly reduced.

OCT Manual Segmentation

Due to the high resolution of the latest generation spectral-domain OCT device used in this study, we were capable of identifying the different retinal layers in transfoveal scans. We manually segmented the retinal layers in horizontal scans through the middle of the fovea and measured the thickness of the different layers (figure 2 A) as previously described [18,30]. The results are summarized in table 1.

The retinal ganglion cell- and inner plexiform layer complex (GCIP) and the inner nuclear layer (INL) were reduced in Wilson's disease patients (M±SD: GCIP: 95.5±0.8 μm, INL: 38.9±3.6 μm) compared with controls (M±SD: GCIP: 99.8±0.8 μm, INL: 44.1±0.5 μm) (figure 2B–C).

We observed no significant differences in the thickness of the mean outer plexiform layer (M±SD: OPL: controls 33.9±0.8 μm, Wilson's disease 36.2±0.7 μm) or the outer nuclear layer (M±SD: ONL: controls: 106±1.3 μm, Wilson's disease: 106±1.4 μm) (figure 2D–E).

Visual Evoked Potentials

The N75 and P100 latencies of the VEPs were significantly prolonged in our Wilson's disease patients (M±SD: N75:80.3 ms ±8.3, P100:108 ms ±6.8) compared with controls (M±SD:

Table 1. OCT-, clinical- and laboratory parameters.

	Controls Means (±SD)	WD Means (±SD)	Controls Median (IQR)	WD Median (IQR)	p-value	Difference (95% C.I)
Mean RNFL μm	99.6 (±10.4)	**95.3* (±8.8)**	100(91;107)	95(88;99)	**0.0267**	−4.27 (−4.63; −3.92)
Mean total MT μm	321 (±14.81)	**311.3* (±15.8)**	323(312;330)	309(301;317)	**0.0012**	−9.7 (−11.3; −8.1)
GCIP μm	99.8 (±7.1)	**95.6* (±6.8)**	100(96;105)	96(91;101)	**0.0026**	−4.17 (−4.63; −3.71)
INL μm	44.0 (±4.0)	**39.0* (±3.7)**	44(42;47)	39(37;41)	**<0.0001**	−5.04 (−5.29; −4.81)
OPL μm	33.9 (±6.8)	35.8 (±3.9)	32(30;36)	36(33;38)	0.1069	1.86 (1.5;2.22
ONL μm	106.0 (±11.3)	107.0 (±10.6)	107(99;112)	107(100;113)	0.6507	1 (1.7;0.3)
VEP N75 ms	74.0 (±5.5)	**80.3* (±8.3)**	74(72;77)	78(75;85)	**0.0019**	6.37 (7.41;5.32)
VEP P100 ms	103.9 (±5.2)	**108.2* (±6.8)**	103(99;108)	107(104;113)	**0.0111**	4.3 (3.8;5)
VEP N140 ms	141.5 (±10.1)	142.0 (±7.9)	143(134;148)	143(136;148)	0.8482	0.5 (−0.4;1.4)
VEP Amplitude μV	8.1 (±4.3)	8.4 (±3.4)	7(5.7;10.2)	7.8(5.7;11.0)	0.75	0.347 (−0.046;0.739)
Wilson Score		4.5 (±3.5)				
Disease Duration y		15.7 (±10.6)				
Follow up time y		9.8 (±5.7)				
Serum Cu^{2+}, mg/l		0.35 (±0.27)				
Cu^{2+}in 24 h urin mg/d		0.30 (±0.69)				
Caeruloplasmin mg/dl		8.1 (±8.5)				
Age y	42.6 (±13.2)	40.2 (±13.6)	45(31;53)	42(28;49)	0.776	
Sex male/female	29/35	18/24				

The means (± standard deviation), the p-values and the mean difference from Wilson's disease to controls with a 95% confidence interval (95% C.I.) are indicated for the acquired parameters. The abbreviations are as follows: RNFL = peripapillary retinal nerve fibre layer thickness in μm, MT = macular thickness in μm, GCIP = retinal ganglion cell layer and inner plexiform layer measured together in μm, INL = inner nuclear layer in μm, OPL = outer plexiform layer in μm, ONL = outer nuclear layer in μm. Means that significantly differed from the control group are in bold and marked with an asterisk ($p<0.05$, two-tailed t-test).

N75:74 ms ±5.5, P100:104 ms ±5.2) while the N140 latency and the amplitude remained unchanged (M±SD: controls N140:142 ms ±10, amplitude: 8.1 μV ±4.3; Wilson's disease: N140 142 ms ±7.9, amplitude: 8.4 μV ±3.4). Therefore the shape of the VEP curves of Wilson's disease patients appeared compressed (Figure 3).

Subgroup Analysis of Treatment Groups

A subgroup analysis revealed no significant differences between patients treated with D-penicillamine, trientine, or tetrathiomolybdate for any OCT or VEP parameter (ANOVA, Tukey's post hoc test).

Correlations

In our Wilson's disease patients, the RNFL thickness correlated positively with the mean total macular thickness ($p = 0.0031$, $r = 0.44$, Pearson, figure 4 A) and GCIP thickness ($p = 0.0141$, $r = 0.35$, Pearson, figure 4 B). The mean macular thickness of Wilson's disease patients correlated positively with the thickness of all of the macular layers except for the OPL (all $p<0.05$, GCIP: $p<0.0001$, $r = 0.67$; INL: $p = 0.0008$, $r = 0.51$; ONL: $p = 0.0008$; $r = 0.47$, Pearson, figure 4 C–E). For the manually segmented paramacular layers, we observed weak but significant positive correlations between the thickness of the GCIP and INL ($p = 0.0398$, $r = 0.32$, Pearson, figure 4 F) and between the INL and ONL ($p = 0.0389$, $r = 0.33$, Pearson, figure 4 G).

A thinner RNFL, macular thickness and GCIP appeared to be associated with longer P100 and N75 latencies and lower VEP amplitudes. However, only ONL thickness and N75 latency were significantly correlated ($p = 0.0073$, Pearson $r = 0.50$, figure 4 H) and the correlation was actually positive. Of note is that the ONL was not altered in Wilson's disease patients compared with controls. We observed no significant correlation between the clinical Wilson score or the time since diagnosis of the disease and the thickness of any retinal layer or with any VEP parameter. Additionally, the Wilson score did not correlate with the time since diagnosis (Spearman).

An analysis of the laboratory parameters of our patients revealed weak positive correlations of both the N75 latency and the P100 latency with the concentrations of copper and caeruloplasmin in serum (N75: $p = 0.0046$ and $p = 0.0188$ respectively, both $r = 0.52$, Pearson, figure 5 A+B; P100: $p = 0.0052$ and, $p = 0.0207$ respectively, Pearson $r = 0.52$ and $r = 0.45$ respectively figure 5 C+D).

As all correlations of VEP parameters were very much influenced by one outlier with a N75 latency of 109 ms and a P100 latency of 130 ms, we recalculated the correlations again after removing this patient from the analysis (dotted lines in figure 4 H and 5 A–D). Without the outlier, the correlations with VEP parameters were not significant whereas P100 and N75 still differed significantly in the group comparison between Wilson's disease and controls (t-test, $p = 0.0019$ and $p = 0.0182$, respectively).

The mean OPL thickness was weakly but significantly correlated with the concentrations of copper ($p = 0.0181$, $r = 0.36$, Pearson Figure 5 E) and caeruloplasmin in serum ($p<0.05$, $r = 0.32$, Pearson, figure 5 F). The copper concentration in 24 h urine showed a weak positive correlation with the clinical Wilson score ($p = 0.0402$, $r = 0.37$, Spearman, figure 5 G) and a stronger positive correlation with the caeruloplasmin concentration in serum ($p<0.0001$, $r = 0.86$, Pearson, Figure 5 H).

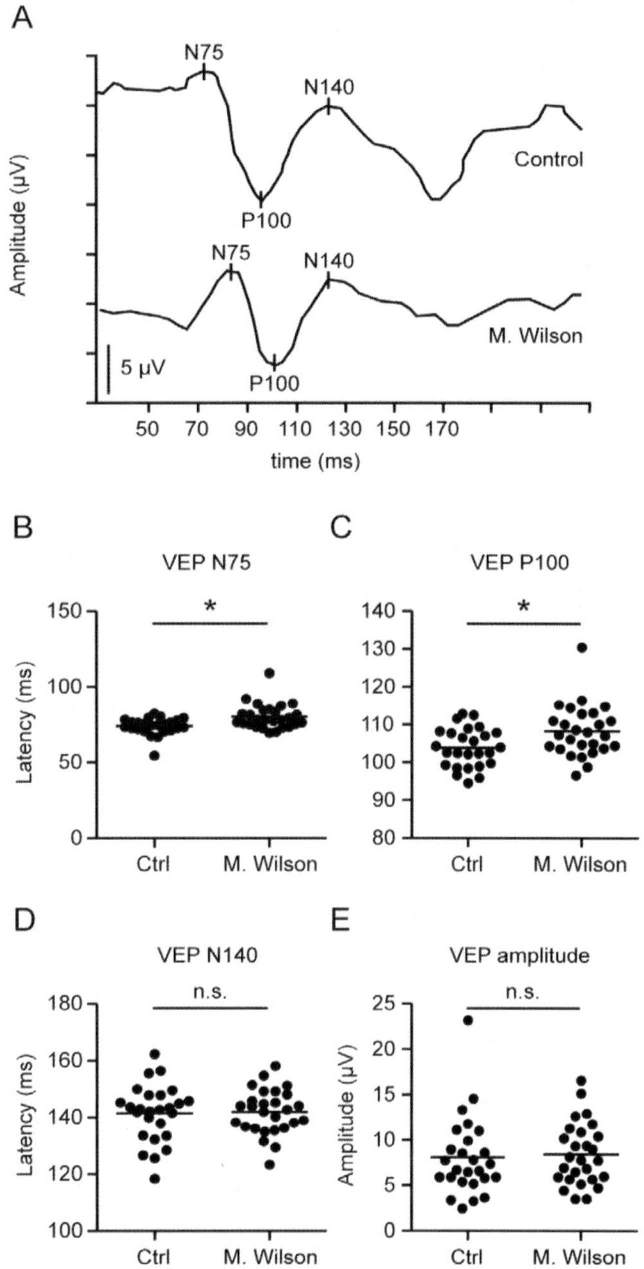

Figure 3. Visual evoked potentials: N75 and P100 latencies are prolonged in Wilson's disease. A Representative VEP curves of Wilson's disease patients and controls are displayed. **B–E** Scatter plots of the mean VEP parameters. Each point represents the mean of the two eyes of one patient. The mean of all patients is indicated by a horizontal bar. Significant differences are indicated by asterisks ($p<0.05$, two-tailed t test); non-significant differences are indicated as n.s.

Visual acuity was above 80% in all patients and correlated significantly only with N75 and P100 VEP latency (Pearson: $p=0.038$, $r=-0.53$, and $p=0.030$, $r=-0.56$ respectively).

As we performed multiple correlations, we used a Bonferroni correction in a post hoc analysis to obtain a more conservative measure, reducing the risk of false positive results while increasing the risk of false negatives. After Bonferroni correction, only the correlations of mean total macular thickness with GCIP ($p<0.0024$), INL ($p=0.0192$), and ONL ($p=0.0192$) and of copper in urine with caeruloplasmin in serum ($p<0.0024$) remained significant.

The clinical and laboratory parameters may influence VEP- and OCT parameters. We therefore performed a multivariate correlation analysis adjusting for age, sex, the clinical disease score and the concentrations of caeruloplasmin in serum and of copper in serum and urine. When controlling for these variables, macular thickness was significantly correlated with RNFL ($p=0.002$, $r=0.67$), GCIP ($p=0.001$, $r=0.72$), INL ($p=0.020$, $r=0.50$) and ONL ($p=0.025$, $r=0.51$). RNFL was correlated with GCIP ($p=0.005$, $r=0.611$), INL ($p=0.028$, $r=0.50$) and ONL ($p=0.025$, $r=0.511$).

To test if any of the clinical parameters had influence on the retinal changes observed, we performed a linear regression based approach, analyzing the effects of age, clinical score, sex, caeruloplasmin in serum, and copper in serum and urine on macular thickness as the main retinal parameter in our patients. Of these parameters only sex had a significant ($p=0.026$) effect with a corrected ß-coefficient of 37%. A further comparison revealed that in our collective, males indeed had a thicker macular thickness than females ($p=0.02$ t-test; M±SD: males: 307.8 µm ±13.9, females: 318.3 µm ±16.5). In the control cohort, in contrast, we observed no difference in macular thickness between males and females ($p>0.05$, t-test, M±SD: males: 324.1 µm ±13.5, females: 318.9 µm ±15.4).

Discussion

We were able to reproduce previously reported findings [10,11,14–16] that indicate that in Wilson's disease, VEP latencies are delayed. We believe that the prolonged P100 latencies are likely to reflect a slowed conduction velocity of the visual tract caused by copper deposits. A structural analysis of the retina by OCT revealed reduced thickness of the RNFL, total macula and GCIP, clearly indicating pathological changes to the retinal ganglion cells and their axons in the retina. In line with previous publications [12], the VEP amplitudes of Wilson's disease patients were unchanged compared with controls. However, in Wilson's disease patients, low VEP amplitudes tended to be associated with thinner RNFL, GCIP and total macular thickness, although these correlations failed to reach significance. In other diseases such as multiple sclerosis, the VEP amplitude is reported to correlate with the RNFL thickness [31]. It is possible that the extent of axonal loss in Wilson's disease patients was not sufficient to significantly reduce the VEP amplitude. However, these findings indicate that OCT may be a more sensitive parameter of axonal loss in Wilson's disease than VEP amplitudes.

To our knowledge, no histopathological studies analyzing the retinae of patients with Wilson's disease have been reported, so the exact mechanisms of retinal degeneration in these patients remain unclear. However, the reduction of RNFL thickness in Wilson's disease reflects degeneration of the retinal ganglion cell axons and degeneration of the retinal ganglion cells themselves and is likely to account for the observed reduced thickness of the GCIP complex. Neuronal degeneration as a consequence of axonal damage due to copper deposition along the optic nerve and tract is a plausible explanation for these observations. The prolonged N75 and P100 latencies of VEPs indicate a slowed conduction of the visual tract due to the copper depositions themselves or secondary demyelination. The observed reduction of the total macular thickness can be attributed to the thinning of the RNFL and GCIP, which make up approximately one-third of the total thickness at the

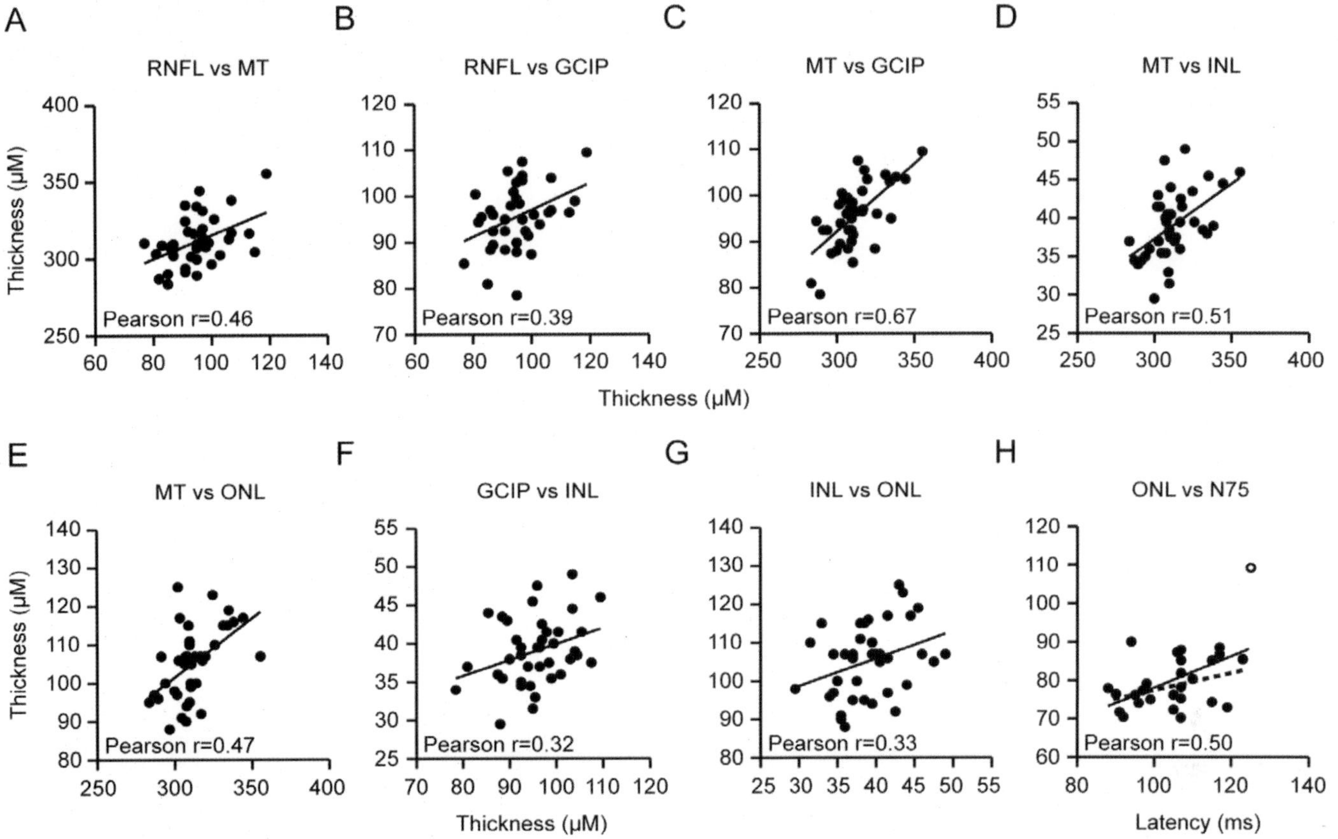

Figure 4. Correlations between layers. A–H The significant correlations between the thickness of the different retinal layers and the VEP parameters of the patients' left eyes are displayed and the Pearson r is indicated ($p<0.05$, Pearson). **H** The continuous lines resemble the linear regression including, and the dotted lines excluding, an outlier with beginning hepatic failure (the outlier is marked as unfilled dot, Pearson r is indicated considering the outlier).

paramacular points of measurement. In line with this observation, RNFL, GCIP and total macular thickness correlated positively.

However, the reduction of the INL thickness that we observed in our Wilson's disease patients cannot be explained as a direct consequence of copper depositions on the retrobulbar visual pathway. Either the reduction of the INL thickness is caused by a direct retinal pathology such as retinal copper deposition or it is a secondary consequence of the degeneration of the retinal ganglion cells, e.g. the bipolar cells from this layer degenerate because they can no longer signal to the degenerated retinal ganglion cells. Similar mechanisms of retrograde transsynaptic degeneration have been postulated for retinal ganglion cells in patients with hemianopia due to retrogeniculate lesions [32,33].

It is not clear whether the treatment of our patients had any effect on the visual system or the retinal morphology. Changes of the retinal pigment epithelium under penicillamine therapy have been described in a case report from 1978 [34]. However, even though penicillamine is the most common treatment for Wilson's disease, to our knowledge no other case of retinopathy induced by penicillamine or the other chelating agents has been reported. Furthermore, we observed no difference in any retinal parameter between patients treated with penicillamine, thrientine, or tetrathiomolybdate. We therefore do not believe that the changes of the retinal and VEP parameters are a consequence of the treatment. Of note is that most patients began their therapy with penicillamine and were later switched to another therapy due to systemic side effects, none of which involved the visual system.

Unexpectedly, we observed no significant correlations between the VEP and the OCT parameters in Wilson's disease patients. Only the ONL thickness, which was unchanged in Wilson's disease patients, actually correlated positively with the N75 latency. The fact that the N75 and P100 latencies correlated positively with the copper and caeruloplasmin concentrations in serum suggests that the VEP latencies may possibly be directly influenced by the current copper metabolism status at the time of examination. On the other hand, the OCT parameters that were altered in Wilson's disease patients did not correlate with the laboratory parameters. So the thicknesses of the RNFL, GCIP, INL and total macula may be stable parameters reflecting long-term neuronal degeneration in these patients. A longitudinal analysis of these parameters is underway and will clarify this theory.

Of note is that P100 and N75 VEP -latencies were the only parameters to correlate with visual acuity as a direct measure of functional deficit.

It should be mentioned, however, that the correlations with the VEP parameters were mainly due to an outlier with a N75 latency of 109 ms and a P100 latency of 130 ms. When this outlier was removed from the analysis, none of the correlations with N75 or P100 remained significant. This was a patient who presented central serous retinopathy of his right eye, so only his left eye was included in the study. He did not report vision problems with his left eye and the ophthalmologic examination revealed no pathology of the left eye, with a corrected visual acuity of 90%.

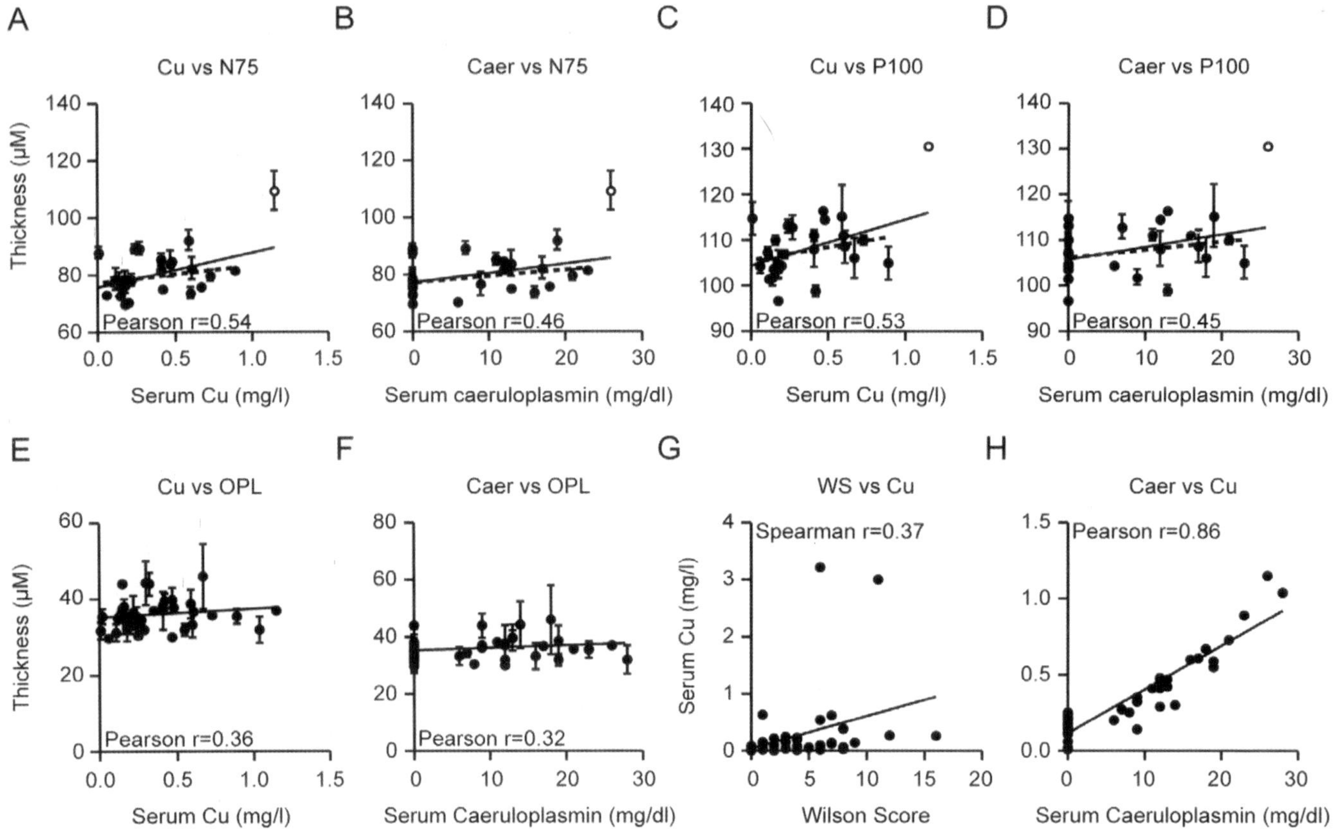

Figure 5. Correlations between layers, VEP parameters and laboratory. A–H The significant correlations between the laboratory parameters and the mean thickness of the retinal layers and VEP parameters of both eyes are shown and the Pearson or Spearman r is indicated ($p<0.05$ including the outlier, all comparisons were made using a Pearson analysis except for the Wilson Score, which was analyzed using a Spearman analysis). **A–D** The continuous lines resemble linear regressions including, and the dotted lines excluding, an outlier with beginning hepatic failure (the outlier is marked as unfilled dot, Pearson r is indicated considering the outlier).

However, the laboratory parameters were indicative of a beginning hepatic failure, with changes of the liver parameters, and he was later diagnosed with a hepatocellular carcinoma. It is possible that changes of the visual pathway due to the hepatic failure, which were not accessible to the ophthalmologic exam, accounted for the prolonged VEP latencies in this patient. The case of this patient stresses the fact that marked changes in VEP latencies can be indicative of a beginning hepatic encephalopathy {Zamir, 2002 #422} and should prompt further investigations.

We observed no correlation between the OCT parameters and visual acuity using Snellen charts. To analyze the functional consequence of the structural changes observed, studies using more sensitive parameters such as analysis of the flicker fusion threshold or low contrast letter recognition are warranted.

When discussing the results of the correlations performed in our study, one must bear in mind that even though the single correlations may be significant with a $p<0.05$, the overall risk of a type I error (false positive result) increases with the number of correlations. Thus, the significant correlations should be interpreted with caution and ideally verified with an independent study. To obtain a more conservative measure of correlation we therefore performed Bonferroni corrections, though this simultaneously increased the risk of a type II error (false negative result). After the Bonferroni correction, only the correlations between macular thickness with GCIP, INL and ONL and between urine copper and serum caeruloplasmin remained significant, which is not astonishing as the macular thickness is greatly influenced by these layers and urine copper and serum caeruloplasmin concentrations are closely linked.

Using a linear regression based approach, we identified age as the only significant influence on macular thickness as the major retinal parameter, with female sex being associated with thinner macular thickness. Males and females did not differ in age, excluding an age-related artifact. Although a higher macular thickness in males compared to females has been reported before [35–37], the macular thickness in our control cohort did not differ between males and females. A possible explanation for the differences observed in our patients could be that the small differences between men and women, which are most likely hormone mediated, may be accentuated by the elevated copper levels in Wilson's disease. The fact that the laboratory parameters did not serve as predictors for retinal degeneration measured by macular thickness is not at all astonishing as all patients were under therapy.

We believe that analyzing the retinal layers using OCT can provide valuable information on the ongoing neuronal degeneration in Wilson's disease and that longitudinal evaluations are suitable for monitoring these patients. OCT and VEPs appear to be ideal tools for treatment trials and for evaluating the long-term efficacy of treatment during routine consultations. However, the manual segmentation algorithm for analysis of the deeper retinal layers used in this study is laborious and therefore not very feasible for the clinical routine. Some clinical trials have already applied fully automated segmentation techniques [17,21,38] that will soon be available for a wider public and may allow analysis of the deeper retinal layers in routine clinical practice.

Author Contributions

Conceived and designed the experiments: PA HH AM. Performed the experiments: PA AKM EC DF MR HH. Analyzed the data: PA AKM MR HH AM GG HPH. Contributed reagents/materials/analysis tools: HPH GG. Wrote the paper: PA AM OA HPH. Revised the manuscript: HPH GG OA MR.

References

1. Bearn AG (1953) Genetic and biochemical aspects of Wilson's disease. Am J Med 15: 442–449.
2. Cumings JN (1948) The copper and iron content of brain and liver in the normal and in hepato-lenticular degeneration. Brain 71: 410–415.
3. de Bie P, Muller P, Wijmenga C, Klomp LW (2007) Molecular pathogenesis of Wilson and Menkes disease: correlation of mutations with molecular defects and disease phenotypes. J Med Genet 44: 673–688.
4. Das SK, Ray K (2006) Wilson's disease: an update. Nat Clin Pract Neurol 2: 482–493.
5. Mufti AR, Burstein E, Csomos RA, Graf PC, Wilkinson JC, et al. (2006) XIAP Is a copper binding protein deregulated in Wilson's disease and other copper toxicosis disorders. Mol Cell 21: 775–785.
6. Riordan SM, Williams R (2001) The Wilson's disease gene and phenotypic diversity. J Hepatol 34: 165–171.
7. Ala A, Walker AP, Ashkan K, Dooley JS, Schilsky ML (2007) Wilson's disease. Lancet 369: 397–408.
8. Singh P, Ahluwalia A, Saggar K, Grewal CS (2011) Wilson's disease: MRI features. J Pediatr Neurosci 6: 27–28.
9. Sinha S, Taly AB, Ravishankar S, Prashanth LK, Venugopal KS, et al. (2006) Wilson's disease: cranial MRI observations and clinical correlation. Neuroradiology 48: 613–621.
10. Arendt G, Hefter H, Stremmel W, Strohmeyer G (1994) The diagnostic value of multi-modality evoked potentials in Wilson's disease. Electromyogr Clin Neurophysiol 34: 137–148.
11. Das M, Misra UK, Kalita J (2007) A study of clinical, MRI and multimodality evoked potentials in neurologic Wilson disease. Eur J Neurol 14: 498–504.
12. Satishchandra P, Ravishankar Naik K (2000) Visual pathway abnormalities Wilson's disease: an electrophysiological study using electroretinography and visual evoked potentials. J Neurol Sci 176: 13–20.
13. Topcu M, Topcuoglu MA, Kose G, Nurlu G, Turanli G (2002) Evoked potentials in children with Wilson's disease. Brain Dev 24: 276–280.
14. Ilic TV, Svetl M, Petkovic S, Kostic VS (2005) [Multimodal evoked potential abnormalities in patients with Wilson's disease]. Srp Arh Celok Lek 133: 331–337.
15. Hsu YS, Chang YC, Lee WT, Ni YH, Hsu HY, et al. (2003) The diagnostic value of sensory evoked potentials in pediatric Wilson disease. Pediatr Neurol 29: 42–45.
16. Satishchandra P, Swamy HS (1989) Visual and brain stem auditory evoked responses in Wilson's disease. Acta Neurol Scand 79: 108–113.
17. Saidha S, Syc SB, Ibrahim MA, Eckstein C, Warner CV, et al. (2011) Primary retinal pathology in multiple sclerosis as detected by optical coherence tomography. Brain 134: 518–533.
18. Albrecht P, Ringelstein M, Mueller A, Keser N, Dietlein T, et al. (2012) Degeneration of retinal layers in multiple sclerosis subtypes quantified by optical coherence tomography. Mult Scler. 2012 Oct;18(10): 1422–9. Epub 2012 Mar 2.
19. Brandt AU, Zimmermann H, Kaufhold F, Promesberger J, Schippling S, et al. (2012) Patterns of Retinal Damage Facilitate Differential Diagnosis between Susac Syndrome and MS. PLoS One 7: e38741.
20. Gelfand JM, Goodin DS, Boscardin WJ, Nolan R, Cuneo A, et al. (2012) Retinal Axonal Loss Begins Early in the Course of Multiple Sclerosis and Is Similar between Progressive Phenotypes. PLoS One 7: e36847.
21. Seigo MA, Sotirchos ES, Newsome S, Babiarz A, Eckstein C, et al. (2012) In vivo assessment of retinal neuronal layers in multiple sclerosis with manual and automated optical coherence tomography segmentation techniques. J Neurol.
22. Syc SB, Saidha S, Newsome SD, Ratchford JN, Levy M, et al. (2012) Optical coherence tomography segmentation reveals ganglion cell layer pathology after optic neuritis. Brain 135: 521–533.
23. Walter SD, Ishikawa H, Galetta KM, Sakai RE, Feller DJ, et al. (2012) Ganglion cell loss in relation to visual disability in multiple sclerosis. Ophthalmology 119: 1250–1257.
24. Warner CV, Syc SB, Stankiewicz AM, Hiremath G, Farrell SK, et al. (2011) The impact of utilizing different optical coherence tomography devices for clinical purposes and in multiple sclerosis trials. PLoS One 6: e22947.
25. Galetta KM, Calabresi PA, Frohman EM, Balcer LJ (2011) Optical coherence tomography (OCT): imaging the visual pathway as a model for neurodegeneration. Neurotherapeutics 8: 117–132.
26. Hefter H, Arendt G, Stremmel W, Freund HJ (1993) Motor impairment in Wilson's disease, I: Slowness of voluntary limb movements. Acta Neurol Scand 87: 133–147.
27. Roberts EA, Schilsky ML (2008) Diagnosis and treatment of Wilson disease: an update. Hepatology 47: 2089–2111.
28. Nassif N, Cense B, Park BH, Yun SH, Chen TC, et al. (2004) In vivo human retinal imaging by ultrahigh-speed spectral domain optical coherence tomography. Opt Lett 29: 480–482.
29. Tewarie P, Balk L, Costello F, Green A, Martin R, et al. (2012) The OSCAR-IB consensus criteria for retinal OCT quality assessment. PLoS One 7: e34823.
30. Albrecht P, Muller AK, Sudmeyer M, Ferrea S, Ringelstein M, et al. (2012) Optical coherence tomography in parkinsonian syndromes. PLoS One 7: e34891.
31. Klistorner A, Arvind H, Nguyen T, Garrick R, Paine M, et al. (2009) Multifocal VEP and OCT in optic neuritis: a topographical study of the structure-function relationship. Doc Ophthalmol 118: 129–137.
32. Jindahra P, Petrie A, Plant GT (2009) Retrograde trans-synaptic retinal ganglion cell loss identified by optical coherence tomography. Brain 132: 628–634.
33. Mehta JS, Plant GT (2005) Optical coherence tomography (OCT) findings in congenital/long-standing homonymous hemianopia. Am J Ophthalmol 140: 727–729.
34. Dingle J, Havener WH (1978) Ophthalmoscopic changes in a patient with Wilson's disease during long-term penicillamine therapy. Ann Ophthalmol 10: 1227–1230.
35. Song WK, Lee SC, Lee ES, Kim CY, Kim SS (2010) Macular thickness variations with sex, age, and axial length in healthy subjects: a spectral domain-optical coherence tomography study. Invest Ophthalmol Vis Sci 51: 3913–3918.
36. Wagner-Schuman M, Dubis AM, Nordgren RN, Lei Y, Odell D, et al. (2011) Race- and sex-related differences in retinal thickness and foveal pit morphology. Invest Ophthalmol Vis Sci 52: 625–634.
37. Wexler A, Sand T, Elsas TB (2010) Macular thickness measurements in healthy Norwegian volunteers: an optical coherence tomography study. BMC Ophthalmol 10: 13.
38. Yang Q, Reisman CA, Chan K, Ramachandran R, Raza A, et al. (2011) Automated segmentation of outer retinal layers in macular OCT images of patients with retinitis pigmentosa. Biomed Opt Express 2: 2493–2503.

Loss of Polycystin-1 Inhibits Bicc1 Expression during Mouse Development

Peiwen Lian[1,2], Ao Li[1,2], Yuan Li[1], Haichao Liu[1], Dan Liang[2], Bo Hu[2], De Lin[4], Tang Jiang[5], Gilbert Moeckel[6], Dahui Qin[7], Guanqing Wu[1,2,3*]

1 Division of Translational Cancer Research and Therapy, State Key Laboratory of Molecular Oncology, Cancer Hospital and Institute, Chinese Academy of Medical Sciences and Peking Union Medical College, Beijing, China, **2** Department of Medicine, Vanderbilt University, Nashville, Tennessee, United States of America, **3** Department of Cell & Developmental Biology, Vanderbilt University, Nashville, Tennessee, United States of America, **4** Department of Biochemistry, Vanderbilt University, Nashville, Tennessee, United States of America, **5** Department of Medicine, First Affiliated Hospital, Sun Yat-sen University, Guangzhou, China, **6** Department of Pathology, Yale University School of Medicine, New Haven, Connecticut, United States of America, **7** Department of Pathology, Moffitt Cancer Center, Tampa, Florida, United States of America

Abstract

Bicc1 is a mouse homologue of *Drosophila Bicaudal-C* (*dBic-C*), which encodes an RNA-binding protein. Orthologs of *dBic-C* have been identified in many species, from *C. elegans* to *humans. Bicc1*-mutant mice exhibit a cystic phenotype in the kidney that is very similar to human polycystic kidney disease. Even though many studies have explored the gene characteristics and its functions in multiple species, the developmental profile of the *Bicc1* gene product (Bicc1) in mammal has not yet been completely characterized. To this end, we generated a polyclonal antibody against Bicc1 and examined its spatial and temporal expression patterns during mouse embryogenesis and organogenesis. Our results demonstrated that Bicc1 starts to be expressed in the neural tube as early as embryonic day (E) 8.5 and is widely expressed in epithelial derivatives including the gut and hepatic cells at E10.5, and the pulmonary bronchi at E11.5. In mouse kidney development, Bicc1 appears in the early ureteric bud and mesonephric tubules at E11.5 and is also expressed in the metanephros at the same stage. During postnatal kidney development, Bicc1 expression gradually expands from the cortical to the medullary and papillary regions, and it is highly expressed in the proximal tubules. In addition, we discovered that loss of the *Pkd1* gene product, polycystin-1 (PC1), whose mutation causes human autosomal dominant polycystic kidney disease (ADPKD), downregulates Bicc1 expression *in vitro* and *in vivo*. Our findings demonstrate that Bicc1 is developmentally regulated and reveal a new molecular link between *Bicc1* and *Pkd1*.

Editor: Joseph Devaney, Children's National Medical Center, United States of America

Funding: This work was supported by the National Institutes of Health of the USA (RR033682) to G.W and by National 973 program (2012CB517700) (2011EG150311) (81173114) (81072688). The funders had no role in study design, data collection and analysis, decision to publish, or preparation of the manuscript.

Competing Interests: The authors have declared that no competing interests exist.

* E-mail: guanqing.wu@vanderbilt.edu

These authors contributed equally to this work.

Introduction

Studies of animal mutant models for polycystic kidney disease (PKD) and of human PKD patients have identified more than 20 genes whose mutations can induce PKD phenotypes [1,2,3]. The continued study of these cyst-associated genes and their products will help elucidate the disease mechanism of human inherited polycystic kidney diseases, such as autosomal dominant and recessive PKD (ADPKD and ARPKD).

Bicc1 is a mouse homologue of *Drosophila Bicaudal-C* (*dBic-C*), the orthologs of which are much conserved in many species, from *C. elegans* to *humans* [4,5,6,7,8]. Loss of *dBic-C* in *Drosophila* disrupts the direction of anterior follicle cell migration and affects anterior-posterior patterning, so that the resulting embryos lack heads and exhibit duplicated posterior segments instead [9,10]. The *Xenopus* homologue of *Bicaudal-C* (*xBic-C*) is one of the few molecules that, when microinjected ectopically, causes endoderm formation in the absence of mesoderm induction [11]. Knockdown of the zebrafish homologue of *Bicaudal-C* (*zBic-C*) induces cystic kidneys *in vivo* [12].

The gene product of *Bicc1* (Bicc1) contains several conserved N-terminal KH domains and a conserved C-terminal SAM domain [13]. The KH domains bind target mRNAs [4]. Recent studies indicated that the KH domains enable Bicc1 to recruit specific miRNA precursors and associate with Dicer, to guide these nascent miRNAs to anchor their target mRNAs. The SAM domain is nonessential for mRNA binding, but it is required for the transfer of Bicc1-targeted mRNAs to P-body-associated AGO proteins for silencing [14]. Therefore, the gene product Bicc1 is thought to be an RNA-binding molecule that functions to regulate diverse proteins at the post-transcriptional level.

To study the functional role of Bicc1, some chemically-induced or natively occurring *Bicc1*-mutant mouse models (*jcpk* and *bpk*) have been identified and several gene-targeting mouse models have been established [5,6,15,16,17]. Although *Bicc1* mutations in these models result from different mutant Bicc1 proteins, all the models exhibit cystic phenotypes in the kidney that are very similar to human polycystic kidney disease. These mouse models can provide insight into the functional roles of Bicc1 during mouse development. Even though gene expression of *Bicc1* during mouse development has been previously reported [5,6,9,14], the developmental profiles of Bicc1 protein during mammalian development remain uncharacterized. Here we generated a polyclonal antibody against Bicc1 and used it to examine the distribution patterns of Bicc1 during mouse embryogenesis and organogenesis. In addition, we investigated the molecular relationship of Bicc1 to other human cystoproteins and discovered that loss of polycystin-1 (PC1), the gene product of *Pkd1*, whose mutation causes human ADPKD, reduced Bicc1 expression *in vitro* and *in vivo*. Our findings demonstrate that Bicc1 is developmentally regulated and indicate that its normal function may require normal PC1 expression.

Materials and Methods

Antibodies and reagents

A pGEX3 GST expression vector (Amersham) was used as the backbone for producing Bicc1 GST-fusion proteins. The cDNA of mouse Bicc1 (Q711-D858) was inserted in-frame into the vector. The mBicc1-fused plasmid was used to transform Rosetta host cells (Novagen) to produce the GST-fusion antigen. The antigen was subcutaneously injected into New Zealand white rabbits, at 0.5 mg per injection. The anti-mBicc1 serum (mBicc1p) was generated as reported in our previous studies [18]. All the antisera product and the preimmune serum (Pre-IM) were affinity-purified before performing experiments.

The following antibodies, staining materials, and reagents were used: anti-HA, and anti-Flag, anti-β-actin, and DAPI (Sigma-Aldrich Inc.); anti-Tamm-Horsfall glycoprotein antibody (THG) (Applied Biological Materials Inc.); fluorescein *lotus tetragonolobus* lectin (LTL) (Vector Laboratories); anti-Aquaporin-2 (AQP2) antibodies (Abcam Inc.); anti-GST antibody and pBABE-Puro retroviral vector (Cell Biolabs Inc.); pCMV-tag4 expression vector (Stratagene Inc.); pSico Lentiviral vector system (Addgene Inc.).

Mouse strains

Our *Pkd2*, *Pkd1*, and *Pkhd1* mutant mice were described in detail previously [19,20,21]. All the mouse models used in this study were backcrossed (over 10 times) to the *C57BL/6* inbred background. The animal protocol was approved by Vanderbilt University Institutional Animal Care and Use Committee (Permit Number: M/12/143).

Western blotting and quantitative PCR

Western blot analyses were performed using protocols similar to those described previously [18,22]. Briefly, proteins from cultured cells or tissues were extracted in lysis buffer (0.5% NP-40, 5% Sodium deoxycholate, 50 μM NaCl, 10 μM Tris-HCl (pH 7.5), 1% BSA), homogenized and centrifuged. Protein samples were solubilized in protein loading buffer and denatured by boiling. The samples were electrophoresed in 10% SDS-PAGE gels. The membranes were incubated with 5% milk at room temperature for one hour and blotted with mBicc1p antibody at room temperature for 4 hours and then were incubated with peroxidase-conjugate secondary antibodies (Sigma) and detected with enhanced chemiluminescence (ECL) (Amersham).

Quantitative PCR was performed using the iCycler iQ Real-Time PCR Detection System with the iQ SYBR Green Supermix kit (Bio-Rad). The *Pkd1* primers were (forward) 5′-GCT AAG CTA CAC TTC TCC TTT ATC CG-3′ and (reverse) 5′-ACT TCT TGG CAT CTT TCA TCC CAC-3′. The *Pkd2* primers were (forward) 5′-GCG TGG TAC CCT CTT GGC AGT T-3′ and (reverse) 5′-CAC GAC AAT CAC AAC ATC C-3′. The *Pkhd1* primers were (forward) 5′-CAA ATG CCA CAG CCC AAC AG-3′ and (reverse) 5′-CAG AAT GGT TAG GGG TGG GA-3′.

Histology, immunofluorescence (IF), immunohistochemistry (IHC), and confocal microscopy

The detailed procedures used for histology, IF, and IHC staining were published previously [18,23]. For the microscopic analysis, a Zeiss Axioplan 2IE research microscope and a Zeiss Axiovert 200 inverted microscope system with 10×, 20×, and 40× objectives were used.

Renal epithelial cell lines and their cultures

Mouse inner medullary collecting duct (IMCD) cells were cultured using the conditions described in the American Type Culture Collection manual. IMCD cells with *Bicc1*-silencing ($IMCD^{shC4C}$) were reported in our previous study [24].

To generate *Bicc1*-overexpressed stable cell line ($IMCD^{Bicc1}$), we initially used Bicc1-pCMV-Tag4 clone (Fig. 1B) as backbone to insert mouse *Bicc1* ORF cDNA into LZRS-GFP vector (Addgene). Resulting LZRS-GFP-Bicc1-flag vector and pBABE-puro vector (Addgene) were co-transfected into HEK293 cells. At time points of cultured 48 and 72 hours, the viral-transfected supernatant was separately harvested and filtered with a 45 uM syringe filter. The 48 hour filtered supernatants were added on subconfluent cultured IMCD cells. After 24 hours, the infection was repeated with the 72 hour viral supernatants. One day later, puromycin was added for cell selection. Through a week Puromycin-selected culture, the remaining cells were resuspended and seeded on 100 mm culture plates (Costar) at a cell density of 1000 per plate. Once Puromycin-selected colonies formed, single colonies were picked and expend the colony into 24-well plates (Costar). A cloned cell line with *Bicc1*-overexpression, $IMCD^{Bicc1}$, was identified by RT-PCR and confirmed by western blot analysis.

The null-*Pkd2* (E8) cell line, its maternally-derived *Pkd2* heterozygous (D3) cell line, the null-*Pkhd1* (M10H2) line, and its littermate-derived wildtype (W10B2) cell line were also described in our previous studies [23,25].

The cells from null-*Pkd1* and its littermate-derived wildtype mice were generated by an approach similar to that reported in our previous studies [23,25]. Briefly, the kidneys from E16.5 $Pkd1^{-/-}$ and wildtype littermate embryos with the *C57BL/6* congenic background were finely minced with a scalpel, and the minced tissue was incubated with 0.5% collagenase type IV at 37°C for 45 minutes and pipetted vigorously. The undigested tissue was removed by filtration through a 40 μm mesh filter. The remaining single cells and small organoids were washed three times with PBS containing 5 mM glucose. The cells were then incubated with 10 μg/ml biotinylated *Dolichos biflorus* agglutinin (DBA) (Vector, B-1035) at 4°C for 60 minutes. The cells were then washed again with PBS followed by incubation with 50 μl CELLectin Biotin binder Dynabeads (Dynal Biotech) at 4°C for 30 minutes. Since Dynabeads are superparamagnetic polystyrene beads, the incubated mixtures were then washed twice with PBS containing 5 mM glucose, using a magnetic rack. The cells were eluted with release buffer (Dynal Biotech) and were plated on 24-well dishes with LHC-9 Medium (Gibco) under 5% CO_2 at 37°C overnight. The cells were then transferred to culture medium containing 5 units/ml murine IFN-γ (Peprotech Inc.), which was changed every other day, and placed in a 33°C incubator for at least 10 cell passages. The culture medium was then switched to 10% FCS DMEM/F12 (1:1) (Gibco), and the cells were cultured for at least another 10 cell passages under the same culture conditions. Since the isolated collecting duct cells were not further cloned, the pool of cells (pool cells) was used for the current study.

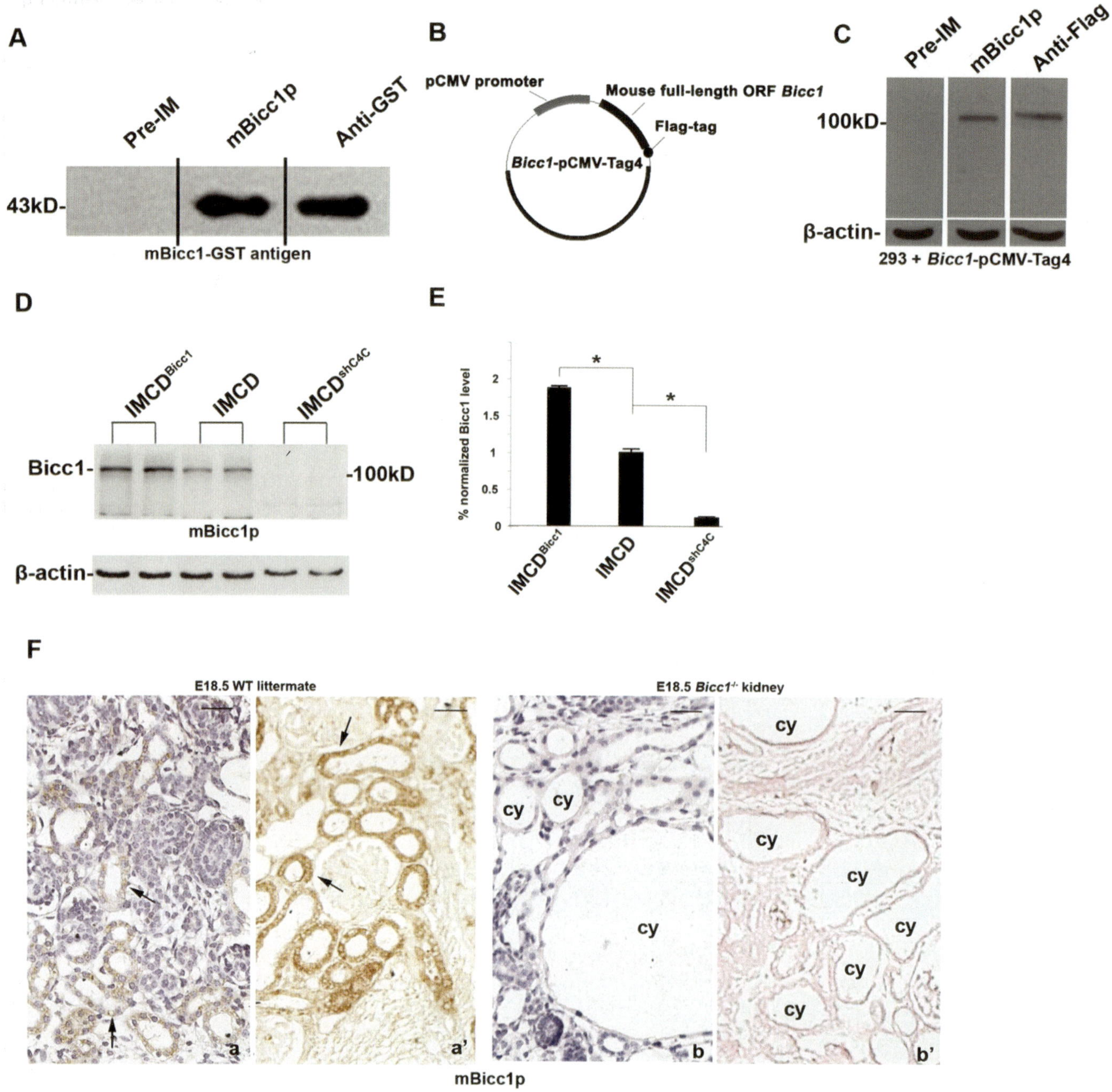

Figure 1. Specificity of the polyclonal antiserum mBicc1p for Bicc1. (A) The mBicc1-GST antigen was subjected to western blot analysis with the antibodies shown. The anti-Bicc1 (mBicc1p) and anti-GST antibodies, but not the preimmune serum (Pre-IM), recognized the mBicc1-GST antigen of the expected size (43 kD). (B) Schematic representation of the *Bicc1*-pCMV-Tag4 expression vector constructed by inserting the full-length ORF of *Bicc1* into Flag-tagged pCMV-Tag4. (C) *Bicc1*-pCMV-Tag4-transfected HEK293 cell lysates were subjected to western blot analysis with the antibodies shown. The anti-Bicc1 (mBicc1p) and anti-GST antibodies but not the Pre-IM recognized the *Bicc1*-pCMV-Tag4 protein of the expected size (~110 kD). (D) Western analysis of duplicated protein lysates from wildtype, *Bicc1*-silenced ($\text{IMCD}^{\text{shC4C}}$), and *Bicc1*-overexpressed IMCD cells ($\text{IMCD}^{\text{Bicc1}}$) were blotted with the mBicc1p antibody. Compared to the wildtype control, the immunoreactivity was significantly increased in *Bicc1*-overexpressed IMCD cells and was almost not detected in the *Bicc1*-silenced cells. (E) Normalized quantitative analysis of the densitometry values of the western analyses. Compared to wildtype IMCD and *Bicc1*-silenced IMCD ($\text{IMCD}^{\text{shC4C}}$) cells, *Bicc1*-overexpressed IMCD ($\text{IMCD}^{\text{Bicc1}}$) cells showed significantly increased Bicc1 expression (*$P<0.05$). (F) Immunohistochemistry (IHC) staining of Bicc1 protein in the kidneys of E18.5 $Bicc1^{-/-}$ and its wildtype littermates. Positive staining (arrows) were showed in the wildtype kidney (a), while no obvious positive staining was seen in the E18.5 $Bicc1^{-/-}$ kidney (b). (a'–b') Corresponding areas of a–b were stained by Bicc1p IHC without counterstaining. Data presented are representative of two to three independently replicated experiments. "cy" = renal cysts. Bars: 25 μm in F.

Pkd1$^{-/-}$ pool cells with PC1-CT expression were produced by pSico Lentiviral vector system (Addgene) in which the entire human *PKD1* COOH-terminus was (V4102-R4278) constructed. Recombinant viruses were packaged and amplified on a large scale in HEK293 cells. Lentiviral particles were purified and infected *Pkd1*$^{-/-}$ pool cells following the introduction of the manufacturer.

Before being used in any cell-based assays, all the established cell lines were cultured under non-permissive conditions (37°C without IFN-γ) for at least three days to turn off the SV40 transgene activity.

Statistics

All biochemical assays were repeated at least three times. Statistical analysis was performed where appropriate using the Student's t-test or one-way analysis of variance (ANOVA) followed by Tukey's Multiple Comparison Test. Differences with P-values <0.05 were considered statistically significant.

Results

Generation and characterization of anti-Bicc1 antiserum

A purified mouse Bicc1-GST fusion protein (mBicc1), encoding residues Q711 to D858 of Bicc1, was used to produce a rabbit polyclonal antiserum (mBicc1p) against the *Bicc1* gene product, Bicc1. The antiserum was generated and affinity-purified as described in our previous studies [18].

To test the specificity of mBicc1p, we performed western blot analyses of the antigen using the Pre-IM, mBicc1p, or an anti-GST antibody. No immunoreactive band was seen with Pre-IM, although strong positive bands of the expected size (~43 kD) were detected with mBicc1p and the anti-GST antibody (Fig. 1A). The mBicc1p-positive band could be competed away with the mBicc1-GST antigen (data not shown), suggesting that the mBicc1p antiserum was specific for Bicc1.

To further confirm the specificity, we constructed a *Bicc1*-expression vector *Bicc1*-pCMV-Tag4, in which a Flag-tag was fused in-frame with the full-length ORF *Bicc1* cDNA (Fig. 1B). Western analyses showed that the transient transfection of HEK293 cells with *Bicc1*-pCMV-Tag4 yielded bands of the expected size (~110 kD) that were immunoreactive with the mBicc1p and anti-Flag antibodies, but not with Pre-IM (Fig. 1C). We also used the mBicc1p antiserum to detect Bicc1 in lysates of IMCD cells, the stably *Bicc1*-overexpressed cell line IMCD$^{\text{Bicc1}}$ and the *Bicc1*-silencing stable cell line IMCD$^{\text{shC4C}}$ [24]. The ~110-kD Bicc1 band was readily detected in wildtype IMCD cells and highly strong band was showed in the IMCD$^{\text{Bicc1}}$ cells, whereas almost no band was seen in the IMCD$^{\text{shC4C}}$ cells (Fig. 1D–E).

In addition, renal tissues from *Bicc1* knockout mice were also used for testing the specificity of mBicc1p antiserum. Strong immunohistochemistry (IHC) staining can be observed in E18.5 wildtype kidney, while there is no positive staining in its *Bicc1*$^{-/-}$ littermate (Fig. 1F). These results strongly indicated that the mBicc1p antiserum was specific for Bicc1.

Bicc1 expression during mouse development

To elucidate the patterns of Bicc1 protein expression during embryogenesis and primary organogenesis in mammals, mBicc1p was used for IHC analyses in developing mouse tissues. We found clear positive staining in the epithelial cells of the neural tube on embryonic day 8.5 (E8.5) (Fig. 2A), and then in the myocardial wall of the heart at E9.5 (Fig. 2B). By E10.5, the epithelial cells in the primordial gut and immature hepatocytes in the liver exhibited positive staining in their cytosol (Fig. 2C–D). By E11.5, Bicc1 expression was seen in the epithelia of the main bronchi, aorta, and early ureteric bud and mesonephric tubules, as the bud penetrated into the metanephrogenic mesenchyme (Fig. 2E–G). Clear positive staining continued to be observed in the renal comma-shaped body and the S-shaped body by E12.5 (Fig. 2H). At this stage, strong positive immunoreactivity could also be seen in the pancreatic primordium and posterior root ganglions (Fig. 2I–J). At E16.5, strong Bicc1 expression was observed in fasciculated cells in the developing adrenal cortex and in olfactory cells (Fig. 2K–L). By E16.5, the Bicc1 expression appeared to decrease in the cardiomyocytes and primordial gut (data not shown). The finding of Bicc1 protein profiling highly coincides with the studies by *Bicc1* mRNA in situ hybridization [5,6,9].

Expression of Bicc1 in the postnatal mouse kidneys

Using the mBicc1p antibody, we next performed IHC analyses of the kidneys in newborn mice. Bicc1-positive staining was predominantly observed in the developing tubules of the kidney (Fig. 2M). By the age of 1 month, the Bicc1 expression was concentrated at the juxta-medullary region, with relatively weak expression in the cortical and medullary regions (Fig. 2N). At 3 months, although staining pattern was similar to that seen at 1 month, increased Bicc1 expression was seen over the cortical region of the kidney (Fig. 2O). At 6 months, the Bicc1 expression also extended into the medullary region (Fig. 2P). We also examined the kidneys of 9- and 12-month-old mice with the same antibody, but found no significant Bicc1 expression changes. The staining was mainly seen in the cytoplasm of the positive cells, suggesting that Bicc1 has a cytosolic distribution *in vivo* (Fig. 2M–P). Collectively, these results showed that Bicc1 expression is regulated during renal development.

Bicc1 is expressed in multiple nephron segments of the adult mouse kidney

The nephron segments with positive mBicc1p staining were identified by costaining with *Lotus tetragonolobus* lectin (LTL) for the proximal tubules (PT), Tamm-Horsfall glycoprotein (THG) for the medullary thick ascending limb of Henle (LH) and distal tubules (DT) [20,26], and anti-Aquaporin-2 (AQP2) antibodies for the collecting ducts (CD). We examined the immunocytochemical distribution of Bicc1 in paraffin-embedded sections of wildtype adult kidneys. The Pre-IM from the same rabbit used to generate mBicc1p was used as the negative staining control (Fig. 3A). Under these conditions, Bicc1 showed diffuse cytoplasmic staining and was strongly co-expressed with the marker for epithelial cells of the proximal convoluted tubules (Fig. 3B), and distal tubules (Fig. 3C). Relatively weak-positive labeling was also seen in the collecting ducts of the adult kidneys (Fig. 3D). These results suggested that, although it is detected in all the nephronic segments, Bicc1 is highly expressed in the epithelial cells of the proximal convoluted tubules, which are derived from the metanephros, coincides with the previous report that this protein is co-expressed with proximal convoluted tubules of the kidney [14].

Loss of *Pkd1* downregulates the Bicc1 expression *in vitro*

To explore the molecular relationship between *Bicc1* and the other known human ADPKD and ARPKD causal genes, *Pkd1*, *Pkd2*, and *Pkhd1*, we first examined the *Bicc1* mRNA levels in *Pkd1*$^{-/-}$, *Pkd2*$^{-/-}$, or *Pkhd1*$^{-/-}$ cells using qPCR and compared them to the levels in their littermate-generated wildtype counterparts [23,25]. Interestingly, only the cells lacking *Pkd1* exhibited a significant downregulation of *Bicc1* (Fig. 4A), suggesting that the loss of *Pkd1* inhibits *Bicc1* gene expression. To confirm this finding,

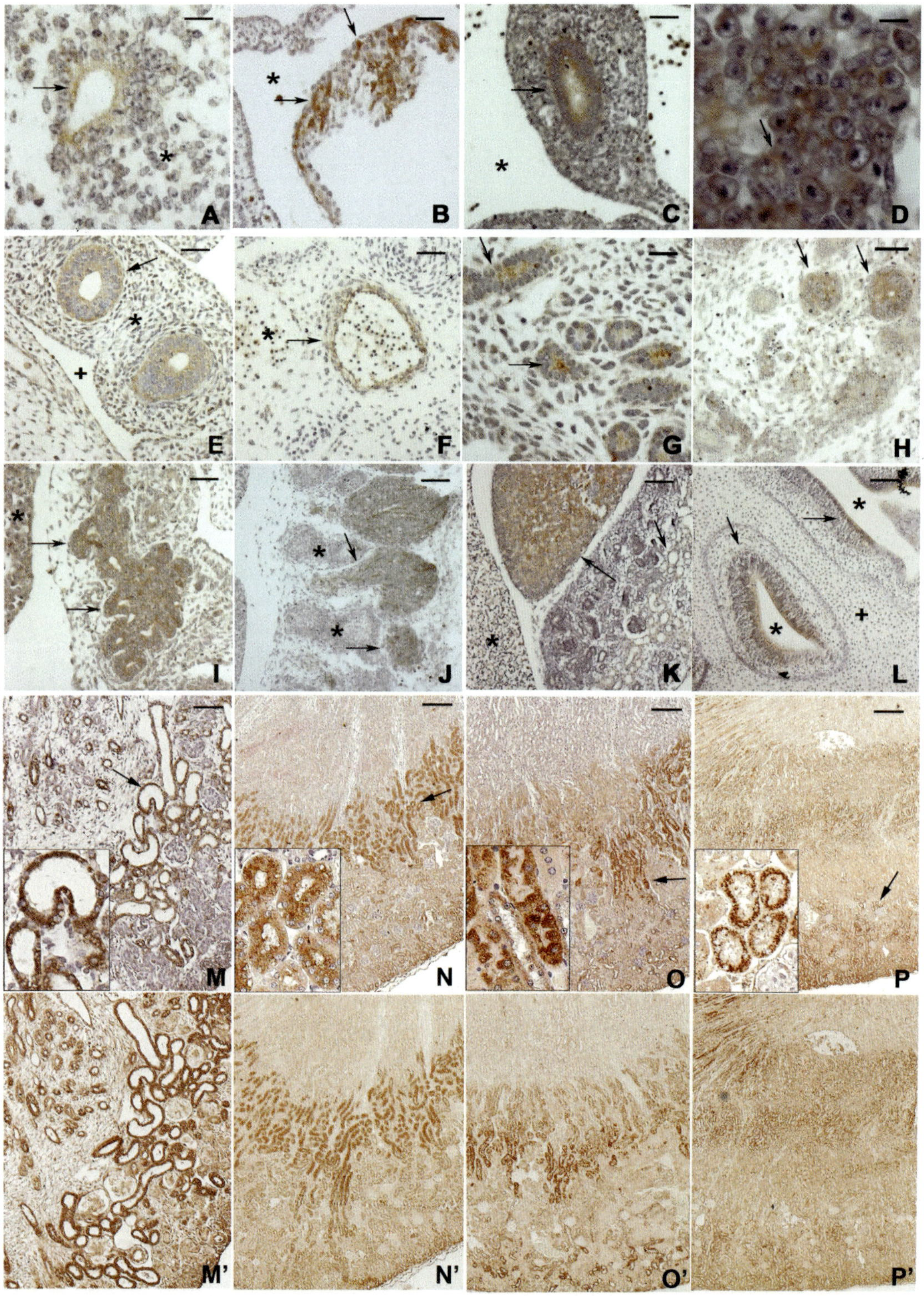

Figure 2. Expressional profiles of Bicc1 protein during embryogenesis and kidney development. By immunohistochemistry (IHC) staining (n≥3), (A) positive labeling is observed in the neural tube (arrow) at E8.5, * indicates the perineural tube mesenchymal tissue; (B) cardiomyocytes in the myocardial wall (arrows) at E9.5, * indicates the pericardio-peritoneal canal; (C) the primordial gut (arrow), * indicates the peritoneal cavity at E10.5; (D) immature hepatocytes (arrow) at E10.5; (E) epithelia of the main bronchi (arrows), + indicates the pericardio-peritoneal canal and * indicates the lung bud tissue; (F) the aortic wall (arrow), * indicates the cardinal vein; and (G) early ureteric bud (lower arrow)/mesonephric duct (upper arrow) at E11.5; (H) the renal comma-shaped body (arrows), (I) epithelia of the pancreatic primordium (arrows), * indicates hepatic tissue and (J) the posterior root ganglions at E12.5, * indicate vertebral bodies. Bicc1 appeared in (K) the adrenal cortex (lower arrow) and cortex of the kidney (upper arrow), * indicates the liver at E16.5; (L) olfactory epithelia (arrows) at E16.5, + indicates the primordial turbinate bone and * indicate the nasal cavities. (M) IHC with mBicc1p antiserum showed positive labeling (arrow) in the newborn mouse kidney. (N) In the 1-month-old kidney, positive staining (arrow) was observed in the juxta-medullary region of the kidney. (O) In the 3-month-old kidney, clear-cut Bicc1 expression (arrow) was seen a similar region of the kidney, but some positive labeling also appeared over the cortical region. (P) Besides of the juxta-medullary and

cortical regions, positive labeling also extended to the medullary regions in the 6-month-old kidney. All high-power positive images were from the arrow-pointed regions and placed on the left-lower corners of M–O. (M′–P′) showed IHC labeling without counterstaining for the corresponding regions of M–O, respectively. Bars: 10 μm in D; 20 μm in A, C, G–H; 25 μm in E and I; 50 μm in B, F, J–L; 100 μm in M; 150 μm in N–O; 300 μm in P.

we used the mBicc1p antibody in western blots of cell lysates from the littermate-derived, paired cell lines $Pkd2^{+/-}$(D3)/$Pkd2^{-/-}$(E8) [23], wildtype (W10B2)/$Pkhd1^{-/-}$(M10H2) [25], or wildtype/ $Pkd1^{-/-}$. We found no differences in Bicc1 expression between the lysates of the $Pkd2^{+/-}$/$Pkd2^{-/-}$ and wildtype/$Pkhd1^{-/-}$ cells (Fig. 4B–C). By comparison, however, there was a marked decrease in Bicc1 expression in the lysates of the $Pkd1^{-/-}$ cells (Fig. 4D). The mRNA and western results together indicated that $Pkd1^{-/-}$ cells had approximately half the Bicc1 levels of their wildtype littermates (Fig. 4A, E), and suggested that both the mRNA and protein of *Bicc1* are downregulated by the lack of *Pkd1*.

To further validate this finding, we have restored the entire human PC1 COOH-terminus (PC1-CT) into $Pkd1^{-/-}$ cells by lentivirus system to determine if re-expression of PC1 can rescue the downregulation of Bicc1 in the null-*Pkd1* cells. The western blots of cell lysates from the littermate-derived cell lines: wildtype, and $Pkd1^{-/-}$, as well as $Pkd1^{-/-}$ cells transfected with the PC1-pSico vector ($Pkd1^{-/-}$+PC1-CT) showed that downregulation of Bicc1 of $Pkd1^{-/-}$ cells can be significantly rescued (Fig. 4F–G). This result strongly demonstrates that downregulation of Bicc1 expression in the *Pkd1* deficient cells is due to loss of PC1.

Mice with null-*Pkd1* alleles also exhibit Bicc1 downregulation

To validate this finding *in vivo*, we performed IHC with mBicc1p using embryonic kidneys from wildtype, *Pkd1*, *Pkd2*, or *Pkhd1* mice. Compared to wildtype, the Bicc1 expression was significantly decreased in the kidney of the $Pkd1^{-/-}$ littermates at E14.5 (Fig. 5Aa *vs.* b). However, the Bicc1 expression levels in E14.5 kidneys of $Pkhd1^{-/-}$ and $Pkd2^{-/-}$ mice seem similar to their wildtype littermates (Fig. 5Ac *vs.* d and Fig. 5Ae *vs.* f).

Finally, we have also performed western analyses from tissue lysates of E14.5 null-*Pkd2*, null-*Pkd1* and null-*Pkhd1* embryos, and their wildtype-littermates as well. Compared to wildtype, Bicc1 is also significantly downregulated in the null-*Pkd1* tissues. However, there are no any Bicc1 expression changes between the tissue lysates with and without *Pkd2* and *Pkhd1* (Fig. 5B–C). These *in vivo* results provide further evidence that the loss of *Pkd1* downregulates Bicc1 expression.

Discussion

Studies using chemically-induced or natively occurring *Bicc1*-mutant mouse models (*jcpk* and *bpk*) and other *Bicc1*-gene-targeted mouse models have recently demonstrated that the disruption of *Bicc1* can induce polycystic kidney disease with phenotypes very similar to human ADPKD [5,6,17]. Although gene expression of *Bicc1* during mouse development has been previously reported [5,6,9,14], the characteristics of *Bicc1* gene product, Bicc1, during embryogenesis and organogenesis in mammals has not been completely explored. In this study, we generated a new polyclonal antibody, mBicc1p, against the *Bicc1* gene product, Bicc1, and used it to study the expression of Bicc1 during mouse development. By using this antibody, we also discovered that the loss of *Pkd1* downregulates Bicc1 expression *in vitro* and *in vivo*, revealing a molecular relationship between *Bicc1* and *Pkd1*, a known causal gene for human ADPKD. Our findings demonstrate that Bicc1 expression is developmentally regulated and that its normal function may require PC1 expression.

To investigate the functional role of Bicc1 during mammalian development, several studies have examined mouse *Bicc1* gene expression patterns using *in situ* mRNA hybridization [6,9]. By whole-mount *in situ* hybridization, *Bicc1* mRNA expression is first detected at the rostral tip of the primitive streak around E7.5 and in neural tissues at E8.5. At E13.5, strong *Bicc1* mRNA labeling is detected in the bone, heart, and lung tissues. In mouse kidney development, *Bicc1* mRNA is detected at the mesonephros and the first branch of the ureteric bud tree at E11.5, and then at the metanephros and the comma- and S-shaped bodies at E13.5. At birth, *Bicc1* mRNA is mainly seen in the proximal tubules of the

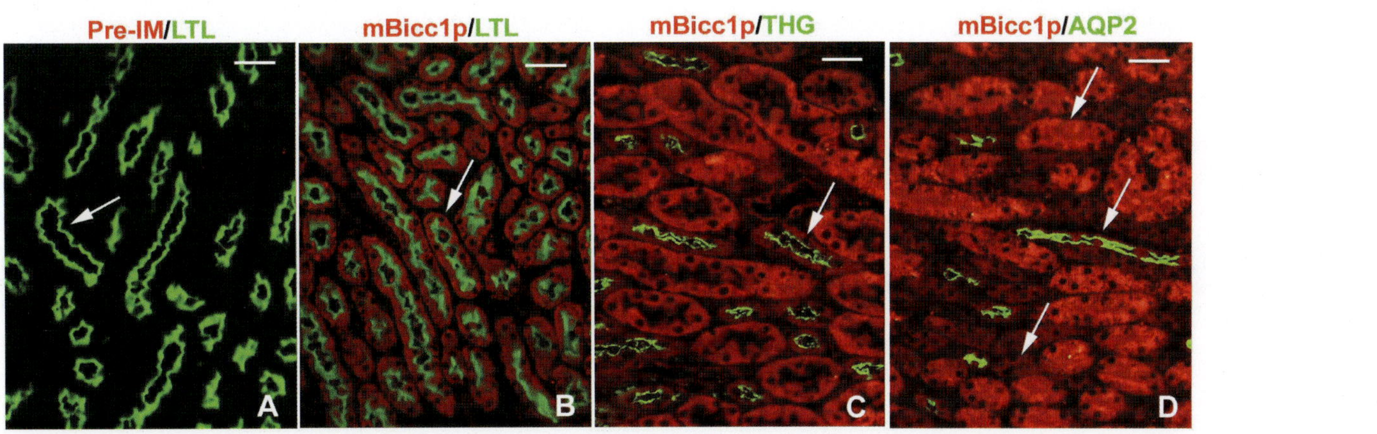

Figure 3. Bicc1 expression in renal nephrons. Double immunofluorescence staining with mBicc1p and nephronic markers (LTL, THG, and AQP2) in paraffin-embedded sections of adult wildtype mouse kidneys (n≥5). (A) The Pre-IM was used as a negative staining control. (B) Bicc1 (red) was co-expressed with LTL (green) in the epithelial cells of the renal proximal tubules; (C) Bicc1 (red) was also co-expressed with THG (green) in the epithelial cells of the Henle's thick ascending limbs; (D) With mBicc1p staining (red), Bicc1 was highly expressed in the renal proximal tubules (top arrow) and weakly expressed in the collecting ducts (lower arrow). mBicc1p co-staining with the anti-AQP2 antibody (green) showed weakly co-expression of Bicc1 and AQP2 in the epithelial cells of the collecting ducts (middle arrow). Bar: 30 μm in A–D.

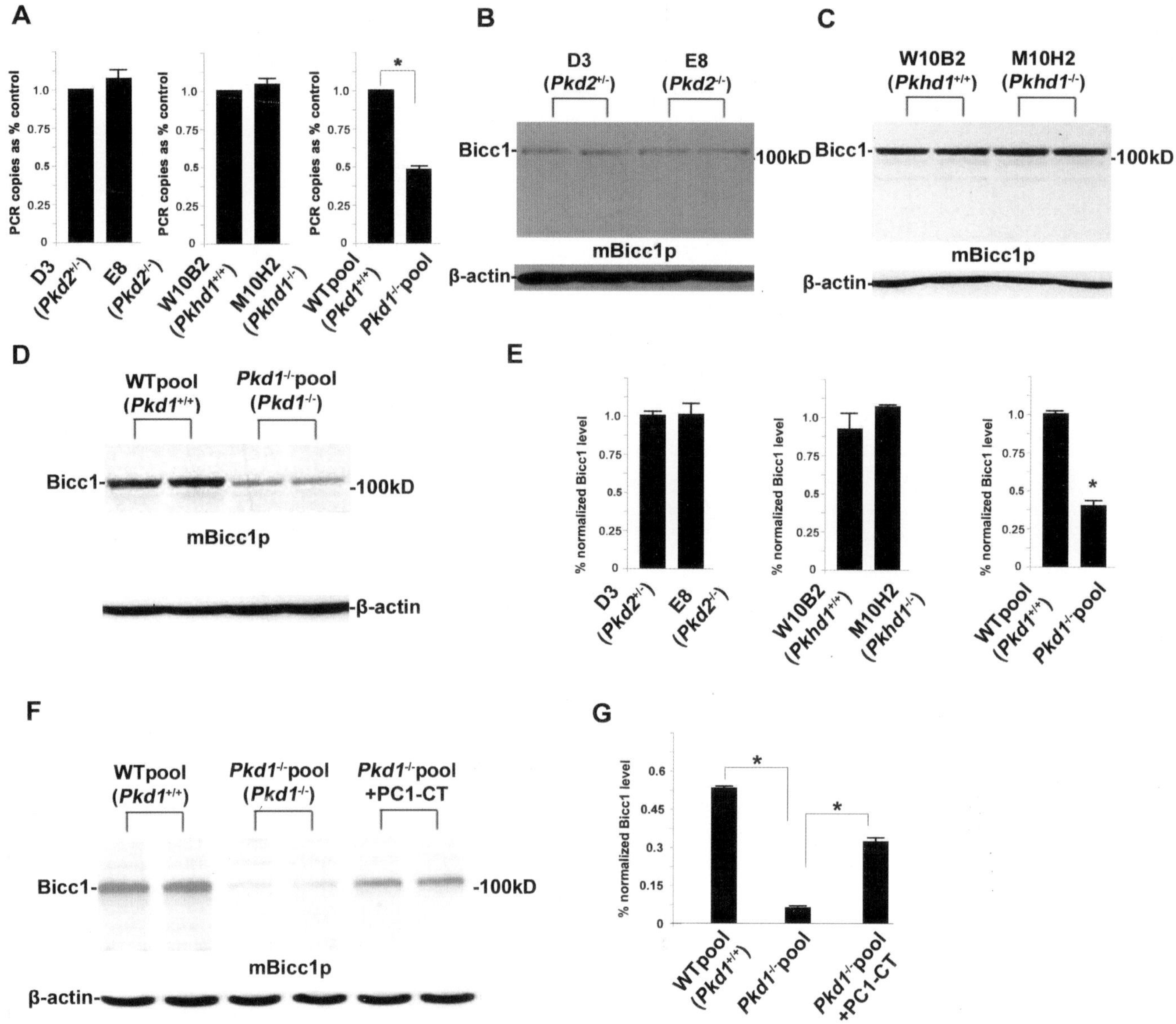

Figure 4. Loss of PC1 downregulates Bicc1 expression *in vitro.* (A) qPCR analysis of cultured cell lines with or without *Pkd1*, *Pkd2*, or *Pkhd1* showed no change in the *Pkd2* or *Pkhd1* mRNA expression, while *Bicc1* was significantly downregulated in the cells lacking *Pkd1* compared to the wildtype control (*P<0.05) (n = 3). (B) Western blot analysis of protein lysates from null-*Pkd2* cells (E8) and *Pkd2*-heterozygous cells (D3) using the mBicc1p antibody suggested that PC2 loss did not affect Bicc1 expression. (C) Similar western blots for null-*Pkhd1* cells (M10H2) and *Pkhd1*-wildtype cells (W10B2) showed that loss of *Pkhd1* also did not affect Bicc1 expression. (D) Western blot analysis for the null-*Pkd1* cells and their wildtype littermate cells showed that loss of *Pkd1* markedly downregulated the Bicc1 protein expression. (E) Normalized quantitative analysis of the densitometry values of the western analyses. Compared to null-*Pkd2* or -*Pkhd1* cells, only the null-*Pkd1* cells showed significantly reduced Bicc1 expression (*P<0.05). (F) With the wildtype littermate cell control, western blot analyses for the null-*Pkd1* pool cells and their PC1-CT transfected cells showed that the restoration of PC1 COOH-terminus markedly rescued the downregulation level of Bicc1 expression in the null-*Pkd1* cells. (G) Normalized quantitative analysis of the densitometry values of the western analyses. Compared to the null-*Pkd1* cells, the cells with PC1-CT transfection can partially restored Bicc1 expression in the null-*Pkd1* cells (*P<0.05). Data presented are representative of two to three independently replicated experiments.

mouse kidney. These *Bicc1* mRNA patterns and tissue distributions highly correspond to our findings with anti-Bicc1 antibody staining, further demonstrating the specificity of the mBicc1p antibody for Bicc1, and supporting protein expression profile described in this study.

Primary cilia are found on diverse cell types ranging from fibroblasts to epithelia [27]. These cilia are generally thought to function as extracellular sensors, for regulating cell behavior [28]. Many human and rodent cystoproteins, the mutants of which cause PKD phenotypes, have been reported to co-localize with the primary cilium/basal bodies of renal epithelia [1,29]. However, previous reports indicate that Bicc1 was distributed to the P-bodies of renal epithelial cells [5,6,14]. This novel subcellular localization of Bicc1 indicated that the primary cilium/basal bodies in renal epithelial cells may not be the only targeted organelle for cystogenesis of the kidney.

We recently established stable IMCD (mouse inner medullary collecting duct) cell lines, in which *Bicc1* is silenced by short hairpin

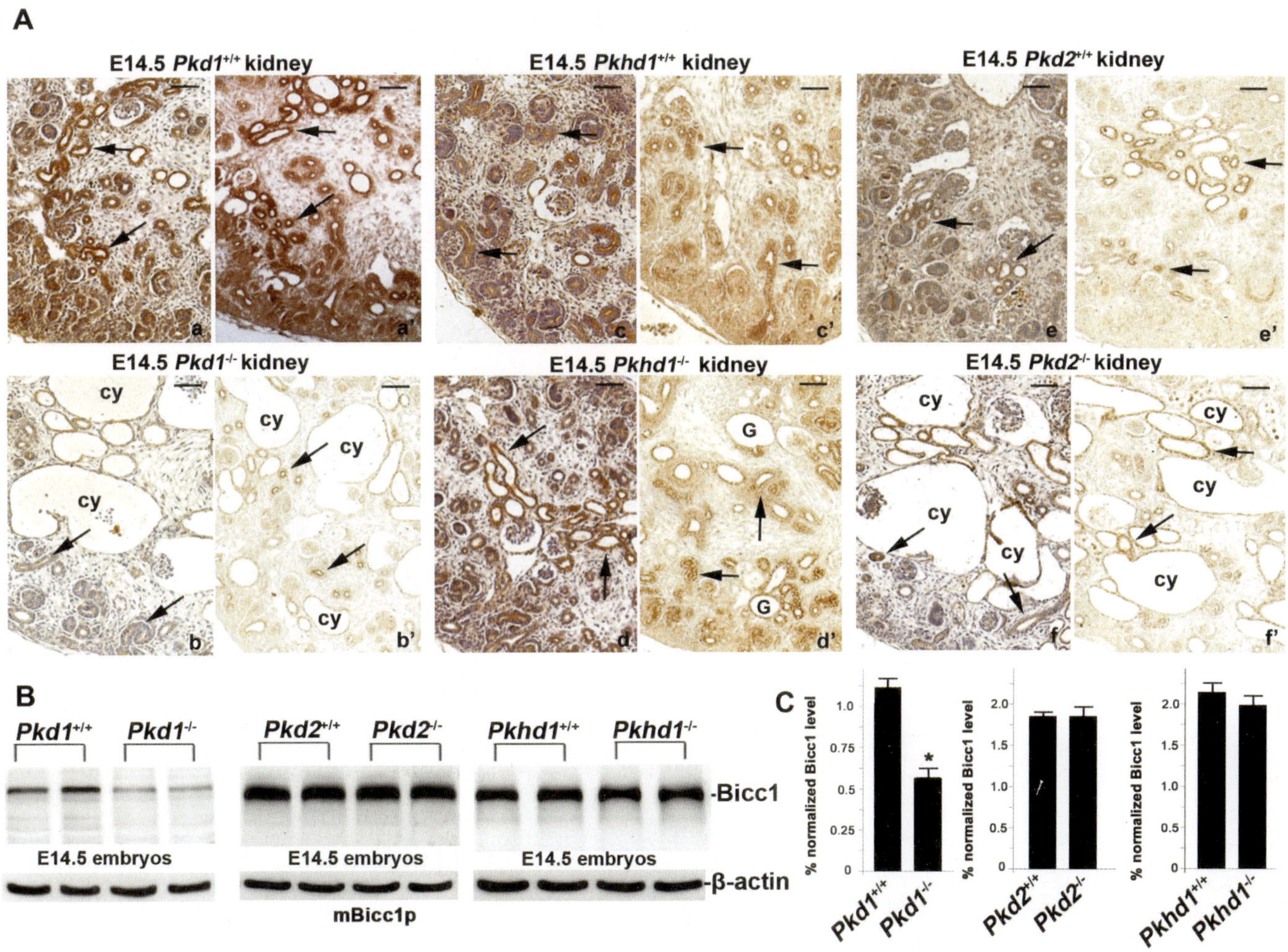

Figure 5. Loss of PC1 downregulates Bicc1 expression *in vivo*. (A) Positive mBicc1p IHC staining (arrows) in the mouse embryonic kidneys. The E14.5 wildtype (a) and its littermate *Pkd1*$^{-/-}$ (b) kidneys were stained by mBicc1p antibody (n≥3). In comparisons of kidney tissues with and without *Pkd1*, the null-*Pkd1* kidney showed significantly reduced Bicc1 expression. However, there are no Bicc1 expressional difference between the age-matched wildtype (c and e) and their littermate *Pkhd1*$^{-/-}$ (d) or littermate *Pkd2*$^{-/-}$ (f) kidneys, respectively. "cy" = renal cysts; "G" = glomerulus. (B) Compared to its wildtype littermate, western blot of duplicated tissue lysates from E14.5 embryos showed that loss of PC1 markedly downregulates Bicc1 protein level (left panel). A similar western blot showed equal immunoreactivities between the tissue lysates from E14.5 *Pkd2*$^{-/-}$ and its wildtype littermate (middle panel) and between the E14.5 *Pkhd1*$^{-/-}$ and its littermate wildtype embryos (n≥3). β-actin for protein loading control. (C) Normalized quantitative analysis of densitometry values of the western analyses. Compared tissues with and without *Pkd1*, *Pkd2* or *Pkhd1*, only null-*Pkd1* tissue shows significantly reduced Bicc1 expression (*$P<0.05$). Bars: 50 μm in A.

RNA (shRNA) expression. Our previous results showed that the inhibition of Bicc1 disrupts normal tubulomorphogenesis and induces the cystogenesis of IMCD cells grown in three-dimensional culture [24]. These cells also have a significant defect in E-cadherin-based cell-cell adhesion, along with abnormalities in actin cytoskeletal organization, cell-extracellular matrix interactions, ciliogenesis, and cell proliferation/apoptosis. Interestingly, these defects are also seen in epithelial cells lacking *Pkd1* and *Pkd2*, mutations that can cause human ADPKD [23,30,31]. We therefore assume that the cystogenesis resulting from the downregulation of *Bicc1* may be associated with a disruption in the normal *Pkd1* or *Pkd2* expression.

As predicted, a recent study demonstrated that the absence of *Bicc1* in cells promotes miR-17's binding to the 3′UTR of *Pkd2* and disrupts the stability of the *Pkd2* mRNA [6]. This finding indicates that *Bicc1* acts as a posttranscriptional factor upstream of *Pkd2* and reveals the molecular relationship between *Bicc1* and *Pkd2*, a causal gene of human ADPKD. In the present study, we showed that another human ADPKD causal gene, *Pkd1*, is involved in the regulation of *Bicc1* expression *in vitro* and *in vivo*. This finding indicates that *Bicc1* is not only associated with *Pkd2*, but also with *Pkd1* expression. The association between Bicc1 and polycystins implies that a disruption of *Bicc1* induces cystic phenotypes through the polycystin pathway.

In summary, we have newly generated a polyclonal antibody, mBicc1p, that is specific for the *Bicc1* gene product Bicc1. Using this antibody, we demonstrated the developmental profile of Bicc1 protein during embryogenesis and organogenesis in mammals. We found that the Bicc1 protein is expressed as early as E8.5 in the mouse neural tube and appears at the ureteric bud and nephronic tubules by E11.5. After birth, Bicc1 expression extends into the proximal tubules of the kidney, and thereby is predominately expressed in this nephron segment. Moreover, we discovered that normal Bicc1 expression requires PC1 expression. These findings together indicate that Bicc1 is a key protein for embryogenesis and organogenesis in mammals and uncover a new molecular link between *Biccl* and *Pkd1*, whose mutation causes human ADPKD.

Acknowledgments

We greatly thank Drs. Oliver Wessely at Cleveland Clinic Foundation and Daniel Constam at Ecole Polytechnique Fédérale de Lausanne (EPFL), School of Life Sciences, Bâtiment SV kindly provides *Biccl* knockout embryos.

Author Contributions

Conceived and designed the experiments: GW. Performed the experiments: PL AL YL HL D. Liang BH D. Lin. Analyzed the data: TJ GM DQ GW. Contributed reagents/materials/analysis tools: PL AL YL HL D. Liang BH D. Lin. Wrote the paper: GM DQ GW.

References

1. Harris PC, Torres VE (2009) Polycystic kidney disease. Annu Rev Med 60: 321–337.
2. Torres VE, Harris PC (2009) Autosomal dominant polycystic kidney disease: the last 3 years. Kidney Int 76: 149–168.
3. Wilson PD, Goilav B (2007) Cystic disease of the kidney. Annu Rev Pathol 2: 341.
4. Bouvrette DJ, Price SJ, Bryda EC (2008) K homology domains of the mouse polycystic kidney disease-related protein, Bicaudal-C (Bicc1), mediate RNA binding in vitro. Nephron Exp Nephrol 108: e27–34.
5. Maisonneuve C, Guilleret I, Vick P, Weber T, Andre P, et al. (2009) Bicaudal C, a novel regulator of Dvl signaling abutting RNA-processing bodies, controls cilia orientation and leftward flow. Development 136: 3019–3030.
6. Tran U, Zakin L, Schweickert A, Agrawal R, Doger R, et al. (2010) The RNA-binding protein bicaudal C regulates polycystin 2 in the kidney by antagonizing miR-17 activity. Development 137: 1107–1116.
7. Kraus MR, Clauin S, Pfister Y, Di Maio M, Ulinski T, et al. (2012) Two mutations in human BICC1 resulting in Wnt pathway hyperactivity associated with cystic renal dysplasia. Hum Mutat 33: 86–90.
8. Zhou L, Dai B, Wu G (2008) Molecular Characteristics and Functions of Bicaudal-C. Int J Genet 31: 432–435.
9. Wessely O, Tran U, Zakin L, De Robertis EM (2001) Identification and expression of the mammalian homologue of Bicaudal-C. Mech Dev 101: 267–270.
10. Mahone M, Saffman EE, Lasko PF (1995) Localized Bicaudal-C RNA encodes a protein containing a KH domain, the RNA binding motif of FMR1. EMBO J 14: 2043–2055.
11. Wessely O, De Robertis EM (2000) The Xenopus homologue of Bicaudal-C is a localized maternal mRNA that can induce endoderm formation. Development 127: 2053–2062.
12. Bouvrette DJ, Sittaramane V, Heidel JR, Chandrasekhar A, Bryda EC (2010) Knockdown of bicaudal C in zebrafish (Danio rerio) causes cystic kidneys: a nonmammalian model of polycystic kidney disease. Comp Med 60: 96–106.
13. Chen T, Damaj BB, Herrera C, Lasko P, Richard S (1997) Self-association of the single-KH-domain family members Sam68, GRP33, GLD-1, and Qk1: role of the KH domain. Mol Cell Biol 17: 5707–5718.
14. Piazzon N, Maisonneuve C, Guilleret I, Rotman S, Constam DB (2012) Bicc1 links the regulation of cAMP signaling in polycystic kidneys to microRNA-induced gene silencing. J Mol Cell Biol.
15. Flaherty L, Bryda EC, Collins D, Rudofsky U, Montogomery JC (1995) New mouse model for polycystic kidney disease with both recessive and dominant gene effects. Kidney Int 47: 552–558.
16. Nauta J, Sweeney WE, Rutledge JC, Avner ED (1995) Biliary epithelial cells from mice with congenital polycystic kidney disease are hyperresponsive to epidermal growth factor. Pediatr Res 37: 755–763.
17. Cogswell C, Price SJ, Hou X, Guay-Woodford LM, Flaherty L, et al. (2003) Positional cloning of jcpk/bpk locus of the mouse. Mamm Genome 14: 242–249.
18. Zhang MZ, Mai W, Li C, Cho SY, Hao C, et al. (2004) PKHD1 protein encoded by the gene for autosomal recessive polycystic kidney disease associates with basal bodies and primary cilia in renal epithelial cells. Proc Natl Acad Sci U S A 101: 2311–2316.
19. Wu G, Markowitz GS, Li L, D'Agati VD, Factor SM, et al. (2000) Cardiac defects and renal failure in mice with targeted mutations in Pkd2. Nat Genet 24: 75–78.
20. Wu G, Tian X, Nishimura S, Markowitz GS, D'Agati V, et al. (2002) Trans-heterozygous Pkd1 and Pkd2 mutations modify expression of polycystic kidney disease. Hum Mol Genet 11: 1845–1854.
21. Kim I, Fu Y, Hui K, Moeckel G, Mai W, et al. (2008) Fibrocystin/polyductin modulates renal tubular formation by regulating polycystin-2 expression and function. J Am Soc Nephrol 19: 455–468.
22. Kim I, Li C, Liang D, Chen XZ, Coffy RJ, et al. (2008) Polycystin-2 expression is regulated by a PC2-binding domain in the intracellular portion of fibrocystin. J Biol Chem 283: 31559–31566.
23. Kim I, Ding T, Fu Y, Li C, Cui L, et al. (2009) Conditional mutation of Pkd2 causes cystogenesis and upregulates beta-catenin. J Am Soc Nephrol 20: 2556–2569.
24. Fu Y, Kim I, Lian P, Li A, Zhou L, et al. (2010) Loss of Bicc1 impairs tubulomorphogenesis of cultured IMCD cells by disrupting E-cadherin-based cell-cell adhesion. Eur J Cell Biol 89: 428–436.
25. Hu B, He X, Li A, Qiu Q, Li C, et al. (2011) Cystogenesis in ARPKD results from increased apoptosis in collecting duct epithelial cells of Pkhd1 mutant kidneys. Exp Cell Res 317: 173–187.
26. Kokot F, Dulawa J (2000) Tamm-Horsfall protein updated. Nephron 85: 97–102.
27. Wheatley DN (1995) Primary cilia in normal and pathological tissues. Pathobiology 63: 222–238.
28. Pazour GJ, Witman GB (2003) The vertebrate primary cilium is a sensory organelle. Curr Opin Cell Biol 15: 105–110.
29. Yoder BK (2007) Role of primary cilia in the pathogenesis of polycystic kidney disease. J Am Soc Nephrol 18: 1381–1388.
30. Boletta A, Qian F, Onuchic LF, Bhunia AK, Phakdeekitcharoen B, et al. (2000) Polycystin-1, the gene product of PKD1, induces resistance to apoptosis and spontaneous tubulogenesis in MDCK cells. Mol Cell 6: 1267–1273.
31. Streets AJ, Wagner BE, Harris PC, Ward CJ, Ong AC (2009) Homophilic and heterophilic polycystin 1 interactions regulate E-cadherin recruitment and junction assembly in MDCK cells. J Cell Sci 122: 1410–1417.

Permissions

All chapters in this book were first published in PLOS ONE, by The Public Library of Science; hereby published with permission under the Creative Commons Attribution License or equivalent. Every chapter published in this book has been scrutinized by our experts. Their significance has been extensively debated. The topics covered herein carry significant findings which will fuel the growth of the discipline. They may even be implemented as practical applications or may be referred to as a beginning point for another development.

The contributors of this book come from diverse backgrounds, making this book a truly international effort. This book will bring forth new frontiers with its revolutionizing research information and detailed analysis of the nascent developments around the world.

We would like to thank all the contributing authors for lending their expertise to make the book truly unique. They have played a crucial role in the development of this book. Without their invaluable contributions this book wouldn't have been possible. They have made vital efforts to compile up to date information on the varied aspects of this subject to make this book a valuable addition to the collection of many professionals and students.

This book was conceptualized with the vision of imparting up-to-date information and advanced data in this field. To ensure the same, a matchless editorial board was set up. Every individual on the board went through rigorous rounds of assessment to prove their worth. After which they invested a large part of their time researching and compiling the most relevant data for our readers.

The editorial board has been involved in producing this book since its inception. They have spent rigorous hours researching and exploring the diverse topics which have resulted in the successful publishing of this book. They have passed on their knowledge of decades through this book. To expedite this challenging task, the publisher supported the team at every step. A small team of assistant editors was also appointed to further simplify the editing procedure and attain best results for the readers.

Apart from the editorial board, the designing team has also invested a significant amount of their time in understanding the subject and creating the most relevant covers. They scrutinized every image to scout for the most suitable representation of the subject and create an appropriate cover for the book.

The publishing team has been an ardent support to the editorial, designing and production team. Their endless efforts to recruit the best for this project, has resulted in the accomplishment of this book. They are a veteran in the field of academics and their pool of knowledge is as vast as their experience in printing. Their expertise and guidance has proved useful at every step. Their uncompromising quality standards have made this book an exceptional effort. Their encouragement from time to time has been an inspiration for everyone.

The publisher and the editorial board hope that this book will prove to be a valuable piece of knowledge for researchers, students, practitioners and scholars across the globe.

List of Contributors

Nathalie Itzhar, Philippe Dessen, Saloua Toujani, Nathalie Auger and Alain Bernheim
Institut de la Santé et de la Reherche Médicale U985, Génétique des tumeurs, Institut Gustave Roussy, Villejuif, France

Nathalie Itzhar, Philippe Dessen, Saloua Toujani and Nathalie Auger and Alain Bernheim
Université Paris XI, Paris Sud, Orsay, France

Nathalie Itzhar, Nathalie Auger, Vladimir Lazar, Véronique Saada, Anelyse Bennaceur and Alain Bernheim
Molecular Pathology, Villejuif, France

Philippe Dessen Catherine Richon and Vladimir Lazar
Institut Gustave Roussy, Functional Genomics Unit, Institut Gustave Roussy, Villejuif, France

Claude Preudhomme
Department of Hematology, Centre de Biologie-Pathologie, Centre Hospitalier Régional Universitaire de Lille, Lille, France

Véronique Saada, Anelyse Bennaceur, Jean Henri Bourhis and Stéphane de Botton
Department of Hematology, Institut Gustave Roussy, Villejuif, France

Ding-Bang Chen, Li Feng, Xiu-Ling Liang and Xun-Hua Li
Department of Neurology, First Affiliated Hospital, Sun Yat-sen University, Guangzhou, China

Xiao-Pu Lin
Nanfang Hospital, Southern Medical University, Guangzhou, China

Wei Zhang and Fu-Rong Li
Laboratory Animal Centre, Sun Yat-sen University, Guangzhou, China

Jayeeta Ghose, Eashita Das and Nitai P. Bhattacharyya
Crystallography and Molecular Biology Division, Saha Institute of Nuclear Physics, Kolkata, West Bengal, India

Mithun Sinha
Structural Genomics Division, Saha Institute of Nuclear Physics, Kolkata, West Bengal, India

Nihar R. Jana
Division of Cellular and Molecular Neuroscience, National Brain Research Centre, Manesar, Haryana, India

Kenneth I. Ataga, Payal Desai, Susan Jones, John Delaney, Dell Strayhorn and Nigel S. Key
Division of Hematology/Oncology, University of North Carolina, Chapel Hill, North Carolina, United States of America

Julia E. Brittain
Department of Biochemistry and Biophysics, University of North Carolina, Chapel Hill, North Carolina, United States of America

Ryan May
Department of Biostatistics, University of North Carolina, Chapel Hill, North Carolina, United States of America

Alan Hinderliter
Division of Cardiology, University of North Carolina, Chapel Hill, North Carolina, United States of America

Jacqueline N. Milton, Paola Sebastiani, Nadia Solovieff and Stephen W. Hartley
Department of Biostatistics, Boston University School of Public Health, Boston, Massachusetts, United States of America

Daniel A. Dworkis, Clinton T. Baldwin, Martin H. Steinberg and Elizabeth S. Klings
Department of Medicine, Boston University School of Medicine, Boston, Massachusetts, United States of America

Elizabeth S. Klings
The Pulmonary Center, Boston University School of Medicine, Boston, Massachusetts, United States of America

Pallav Bhatnagar and Dan E. Arking
McKusick-Nathans Institute of Genetic Medicine, Johns Hopkins University School of Medicine, Baltimore, Maryland, United States of America

James F. Casella and Emily Barron-Casella
Department of Pediatrics, Division of Pediatric Hematology, Johns Hopkins University School of Medicine, Baltimore, Maryland, United States of America

Christopher J. Bean and W. Craig Hooper
Clinical and Molecular Hemostasis Laboratory Branch, Division of Blood Disorders, National Center on Birth Defects and Developmental Disabilities, Centers for Disease Control and Prevention, Atlanta, Georgia, United States of America

Michael R. De Baun
Vanderbilt School of Medicine, Nashville, Tennessee, United States of America

Melanie E. Garrett, Karen Soldano, Marilyn J. Telen and Allison Ashley-Koch
Department of Medicine, Duke University Medical Center, Durham, North Carolina, United States of America

Mark T. Gladwin
Division of Pulmonary, Allergy and Critical Care Medicine and the Vascular Medicine Institute, University of Pittsburgh, Pittsburgh, Pennsylvania, United States of America

Ying Sun, Huimin Ran, Benjamin Liou, Brian Quinn, Matt Zamzow and Gregory A. Grabowski
The Division of Human Genetics, University of Cincinnati College of Medicine, Cincinnati, Ohio, United States of America

Wujuan Zhang and Kenneth D. R. Setchell
The Division of Pathology and Laboratory Medicine, Cincinnati Children's Hospital Medical Center, University of Cincinnati College of Medicine, Cincinnati, Ohio, United States of America

Ying Sun, Huimin Ran, Benjamin Liou, Brian Quinn, Matt Zamzow, Wujuan Zhang, Kenneth D. R. Setchell and Gregory A. Grabowski
The Department of Pediatrics, University of Cincinnati College of Medicine, Cincinnati, Ohio, United States of America

Jacek Bielawski, Kazuyuki Kitatani and Yusuf A. Hannun
The Department of Biochemistry and Molecular Biology, Medical University of South Carolina, Charleston, South Carolina, United States of America

Kazuyuki Kitatani
The Department of Clinical Laboratory, Tottori University Hospital, Tottori University, Yonago, Japan

Lawrence W. Gray, Venkata S. Pendyala, Abigael Muchenditsi and Svetlana Lutsenko
Department of Physiology, Johns Hopkins University, School of Medicine, Baltimore, Maryland, United States of America

Fangyu Peng
Department of Radiology, University of Texas Southwestern Medical Center, Dallas, Texas, United States of America

Shannon A. Molloy and Jack H. Kaplan
Department of Biochemistry and Molecular Genetics, University of Illinois at Chicago, Chicago, Illinois, United States of America

Otto Muzik
Carman and Ann Adams Department of Pediatrics and Department of Radiology, Wayne State University, School of Medicine, Detroit, Michigan, United States of America

Jaekwon Lee
Redox Biology Center, Department of Biochemistry, University of Nebraska, Lincoln, Nebraska, United States of America

Marie D. Burdick, Brett A. Strieter, Ling Liu, Borna Mehrad, C. Edward Rose, Jr. and Robert M. Strieter
Department of Medicine, Division of Pulmonary and Critical Care Medicine, The University of Virginia School of Medicine, Charlottesville, Virginia, United States of America

Joshua J. Field
Blood Center of Wisconsin, Blood Research Institute, Milwaukee, Wisconsin, United States of America

Michael R. De Baun
Departments of Pediatrics and Medicine, Division of Hematology and Oncology, Vanderbilt University School of Medicine, Nashville, Tennessee, United States of America

Joel Linden
La Jolla Institute for Allergy and Immunology, La Jolla, California, United States of America

Carles Garcia-Linares, Jaume Mercadé, Bernat Gel, Josep Biayna, Ernest Terribas and Eduard Serra
Institute of Predictive and Personalized Medicine of Cancer (IMPPC), Badalona, Barcelona, Spain

Conxi Lázaro
Programa de Diagnòstic Molecular de Càncer Hereditari, Laboratori de Recerca Translacional, Institut Català d'Oncologia (ICO) - IDIBELL, L'Hospitalet de Llobregat, Barcelona, Spain

Joost Schulte, Katharine J. Sepp and J. Troy Littleton
Department of Biology, Department of Brain and Cognitive Sciences, The Picower Institute for Learning and Memory, Massachusetts Institute of Technology, Cambridge, Massachusetts, United States of America

Chaohong Wu and Pengyu Hong
Department of Computer Science, National Center for Behavioral Genomics, Brandeis University, Waltham, Massachusetts, United States of America

Deborah A. Altomare, Craig W. Menges, Jinfei Xu, Jianming Pei, Lili Zhang, Ara Tadevosyan, Erin Neumann-Domer, Zemin Liu, Andres J. Klein-Szanto and Joseph R. Testa
Cancer Biology Program, Fox Chase Cancer Center, Philadelphia, Pennsylvania, United States of America

Michele Carbone
Thoracic Oncology Program, Cancer Research Center of Hawaii, University of Hawaii, Honolulu, Hawaii, United States of America

Ilse Chudoba
MetaSystems, Altlussheim, Germany

Marina Antelo, Ana Cabanne, Mario Edmundo Barugel and Enrique Luis Roca
Oncology and Pathology Sections, Hospital of Gastroenterology "Dr. C. B. Udaondo", Buenos Aires, Argentina

Francesc Balaguer, Yan Shen, Keun Hur, Masanobu Takahashi, Mildred Arnold and C. Richard Boland and Ajay Goel
Department of Internal Medicine, Division of Gastroenterology, Charles A. Sammons Cancer Center and Baylor Research Institute, Baylor University Medical Center, Dallas, Texas, United States of America

Francesc Balaguer, Leticia Moreira, Maria Dolores Giraldez and Sergi Castellvi-Bel
Department of Gastroenterology, Hospital Clínic, Centro de Investigación Biomédica en Red de Enfermedades Hepáticas y Digestivas (CIBERehd), Institut d'Investigacions Biomediques August Pi i Sunyer (IDIBAPS), University of Barcelona, Barcelona, Catalonia, Spain

Jinru Shia
Department of Pathology, Memorial Sloan Kettering Cancer Center, New York, New York, United States of America

Luis Bujanda
Department of Gastroenterology, CIBERehd, University of Country Basque, Donostia Hospital, San Sebastián, Spain

Montserrat Andreu
Deparment of Gastroenterology, Hospital del Mar, Barcelona, Spain

Xavier Llor
Department of Medicine and Cancer Center, University of Illinois at Chicago, Chicago, Illinois, United States of America

Rodrigo Jover
Gastroenterology Unit, Hospital General Universitario, Alicante, Spain

David C. Butler and Anne Messer
Wadsworth Center, New York State Department of Health, Albany, New York, United States of America
Department of Biomedical Sciences, University at Albany, Albany, New York, United States of America

Anna Bobrowska and Gillian P. Bates
Department of Medical and Molecular Genetics, King's College London, London, United Kingdom

Paolo Paganetti
Novartis Institutes for BioMedical Research, Neuroscience Discovery, Basel, Switzerland

Patrick Matthias
Friedrich Miescher Institute for Biomedical Research, Novartis Research Foundation, Basel, Switzerland

Marly A. Cardoso
Department of Nutrition, School of Public Health, University of São Paulo, São Paulo, Brazil

Kézia K.G. Scopel
Department of Parasitology, Immunology and Microbiology, Federal University of Juiz de Fora, Juiz de Fora, Minas Gerais, Brazil

Pascoal T. Muniz
Department of Health Sciences, Federal University of Acre, Rio Branco, Acre, Brazil

Eduardo Villamor
Departments of Environmental Health Sciences and Epidemiology, University of Michigan School of Public Health, Ann Arbor, Michigan, United States of America

Marcelo U. Ferreira
Department of Parasitology, Institute of Biomedical Sciences, University of São Paulo, São Paulo, Brazil

Nai-Kuei Huang, Wan-Ping Chen, Yuh-Chiang Shen and Yun-Lian Lin
National Research Institute of Chinese Medicine, Taipei, Taiwan

Jung-Hsin Lin
Division of Mechanics, Research Center for Applied Sciences, Academia Sinica, Taipei, Taiwan

Jung-Hsin Lin, Jiun-Tsai Lin, Hui-Mei Chen, Hsing-Lin Lai, Yu-Shuo Wu, Chen Chang and Yijuang Chern
Institute of Biomedical Sciences, Academia Sinica, Taipei, Taiwan

Jung-Hsin Lin, Eric Minwei Liu and Chun-Jung Lin
School of Pharmacy, National Taiwan University, Taipei, Taiwan

Chia-I Lin, Jhih-Bin Chen, Chieh-Wen Yang and Jim-Min Fang
Department of Chemistry, National Taiwan University, Taipei, Taiwan

Jim-Min Fang
The Genomics Research Center, Academia Sinica, Taipei, Taiwan

Li Zou, Qi Wang, Yang Yang, Haibing Xiao, Lei Chang, Ding Xia and Hua Xu
Department of Urology, Tongji Hospital, Tongji Medical College, Huazhong University of Science and Technology, Wuhan, China

Rong Zhong, Jiao Lou, Xuzai Lu, Juntao Ke, Ti Zhang and Yu Sun
Department of Epidemiology and Biostatistics and MOE Key Lab of Environment and Health, School of Public Health, Tongji Medical College, Huazhong University of Science and Technology, Wuhan, China

Jiahong Xia
Department of Cardiovascular Surgery, Union Hospital, Huazhong University of Science and Technology, Wuhan, China

Li Liu
Department of Epidemiology and Biostatistics, School of Public Health, Guangdong Pharmaceutical University, Guangzhou, China

Yongping Cui
Key Laboratory of Cellular Physiology, Ministry of Education, Shanxi Medical University, Taiyuan, Shanxi, China

Dongping Chen, Yiyi Ma, Xueqi Wang, Shengqiang Yu, Lin Li, Bing Dai, Zhiguo Mao, Lijun Sun, Chenggang Xu, Shu Rong, Mengjun Tang and Changlin Mei
Kidney Institute, Department of Nephrology, Shanghai Changzheng Hospital, Second Military Medical University, Shanghai, P. R. China

Hongbo Zhao, Hongchao Liu and Shiyuan Liu
Department of Radiology, Shanghai Changzheng Hospital, Second Military Medical University, Shanghai, P. R. China

Andreas L. Serra and Rudolf P. Wüthrich
Division of Nephrology, University Hospital, Zürich, Switzerland

Nicole Graf
Graf biostatistics, Winterthur, Switzerland

Laura García-Ortí, Ion Cristó bal, Cristina Cirauqui, Nerea Marcotegui, Remedios Castello-Cros and María D. Odero
Division of Oncology, Center for Applied Medical Research (CIMA), University of Navarra, Pamplona, Spain

Ion Cristóbal, María J. Calasanz and María D. Odero
Department of Genetics, University of Navarra, Pamplona, Spain

Elisabet Guruceaga
Unit of Proteomics, Genomics and Bioinformatics, Center for Applied Medical Research (CIMA), University of Navarra, Pamplona, Spain

Philipp Albrecht, Ann-Kristin Müller, Marius Ringelstein, Eva Cohn, Orhan Aktas, Hans-Peter Hartung, Harald Hefter and Axel Methner
Department of Neurology, Medical Faculty, Heinrich-Heine University, Düsseldorf, Germany

David Finis and Gerd Geerling
Department of Ophthalmology, Medical Faculty, Heinrich-Heine University, Düsseldorf, Germany

Peiwen Lian, Ao Li, Yuan Li, Haichao Liu and Guanqing Wu
Division of Translational Cancer Research and Therapy, State Key Laboratory of Molecular Oncology, Cancer Hospital and Institute, Chinese Academy of Medical Sciences and Peking Union Medical College, Beijing, China

Peiwen Lian, Ao Li, Dan Liang, Bo Hu and Guanqing Wu
Department of Medicine, Vanderbilt University, Nashville, Tennessee, United States of America

Guanqing Wu
Department of Cell and Developmental Biology, Vanderbilt University, Nashville, Tennessee, United States of America

De Lin
Department of Biochemistry, Vanderbilt University, Nashville, Tennessee, United States of America

Tang Jiang
Department of Medicine, First Affiliated Hospital, Sun Yat-sen University, Guangzhou, China

Gilbert Moeckel
Department of Pathology, Yale University School of Medicine, New Haven, Connecticut, United States of America

Dahui Qin
Department of Pathology, Moffitt Cancer Center, Tampa, Florida, United States of America

Index

A

aCGH, 1, 3, 6-7, 9-11, 19, 21, 133, 136
Acute Chest Syndrome, 58-60, 62-64, 66, 99
Acute Myeloid Leukemia, 21-22, 213, 221
Adenosine Transporter, 180-181, 183
Adenosinergic System, 180-181, 184
Adjusted Prevalence Ratios, 172, 174-175
Allele Copy-number, 110, 112
Allelic Imbalances (AIS), 110
Autosomal Dominant Polycystic Kidney Disease (ADPKD), 202, 230

B

Bdnf, 161-162, 166, 168-171, 183, 185, 187, 190-191
Bicc1, 230-238
Blood-brain Barrier (BBB), 23

C

Cag Trinucleotide, 161, 180
Carcinogenesis., 149, 213
Cdkn2a/arf Locus, 132-134, 136
Chaperone, 37, 43, 52, 56, 77, 86-87, 131, 170
Cholelithiasis Risk, 67-68, 74
Coagulation Activation, 58, 60-61, 63, 65-66
Colorectal Cancer, 16, 75, 98, 118, 138, 144-145, 148-149, 193-194, 196, 199-201
Conventional Cytogenetics, 1
Copy Number Variations (CNV), 5, 213
Ctr1, 23-24, 26-28, 30-35, 89-90, 92-96, 98
Cytotoxic Therapy, 1

D

De Novo Aml, 1, 216
Dermal Neurofibromas, 110-111, 113
Drosophila, 119-120, 122, 124-125, 128-131, 150, 155, 160, 162, 168, 170-171, 230

E

Estimated Glomerular Filtration Rate (EGFR), 202, 212
Etoposide, 1, 125, 131, 133, 135

F

Fibrocytes, 99-109

G

G6pd, 172-174, 176-178

H

Hdac6 Knock-out, 161-163, 166-170
Hemolysis, 58, 60, 62, 65-67, 73-75, 106, 177
Hemolytic Anemias, 67, 73
Hepatic Copper, 36, 89, 91, 94-96, 98, 222
Human Adenosine, 188, 190
Huntington's Disease (HD), 37, 119, 150, 161, 180
Hypercoagulability, 58, 63, 65-66
Hypomethylation, 138-139, 142, 145-146, 148-149

I

Isofagomine, 77, 87

L

Luciferase Assays, 54-55, 220
Lynch Syndrome, 138-142, 145-149, 193, 195-196, 198-201

M

Malignant Mesothelioma, 132, 135, 137
Microparticle-associated Tissue Factor (MPTF), 58
Microsatellite Multiplex Pcr Analysis (MMPA), 110, 116
Mir-146a, 37-38, 40, 43-46, 48-56
Mrna Arrays, 213-215

N

Necrosis, 58, 60, 63-64, 89-91, 96, 222
Neurodegenerative Disorder, 119, 150, 161
Neuronopathic Gaucher Disease, 77, 87
Neurotoxicity, 24, 56, 119, 124, 128, 160, 171, 187, 192
Nf1, 12, 15, 20-22, 111, 113-115, 117-118, 213-221

O

Oligonucleotide, 3, 5, 22, 221
Oxidative Stress, 23, 34, 36, 56, 89

P

P16(INK4A), 132-134, 137
P-aml, 1-5, 8-12, 16, 18-21
Penicillamine (PA), 23, 34
Pet-ct, 89-90, 92, 95-98
Polycystin-1, 202, 230-231, 238

R

Rela/nfkb, 37-40, 43, 45, 47-53

Rna Extraction, 54, 57, 169
Rnai Suppressor Screens, 119, 121
Rs3802842,, 193-194, 200

S
Scfv-6e-pest, 153, 156
Serum Vegf-d, 252-253, 255-258
Sickle Cell Anemia, 63, 66-68, 73-75, 108
Sickle Cell Lung Disease, 99, 106
Single Nucleotide Polymorphisms, 67, 71-72, 193
Sirolimus, 131
Sporadic Mss, 138, 142, 145
Strongyloides Stercoralis, 174, 176

T
T-aml, 1-3, 5-6, 9-12, 16, 18-20
Thrombocyte, 202, 205-206, 208, 210-211
Total Bilirubin, 59-62, 67-71, 73-74
Total Kidney Volume (TKV), 202
Trichuris Trichiura, 174, 176
Trinucleotide, 150, 161, 170, 180, 191
Tubulin Acetylation, 161-162, 164-165, 167-171

V
Visual Evoked Potentials (VEPS), 222-223

W
Wilson Disease (WD), 23